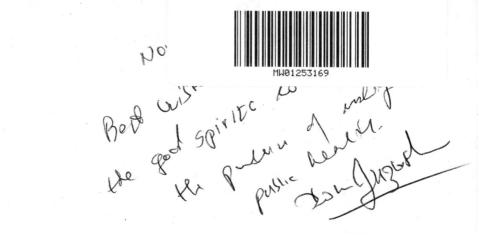

A HISTORY OF PUBLIC HEALTH IN ALBERTA, 1919–2019

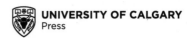
UNIVERSITY OF CALGARY
Press

A HISTORY OF PUBLIC HEALTH IN ALBERTA, 1919-2019

Lindsay McLaren
Donald W. M. Juzwishin
Rogelio Velez Mendoza

© 2024 Lindsay McLaren, Donald W. M. Juzwishin, and Rogelio Velez Mendoza

University of Calgary Press
2500 University Drive NW
Calgary, Alberta
Canada T2N 1N4
press.ucalgary.ca

All rights reserved.

This book is available in an Open Access digital format published under a CC-BY-NCND 4.0 Creative Commons license. The publisher should be contacted for any commercial use which falls outside the terms of that license.

LIBRARY AND ARCHIVES CANADA CATALOGUING IN PUBLICATION

Title: A history of public health in Alberta, 1919-2019 / Lindsay McLaren, Donald W. M. Juzwishin, Rogelio Velez Mendoza.
Names: McLaren, Lindsay, author. | Juzwishin, Donald W. M. (Donald William Moore), 1953- author. | Mendoza, Rogelio Velez, author.
Description: Includes bibliographical references and index.
Identifiers: Canadiana (print) 20240403134 | Canadiana (ebook) 20240403185 | ISBN 9781773855455 (softcover) | ISBN 9781773855448 (hardcover) | ISBN 9781773855486 (EPUB) | ISBN 9781773855479 (PDF) | ISBN 9781773855462 (Open Access PDF)
Subjects: LCSH: Public health—Alberta—History—20th century. | LCSH: Public health—Alberta—History—21st century.
Classification: LCC RA450.A4 M35 2024 | DDC 362.1097123—dc23

The University of Calgary Press acknowledges the support of the Government of Alberta through the Alberta Media Fund for our publications. We acknowledge the financial support of the Government of Canada. We acknowledge the financial support of the Canada Council for the Arts for our publishing program.

 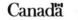

Printed and bound in Canada by Imprimerie Gauvin
⟳ This book is printed on Enviro paper

Copyediting by Rhonda Kronyk
Cover image: "Corner of Round and Ford Streets, Lethbridge, Alberta." [ca. 1912], (CU1172838) by Unknown. Courtesy of Glenbow Library and Archives Collection, Libraries and Cultural Resources Digital Collections, University of Calgary.
Cover design, page design, and typesetting by Melina Cusano

Contents

List of Figures

List of Tables

Abbreviations

GDP	Gross Domestic Product
MLA	Minister of the Legislative Assembly
NDP	New Democratic Party
PC	Progressive Conservative Party
RCMP	Royal Canadian Mounted Police
SC	Social Credit Party

Acknowledgements

We gratefully acknowledge funding support from the Government of Alberta through the Alberta Historical Resources Foundation (File # R-1808-18F and File # R-1725-15F), the Canadian Institutes of Health Research (Funding Reference Numbers CPP-137907, TLB-162870, PJT-156258), and Alberta Innovates Health Solutions (Record # 201400593).

We extend sincere appreciation to the following individuals, who generously shared their time and expertise in making this book better (listed alphabetically by last name): Jacen Abrey, Ella Arcand, Farah Bandali, Chris G. Buse, Jason Cabaj, Kevin Cowan, Maureen Devolin, Sandra Dewar, Warren Elofson, Herb Emery, Rafael Figueiredo, Brent Friesen, Suzanne Galesloot, Cathy Gladwin, Jenny Godley, Les Hagen, Bonnie Healy, Ken Hoffer, Chris Hosgood, Marianne Howell, Lene W. Jorgensen, Don Junk, Nathalie Lachance, Bonnie Lashewicz, Eunice Louis, Jack Lucas, Kelsey Lucyk, Wanda Martin, Karen Mills, Morgan Mouton, Richard Musto, Brian Pickering, G. Barry Phillips, Gerry Predy, Kim Raine, Sandra M. Reilly, Ardene Robinson Vollman, Margaret Russell, Chris Sarin, Jim Talbot, Charles Weaselhead, Douglas R. Wilson, Ruth Wolfe, Sharon Yanicki, and Kue Young. We also thank the team at University of Calgary Press for their consistent support; our talented and thoughtful editor, Rhonda Kronyk; and the two anonymous reviewers for highly constructive comments.

What Is Public Health, and Why Does It Matter?

Lindsay McLaren, Donald W.M. Juzwishin and Frank W. Stahnisch

> *Public Health:* "*The science and art of preventing disease, prolonging life, and promoting physical health and efficiency through organized community efforts.*"
>
> — Charles-Edward Winslow,
> "The Untilled Fields of Public Health," 1920.[1]

Introduction

The immediate impetus for this book, which considers a century of public health in the province of Alberta, is an opportunity to recognize the centenary of the 1919 provincial act that established Alberta's first department of public health.[2] However, that impetus belies several other complex and contested aspects of public health that we seek to explore. First, lying beneath the seemingly straightforward definition with which we open this chapter is our recognition that, while public health is often celebrated for its achievements in improving health status and conditions of populations,[3] those achievements are accompanied, and sometimes undermined, by significant challenges and tensions. For example, the oftentimes blunt and colonial nature of public health measures, which underlies their leverage for population-wide impact, can also — in interaction with socio-political context — create and perpetuate conditions of inequity and exclusion (see for example chapters 1, 3, 7, and 9).[4]

Second, and as described in more detail in this introduction and throughout the book, public health today faces important challenges: it is widely misunderstood (e.g., it is frequently conflated with publicly funded medical care), and there are tensions within the field, including between scholarly communities with a critical orientation and practitioner communities who may be more aligned with a biomedical perspective.[5] These challenges limit the field's ability to mobilize as a collective toward creating conditions for population well-being and health equity, and they provide a strong rationale indeed for reflecting on public health's scope, developments, achievements, and failures in the province's past.

To signal our concern with these challenges and our commitment to advancing a coherent vision for the future, we conceptualize public health as a field of applied practice and scholarly inquiry that brings unique elements to understanding and improving health and well-being. Distinct from the individualized and often reductive orientation of biomedicine and other aspect of health care, public health is characterized by a focus on populations as collectives. Also, rather than focusing on treatment or management of people's illnesses when they are sick, public health emphasizes keeping people healthy in the first place through prevention, health promotion, and thinking about "upstream" or root causes of poor health and health inequity.[6] Moreover, in line with its intersections with social sciences,[7] public health activities are — or should be — conceptually anchored in critical perspectives that are concerned with collective and structural processes that shape well-being and health equity and aim to "speak truth to power."[8] This includes — but is not limited to — illuminating and demonstrating leadership around the pernicious effects on population well-being and health equity of medicalization (i.e., the processes by which problems that result from large-scale social forces and political decisions are reductively treated as individual-level problems amenable to technical or individualized solutions) and neoliberal capitalism (i.e., the dominant global political economic system since the early 1980s, characterized by aggressive pursuit of the capitalist vision of protecting and accumulating private wealth through policies such as deregulation of industry and labour markets, austerity and privatization of public services, and trade liberalization).[9]

We are fortunate, in this project, to draw and build on many existing contributions. However, a consolidated history from a contemporary vantage point that takes a broad vision of public health is scarce, and our aim with this book is to begin to address that gap. Perhaps the most wide-ranging history of public health in Alberta is the 1982 publication by Adelaide Schartner titled *Health Units of Alberta*,[10] which was a celebratory effort by the Health Unit Association of Alberta on the fiftieth anniversary of the creation of health units in the province. That work analyzed local health boards, district nursing, and the activities of health units since the 1930s. However, it did not expand on efforts outside of health unit administration and structure. In 1984, public health physician Gerald Predy wrote a brief history of public health in Alberta, published in the *Canadian Journal of Public Health* as part of a historical issue commemorating the journal's seventy-fifth anniversary.[11] Predy's overview includes health concerns, demographic and economic circumstances, legislative changes and other public health efforts, and the professional public health workforce, in Alberta; the main limitation is its brevity of two pages.

Other important published historical accounts include, but are not limited to, publications by former Deputy Minister of Health of Alberta, Malcolm Bow, and indeed many papers published in what is now called the *Canadian Journal of Public Health* (see Appendix A). Bow's papers, including "The History of the Department of Public Health of Alberta" from 1935; and "Public Health Yesterday, To-Day, and To-Morrow" from 1937; coupled with later publications such as 1959's "The Alberta Department of Public Health" by A. Somerville, Alberta's then deputy minister of health, provide insights into major health problems at the time and the nature and extent of Alberta's societal response, as well as public health's origins in a largely medical practice.[12] As one example of early provincial attention to some forms of health inequality, intersecting with economic development in a province in its early stages of governance, Bow pointed out in 1935 that unequal access to preventive services had resulted from some areas of the province developing rapidly, while "pioneer conditions [were] still to be found in many others."[13]

More recent works include 1994's *Public Health: People Caring for People* by Edmonton writer Bill Carney, prepared for the Health Unit Association of Alberta,[14] which acknowledges Schartner's *Health Units of Alberta* as a key source; 2007's *A Century of Public Health Services in Alberta* written by Alberta social worker and historian Baldwin Reichwein for the Alberta Public Health Association, which gives an overview of public health services in the province organized into social and economic epochs;[15] and our own project, 2017's *Public Health Advocacy: Lessons Learned from the History of the Alberta Public Health Association*, which served as a starting point for this project.[16] In addition to these provincial works are historical overviews of local public health authorities and activities within Alberta's cities — especially Edmonton and Calgary[17] — and recent work with a national scope, such as 2010s *This is Public Health: A Canadian*

History by Christopher Rutty and Sue C. Sullivan, which commemorates the centenary of the Canadian Public Health Association.[18]

We have opportunity, through this project, to update these important works and to consider them from a contemporary perspective characterized by, among other things, increasing attention — in theory if not in practice — to significant and entrenched forms of social inequities in health;[19] emergent public health concerns such as intensification of climate change and ecological degradation (see Chapter 8),[20] the opioid crisis (see Chapter 7 where we share the Kainai Nation's community response to this issue),[21] and the COVID-19 pandemic (see Chapter 14);[22] a broad and diverse public health community that includes scholars, activists, practitioners, and members of publics; and a socio-political environment that, as described in this introduction and throughout the book, is increasingly unfriendly to the public's health.

What Is Public Health?

The overall objective of this volume is to commemorate, critique, and learn from Alberta's public health history. By doing so, we aspire to articulate the contours of a public health that, as a discipline and field of practice, is positioned to address contemporary health concerns and their determinants.[23] A historical approach is well suited to this task, because it theoretically allows for the identification of core, enduring features of public health. Being able to identify and articulate those core features is critical if public health is to remain a relevant societal institution through significant demographic, social, political, economic, epidemiologic, and technological trends that characterize its past, present, and future.[24]

What are public health's core features? Writing in 1920, American bacteriologist and public health expert Charles-Edward Winslow offered "a tentative, if necessarily imperfect, formulation of the scope and tendencies of the modern public health campaign," from which one can begin to glean core features.[25] In addition to a focus on communities or populations, rather than individuals (which he aligned with "private medicine"), Winslow viewed public health as concerned with prevention, arguing that: "medical knowledge has generally been applied only when disease has gone so far that the damage is irremediable. Medical knowledge will be highly effective only when applied in the incipient stages of disease."[26]

Additionally, Winslow recognized the importance of social and economic determinants of health: "we come sooner or later to a realization of the fact that education and medical and nursing service, while they can accomplish much, cannot cope successfully with the evil effects of standards of living too low to permit the maintenance of normal physical health."[27] Acknowledging the implications of that knowledge, he further stated: "If an initially normal family cannot gain a livelihood adequate for its minimum physical needs, there is evidently *a problem of social readjustments which our nation must face*" [emphasis added], thus speaking to the need for societal solutions to population health problems.

Nearly 100 years later, the Canadian Public Health Association identified similar core elements for public health, including concern with maintaining and improving (e.g., through promotion, protection, and prevention) the health of populations, key principles of social justice and equity, and attention to addressing underlying social, economic, political, ecological, and colonial determinants of health, along with evidence-informed policy and practice.[28] A newer emphasis on maintaining and improving health, as distinct from preventing illness as articulated by Winslow, reflects historically significant interim occurrences such as the 1946 Constitution of the World Health Organization,[29] the Health Field concept contained in the 1974 report, *A New Perspective on the Health of Canadians*,[30] and the 1986 *Ottawa Charter for Health Promotion* (see Chapter 10).[31] These documents, and others, signal a shift, at least in theory, toward a more holistic conceptualization of health that includes not only illness or its absence, but also well-being (social, emotional, spiritual), and recognition that medicine and health care are only partial options for maintaining and improving the health of populations.

Public health's emphasis on improving health and well-being among populations via attention to upstream social determinants of health introduces an additional core feature of the field and of this book — namely, power and politics. In the introduction to her important, and still highly relevant, 1988 book, *Hidden Arguments: Political Ideology and Disease Prevention Policy*, University of Arizona professor Sylvia Noble Tesh argues that "behind debates about such questions as the toxicity of environmental pollutants, the hazards of smoking, and the health effects of cholesterol lie other, hidden arguments. These arguments are more fundamental: What is the legitimate source of knowledge? What is the nature of human beings? And what is the ideal structure of society?"[32] American historian of public health, Dorothy Porter, speaks to the enduring importance of these considerations in her 1999 volume where she said, "the concern with collective social action involves an analysis of the structural operation of power, which makes the political implications of population health in different periods and in different societies a persistent theme."[33] That is, although the details of power and politics may take different forms depending on time and place, their importance to our field persists. Finally, American author Deborah Stone in her book *Policy Paradox: The Art of Political Decision Making* emphasizes that how problems are identified and defined is determined by those in power, those who have the authority to make decisions and policy, thus prompting the importance of asking questions such as: "Who is given the right to make decisions about the problem? Whose voice counts, both for choosing leaders and for choosing policies? Who is subordinated to whom? What kind of internal hierarchy is created? Who is allied to whom? How does the authority structure create loyalties and antagonisms among members of the community?"[34] One of our goals in the succeeding chapters is to keep a critical eye on structures and relationships and their intersections with public health priorities and activities.

Despite this identification of core features and principles that have endured over time, public health is a term that is frequently misunderstood. It is often conflated with publicly funded medical care, which dilutes its unique emphasis on root causes of population-level health problems and health inequities. Public health is moreover often reduced in scope and substance to singular elements such as immunization, the opioid crisis, or communicable disease outbreaks.[35] The COVID-19 pandemic is a case in point: although the pandemic has thrust public health into the spotlight, it has perpetuated a narrow, technical, and individualized version of public health, focused on physical illness and characterized by communicable disease control, and led by medical practitioners in the health care system.[36]

Furthermore, even within the public health community, including practitioners, academics, and activists, there are different perspectives on public health that differ importantly in structure and scope.[37] A narrower perspective focuses on the formal public health system and its institutional parameters, including delivery of public health services by health authorities; while another, broader, perspective embraces root causes of poor health and health inequities embodied in systems and structures that extend far beyond the formal health sector. Taking a narrower view of public health has the advantages of making the term more readily definable and having existing institutional (e.g., legal and governance) structures.[38] Its primary disadvantage — and this is a significant criticism — is its limited scope and usually uncritical nature.[39] As scholars in critical public health and health promotion traditions have long recognized, foundations of population health are social and political in nature and demand an intersectoral and interdisciplinary approach coupled with deep reflexivity and humility, including epistemic humility, to tackle entrenched forms of power that underpin social and health inequities.[40] These considerations demand a broader conceptualization of public health. Yet, any concept — including public health — that is too broad risks being useless. Although different perspectives on public health can be a strength for the field, it can also create fracture and lack of unity, especially if — as described in this introduction — public health is "weakening."[41]

This question of "how broad the mandate" should be for public health, which has been described as "timeless,"[42] presents important challenges for this book and for the field more broadly. For example, on a practical level, a narrower versus broader conceptualization of public health has implications for identifying which government departments are relevant to public health, or for deciding what should be included or excluded in public health spending.[43] Beyond these practical decisions, the question of the scope of public health has deeper implications. With the future well-being of all populations in mind, do we want to continue to focus on current public health programs and services and their institutional parameters (a narrower version of public health)? Or do we want to focus on the ultimate aims of public health — population well-being and health equity — and use that broader aim to shape what we do as a society, including the messiness of boundaries that comes with it?

Why Do This Now?

The year 2019 marked the centenary of the 1919 act that led to the establishment of Alberta's first provincial Department of Public Health.[44] Alberta was the second province in Canada to establish such a department, following New Brunswick in 1918. The federal government also introduced a Department of Health in 1919.[45] Anniversaries provide an opportunity to reflect and learn from our past, toward strengthening our future.

The mere year of 1919 is of course not the beginning of public health in Alberta. As discussed elsewhere in this book (e.g., Chapter 4), public health activities in the area predated the formal creation of the province.[46] As with many foundational dates in the wider history of social movements, we could have chosen to commemorate various earlier occurrences or pieces of legislation; for example, Alberta's first Public Health Act or its Vital Statistics Act, which were passed in 1907,[47] or the signing of Treaties 6, 7, or 8 in the late nineteenth century, which brought devastating implications for the well-being of Indigenous communities that persist to this day (see also Chapter 7).[48]

We singled out the 1919 act because it has features that make it interesting and relevant as a starting point for historical study. First, prior to 1919 — in the first fourteen years of the province[49] — formal public health activities in Alberta were housed under various departments and ministries, including the Attorney General, Agriculture, and Municipal Affairs.[50] The year 1919 marked the establishment of a provincial department devoted specifically to public health, signifying public health's importance to at least some in Alberta at that time. Second, the wording of the 1919 act communicates a consolidation of public health under one umbrella; for example, "All that part of the administration of the government of the province, which relates to public health."[51] This provides an opportunity for insights around why this centralization occurred and to what end, including from a contemporary vantage point anchored in a broad vision of public health.[52]

The Current State of Public Health in Canada and Alberta

While the centenary of the 1919 Public Health Act provides a convenient opportunity for historical reflection, the substantive impetus for our project concerns the state of public health in Canada and Alberta. First, contemporary national discourse suggests that public health is weakening. Quite recent scholarly and review commentaries by public health professors and practitioners Louise Potvin (Université de Montréal), Ak'ingabe Guyon (Université de Montréal), and Trevor Hancock (Prof. Emer., University of Victoria) for instance have identified important trends across Canada.[53] Within the formal public health sector, emphasized in the narrower version of public health, these include a downgrading of the status of public health activities within health authorities, eroding the independence of medical officers of health (for example, the arbitrary dismissal of medical officers of health who "speak truth to power" on matters of public health concern),[54] decreasing funding, and limiting or diluting the scope of public health. This latter trend includes instances where public health departments or activities are combined with primary or community care in such a way that, problematically, community and population-level public health responsibilities are displaced by individually-focused clinical tasks.

Moreover, there are indications of resistance to a broader version of public health that is concerned with upstream determinants of well-being and health equity. As reported by Potvin in her editorial, "Canadian Public Health Under Siege," a 2014 *Globe and Mail* column asserted that, "it is not the job of public health to have an opinion on taxes, economic policy, free trade or corporate control," arguing instead that public health should limit itself to a narrow focus on communicable disease prevention and control.[55] The important role of the popular press in shaping (i.e., limiting) the contours of public health is supported by scholarly work demonstrating that mainstream media coverage of "health" in Canada is dominated by topics related to medical care (e.g., service provision, service delivery, management, regulation) and only very infrequently considers social determinants of health.[56] This is a significant challenge that must be overcome to realize a broad public health vision.

In terms of whether public health has been weakened by inadequate funding, this is another dimension that is complicated by the existence of different definitions of public health. On the one hand, it is clear from available data that although spending on medical care in Canada is significant, spending on formal public health activities, as a component of medical care spending, constitutes only a very small proportion of those costs. For example, according to the Canadian Institute for Health Information, total health care expenditure in Canada in 2019 was estimated at $264.4 billion, or $7,068 per Canadian, corresponding to 11.6 percent of Canada's gross domestic product (GDP), up from 7 percent of GDP in 1975.[57] Public health, defined by the Canadian Institute for Health Information as "expenditures for items such as food and drug safety, health inspections, health promotion activities, community mental health programs, public health nursing, measures to prevent the spread of communicable disease and occupational health to promote and enhance the safety at the workplace in public sector agencies," constituted 5.4 percent of those expenditures.[58]

Focusing on Alberta in particular, Figure 0.1 presents annual provincial government per capita health expenditure from 1975 to 2019,[59] for two spending categories as defined by the Canadian Institute for Health Information : 1) public health and — as a contrast — 2) hospitals, which is the largest health spending category:[60]

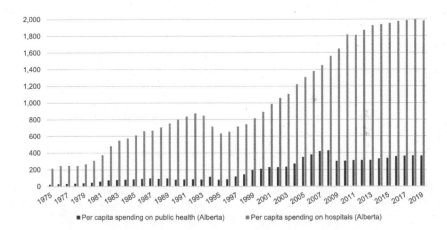

■ Per capita spending on public health (Alberta)   ■ Per capita spending on hospitals (Alberta)

Fig. 0.1: Annual provincial government per capita health expenditure in current dollars for 1) public health (black bars) and 2) hospitals (grey bars), Alberta, 1975 to 2019.

Source: Canadian Institute for Health Information, Open data on health spending (modifiable data set that can be freely used). Available at: https://www.cihi.ca/en/national-health-expenditure-trends-1975-to-2019 (scroll down to "Health spending data tables"; Table D4: Provincial/territorial government expenditures; Table D.4.9.3 Provincial government per capita health expenditure by use of funds in current dollars, Alberta, 1975 to 2019).

The figure illustrates that per capita spending on both public health (as defined above) and hospitals in Alberta has increased over time; however, the amount spent on hospitals is consistently much higher than that spent on public health. Figure 0.2 shows relative spending on public health in Alberta, that is, the annual provincial government spending on public health, as a percent of total health expenditure, 1975 to 2019.

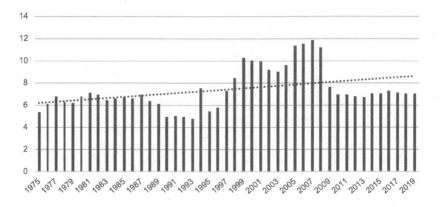

Fig. 0.2: Annual percentage of provincial government health expenditure on public health for Alberta, 1975 to 2019.

Source: Canadian Institute for Health Information, Open data on health spending (modifiable data set that can be freely used). Available at: https://www.cihi.ca/en/national-health-expenditure-trends-1975-to-2019 (scroll down to "Health spending data tables"; Table D4: Provincial/territorial government expenditures; Table D.4.9.2 Percentage distribution of provincial government health expenditure by use of funds, Alberta, 1975 to 2019).

The figure shows that, during the 1975 to 2019 period, the relative spending on public health in Alberta ranged from approximately 5 percent (early 1990s) to almost 12 percent (2007) of total health spending. Some variation is evident, including that which coincides with significant changes to health care system governance in the 1990s (health care regionalization) and early 2000s (transition from regional health authorities to Alberta Health Services).[61] Overall, however, the modest trend over time in terms of percent of health spending on public health has been upward, not downward, in Alberta.

The story told by these spending data, however, is incomplete. From a social determinants of health point of view (embraced by a broad definition of public health), the primary determinants of health and well-being are economic and social conditions, which reflect public policy decisions including spending out-side of health care. Yet, spending in ministries outside of health is not typically included in estimates of public health spending. This is an important omission.[62] For example, based on an analysis of provincial spending data from 1981 to 2011, professor Daniel Dutton and colleagues demonstrated a positive association between social spending (i.e., spending in social service sectors) and population health outcomes; in fact, social spending was more important to population health outcomes than health care spending.[63] Yet, social spending across provinces in Canada remained at a low and in some cases declining level during this time period, while health care spending increased significantly.

Thus, although public health spending as defined by the Canadian Institute for Health Information has not shown a decreasing trend in Alberta for the period for which data are readily available, government spending on activities that would improve population health and well-being — that is, spending in the social and other public sectors — is low and is declining — especially relative to health care spending — over time. A broader definition of spending that includes social spending better aligns with Winslow's definition of public health with which we opened this chapter: "The science and art of preventing disease, prolonging life, and promoting health and efficiency through organized community efforts,"[64] which necessarily extends beyond the formal health sector. Taking a broad public health perspective, public sector investment in health in Alberta and across Canada is low and has indeed declined over time.

Although a one hundred-year analysis of public health spending in Alberta was not feasible, we have an early glimpse of this issue from the 1939 annual report of the Department of Public Health, in which Deputy Minister of Public Health, Malcolm Bow, made the following comments, with reference to the statement of revenue and expenditure for the 1939–1940 fiscal year [emphasis added]:

> An analysis of this statement shows that the total expenditure for all activities of this Department was $2,600,711.25. The expenditure for the Child Welfare and Mothers' Allowance Branch amounted to $710,811.63. . . . Of the [remainder] [$1,889,959.62], $1,677,366.16 was expended for the maintenance and operation of the various institutions which are under the administration of the Department, for grants to hospitals and homes, and for other forms of what might be termed treatment services; $212,593.46 representing 11.2% of the total budget of the Department, excluding the amounts expended for Child Welfare and Mothers' Allowances, was expended for all other activities, including clinic services, vital statistics, communicable disease control, public health units, general administration and all preventive services. *Thus, out of every dollar expended by the Department, 11.2 [cents] were spent for preventive health activities. The need for the extension of preventive health service, particularly*

in our rural and smaller urban centres is great. No expenditure will
pay larger dividends in ensuring a sound structure of health in this
Province.[65]

Dr. Bow's comments in 1939 illustrate two things: first, that there is a historical legacy of separating social spending (at that time, child welfare and mother's allowance) from health spending, which presents a challenge to a broad version of public health; and second, that spending on preventive health activities relative to treatment services was limited, thus showing early concern about an issue that continues to preoccupy the community today.

What This Book Is, and What It Is Not

This book offers "a" history of public health in Alberta. It was prompted by our observation and concern that public health, as a field of scholarly inquiry and applied practice, is diffuse, divided, and poorly understood. This creates a problem when it comes to mobilizing as a collective to support efforts to improve well-being and health equity in populations. It is also important for our political leaders who are charged with the responsibility of providing conditions to protect and support the health and well-being of all of us.

Anchored in long-standing definitions of public health (i.e., the science and art of preventing disease and promoting health through organized efforts of society) that have yet to be fully realized, we present a work that aims to illustrate contours of the field historically in Alberta. Inevitably, we brought our own experiences and perspectives to this project. These shaped the overall orientation of the book, its largely narrative approach, and the topics and examples we have chosen. Our focus on illustrating a broad version of public health, as discussed above, at times precluded deeper analysis of the episodes covered; this is a trade-off for which we feel some discomfort. We enthusiastically await the efforts of those who follow, to take those deeper and more critical dives while, we hope, retaining a focus on strengthening a coherent vision for the field as a whole.

Consistent with our broad definition of public health, the intended audience for this book is also broad. While we carry no illusions that everyone will agree with our approach, we hope that our efforts to articulate and illustrate contours of our field will resonate in some way with researchers, scholars, activists, practitioners, policy actors, students, and members of publics.

The Chapters Ahead

The book is organized as follows. The first three chapters aim to set the stage for the remainder of the book. Chapter 1 addresses what we view as a fundamental question, namely, who is the public in public health. In Chapter 2, we use an innovative data source — Alberta government throne speeches since 1906 — to shed light on how health and public health have been understood by provincial leadership over time. Chapter 3 considers, from the perspective of historically available statistics, the health — or more accurately, the sickness — of Albertans over time.

In chapters 4 through 7, we consider a range of institutions, sectors, and populations. Chapter 4 focuses on public health governance; it provides a historical overview of legislative and institutional dimensions of public health in the province, anchored in the provincial Public Health Act. Chapter 5 considers the non-profit sector, with a particular focus on the only provincial non-profit organization that is explicitly concerned with public health: the Alberta Public Health Association. Chapter 6 focuses on public health education in the province, with attention to university programs in public health. And in Chapter 7 we share stories about public health from First Nation communities in Treaties 6, 7, and 8.

Chapters 8 through 12 are organized using contemporary public health functions as described by the Public Health Agency of Canada;[66] these include health protection (Chapter 8), disease and injury prevention (Chapter 9), health promotion (Chapter 10), and emergency preparedness and response (Chapter 11), in addition to the social determinants of health (Chapter 12). Each chapter considers a small number of focal topics or examples to illustrate different types of problems and solutions, and how those played out within their socio-historical context.

To anchor the book, chapters were prepared while keeping two questions in mind. The first question, informed by our concerns about the state of public health in Alberta and Canada, asks, what happened, when, and why? Learning from our history, the second question asks how we might work to strengthen public health moving forward. Our final two chapters shed additional light on these questions: Chapter 13 by showcasing a subset of individuals across Alberta's public health history who have publicly contended with these challenges, and Chapter 14 by synthesizing some substantive insights from the volume as a whole. Written during the COVID-19 pandemic, that concluding chapter considers the significant opportunity presented by the pandemic to shape a coherent vision for the future of public health, in Alberta and beyond.[67]

NOTES

1 Charles-Edward Winslow, "The Untilled Fields of Public Health," *Science* 51, no. 1306 (1920), 23.

2 *An Act respecting the Department of Public Health*, Statutes of the Province of Alberta (S.P.A.), 1919, c. 16.

3 Christopher Rutty and Susan C. Sullivan, *This Is Public Health: A Canadian History* (Ottawa, Canadian Public Health Association, 2010), 2.9f; Winslow, "Untilled Fields," 23.

4 Marjorie MacDonald, *Introduction to Public Health Ethics 1: Background* (Montréal, QC: National Collaborating Centre for Healthy Public Policy, 2014), http://www.ncchpp.ca/docs/2014_Ethics_Intro1_En.pdf; Nuffield Council on Bioethics, *Public Health: Ethical Issues* (London: Nuffield Council on Bioethics, 2007), http://nuffieldbioethics.org/wp-content/uploads/2014/07/Public-health-ethical-issues.pdf.

5 Kelsey Lucyk and Lindsay McLaren, "Commentary — Is the Future of 'Population/Public Health' in Canada United or Divided? Reflections from within the Field," *Health Promotion and Chronic Disease Prevention in Canada: Research, Policy and Practice* 37, no. 7 (July 2017), https://www.ncbi.nlm.nih.gov/pmc/articles/PMC5650033/; Lindsay McLaren and Trevor Hancock, "Public Health Matters — but We Need to Make the Case," *Canadian Journal of Public Health* 110, no. 3 (1 June 2019), https://doi.org/10.17269/s41997-019-00218-z; Canadian Network of Public Health Associations (CNPHA), "A Collective Voice for Advancing Public Health: Why Public Health Associations Matter Today," *Canadian Journal of Public Health* 110, no. 3 (2019), https://pubmed.ncbi.nlm.nih.gov/30937728/.

6 Canadian Public Health Association (CPHA), *Public Health: A Conceptual Framework, Canadian Public Health Association Working Paper*, 2nd ed. (Ottawa: CPHA, 2017); McLaren and Hancock, "Public Health Matters."

7 Lori Baugh Littlejohns, Neale Smith, and Louise Townend, "Why Public Health Matters Today More than Ever: The Convergence of Health and Social Policy," *Canadian Journal of Public Health* 110, no. 3 (7 January 2019), https://doi.org/10.17269/s41997-018-0171-1; Lindsay McLaren, "In Defense of a Population-Level Approach to Prevention: Why Public Health Matters Today," *Canadian Journal of Public Health* 110, no. 3 (1 June 2019), https://doi.org/10.17269/s41997-019-00198-0.

8 Michael Harvey, "The Political Economy of Health: Revisiting Its Marxian Origins to Address 21st-Century Health Inequalities," *American Journal of Public Health* 111, no. 2 (22 December 2020), https://doi.org/10.2105/AJPH.2020.305996; Dennis Raphael et al., *Social Determinants of Health: The Canadian Facts*, 2nd ed. (Oshawa: Ontario Tech University Faculty of Health Sciences and Toronto: York University School of Health Policy and Management, 2020), http://www.thecanadianfacts.org/.

9 Ted Schrecker, "What Is Critical about Critical Public Health? Focus on Health Inequalities," *Critical Public Health* 32, no. 2 (15 March 2022), https://doi.org/10.1080/09581596.2021.1905776.

10 Adelaide Schartner, *Health Units of Alberta* (Edmonton: Health Unit Association of Alberta, 1982).

11 Gerald Predy, "A Brief History of Public Health in Alberta," *Canadian Journal of Public Health* 75, no. 5 (1984); John M. Last, "Seventy-five Years On," *Canadian Journal of Public Health* 75, no. 5 (1984).

12 Malcolm R. Bow and F. T. Cook, "The History of the Department of Public Health of Alberta," *Canadian Public Health Journal* 26, no. 8 (1935); Malcolm R. Bow, "Public Health Yesterday, To-Day, and To-Morrow," *Canadian Public Health Journal* 28, no. 7 (1937); A. Somerville and R.D. DeFries, "The Alberta Department of Public Health," *Canadian Journal of Public Health* 50, no. 1 (1959).

13 Bow and Cook. "Department of Public Health," 396.

14 Bill Carney, *Public Health: People Caring for People* (Edmonton: Health Unit Association of Alberta, 1994).

15 Baldwin P. Reichwein, *A Century of Public Health Services in Alberta: Celebrate Success while Remaining Alert to New Threats* (Edmonton: A monograph developed for the Alberta Public Health Association, 2007).

16 Lindsay McLaren, Kelsey Lucyk, and Frank Stahnisch, "Public Health Advocacy: Lessons Learned from the History of the Alberta Public Health Association." Research grant, Alberta Historical Resources Foundation — Heritage Preservation Partnership Program, July 2015–June 2018; Rogelio Velez Mendoza, et al., "The History of the Alberta Public Health Association" (narrative report produced for the Alberta Public Health Association) (Calgary: APHA, 2017), available at www.apha.ab.ca.

17 For example, James M. Howell, "Edmonton Board of Health Celebrates 100 Years — or More," *Canadian Journal of Public Health* 83, no. 4 (1992); Jack Lucas, "Urban Governance Backgrounders for Six Cities (Calgary, Edmonton, Hamilton, Toronto, Vancouver, Victoria) and Five Policy Domains (education, policing, public health, public transit, water supply)," Scholars Portal Dataverse, V1 (2018), doi.org/10.5683/SP/HLKDPK.

18   Rutty and Sullivan, *This Is Public Health.*

19   Alberta Health Services and Calgary Institute for Population and Public Health, *Measuring Health Inequalities: Learning for the Future* (Calgary, 28 February 2011), https://www.albertahealthservices.ca/assets/healthinfo/poph/hi-poph-surv-shsa-measuring-health-inequalitie.pdf; Public Health Agency of Canada, *Reducing Health Inequalities: A Challenge For Our Times* (Ottawa, 2011), http://publications.gc.ca/collections/collection_2012/aspc-phac/HP35-22-2011-eng.pdf; Commission on Social Determinants of Health, *Closing the Gap in a Generation: Health Equity through Action on the Social Determinants of Health*, Final Report of the Commission on Social Determinants of Health (Geneva: World Health Organization, 2008); Truth and Reconciliation Commission of Canada, *Honouring the Truth, Reconciling for the Future, Summary of the Final Report of the Truth and Reconciliation Commission of Canada* (Winnipeg, MB: Truth and Reconciliation Commission of Canada, 2015), www.trc.ca.

20   Canadian Public Health Association, *Global Change and Public Health: Addressing the Ecological Determinants of Health*, Discussion Paper (Ottawa: Canadian Public Health Association, May 2015).

21   Benedikt Fischer, et al., "Non-medical Prescription Opioid Use, Prescription Opioid-related Harms and Public Health in Canada: An Update 5 Years Later," *Canadian Journal of Public Health* 105, no. 2 (2014), https://www.canada.ca/en/public-health/news/2017/09/statement_from_theco-chairsofthefederalprovincialandterritorials.html; "Opioid Reports," Government of Alberta, accessed 20 March 2020, https://www.alberta.ca/opioid-reports.aspx.

22   Theresa Tam, *From Risk to Resilience: An Equity Approach to COVID-19, The Chief Public Health Officer of Canada's Report on the State of Public Health in Canada 2020* (Ottawa: Public Health Agency of Canada, Minister of Health, 2020), https://www.canada.ca/en/public-health/corporate/publications/chief-public-health-officer-reports-state-public-health-canada/from-risk-resilience-equity-approach-covid-19.html.

23   Lindsay McLaren and Trish Hennessy, "A Broader Vision of Public Health," *The Monitor* (January/February 2021), https://www.policyalternatives.ca/publications/monitor/broader-vision-public-health.

24   Robert E. McKeown, "The Epidemiologic Transition: Changing Patterns of Mortality and Population Dynamics," *American Journal of Lifestyle Medicine* 3, no. 1, Suppl (2009); https://www.ncbi.nlm.nih.gov/pmc/articles/PMC2805833/; Paul Weindling, "From Germ Theory to Social Medicine: Public Health, 1880–1930," in *Medicine Transformed: Health, Disease and Society in Europe, 1800–1930*, ed. Deborah Brunton (Manchester: Manchester University Press in association with the Open University, 2004).

25   Winslow, "Untilled Fields," 24.

26   Winslow, "Untilled Fields," 28.

27   Winslow, "Untilled Fields," 29.

28   Canadian Public Health Association (CPHA), *Public Health: A Conceptual Framework.*

29   Constitution of the World Health Organization: Principles (1946), https://www.who.int/about/accountability/governance/constitution; William F. Bynum and Roy Porter, "The World Health Organization and Its Work," *American Journal of Public Health* 98, no. 9 (1 September 2008).

30   Marc Lalonde, "A New Perspective on the Health of Canadians," Government of Canada working paper (Ottawa: Minister of Supply and Services Canada, 1981); Hubert L. Laframboise, "Health Policy: Breaking the Problem Down into more Manageable Segments," *Canadian Medical Association Journal* 108 (3 February 1973).

31   World Health Organization, "Ottawa Charter for Health Promotion: An International Conference on Health Promotion: the Move Towards a New Public Health," November 17–21, 1986, Ottawa, Ontario, Canada, http://www.who.int/healthpromotion/conferences/previous/ottawa/en/index4.html; Trevor Hancock, "The Ottawa Charter at 25," *Canadian Journal of Public Health* 102, no. 6 (2011): 404; Louise Potvin and Catherine M. Jones. "Twenty-five Years after the Ottawa Charter: The Critical Role of Health Promotion for Public Health," *Canadian Journal of Public Health* 102, no. 4 (2011).

32   Sylvia Noble Tesh, *Hidden Arguments: Political Ideology and Disease Prevention Policy* (New Brunswick, N.J.: Rutgers University Press, 1988), 3.

33   Dorothy Porter, *Health, Civilization and the State: A History of Public Health from Ancient to Modern Times* (London: Routledge, 1999), 163–278, 5.

34   Deborah Stone, *Policy Paradox: The Art of Political Decision Making*, Revised Edition (New York: W.W. Norton and Company Inc., 2002), 356.

35   Ruta K. Valaitis et al., "Strengthening Primary Health Care through Primary Care and Public Health Collaboration: The Influence of Intrapersonal and Interpersonal Factors," *Primary Health Care Research & Development* 18, no. 1 (2018); Alberta Public Health Association. "Public Health: Taking It to the Streets." Created in 1993, video, available from the authors; Susan Nall Bales, Andrew Volmert,

and Adam Simon, *Overcoming Health Individualism: A FrameWorks Creative Brief on Framing Social Determinants in Alberta* (FrameWorks Institute, March 2014).

36 Trevor Hancock et al., "There Is Much More to Public Health than COVID-19," *Healthy Debate,* 15 June 2020, https://healthydebate.ca/opinions/more-to-public-health-than-covid.

37 Michael M. Rachlis, "Moving Forward with Public Health in Canada," *Canadian Journal of Public Health* 95, no. 6 (2004), 405; Sutcliffe and others, "Public Health in Canada;" Canadian Network of Public Health Associations (CNPHA), "A Collective Voice for Advancing Public Health; Canadian Public Health Association, *Public Health: A Conceptual Framework.*

38 *An Act respecting Public Health,* S.P.A. 1907, c. 12; Jack Lucas, "Historical Overview: Public Health Governance in Calgary," *Canadian Urban Policy Governance Backgrounders* (2015), http://jacklucas. pennyjar.ca/governance; Jack Lucas, "Historical Overview: Public Health Governance in Edmonton," *Canadian Urban Policy Governance Backgrounders* (2015), http://jacklucas.pennyjar.ca/governance.

39 CNPHA, "A Collective Voice for Advancing Public Health."

40 Commission on Social Determinants of Health, *Closing the Gap in a Generation*; Sarah Whitmee et al., "Safeguarding Human Health in the Anthropocene Epoch: Report of The Rockefeller Foundation-Lancet Commission on Planetary Health," *Lancet* 386, no. 10007 (2015); Truth and Reconciliation Commission of Canada, *Honouring the Truth*; Louise Potvin and Jeff Masuda, "Climate Change: A Top Priority for Public Health," *Canadian Journal of Public Health* 111, no. 6 (1 December 2020), https://doi.org/10.17269/s41997-020-00447-7.

41 Lucyk and McLaren, "Is the Future of "Population/Public Health" in Canada United or Divided?"

42 Michael M. Rachlis, "Moving Forward with Public Health."

43 Lindsay McLaren and Daniel J. Dutton, "The Social Determinants of Pandemic Impact: An Opportunity to Rethink What We Mean by 'Public Health Spending,'" *Canadian Journal of Public Health* 111, no. 4 (1 August 2020), https://doi.org/10.17269/s41997-020-00395-2.

44 *An Act respecting Public Health*, S.P.A., 1907, c. 12.

45 Jasmin H. Cheung-Gertler, "Health Canada," *The Canadian Encyclopedia,* Historica Canada, last edited 5 August, 2014.

46 See for example: Anne Woywitka, "Pioneers in Sickness and in Health," *Alberta History* 49, no. 1 (2000): 16; John Bunn, "Smallpox Epidemic of 1869–70," *Alberta Historical Review* 11 (1963): 18; Eileen M. McNeill, "Women of Vision and Compassion: The Foundation of Health Care in Calgary," *Alberta History* 50, no. 1 (Winter 2002); Janice P. Dickin McGinnis, "A City Faces an Epidemic," *Alberta History* 24, no 4 (1976); Sharon Richardson, "Frontier Health Care: Alberta's District and Municipal Nursing Services 1919 to 1976," *Alberta History* 46, no 1 (1998).

47 *An Act respecting Public Health*, S.P.A., 1907; *Act respecting the Registration of Births, Marriages and Deaths,* S.P.A., 1907, c.13; Bow and Cook, "Department of Public Health."

48 Truth, and Reconciliation Commission of Canada, *Canada's Residential Schools: The History, Part 1, Origins to 1939: The Final Report of the Truth and Reconciliation Commission of Canada,* Vol. 1 (McGill-Queen's Press-MQUP, 2016), http://nctr.ca/reports.php

49 Howard Palmer and Tamara Palmer, *Alberta: A New History* (Edmonton: Hurtig, 1990); Catherine Anne Cavanaugh, Michael Payne and Donald Grant Wetherell, eds., *Alberta Formed, Alberta Transformed* (Edmonton: University of Alberta, 2006).

50 Gerald Predy, "Public Health in Alberta."

51 Predy, "Public Health in Alberta."

52 World Health Organization, *Health in All Policies: Helsinki Statement. Framework for Country Action,* 8th Global Conference on Health Promotion 2013 (Helsinki, 2014), http://www.who.int/healthpromotion/frameworkforcountryaction/en/; "Health in All Policies," Centers for Disease Control and Prevention, last updated 9 June 2016, https://www.cdc.gov/policy/hiap/index.html; Fran Baum et al., "Evaluation of Health in All Policies: Concept, Theory and Application," *Health Promotion International* 29, suppl, 1 (June 2014), https://doi.org/10.1093/heapro/dau032.

53 Ak'ingabe Guyon et al., "The Weakening of Public Health: A Threat to Population Health and Health Care System Sustainability," *Canadian Journal of Public Health* 108, no. 1 (2017); Trevor Hancock, "Erosion of Public Health Capacity Should be a Matter of Concern for All Canadians," *Canadian Journal of Public Health* 109, no. 1 (2018); Louise Potvin, "Canadian Public Health under Siege," *Canadian Journal of Public Health* 105, no. 6 (2014).

54 Brad Mackay, "Firing Public Health MD over pro-Kyoto Comments a No-no, Alberta Learns," *Canadian Medical Association Journal* 167, no. 10 (November 12, 2002).

55 Potvin, "Canadian Public Health under Siege."

56   Michael Hayes et al., "Telling Stories: News Media, Health Literacy and Public Policy in Canada," *Social Science & Medicine* 64, no. 9 (1 May 2007), https://doi.org/10.1016/j.socscimed.2007.01.015; Mike Gasher et al., "Spreading the News: Social Determinants of Health Reportage in Canadian Daily Newspapers," *Canadian Journal of Communication* 32, no. 3 (2007), doi.org/10.22230/cjc.2007v32n3a1724.

57   For the Canadian Institute for Health Information, health expenditure includes "any type of expenditure for which the primary objective is to improve or prevent the deterioration of health status;" including "activities that are undertaken with the direct purpose of improving and maintaining health." The main categories included in health expenditure are hospitals; other institutions, such as residential care types of facilities; physicians; other professionals; drugs; capital; public health; administration; and other health spending, such as research. Canadian Institute for Health Information (CIHI), *National Health Expenditure Trends, 1975 to 2019* (Ottawa: CIHI, 2019), Methodology Notes, https://www.cihi.ca/sites/default/files/document/nhex-trends-narrative-report-2019-en-web.pdf.

58   Canadian Institute for Health Information, *National Health Expenditure Trends.*

59   Expenditure data from 1975 through 2019 are readily available from CIHI, through their *National Health Expenditure Trends* publication. We would like to have included expenditures for the entire period of interest in this volume, however, that exercise is significantly complicated by changes over time in what public health entailed and how those activities are recorded in provincial budgets.

60   The largest spending categories across Canada are hospitals (26.6% for Canada in 2019), drugs (15.3%) and physicians (15.1%), which amounted to almost 60% of total health spending in Canada in 2019. Canadian Institute for Health Information, *National Health Expenditure Trends, 1975 to 2019.*

61   Jack Lucas, "Historical Overview."

62   McLaren and Dutton, "Social Determinants of Pandemic Impact."

63   Daniel J. Dutton et al., "Effect of Provincial Spending on Social Services and Health Care on Health Outcomes in Canada: An Observational Longitudinal Study," *Canadian Medical Association Journal* 190, no. 1 (2018).

64   Winslow, "Untilled Fields," 23.

65   Alberta Department of Public Health, *Annual Report 1939* (Edmonton: Printed by A. Shnitka, King's Printer, 1941), 24–25 [emphasis added].

66   Public Health Agency of Canada, *Core Competencies for Public Health in Canada: Release 1.0* (Ottawa: Her Majesty the Queen in Right of Canada, represented by the Minister of Health, 2008), https://www.phac-aspc.gc.ca/php-psp/ccph-cesp/pdfs/cc-manual-eng090407.pdf.

67   McLaren and Hennessy, "A Broader Vision of Public Health."

Who Is the Public in Public Health?

Erna Kurbegović and Benjamin Sasges (contributed equally)

Introduction

In 1953, at the age of nine, Leilani Muir was admitted to the Provincial Training School for Mental Defectives in Red Deer, Alberta, which provided care and training for persons thought to be "mentally deficient." There was no medical examination upon admittance to the training school, and no evidence was provided by the physicians that Muir was in fact "mentally deficient."[1] Following an inaccurate IQ test, the training school psychiatrist recommended Muir for sterilization, under Alberta's Sexual Sterilization Act. At the age of fourteen, Leilani Muir was sterilized without her consent.[2]

Alberta's eugenics program (operationalized via the Sexual Sterilization Act), administered by the provincial Department of Public Health, was in operation from 1928 until 1972 (see also Chapter 4), and it disproportionately affected marginalized individuals like Leilani Muir, a working class, Irish-Polish, Catholic girl.[3] Sociologists Jana Grekul, Harvey Krahn, and Dave Odynak have demonstrated that the primary targets of the program were certain populations deemed to be "vulnerable," including women, youth, and Indigenous Peoples who often came from lower socio-economic backgrounds.[4] This raises the question of what "public" in public health meant. Was it aimed at certain individuals and not others? Who was it intended to protect? Who was — advertently or inadvertently — included and excluded?

Muir's case provides one of many illustrations that the answers to these questions are complex and that who and what constitutes the public is a construct defined by shifting socio-political tides. For early twentieth-century public health officials, medical professionals, social reformers, and politicians, what constituted the public, was an ideal community shaped by British imperialist notions of race and racial hierarchies. Their ideal community was a white, Anglo-Protestant Canada that prospered not only economically but socially as well. Muir stood on the margins of this imagined community. Her religious and ethnic background was widely perceived as less desirable than those of Anglo-Protestant heritage. Her family was also poor and therefore seen as a burden on the state rather than a productive part of it (see also Chapter 12). As a woman, there were concerns about potential sexual deviances leading to illegitimate births. As a child, she was more a ward of the state than a citizen. Finally, Muir's supposed condition of "mental deficiency" was so broad and subjective as to render it meaningless.[5]

Individuals like Muir were singled out because in nearly every social category they were not what most of the elite elements in society considered "desirable" or "healthy." For them, those labelled as "mentally deficient" did not contribute to the betterment of Canadian society but rather detracted from it. Alberta's eugenics program is a tragic and instructive example of an idealized social construct being used to determine the meaning of public in public health. Public health policies with respect to eugenics were inherently exclusionary. For a field that prides itself on being concerned with upstream determinants of population well-being and health equity, questions about who is — and who is not — considered part of the public in public health are critical ones indeed.

Conceptualizing "the Public"

In this chapter, we explore the idea that the public is a constructed category, reflecting various values and ideologies, and how this has played out in Alberta's public health history. In a wide variety of programs and policies, the socially constituted nature of the public has impacted public health's objectives, implementation, and targets. We illustrate this observation using three examples: first, through the experiences of Leilani Muir and others affected by Alberta's eugenics program; second, through immigration policy in the province; and third, by the framing and deployment of tuberculosis control efforts in Alberta, which marginalized (in fact, aggressively excluded) Indigenous tuberculosis patients in particular.

This chapter contributes to a robust body of contemporary international public health scholarship concerned with defining the public and with paradigms of inclusion and exclusion. For example, in 2007, Marcel Verweij and Angus Dawson wrote the influential paper, "The Meaning of 'Public' in 'Public Health.'" Here, the authors develop the idea that the meaning of the public is not static, but rather a constituency defined by the objectives and aims of a particular health intervention. Therefore, even if the public refers to an indefinite number of people, any given intervention does not necessarily benefit many, or even a majority, of a population.[6] In his 2012 book, *What Makes Health Public?*, John Coggon considers the broad span of political, ethical and legal implications of public health, which in turn prompts a need to recognize the legal structures that are used to turn notions of public health into policy.[7] This critical theorization undergirds the types of analyses done in the present chapter, particularly as it strives to show the ways in which the state constructs public health threats (and their responses) through institutional (including legal) and ethical lenses and means.

There are several examples of how these phenomena play out in the Canadian context. Notably, *Social Determinants of Health*, an edited collection by Dennis Raphael, contains an array of important works, including one by Grace-Edward Galabuzi that delineates and comprehensively deals with the forces that cause social exclusion — and thus poorer health — of various social groups.[8] Ronald Labonté builds on Galabuzi's thesis by cautioning against efforts to correct social exclusion by centering social inclusion and placing blame for exclusion on individuals.[9] Finally, Janet Smylie addresses the ways in which social exclusion affects Indigenous Peoples in particular, focusing on living conditions.[10] In terms of research by Alberta-based scholars, Melanie Rock has considered whether animals, in particular pets, should be included in definitions of the public using data from the City of Calgary. On the discussion of inclusion-exclusion paradigms, Rebecca Haines-Saah demonstrates the phenomenon of "privileged normalization" in marijuana use, whereby media narratives surrounding marijuana use convey greater acceptability of the practice among those with power and status than among those without.[11]

Bringing these various strands together is the concept of intersectionality, which is increasingly incorporated in public health scholarship in Canada and internationally.[12] The lens of intersectionality draws attention to the impacts that structures and processes that create exclusion and marginalization based on intersecting identities like gender, race, Indigeneity, ability, and age have on well-being and health equity. This chapter builds on these ideas by showing how conceptualizations of the public have informed the deployment of public health, particularly through paradigms of inclusion-exclusion, through Alberta's public health history.

Immigration, Public Health, and Exclusion

Ethnicity/race, ability, and class were central to Canada's immigration policy from the late nineteenth century into the early decades of the twentieth century. Although the Immigration Act of 1869 contained very few restrictions regarding entry into Canada, over time federal immigration policy became much more restrictive and excluded immigrants on the basis of their ethnicity, race, and national origin.[13] The federal government sought to attract "desirable" immigrants, primarily those from the British Isles and the United States, and it sought to curtail immigration from "less desirable" areas such as central and eastern Europe and Asia.[14] Yet, the federal colonial campaign to attract farmers to settle the West allowed for approximately three million newcomers to enter Canada by 1914, with the majority arriving from non-Anglo-Saxon countries, including Ukraine, Poland, Germany, and Hungary.[15]

While the influx of immigrants from central and eastern Europe into western Canada brought out nativism and xenophobia among Anglo-Canadians, and led to hostility toward newcomers in general, there was a hierarchy in the desirability of new immigrants.[16] While central and eastern Europeans were viewed relatively favourably in terms of their likelihood of assimilating into Canadian society, the debate over Asian immigration focused on implementing measures to exclude them from entering Canada altogether.[17] Immigration restrictions, particularly the Chinese Immigration Act of 1885 and subsequent amendments, over time reduced the number of Chinese newcomers in Canada.[18]

The discourse over Chinese immigration to Alberta intersected with public health even before Alberta had officially become a province. In 1892, open hostility toward Chinese immigrants resulted in a mass city riot in Calgary, sparked by an outbreak of smallpox that was initially observed in a Chinese man.[19] For the authorities, the case was proof that white Calgarians needed to "remain vigilant against the potential deleterious effects of Asian men on the community."[20] Racial animus on the grounds of health was promulgated through newspapers and state action. For example, the Chinese men who were afflicted with smallpox were treated as deceptive and malevolent in local newspapers, while white patients were treated sympathetically.[21] The Calgarian experience fed into, and was influenced by, national rhetoric that claimed that in "moral, social, and sanitary status, Chinese were below the most inferior standard of Western life."[22] This nativist rhetoric explicitly constructed a threat to public health as being Chinese, and the public as white Anglo-Saxon Calgarians.[23] The demarcation between who was part of the public and who was not extended to conceptualizations of space: as historian Nayan Shah has pointed out, North American conceptualizations of the condition of Chinese homes were that of filth and decay, in sharp contrast to the supposed hygiene and cleanliness of white, Christian homes.[24] The homes and workplaces of Chinese immigrants were sites that were inherently linked with ill health, and their presence needed to be treated, as one would a disease.

In the early decades of the twentieth century, the legacy of othering Asian, in particular Chinese, immigrants continued to be tied with themes of public health.

During the 1920s, the small Chinese population in Calgary and Edmonton was linked with another public health problem, drug consumption.[25] Popularized during the 1920s by Albertan reformers such as Emily Murphy, but present since the beginning of Chinese immigration to Canada, depictions of Chinese immigrants as drug addled menaces to the Canadian way of life permeated the mainstream. In response to the Calgary riots noted above, *The Edmonton Bulletin* published an article called simply "The Chinese," in which the author asserted that Alberta had no responsibility to provide "Christian charity" to those who would "engage in the distribution of opium . . . and the most loathsome forms of vice," character traits seen as distinct to the Chinese people.[26] As also seen with other groups of immigrants, the othering of Chinese immigrants propped up public health policy that — rather than integrate and protect and promote the health of the Chinese immigrants themselves — sought to protect the rest of the public from them. The very idea of a public worth protecting was built around the value of the moral and ethnic character of white Anglo-Saxon Canadians, a definition which firmly excluded the so-called menace that were Chinese immigrants. (A parallel can be made with how Indigeneity in Alberta has been and continues to be linked to alcoholism and drug use; see Chapter 7)

During the interwar period, politicians, physicians, and social reformers in Alberta were concerned about the arrival of "unhealthy" and "defective" immigrants, primarily from central and eastern Europe, to the province. They attributed the spread of infectious diseases and the increase in the "deficiency" of the population to the unhygienic habits and deviant behaviours of the newcomers. The new immigrants were presented as a threat to the well-being of the province and politicians and public health officials were determined to quarantine them, to place them under constant surveillance, or to expel them from the country.[27] As early as 1922, Alberta Liberal MP Charles Stewart informed parliament of the situation in western Canada, particularly Alberta, arguing "that too large a percentage of people who are mentally unfitted to come to this country have been allowed to enter Canada. . . . I know whereof I am speaking," Stewart continued, "because our mental hospital in Alberta has had too large a percentage of people allowed to come to Canada who were mentally unfit."[28] In other words, Stewart implied that Canada's immigration policy was problematic because it allowed "defective" immigrants to enter, settle in Alberta, and become a public charge.

Similar sentiments were expressed by Alberta's Department of Public Health where, in 1924, the Deputy Health Minister, W.C. Laidlaw, wrote to Premier John Brownlee objecting to the "cursory" examination of immigrants, because "under this system only the most obvious cases [of "defective" immigrants] would be detected."[29] The minister wanted more effective procedures in place that would prevent immigrants with mental and physical disabilities, those with criminal tendencies, and those who were likely to become a public charge from entering Alberta. Likewise, Miss Elizabeth Clark from the Nursing Branch of the Department of Public Health forwarded a list of "undesirable" immigrants and immigrant families to Dr. Laidlaw and to the premier arguing that they had passed through the inspection undetected and should be deported. Clark described one newcomer from Germany as suffering from "tubercular glands of the neck," and had informed the Department of Public Health that deportation paperwork had been filed.[30] Historian Barbara Roberts has demonstrated that, according to the statistics provided by the Department of Immigration, deportations peaked during four periods in the first three decades of the twentieth century: 1908–1909, 1913–1914, 1921–1924, and 1929–1930. All these periods represent years of economic recession in Canada. Therefore, those immigrants who were hurt the most by the economic downturn and who had become a public charge were deported.[31]

The concerns over the quality of immigrants in Alberta was also evident in the 1921 report of Alberta's Department of Public Health, which described Ukrainian immigrants as having difficulties assimilating to the Canadian way of life. According to the report, their language, culture, and traditions increased the likelihood of "feeblemindedness" in the family, and their "ignorance" of health and hygiene made them susceptible to the spread of diseases.[32] The Department of Public Health furthermore singled out the living arrangements of central and eastern Europeans as particularly problematic, stating "the foreign element, called collectively Russian although including Galician, Pole and Austrian . . . has no concept of the meaning of the word sanitation."[33] The supposed inability of some immigrants to adapt to Canadian society meant that new immigrants were often under surveillance. For example, according to historian Erica Dyck, inspectors and public health nurses in Alberta conducted home visits in immigrant neighbourhoods to ensure proper hygiene was practised in the home, and sometimes they sought to force sanitary measures on immigrant families if habits remained unchanged.[34] By employing such public health measures, public health officials gained significant knowledge of the living conditions and behaviours in immigrant quarters of the provinces. They presented these living habits as different and even dangerous, and thus helped construct some new immigrants as a threat to the province and as outsiders to the collective idea of the public.

Eugenics and Public Health

Eugenics, including forced sterilization, and public health have often crossed paths. In his work on the history of public health in the United States, historian

Martin Pernick notes that the goals, agendas, and personnel of the eugenics and the public health movements frequently overlapped.[35] Concerns over public health were a key incubator in which horrific eugenic ideas could grow; for example, some in public health turned to eugenics to find solutions to seemingly intractable problems, including poverty, criminality, "mental deficiency," and "feeblemindedness."

Although eugenic theory emerged in Britain in response to the social conditions and concerns over perceived degeneration of the population, eugenic ideas and their aims of "human improvement" gained popularity around the world.[36] The methods by which these goals were realized and implemented varied between and within countries[37] and included so-called positive eugenics, which aimed to encourage the reproduction of individuals with desirable characteristics, and negative eugenics, which discouraged (or, in fact, forcefully prevented) reproduction among individuals with undesirable traits.[38] In Canada, negative eugenics found government health policy manifestations in the provinces of British Columbia and Alberta in the form of sexual sterilization measures. As noted above, Alberta's Sexual Sterilization Act (1928), which fell under the administration of the provincial public health department, allowed for the sterilization of patients in mental institutions, particularly those diagnosed with "mental deficiency."[39] Social and economic changes in Canada during the first decades of the twentieth century provided important context for the act. Many social reformers and politicians were concerned that Canada was becoming less homogenous, and as Erika Dyck suggests, "eugenics offered an appealing solution to the growing problem of social and moral decay by promising to support stricter immigration policies, while focusing on the internal make-up of western Canadian society and even promoting invasive measures to ensure that the so-called unfit members of society were not capable of reproduction."[40]

The concerns over national degeneration, due to the supposed increase in "mental deficiency," were intensified by findings from the Mental Hygiene Surveys conducted by psychiatrists C. K. Clarke and Clarence Hincks. Their survey of the province of Alberta in 1921 revealed that the provincial institutions were overrun with "mental defectives," a term used to describe individuals with intellectual disabilities.[41] As sociologist Gerald V. O'Brien suggests, and as illustrated in the case of Leilani Muir described at the beginning of this chapter, the notion of "mental deficiency" was imprecise and broad, such that its definition could be expanded to include a vast number of behaviours perceived to be deviant, and was often associated with individuals whom society otherwise had already marginalized.[42] Nonetheless, the findings of the Alberta Mental Hygiene survey were taken up by social reformers in the province, particularly the United

Farm Women of Alberta, who raised concerns about "mental deficiency" and lobbied the provincial government to implement measures, such as sexual sterilization, to reduce the numbers of "defective" individuals.[43] By 1928, the campaign would prove successful, as Alberta became the first province in Canada to implement a eugenics program and in fact was considered a pioneer in the British Commonwealth in that regard.[44]

Several scholars studying Alberta's eugenic past have demonstrated that the provincial eugenics program primarily targeted vulnerable individuals including women, young people, new immigrants, and Indigenous Peoples.[45] A central aspect of the provincial eugenics program was its focus on individuals who were constructed as "abnormal" and thus a public health menace. As was evident in Muir's case, socio-economic status, gender, and ethnic background singled people out as ideal candidates for sterilization under the Sexual Sterilization Act.

Tuberculosis and Modes of Exclusion

Our final example of public health examined through the paradigms of inclusion and exclusion is tuberculosis. As historian Katherine McCuaig notes, many reformers and thinkers of the twentieth century believed that "to cure [tuberculosis], one had to cure society."[46] Although that fundamental assumption spurred the mobilization of social and economic resources in the fight against tuberculosis, the question of how to "cure society" brought answers that were explicitly exclusionary, particularly along the lines of class and Indigeneity.[47]

In the early 1900s, various political bodies argued that Alberta was receiving more than its fair share of tubercular patients.[48] Many members of the growing ranks of public health practitioners expressed a sentiment that the Canadian response should be a nationally coordinated and locally deployed system of public health, accompanied by measures to mitigate immigration. The loss of economic productivity was central in the justification of these mobilizing efforts, thus placing tuberculosis at the intersection of public health, public finance, immigration, and race. In this context, it did not take long for narratives to emerge that positioned racialized groups as detrimental to the public's finances as well as to public health. As an illustration concerning tuberculosis, a 1910 editorial in the *Western Canada Medical Journal* stated that not merely immigrants, but those who came to the western provinces hiding their illness, and indeed, hiding the fact that they were poor, cost the country millions of dollars and were a serious concern.[49] In these types of narratives, individuals with tuberculosis were seen as insidious threats to the province, leeching off its finances and infecting its citizens with disease. These concerns were paired with eugenic thought, as in this paradigm an influx of sickly, lower-class citizens would prove detrimental to the racial hygiene of the province.

Inequities within the constructed public are acutely seen when examining the experiences of Indigenous Peoples in Alberta, for whom tuberculosis was yet another reminder of the reality of their existence outside the constructed public. Social exclusion of Indigenous Peoples is the result of a variety of factors, dealt with at length in, for example, the Truth and Reconciliation Commission's reports, but which can be summarized as the workings of colonial apparatuses, including federal and provincial policy arrangements whose goal was coercive assimilation. This often took the form of colonial governments dispossessing Indigenous Peoples of their lands, placing restrictions on their livelihoods, forcing their children into residential schools, and suppressing their cultures (see also Chapter 7).[50] Across levels of government, racialized conceptualizations of Indigenous Peoples as sickly were prominent. Historian Mary Ellen Kelm has demonstrated that from the 1930s onward the perspectives in public health literature shifted from viewing Indigenous Peoples suffering from tuberculosis as "victims of an imported disease to being infectious agents to white populations."[51] In Alberta, for example, the racialized belief that Indigenous Peoples had a genetic predisposition to tuberculosis was commonly accepted among western Canadian medical professionals in the early twentieth century.[52] This characterization was maintained despite long-standing efforts by Indigenous persons themselves to show that economic inequality, poor nutrition, and overcrowded living conditions, all imposed by colonial systems and structures rather than genetics, significantly contributed to ill health.[53]

The misconception that Indigenous Peoples were genetically predisposed to tuberculosis, and were thus a threat to larger society, had significant ramifications in the subsequent years. For example, Indigenous patients were rarely admitted for treatment at provincial sanatoriums.[54] Physician Anne Fanning, director of Tuberculosis Services for Alberta from 1987 to 1995, recalls how at one time during the history of Alberta, there was no place where Indigenous Peoples could receive tuberculosis treatment, although some of the children in the residential schools were cared for in local health units (see Chapter 13).[55] The perceived threats to the (white) public's health led to the establishment of Indian hospitals by the federal government from the 1940s onward.[56] These hospitals were presented as tuberculosis sanatoriums by the federal government but they admitted Indigenous patients suffering from various diseases, ensuring their segregation from the white population.[57] For example, when establishing an Indian Hospital in Edmonton, the Department of Health and Welfare re-assured the mayor of the city that the "the patients would be confined to the institution and it would be better than having '. . . tuberculous Indians wandering about the streets of Edmonton . . . and spreading the disease.'"[58]

A racialized conceptualization of tuberculosis manifested in significant disparities in disease incidence and outcomes. In 1939, Alberta's Department of Public Health recognized that there was "still much to be desired in the Indian tuberculosis problem . . . it appears that no great reduction can be expected in the present Provincial tuberculosis death rate until competent . . . measures are made available to the Indian population."[59] Nonetheless, six years later, in early 1945, the Advisory Committee for the Control and Prevention of Tuberculosis Among the Indians, of which Alberta's deputy health minister was a member, stated that the non-Indigenous death rate from tuberculosis had declined by 39 percent in the fifteen years prior, while the Indigenous death rate had changed very little.[60] In the context of myriad social and colonial determinants of health, this was likely due in part to poor conditions in the Indian hospitals including understaffing and inadequate medical treatment.[61] Indigenous inequities in tuberculosis treatment continued throughout the 1940s;[62] even as Alberta's Department of Public Health was celebrating five years of falling death rates from tuberculosis, the disproportionate burden of deaths in Indigenous Peoples persisted. In 1952, out of 125 deaths from tuberculosis, fifty-two (or approximately 42 percent) were from Indigenous Peoples,[63] even though they only made up approximately 2.3 percent of the Alberta population at the time.[64] In 1956, while the overall death rate from tuberculosis continued to decline, Indigenous Peoples in Alberta still made up nearly a third of all deaths,[65] which in part reflected that they were "in the hands of harried, if not unqualified staff, in crowded and dismal institutions."[66] Recent estimates show that tuberculosis rates among the Indigenous population in Alberta remained very high until the 1960s, at which point they began to decline — first rapidly (until the 1980s), and then more slowly. Despite the decline from the 1960s to the early 2000s, tuberculosis rates among Indigenous populations in Alberta remain higher than in the non-Indigenous population.[67]

Tuberculosis thus provides another illustration of power, resources, opportunities and thus health outcomes being tied to social identity, including racial identity. The constructed nature of the public, which excluded or segmented Indigenous Peoples on colonial, jurisdictional and racist grounds, fostered systemic inequities including differential approaches to prevention and control.

Conclusion

This chapter has illustrated ways in which the public in public health has been constructed throughout Alberta's history. The public has consistently been, implicitly, or explicitly, defined through processes of compartmentalizing, structuring, and conceptualizing a group in ways that contribute to paradigms of inclusion and exclusion. As the consideration of the eugenics program shows, concepts of "mental deficiency" were intimately tied to racial purity, which in turn interacted with socio-economic status to disenfranchise various groups and categorize them as part of the threat. An analysis of immigration further illustrates racialized assumptions about causes of ill health and how the ensuing discourse of social exclusion influenced public policy. And with tuberculosis, some individuals were seen, on the basis of their intersecting social locations of class, race, gender, etc., to be contagions of disease, and therefore morally bankrupt and excluded from particular public services and resources. More extensively, Indigenous Peoples' health concerns were dictated in a unilateral colonial fashion that placed them outside of a broader public, with frailties assigned to them due to their ethnicity that underscored unacceptably paternalistic treatment. In each case, the public was conceived in a distinct way that led to diversions from the idealized norm being treated differently and almost always unfairly.

As acknowledged at the outset of this chapter, considerable work is being done to theorize more equitable ways in which public health can be conceptualized and practised, which necessitates taking into consideration the structures and processes that advantage or disadvantage individuals and groups on the basis of multiple factors (e.g., race, gender, age, Indigenous status, ability), and directing public policy efforts toward redressing the systemic factors that create and perpetuate those inequities. To provide structure to these inquiries within applied public health, the Canadian Public Health Association reminds us of the foundational role of equity in our field.[68] To a certain extent, the very nature of public health — which is concerned with the conditions of the health of a population — carries the risk of being "equal but not equitable." However, this is a challenge to which we must rise if we wish to retain a robust and relevant vision of public health that embraces the social determinants of health in a meaningful and critical way.

NOTES

1   Doug Whalsten, "Leilani Muir versus the Philosopher King: Eugenics on trial in Alberta," *Genetica* 99 (1997).

2   Whalsten, "Leilani Muir," 194–195.

3   Amy Samson, "Eugenics in the Community: The United Farm Women of Alberta, Public Health Nursing, Teaching, Social Work, and Sexual Sterilization in Alberta, 1928–1972" (PhD diss., University of Saskatchewan, 2014), 2, Harvest database, http://hdl.handle.net/10388/ETD-2014-12-1975.

4   Jana Grekul, Harvey Krahn, and Dave Odynak, "Sterilizing the "Feeble-minded": Eugenics in Alberta, Canada, 1929–1972," *Journal of Historical Sociology* 17, no. 4 (2004).

5   The Sexual Sterilization Act (1928) did not explain how "mental deficiency" was conceptualized. Patients were usually deemed to be mentally deficient if they scored below 70 on an IQ test, but sociologist Jana Grekul has demonstrated that "the 'mentally defective' status of people passed by the [Eugenics] Board for sterilization is questionable." This is primarily because some patients were labelled mentally defective despite scoring 70 or higher on the IQ test. Jana Grekul, "The Social Construction of the Feebleminded Threat: Implementation of the Sexual Sterilization Act in Alberta, 1929–1972" (PhD diss., University of Alberta, 2002), 123, ERA [education & research archive] database, https://doi.org/10.7939/r3-5s4e-ez69.

6   See Marcel Verweij and Angus Dawson, "The Meaning of 'Public' in 'Public Health,'" in *Ethics, Prevention, and Public Health*, eds. Angus Dawson and Marcel Verweij (Oxford: Oxford University Press, 2007).

7   See John Coggon, *What Makes Health Public? A Critical Evaluation of Moral, Legal, and Political Claims in Public Health* (Cambridge: Cambridge University Press, 2012).

8   Grace-Edward Galabuzi, "Social Exclusion," in *Social Determinants of Health: Canadian Perspectives*, ed. Dennis Raphael (Toronto: Canadian Scholars Press, 2009).

9   Ronald Labonté, "Social Inclusion/Exclusion and Health: Dancing the Dialect," in *Social Determinants of Health: Canadian Perspectives*, ed. Dennis Raphael (Toronto: Canadian Scholars Press, 2009).

10   Janet Smylie, "The Health of Aboriginal Peoples," in *Social Determinants of Health: Canadian Perspectives*, ed. Dennis Raphael (Toronto: Canadian Scholars Press, 2009).

11   Melanie Rock, "Who or What Is 'the Public' in Critical Public Health? Reflections on Posthumanism and Anthropological Engagements with One Health," *Critical Public Health* 27, no. 3 (2017); Rebecca J. Haines-Saah, et al., "The Privileged Normalization of Marijuana Use — An Analysis of Canadian Newspaper Reporting, 1997–2007," *Critical Public Health* 24, no. 1 (2014).

12   See for example: G.R. Bauer, "Incorporating Intersectionality Theory into Population Health Research Methodology: Challenges and the Potential to Advance Health Equity," *Social Science & Medicine* 110 (2004); Mary Susan Thomson, et al., "Improving Immigrant Populations' Access to Mental Health Services in Canada: A Review of Barriers and Recommendations," *Journal of Immigrant and Minority Health* 17, no. 6 (2015); Olena Hankivsky, *Health Inequities in Canada: Intersectional Frameworks and Practices* (Vancouver: University of British Columbia Press, 2011); Josée Lapalme, Rebecca Haines-Saah, and Katherine L. Frohlich, "More than a Buzzword: How Intersectionality Can Advance Social Inequalities in Health Research," *Critical Public Health* 30, no. 4 (2020).

13   See for example, Ninette Kelley and Michael Trebilcock, *The Making of the Mosaic: A History of Canadian Immigration Policy* (Toronto: University of Toronto Press, 1998).

14   Kelley and Trebilcock, *Making of the Mosaic*.

15   Donald H. Avery, *Reluctant Host: Canada's Response to Immigrant Workers, 1896–1994* (Toronto: McClelland & Stewart, Inc., 1995), 20.

16   See for example, Howard Palmer, *Patterns of Prejudice: History of Nativism in Alberta* (Toronto: McClelland and Stewart Ltd., 1982).

17   Palmer, *Patterns of Prejudice*, 31–32.

18   Valerie Knowles, *Strangers at Our Gates: Canadian Immigration and Immigration Policy, 1540–1990* (Toronto: Dundurn Press, 1992), 136.

19   Palmer, *Patterns of Prejudice*, 21.

20   Kristin Burnett, "Race, Disease, and Public Violence: Smallpox and the (Un)Making of Calgary's Chinatown, 1892," *Social History of Medicine* 25, no. 2 (May 2012), 370.

21   Burnett, "Race, Disease, and Public Violence," 368.

22   Ban Seng Hoe, "Structural Changes of Two Chinese Communities in Alberta, Canada," *Canadian Centre for Folk Culture Studies* 19 (1976): 45.

23   Burnett, "Race, Disease, and Public Violence," 366.

24   Nyan Shah, *Contagious Divides: Epidemics and Race in San Francisco's Chinatown* (London: University of California Press, 2001), 115.

25   Palmer, *Patterns of Prejudice*, 82.

26   "The Chinese," *The Edmonton Bulletin*, 15 August 1892, 4.

27   Erika Dyck, *Facing Eugenics: Reproduction, Sterilization and the Politics of Choice* (Toronto: University of Toronto Press, 2013), 34.

28   Canada. *House of Commons Debates*, 23 May 1922. 14th Parliament, 1st Session: Volume 3, 2145–2146, https://parl.canadiana.ca/view/oop.debates_HOC1401_03/2.

29   Provincial Archives of Alberta, Premier's Office Files, 69.289, roll 433, memorandum from Dr. Laidlaw to Premier Brownlee, 6 November 1924.

30   Letter from Miss E. Clark to Dr. Laidlaw and Premier Brownlee, 10 September 1924, PAA, 69.289, roll 433, premier's office files.

31   Barbara Roberts, *Whence They Came: Deportation from Canada, 1900–1935* (Ottawa: University of Ottawa Press, 1988), 47–48.

32   Dyck, *Facing Eugenics*, 44.

33   Cited in Dyck, *Facing Eugenics*, 45.

34   Dyck, *Facing Eugenics*, 45.

35   Martin Pernick, "Eugenics and Public Health in American History," *American Journal of Public Health* 87, no. 11 (1997): 1767–1768.

36   Eugenics was a term coined by British statistician, Francis Galton (1882–1911) in 1883. See Francis Galton, *Inquiries into Human Faculty and its Development* (London: Macmillan, 1883), 17.

37   Marius Turda, *Modernism and Eugenics* (London: Palgrave Macmillan, 2010), 7.

38   Dorothy Porter, *Health, Civilization, and the State: A History of Public Health from Ancient to Modern Times* (London: Routledge, 1999), 168.

39   *The Sexual Sterilization Act*, Statutes of the Province of Alberta 1928, c. 37, 117–18.

40   Dyck, *Facing Eugenics*, 9.

41   Clarence Hincks. *Mental Hygiene Survey of the Province of Alberta 1921*. [n.p.]: Canadian National Committee for Mental Hygiene, 1921.

42   Gerald V. O'Brien, *Framing the Moron: The Social Construction of Feeble-mindedness in the American Eugenics Era* (Manchester.: Manchester University Press, 2013), 6.

43   For more information about the United Farm Women of Alberta and their eugenics campaign see, A. Naomi Nind, "Solving an 'Appalling' Problem: Social Reformers and the Campaign for the Alberta Sexual Sterilization Act, 1928," *Alberta Law Review* 38, no. 2 (2000); Sheila Gibbons, "'The True [Political] Mothers of Today': Farm Women and the Organization of Eugenics Feminism in Alberta." (Master's thesis, University of Saskatchewan, HARVEST database, 2012), https://harvest.usask.ca/items/f47f616c-7f0a-4c00-82d1-38786f2af9eb.

44   Erna Kurbegović, "Eugenics in Comparative Perspective: Explaining Manitoba and Alberta's Divergence on Eugenics Policy, 1910s to the 1930s" (PhD diss., University of Calgary, 2019), 211, Prism database, http://hdl.handle.net/1880/109868; Amy Samson, "Eugenics in the Community."

45   See for example, Christian, "The Mentally Ill and Human Rights in Alberta;" Jana Grekul, "Sterilization in Alberta, 1928–1972: Gender Matters," *Canadian Review of Sociology* 45, no. 3 (2008); Karen Stote, *An Act of Genocide: Colonialism and the Sterilization of Aboriginal Women* (Winnipeg: Fernwood Publishing, 2015); Erika Dyck, *Facing Eugenics*.

46   Katherine McCuaig, *The Weariness, the Fever, and the Fret* (Montreal: McGill-Queen's University Press, 1999), 8.

47   While including several different examples of social exclusion in this chapter, we are cognizant of Eve Tuck and K. Wayne Yang's powerful reminder that *decolonization is not a metaphor*: Indigenous inequities are different from other forms of inequities, and decolonization is not just another social justice project. Eve Tuck and K. Wayne Yang, "Decolonization is Not a Metaphor," *Decolonization: Indigeneity, Education & Society* 1, no. 1 (2012).

48   McCuaig, *The Weariness*, 17.

49   Editorial. "The Question of Immigration," *Western Canada Medical Journal* 4, no. 7 (July, 1910), 328.

50   Alberta Department of Public Health, *Annual Report 1939* (Edmonton: printed by A. Shnitka, King's Printer, 1941), 21; Maureen Lux, "Beyond Biology: Disease and its Impact on the Canadian Plains Native People, 1880–1930" (PhD diss., Simon Fraser University, 1996), 343, Summit Research Repository, https://summit.sfu.ca/item/7012; see, for instance: Truth and Reconciliation Commission of Canada, *Honouring the Truth, Reconciling for the Future, Summary of the Final Report of the Truth*

and *Reconciliation Commission of Canada* (Winnipeg, MB: Truth and Reconciliation Commission of Canada, 2015), www.trc.ca.

51   Mary Ellen Kelm, "Diagnosing the Discursive Indian: Medicine, Gender, and the 'Dying Race,'" *Ethnohistory* 52, no. 2 (Spring 2005), 381.

52   R. C. Ferguson and R. G. Ferguson, "Activities in a Province-Wide Programme for the Control of Tuberculosis," *Canadian Public Health Journal* 26, no. 3 (March 1935), 134.

53   Maureen Lux, "Care for the 'Racially Careless': Indian Hospitals in the Canadian West, 1920–1950s," *Canadian Historical Review* 91, no. 3 (September 2010), 273, 344; Lux, "Beyond Biology," 344.

54   Maureen Lux, *Separate Beds: A History of Indian Hospitals in Canada, 1920s–1980s* (Toronto: University of Toronto Press, 2016), 11; Lux, "Care for the 'Racially Careless,'" 420.

55   Anne Fanning, interview by Don Juzwishin and Rogelio Velez Mendoza, 30 August 2018.

56   Lux, *Separate Beds*, 9–10.

57   Lux, *Separate Beds*, 10.

58   Lux, "Beyond Biology," 382.

59   Lux, "Care for the 'Racially Careless.'"

60   Lux, "Beyond Biology," 379.

61   Lux, *Separate Beds*, 103.

62   Alberta Department of Public Health, *Annual Report 1947* (Edmonton: printed by A. Shnitka, King's Printer, 1949), 25.

63   Alberta Department of Public Health, *Annual Report 1952* (Edmonton: printed by A. Shnitka, King's Printer, 1954).

64   This approximation comes from the 1951 Statistics Canada long-form census. According to the 1951 Census Table 34: "Population by origin and sex, for counties and census divisions," Alberta had a total population of 939,501, of which 21,210 (approx. 2.3%) responded to the census question as having "Indian and Eskimo" origin. It is important to emphasize that estimates of the Indigenous population in Canada depend on the source, and different data collection methods impact the estimates. For example, the numbers reported by Statistics Canada from the long-form census "comprise all persons who self-identify as having Aboriginal ancestry and/or Aboriginal identity." This is different from the estimates from the Indian Register administered by Indigenous and Northern Affairs Canada (INAC). Prior to the 1985 enactment of Bill C-31, *An Act to Amend the Indian Act*, many people were disqualified from receiving their Indian Status and any related rights through forcible enfranchisement. For the census figures see Canada. Dominion Bureau of Statistics, Ninth Census of Canada (Ottawa: King's Printer, 1951), Vol. 1, Table 34. For the difficulties in assessing population see, Frank Trovato, and Laura Aylsworth, "Demography of Indigenous Peoples in Canada," in *The Canadian Encyclopedia*, last edited 17 January 2018, https://www.thecanadianencyclopedia.ca/en/article/aboriginal-people-demography.

65   Alberta Department of Public Health, *Annual Report 1956* (Edmonton: printed by A. Shnitka, King's Printer, 1958), Alberta Department of Public Health, *Annual Report of the Bureau of Vital Statistics*, 3.

66   Lux, *Separate Beds*, 129.

67   Kianoush Dehghani, et al., "Determinants of Tuberculosis Trends in Six Indigenous Populations of the USA, Canada, and Greenland from 1960 to 2014: A Population-Based Study," *Lancet Public Health* 3, issue 3 (6 February 2018), https://doi.org/10.1016/S2468-2667(18)30002-1; Thomas Kovesi, "Respiratory Disease in Canadian First Nations and Inuit Children," *Pediatric Child Health* 17, no. 7 (August–September 2012), 377.

68   See Canadian Public Health Association (CPHA), *Public Health: A Conceptual Framework*, Canadian Public Health Association Working Paper, 2nd ed. (Ottawa: CPHA, 2017).

2

Priorities and Concerns of Provincial Governments: A Historical Public Health Landscape

Lindsay McLaren, Rogelio Velez Mendoza, and Jack Lucas

Introduction

In this chapter, we aim to provide a bird's eye view of the historical landscape of public health in Alberta, from the perspective of successive provincial governments. By "landscape," we mean two things: 1) overall attention to public health, and 2) the ways in which health and public health have been understood, over time, from the government perspective.

As noted in the introduction to this book, a challenge facing public health today is that it is frequently misunderstood. In contrast to its broad definition — which emphasizes population-level well-being and health equity via prevention, promotion, and upstream thinking about root causes — public health, in Canada and elsewhere, is often conflated with publicly funded medical care, and/or reduced to single elements, such as immunization or health behaviour change.[1] A historical analysis can shed light on how the socio-political context has shaped dominant understandings of health and disease causation, and thus public policy responses, such as an increasingly costly health care system that is overwhelmingly focused on acute medical care and technologies. It can also shed light on who is included and who is excluded from the public health community and its activities (see Chapter 1).[2] A historical analysis can furthermore illuminate core features of public health that have permitted the field to endure, even as specific priorities and concerns change. An understanding of those core features is essential if public health is to remain a strong and relevant public institution and policy priority moving forward.

Data Source

How has the public health landscape evolved in Alberta since the province was established in 1905? To answer this question, we draw on a unique and valuable data source that has existed through Alberta's history as a province: government throne speeches.

In keeping with a large international research initiative called the Comparative Agendas Project,[3] we focus in this chapter on policy attention — that is, the extent to which particular topics have been part of the government's policy agenda through time. To capture policy attention, scholars in the Comparative Agendas tradition seek out data sources that allow for systematic analysis of policy agendas over very long spans of time. Throne speeches, which are explicit statements of the government's legislative agenda at the beginning of each legislative session, are ideal documents for this purpose, allowing researchers to understand the relative importance of particular policy topics — in this case, public health — in a government's legislative agenda over time.[4]

To allow for systematic analysis across jurisdictions and over time, researchers in the Comparative Agendas Project have developed a standardized coding scheme in which sentences (or portions of sentences) in a policy document are coded by topic.[5] The data analyzed for this chapter consist of all text from all Alberta government throne speeches from 1906 to 2017, broken down into policy statements (i.e., sentences or sub-sentences, hereafter referred to as quasi-sentences). The full data set contains 14,193 quasi-sentences, spanning 1906–2017. Overall, as shown in Figure 2.1, there is a trend toward longer speeches in recent years. The number of quasi-sentences each year ranges from a low of nine in a war time speech in 1914 to a high of 357 in 1985.[6]

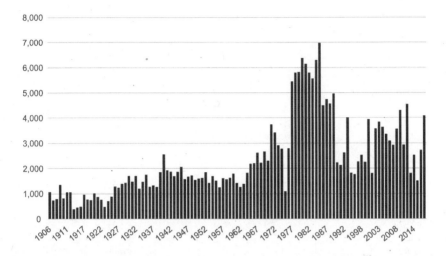

Fig. 2.1: Number of words in Alberta government throne speeches, by year, 1906–2017. The figure excludes years with no throne speech data (1912, 1994, and 2013) and years with more than one speech during the year (1913, 1922, 1945, 1949, 1975, 1989, 2001, 2008, and 2014).

Each quasi-sentence in the data set is coded, according to the single predominant and substantive area, into one major topic code. For the Alberta data set, quasi-sentences were coded using a version of the policy agendas codebook adapted to the Canadian context.[7] The Canadian version contains twenty-five major topic codes (each of which has several subtopic codes), which are shown in Table 2.1 and which provide the broader context for our analysis below.

TABLE 2.1: Major topic codes appearing in the Alberta throne speech data set.

Major topic code	Examples
Macroeconomics	Inflation, prices, and interest rates; Unemployment rate; Monetary supply, federal reserve board, and the treasury
Civil Rights, Minority Issues, and Multiculturalism*	Ethnic minority and racial group discrimination; Gender and sexual orientation discrimination; Age discrimination
Health	Health care reform, health care costs, and availability; Health care funding arrangements; Regulation of prescription drugs, medical devices, and medical procedures
Agriculture & Forestry*	Agricultural trade (international); Government subsidies to farmers and rangers, agricultural disaster insurance; Food inspection and safety
Labour, Employment, and Immigration	Worker safety and protection; Employment training and workforce development; Employee benefits
Education	Higher education; Elementary and secondary education; Education of underprivileged students
Environment	Drinking water safety; Waste disposal; Hazardous waste and toxic chemical regulation, treatment, and disposal
Energy	Nuclear energy and nuclear regulatory commission issues; Electricity and hydroelectricity; Natural gas and oil
Fisheries*	Fish stocks; Economic problems; Foreign fishing
Transportation	Mass transportation and safety; Highway construction, maintenance and safety; Airports, airlines, air traffic control and safety
Law, Crime, and Family Issues	Agencies dealing with law and crime; White collar crime and organized crime; Illegal drug production, trafficking, and control
Social Welfare	Food stamps, food assistance, and nutrition monitoring programs; Poverty and assistance for low-income families; Elderly issues and elderly assistance programs
Community Development and Housing Issues	Housing and community development; Urban economic development and general urban issues; Rural housing and CMHC [Canadian Mortgage and Housing Corporation] housing assistance programs
Banking, Finance, and Domestic Commerce	Canadian banking system and financial institution regulation; Securities and commodities regulation; Consumer finance, mortgages, and credit cards
Defence	Canadian and other defense alliances; Military intelligence, CSIS, Espionage; Military readiness, coordination of armed services air support and sealift capabilities, and national stockpiles of strategic materials
Space, Science, Technology and Communications	Canadian Space Agency; Commercial use of space, satellites; Science technology transfer, international scientific cooperation
Foreign Trade	Trade negotiations, disputes, and agreements; Export promotion and regulation; International private business investment
International Affairs and Foreign Aid	Foreign aid; International resources exploitation and resources agreement; Development countries issues
Government Operations	Government efficiency and bureaucratic oversight; Postal service issues; Government employee benefits

Table 2.1: (*continued*)

Major topic code	Examples
Public Lands and Water Management	National parks, memorials, historic sites, and recreation; Natural resources, public lands, and forest management; Water resources development and research
Culture and Entertainment	National culture and heritage issues; Sports
Provincial and Local Government Administration	Provincial and municipal government administration
Intergovernmental Relations & Trade*	Fiscal arrangements – social programs; Inter-provincial trade – agricultural; Regional development arrangements and programs
Constitutional and National Unity Issues*	Constitutional issues, e.g., issues relating to the division of powers, the patriation of the Constitution, or various elements of the Constitution
Native Affairs*	First Nations organizations; socio-economic conditions of First Nations; cultural preservation; treaties and negotiations.

Note: Those codes that were newly developed to reflect the Canadian context are denoted with asterisks.

Findings: Policy Attention to Health, Public Health, and Prevention in Alberta Government Throne Speeches, 1906–2017

One of the twenty-five major topic codes assigned to the throne speech data is health, and that was our starting point. Within the data set, we first examined the rise and fall of health — as a broad concept, as well as specific elements — as a topic of policy attention in the Alberta legislature. We then considered how concepts of public health, followed by prevention (based on public health's stated focus on prevention, rather than treatment, of health problems), appeared in the speeches over time. As presented next, our findings shed light on subtle but important shifts in how these terms have been used and understood by Alberta's provincial government, with implications for the field of public health and for the health and well-being of Albertans.

Health

In the Alberta throne speech data set, there were 1,125 quasi-sentences coded under health (major topic code 3), representing approximately 8 percent of the full data set. As with all major topic codes, the health code is broad and includes anything to do with health, medicine, well-being, illnesses, and health interventions.[8]

TRENDS OVER TIME IN POLICY ATTENTION TO HEALTH

Figure 2.2 illustrates trends over time in the proportion of all Alberta throne speech quasi-sentences that were coded under the health major topic code.

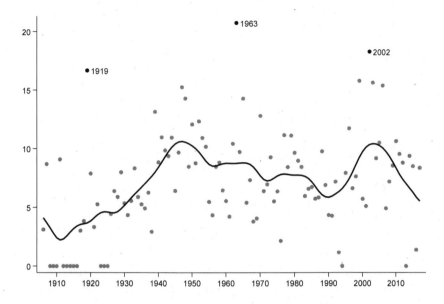

Fig. 2.2: Trends over time in the percent of all Alberta throne speech quasi-sentences coded as health (major topic code 3), 1906–2017 (lowess plot).[9]

One can see from Figure 2.2 that health, broadly conceived, occupied a relatively higher proportion of the throne speech entries during two periods: first, the post-WWII decades (late 1940s), and second, the decades following health system regionalization in Alberta (late 1990s and early 2000s). By considering the content of the speeches, one can shed light on these trends.

First, the throne speeches indicate that the post-WWII decades, under the Social Credit (SC) leadership of Ernest Manning, were a period of growth and expansion for health. The Manning government's 1946 speech opened by stating that "the Provincial Department of [Public] Health has prepared a comprehensive post-war program designed to improve the health conditions of our people."[10] Throughout the late 1940s and early 1950s, speeches made frequent reference to building or expanding health-related infrastructure. Examples include efforts to expand the public health workforce, protect health care workers, provide preventive health services in rural areas, and address particular diseases.

> A training school will be opened to provide facilities for field training of physicians, public health nurses and sanitary inspectors. (1946)[11]

Services safeguarding the health of workers in industry will be advanced through a survey of the industrial hazards and a study of diseases peculiar to the workers in various industries. (1948)[12]

Legislation also will be introduced providing for the establishment, administration and services of Rural Health Units. (1951)[13]

You will be asked to approve the emergent actions taken by my Government to relieve the financial burden of those afflicted by the severe epidemic of poliomyelitis . . . to provide adequate facilities for the care of those afflicted. (1954)[14]

Second, the period of the late 1990s and early 2000s was also an active one in terms of policy attention to health in Alberta, based on the throne speech content (Figure 2.2). This period aligns with regionalization of health services in Alberta (see Chapter 4). Under the Progressive Conservative leadership of Ralph Klein, throne speech references to health during that period suggested a strong focus on health care, with an emphasis — not surprising in the neoliberal period — on efficiency, privacy, and individualized diagnostic and treatment-oriented activities.

Initiatives to improve patient care and ensure an efficient system will include a pilot project using health smart cards. (1996)[15]

It will introduce new legislation to protect information related to Albertans' personal health. (1999)[16]

Government will increase access to essential services by . . . reducing waiting times for surgeries and diagnostic procedures. (2000)[17]

In addition to these broader periods, policy attention to health was especially prominent in the throne speeches in three individual years (see outlier high points in Figure 2.2): 1919 (16.7 percent of speech quasi-sentences that year), 1963 (20.8 percent), and 2002 (18.3 percent). First, references to health in the 1919 speech, from the Liberal government of Premier Charles Stewart, focused entirely on influenza and efforts taken to address it.

The epidemic of influenza from which the Province suffered in the latter part of 1918 has been, I regret to say, uncommonly severe, particularly in the more sparsely unsettled sections of the province.

. . . This experience brings clearly to view the need of further health and sanitation laws and regulations throughout the province.[18]

These statements foreshadowed both the creation of the provincial Department of Public Health in 1919,[19] and an amendment to Alberta's Public Health Act that expanded the list of communicable diseases, over which the provincial board had authority, to include influenza.[20]

Second, in 1963, Premier Ernest Manning's SC government focused on broadening access to public health and health care services and expanding infrastructure:

> To further improve the province's extensive public health services, amendments will be introduced to The Health Unit Act and The Treatment Services Act.
>
> A 100-bed hospital-school for multiple-handicapped children will be constructed in Edmonton.[21]

The context of Manning's comments included important milestones in health policy in Alberta, including the 1965 *Report of the Special Legislative and Lay Committee Inquiring into Preventive Health Services*[22] and the province's transition to national medical insurance in 1969.[23]

The third single-year peak in Figure 2.2 is 2002, corresponding to the government of Premier Ralph Klein (Progressive Conservative). Klein's government acknowledged the broader determinants of health.

> When Albertans speak about health, they don't only mean services provided in hospitals or prescription drugs or ambulance services. . . . They know that people's health status is affected by their lifestyles, their socioeconomic status, their education, their sense of inner security and external security, their feeling of being part of a larger community, their access to jobs and safe and healthy foods and cultural experiences, and by many other factors that exceed the scope of the conventional health system.[24]

Although these comments appear to align with trends at the time toward greater attention to the social determinants of health,[25] with few exceptions[26] Klein's subsequent comments betray alignment with a biomedical and behavioural view of health, characterized by emphasis on individualized lifestyle and health care, and are thus contrary to a public health perspective. For example, intentions identified for the coming year included to "launch a campaign to give Albertans reliable health information and encourage them to make healthy lifestyle choices;" to "work with physicians and health authorities to explore new options in physician compensation;" and to expand "the pharmaceutical information network to improve drug therapy and reduce costs."[27]

POLICY ATTENTION TO SUBCONCERNS WITHIN HEALTH, OVER TIME

To get a better sense of how health was described over time in the throne speeches, we developed subtopic codes for the quasi-sentences coded within health as a major topic.[28] The sub-codes are described in Table 2.2. They are:

- establishment or construction of facilities or infrastructure (treatment-oriented, e.g., hospitals);
- non-insured health services (treatment-oriented, e.g., pharmaceuticals);
- prevention, protection, promotion, core public health functions;
- costs and financing;
- major or inter-jurisdictional health care reform;
- treatment-, curative-, or management-oriented health care;
- health status assessment;
- health professionals, the health workforce;
- research; and
- general, other, or generic.

TABLE 2.2: Subtopic coding that we developed and applied to Alberta throne speech quasi-sentences coded as Health (major topic 3).

Sub-topic label	Sub-topic details / examples
Establishment or construction of treatment-oriented health facilities or health services delivery infrastructure (sub-code 310)	• Buildings (e.g., hospitals, clinics) • New technologies e.g., robotics • Could be general or issue-/population-specific. (e.g., hospital, children's hospital, alcohol rehabilitation facility) • Includes electronic infrastructure, e.g., electronic medical records, software systems to ensure patient privacy • Laboratory
Non-insured health services (treatment-oriented) (sub-code 315)	• Prescription drugs/pharmaceuticals • Other services – e.g., dentistry, optometry etc.

Prevention / protection / promotion / core public health functions (sub-code 320)	• Preventive health services
	  - Major - Preventive health services reform – e.g., legislation to establish health units; reforming the health system to be more prevention-oriented
	  - More minor aspects of preventive health services
	• Creation of a single health unit
	• Prevention more generally
	  - Primary or secondary
	• Public health more generally, unless there is indication that it is not prevention-oriented
	• Specific prevention initiatives e.g., immunization, 'healthy living', health promotion, health education
	• Includes specific populations & issues, if statement is prevention/ oriented
	• If a statement includes "prevention and treatment" or "prevention and control", *with no indication of which is privileged*, then code it as 320.

Costs and financing – anything related to money and the health care system (other than federal transfers) (sub-code 330)	• Should have an element of substance/specificity, versus e.g., "we will make health care more efficient" which would be 300. • Cost burden of health care system / services / technologies • Premiums • Grants – to fund services • Insurance (unless statement is about change/reform, in which case it would be 340) • Funding for workforce and research would be coded as 380 or 390 respectively

High-level / inter-jurisdictional / major health care reform (sub-code 340)	• Federal-provincial issues, including Canada Health Act
	• Other major reforms of similar scale, to do with coverage / insurance
	  - E.g., free health care coverage for certain groups
	• Major periods in the evolution of health service delivery
	  - E.g., establishment of new Ministry or Department signifying shift in priorities or focus
	  - Regionalization (shift to regional health authorities)
	• Federal transfers

Sub-topic label	Sub-topic details / examples

Other health care (treatment/ curative or management-oriented) (sub-code 350)	• Should have an element of substance/specificity, versus e.g., "we will improve service delivery" which would be 300.
	• More minor reforms, with some specificity, to improve the health system.
	• Specific statements about service delivery
	   - E.g., tobacco, alcohol, home care, cancer
	• Important new strategic initiatives
	   - E.g., mental health, home care, cancer, addictions
	• Specific promises – e.g., we will create an emergency response plan for communicable disease emergencies

Health status of the population / large-scale threats to health / surveillance (sub-code 370)	• E.g., # of youth drinking • E.g., substance abuse impact on families • Could be specific (above) or general – e.g., securing the health of the population • General and specific health surveys (unless framed as research, in which case code as 390, or unless it is a survey or study that is part of making a specific improvement to health services, in which case code as 350)
Health professionals / the health workforce (sub-code 380)	• Includes allocating funds to train new staff • Training programs for health professionals - E.g., new nursing school
Research (sub-code 390)	• Health research • Medical research • Includes funding for research
General / leftover / generic (sub-code 300)	• Non-substantive / vague • E.g., health care is important • Generic comments about health care – e.g., strong, accountable, flexible health care system • Generic problems about health care – e.g., fix the inefficiencies in our health care system

Overall, between 1906 and 2017, the three most common health sub-topics were establishment or construction of treatment-oriented facilities or infrastructure (18.9 percent of all health sub-topics), and treatment-, curative-, or management-oriented health care (24.4 percent), along with the less informative general, other, or generic (20.4 percent). In contrast, prevention, protection, promotion, and core public health functions were less common, representing 11.7 percent of all health quasi-sentences.

Trends over time for select sub-codes are shown in Figure 2.3.

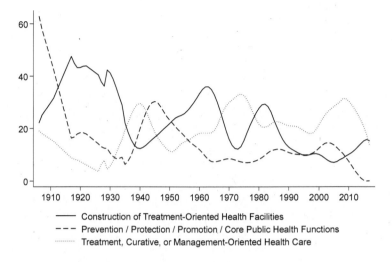

Construction of Treatment-Oriented Health Facilities
– – – Prevention / Protection / Promotion / Core Public Health Functions
·········· Treatment, Curative, or Management-Oriented Health Care

Fig. 2.3: Trends over time in the percent of health quasi-sentences from the Alberta throne speeches coded under three sub-codes: Establishment or construction of treatment-oriented facilities or infrastructure (solid line); Prevention, protection, promotion, core public health functions (dashed line); and Treatment, curative, or management-oriented health care (dotted line), 1906–2017 (lowess plot).

First, one can see from Figure 2.3 that reference to the sub-category establishment or construction of treatment-oriented facilities or infrastructure (solid line) shows a gradual decline over time. An early prominence of this sub-code reflects attention to infrastructure and facilities in the context of a new and growing province, such as an institution for "the relief of the mentally afflicted" at Ponoka (1911), a system of travelling clinics (1927), and hospitals for tubercular patients (1931). During the late 1940s through the early 1960s, infrastructure-related policy attention was focused on mental health (e.g., a mobile mental hygiene clinic to serve the northern areas of the province, 1948), tuberculosis (e.g., the Aberhart Memorial Sanatorium, completed in 1952), polio (e.g., addition of a poliomyelitis unit to the University Hospital in Edmonton, 1954), and physical disability (e.g., facilities for the treatment and education of children with physical disabilities, 1963). Finally, the 1970s and 1980s were diverse with respect to the sub-category establishment or construction of treatment-oriented facilities or infrastructure, but Alberta throne speech content indicated policy attention to building or expanding facilities for seniors, such as extended care facilities and nursing homes; rehabilitation centres for alcohol and drug dependence; and a variety of specialized services for patients with cancer (e.g., diagnostic radiology) and cardiovascular illnesses (e.g., catheterization laboratories). The rise of this construction sub-code in the late 1970s and early 1980s illustrates the Progressive Conservative policy, under Premier Peter Lougheed, of "modernizing the province," including building key infrastructure such as hospitals, during a period of significant economic growth in Alberta.[29]

Second, Figure 2.3 shows that relative attention to the sub-code prevention, protection, promotion, and core public health functions (dashed line) has gradually decreased over time, while treatment-, curative-, or management-oriented health care (dotted line) has shown a gradual increase. The greater policy attention to prevention and other core public health functions early in the period reflects items such as early iterations of the Public Health Act,[30] medical inspection of children in schools and public health nursing,[31] prevention of the spread of infectious diseases,[32] prevention-oriented health units,[33] and maternal and child health and welfare.[34] We further explore the shifting focus and meaning of references to prevention and public health over time below.

Public Health

Another way to glean insight into how public health is understood and referenced over time is to search within the quasi-sentences coded as health (major topic 3) for the phrase "public health." There was a total of just fifty-eight occurrences of the term, and interesting trends are apparent, as shown in Figure 2.4.

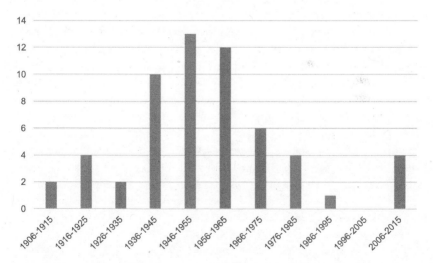

Fig. 2.4: Number of times "public health" is mentioned, in Alberta throne speech quasi-sentences coded as health (major topic code 3), by decade, 1906–2017. (It was necessary to group multiple years together because of low numbers within individual years. The decade grouping used here is arbitrary.)

Figure 2.4 shows that, although the overall numbers were low, there were some periods when public health was mentioned consistently (at least once in nearly every throne speech), such as the mid-1940s to the mid-1960s. In other periods, public health was mentioned infrequently or not at all. Looking at the year-by-year counts (not shown), public health was not mentioned at all in Alberta throne speeches between 1908 and 1917 (ten years), between 1976 and 1983 (eight years), and, for the lengthy nineteen-year period between 1988 and 2006.

REFERENCE TO PUBLIC HEALTH IN GOVERNMENT THRONE SPEECHES: ALBERTA'S EARLY DECADES

Examining the content and context in which public health was mentioned sheds further light on these patterns. The first instance was in 1906 by Premier Alexander C. Rutherford's Liberal government. From 1870, when the Northwest Territories entered Canadian confederation, until 1905, the territory now known as Alberta was governed as part of the Territories, and public health activities were administered under the territorial Public Health Ordinance.[35] Rutherford's government was lamenting the limitations of the Northwest Territories' Public Health Ordinance. They spoke of the need for Alberta to have its own law to govern "every phase of public health and sanitation;" Alberta's first Public Health Act was passed in 1907.[36]

The term "public health" did not appear again in the throne speeches until 1918; not surprisingly, this was in the context of the 1918/19 influenza epidemic and aftermath as illustrated by speech excerpts noted above from the Stewart government. In 1920, Stewart's government provided an update on the new Department of Public Health, including that financial provision had been made for "such important matters as child welfare, medical inspection of children in schools, public health nursing . . . [and] the establishment of municipal hospitals."[37] By 1922, Alberta had a new provincial government, under Premier Herbert Greenfield of the United Farmers of Alberta, which promised "earnest consideration" of public health by that government, "not only from the preventive but also from the curative standpoint."[38] Seven years later, the government of subsequent United Farm Worker Premier John E. Brownlee spoke of an important provision to establish District Health Units that would serve "to supplement remedial measures by preventive and safeguarding methods,"[39] and an amendment to the Public Health Act to permit that initiative.[40]

The depression-era conditions of the 1930s led Premier William Aberhart's SC government to announce that there would be "some consideration" given to the revision and improvement of public health services and programs, "notwithstanding the necessity for rigid economy due to falling revenues."[41] Aberhart's government, which spoke of public health and prevention on several occasions throughout its tenure, later made more specific statements about strengthening public health services, including:

> [Providing] additional nursing services . . . to outlying areas remote from medical and hospital facilities.[42]

> [Proposing] to go forward with the organization of additional full-time health units until all districts in the Province have been given the advantage of modern preventive Public Health Service.[43]

PUBLIC HEALTH – THE MANNING YEARS

During Premier Ernest C. Manning's Social Credit government's lengthy time in office (1943 to 1968) there were many references to public health, suggesting that this was a topic of some importance to this administration. Across Manning's tenure, which coincided with a recovery from the economic depression of the 1930s, throne speech statements about public health were about growth and expansion of services, staff, and facilities. However, partly because of the sheer length of time in office, one can see during his tenure a shift in the focus and nature of his statements about public health.

From the mid-1940s through the mid-1950s, the Manning government's statements were heavily focused on the expansion of preventive programs and services throughout the province, which was part of his vision of a "post war public health program." One statement proposed "a complete preventive public health program [that would permit Alberta to] continue in its position of leadership in the field of public health in Canada."[44] This expansion involved the establishment or expansion of facilities and infrastructure (e.g., additional health units[45] and travelling clinics[46]); training of health personnel (e.g., a training centre for public health nurses and sanitary inspectors[47] and grants to "assist and encourage young women to enter the nursing profession"[48]); other facilities (e.g., a branch of the provincial laboratory in Central Alberta[49]); and other initiatives, such as funding to purchase the polio vaccine[50] and regulations to control hazards associated with radiation.[51]

In 1958, Manning announced an "important change . . . in the field of public health" that would be considered, namely, "the statutory and financial provisions necessary to put into operation . . . a comprehensive hospitalization program designed to fit into the national program in which the federal government proposes to participate at a later date."[52] Although Manning's speeches had mentioned hospitals before, the 1958 speech, with its focal topic of subsidized hospital services, seemed to signal a shift in what public health meant or entailed. That is, prior to 1958, public health as described in Alberta throne speeches included a range of activities and services, of both a preventive and curative orientation, with primary prevention and health protection activities featuring prominently. Starting around 1958, the meaning of "public health," as used in the Alberta legislature, started to drift downstream.

For instance, the Manning government's statements about improvements and expansion to "public health" in 1959 and 1961 include provision of hospital care for those with chronic illness, early treatment for children with mental illness, expansion of services for people with diabetes, rheumatic fever, and other illnesses, construction of a new provincial hospital and diagnostic and referral centre in Calgary, and facilities for treatment and education of children with physical disabilities.[53]

Subsequent announcements focused on establishing a University of Alberta Hospital Foundation, whose funds in 1962 would be used to "augment teaching and clinical research"[54] including:

[Co-operating with the medical profession] to develop and implement a program of voluntary prepaid medical services.[55]

Establish[ing] a comprehensive program of nursing home care. [56]

Extend[ing] the benefits under the Alberta hospital plan to include out-patient service at hospitals throughout the province.[57]

Propos[ing] the establishment of a Western Canada Heart Institute and a centre for neurological, renal, endocrine and sensory organ disease, in which the most up-to-date diagnostic, research, and treatment services will be available to our people.[58]

Improv[ing] and simplify[ing] the subsidized health care insurance under the Alberta Health Plan.[59]

Overall, these statements reveal a version of public health, characterized by a focus on treatment, management, and rehabilitation for individuals experiencing illness and on enhancing clinically oriented infrastructure (e.g., diagnosis and treatment); as well as the insurance to support people in accessing those services and activities. Although the Manning government's throne speeches were not devoid of reference to prevention, they were in the minority during the later years of his tenure (see also the analysis of the sub-code prevention below).

Closing out the Social Credit era was the shorter tenure of Premier Harry Strom (1968–1971), whose throne speeches included only one explicit mention of public health. In 1970, his government's speech included the following statement: "in other fields of public health, you will be asked to consider legislation for the establishment of a commission on alcohol and drug abuse."[60] The focal topic of the proposed legislation as well as the activities envisioned — for example, an educational film on drug misuse — may be seen in hindsight as a sign of a troubling shift toward the individualized and morally infused orientation to health ushered in by the neoliberal era.

PUBLIC HEALTH — THE POST-MANNING YEARS

Perhaps most notable about Premier Peter Lougheed's administration, from the point of view of public health, is how infrequently they mentioned the topic in their throne speeches, considering the length of tenure. During Lougheed's fourteen years in office (1971–1985), his government's speeches mentioned "public health" only five times, and in fact, one of the longest gaps in Alberta's history in this regard, 1976 to 1983 (Figure 2.4) was during Lougheed's tenure.

The Lougheed government's statements about public health continued earlier threads regarding the need for services in rural or isolated communities, and in 1973 he proposed three new programs to help redress this imbalance: speech therapy services, a mobile dental program, and efforts to enable health units to provide improved services to those with mental and physical disabilities.[61] That same speech referenced initiatives related to drug benefits for seniors, the Alberta Health Care Insurance Plan premium subsidy, and significant amendments to The Nursing Homes Act. Finally, they made reference, in the context of public health, to physical fitness, including their government's "concern for the health and fitness of Albertans . . . [and the development of] programs aimed at encouraging people of all ages to participate in enjoyable fitness activities."[62] In the 15 March 1984 throne speech, Lougheed's government announced a proposed new Public Health Act, which would constitute a substantial revision from the previous versions (see Chapter 4).[63]

In 1987, the throne speech of the Progressive Conservative government of Don Getty announced expansion of the province's immunization program to include haemophilus influenza B, described as "a disease which causes meningitis and other serious infections."[64] Although Getty's speech mentioned other activities and initiatives related to health more broadly, immunization was explicitly connected with public health, thus illustrating the strength of public health's historical ties to physical (and especially communicable) illness, including the embodiment of those ties in Alberta's Public Health Act.

Following Getty, during the nineteen-year period from 1988 to 2006, "public health" was not mentioned in the throne speeches at all. Premiers during this time were Getty (until 1992) and Ralph Klein (1992–2006). The next mention of public health came in 2006, toward the end of Klein's leadership, and was very much focused on health care, when he said, "This session we will set out clear principles to guide the health system, principles that reflect Albertans' values. They will provide a framework for a comprehensive public health system that fulfills government's commitment to provide high-quality health services to all Albertans."[65] This use of "public health," refers to publicly funded health care. The ensuing comments focus on "flexibility and choice" in health care, and a "major offensive in the fight against cancer."[66]

The final mention of "public health" between 1906 and 2017 was by Premier Ed Stelmach's Progressive Conservative government (2006–2011). In their first year in office, Stelmach's government declared that there would be "a sustained focus on wellness, injury reduction, and disease prevention combined with efforts to improve productivity and accountability in health care delivery will provide the framework to ensure a sustainable public health care system."[67] While that statement could conceivably indicate a broad conceptualization of public health as per the pre-Manning years, subsequent comments suggest otherwise. These include a focus on primary health care and self-management of chronic diseases; improved access to support services and treatment for people living in the community with serious mental illness, and their families; a new pharmaceutical strategy, and intentions to expand long-term care capacity, improve standards, and ensure that facilities and supports are available to seniors as the population ages.[68] On the other hand, the Stelmach government's 2009 speech announced an important amendment to the Public Health Act, which was to "lay a solid foundation for improving public health by strengthening the role and authority of the chief medical officer of health in protecting and promoting Albertans' health."[69]

There were no mentions of public health after 2009, which included Premier Allison Redford's (PC) tenure (2011 to 2014), and the early years (2015 to 2017) of Premier Rachel Notley's New Democratic Party (NDP) term. With respect to the value of hindsight and having adequate time to reflect, we decline to comment on these very recent periods, and hope that future analysis will place them in historical context.

Prevention

Because it is so central to public health, our final consideration in this chapter concerns the concept of prevention, including when, how often, and with what meaning the concept was used in the Alberta throne speech data set.

We performed a keyword search of the entire Alberta throne speech data set (i.e., all 14,193 quasi-sentences, from 1906 to 2017) for "prevent" (which captured iterations, such as prevention, preventing, preventive), and found 139 instances. Recognizing that prevention is not unique to health, we first considered how these 139 instances were distributed across the twenty-five major topic codes representing all areas of public policy. In fact, the largest proportion (n=61, 44 percent) occurred in health (major topic code 3), followed by law, crime, and family issues (n=21, 14 percent, major topic code 12; e.g., "implementing new initiatives to prevent family violence"[70]) and social welfare (n-16, 12 percent, major topic code 12; e.g., "preventive social programs are a high priority of my government"[71]). "Prevent" and its iterations occurred fewer than ten times in the other major topic codes. Therefore, across the various policy areas, the concept of prevention was quite strongly aligned with health (which, in itself may help to explain some of the challenges that prompted this volume as a whole; see also Chapter 12), and we restricted our analysis to the health major topic code.

The frequency of reference to "prevent" and its iterations in quasi-sentences coded as health, by decade, is shown in Figure 2.5.

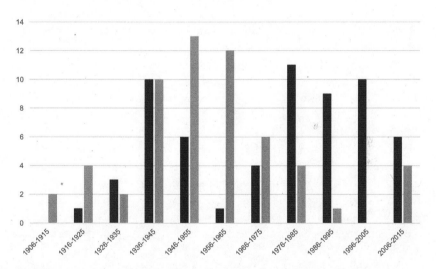

Fig. 2.5: Number of times "prevent" (and iterations) is mentioned, in quasi-sentences coded as health (major topic code 3) in the Alberta throne speech data set, by decade (black bars). References to "public health" (grey bars, from Figure 2.4) are also shown for comparison. (It was necessary to group multiple years together because of low numbers within individual years. The decade grouping used here is arbitrary.)

As seen in Figure 2.5, references to both public health and prevention were infrequent during the early decades; they appeared equally frequently during the decade 1936 to 1945, and thereafter patterns diverged. While references to public health (grey bars) in the throne speeches peaked during the post-WWII years through the 1960s as discussed above, references to prevent (black bars) peaked later, starting in the mid-1970s. This later peak coincided with Canadian and international health trends, including a growing focus on risk factor epidemiology (e.g., the quest to identify, for the purpose of intervention, individual-level risk factors, primarily for chronic diseases); and the health promotion movement (see Chapter 10). Within a context of growing concern about escalating costs of health care, a strong discourse emerged that encouraged individual responsibility for health as a way to contain costs.[72]

OBJECTS OF PREVENTION: WHAT IS TO BE PREVENTED?

Looking at the content of throne speech quasi-sentences about prevention sheds light on how, and with what meaning, the term was used over time. First, not surprisingly, there were shifts in what was to be prevented, with the first half of the twentieth century showing strong attention to preventing the spread of communicable diseases[73] — in general, and specific to certain diseases such as tuberculosis and polio[74] — as well as frequent references to general preventive health services.[75]

Later, a shift is apparent toward a focus on preventing chronic or non-communicable illness and injury. Although the first reference to preventing cancer appeared in 1940, the focus on preventing chronic illness and injury began in earnest in the 1960s and continued for the remainder of the data set (until 2017).[76] In addition to references to illness prevention in general, specific attention was given to alcoholism, mental health problems, cardiac problems, dental problems, injuries, fetal alcohol syndrome, cancer, and risk factors for type 2 diabetes. Among the specific objects of prevention mentioned in this later period, a common one was addictions (variously described using negative language such as "alcoholism," "alcohol and drug abuse," "abuse habits," etc.), which was mentioned in conjunction with prevention at least once during each decade from the 1960s through the early 2000s.

Statements about prevention in the context of communicable disease, while not absent during the second half of the twentieth century, were limited to one reference in 1983 by Lougheed's government, which says, "in the important area of preventive health, modification of the immunization program has extended protection to Alberta children against seven serious diseases, while a program to provide hepatitis B vaccine to patients and workers at risk of exposure to this potentially serious disease has also been introduced."[77] There were two throne speech references to communicable disease prevention by Getty's government, including one in 1987 announcing expansion of the existing public health immunization program, which said that "the introduction of a new vaccine to protect our children against haemophilus influenza B, a disease which causes meningitis and other serious infections . . . will be administered to two-year-olds throughout the province by the 27 local health units."[78] Finally, in 2000, the Klein government announced their intention of "launching a new three-year immunization plan."

APPROACHES TO PREVENTION

An additional way to examine trends over time in illness prevention is to consider what it entails or how it would be achieved. Based on the Alberta throne speech data set, there is some indication of a shift over time in this regard.

During the first half of the twentieth century, policy attention to prevention showed alignment with the concept of primary prevention, namely, intervening before health problems or risk factors occur. That is, activities such as expansions to the scope of health protection activities, via amendments to the Public Health Act, and to preventive health service infrastructure, such as travelling clinics in the 1920s[79] and health units in rural areas in the 1940s and 1950s,[80] represented efforts to reach all Albertans, thus preventing the occurrence of an array of illnesses.

Later, two shifts in emphasis are apparent. First, whereas early in the twentieth century, prevention was often mentioned on its own (e.g., preventing the spread of infectious and contagious diseases or increasing the number of preventive health units), later throne speeches increasingly contained instances where prevention and treatment were mentioned in the same sentence; for example:[81] preventive and treatment services for alcohol dependence; mental health treatment and prevention; prevention, research, and treatment around addictions; addressing the needs of children affected by fetal alcohol syndrome and finding ways to prevent it; and prevention, detection and treatment of cancer. Although a joint focus on efforts to treat or manage illness in those afflicted, and to prevent new cases, is understandable, this subtle shift in framing suggests a gradual, relative reduction in emphasis on prevention over time.

The second shift in emphasis starts in the late 1970s, with references to secondary forms of prevention. In contrast to primary prevention, which aims to prevent occurrence of disease or injury in the population as a whole, secondary prevention is more downstream in that it aims to "arrest the progress and reduce the consequences of disease or injury once established."[82] Examples in the throne speeches include: a provincial plan for cardiac rehabilitation services geared to primary and secondary prevention;[83] plans for a comprehensive service that will emphasize early detection and prevention of mental health-related problems;[84] greater emphasis on preventing illness and injury through a metabolic screening program for newborns;[85] prevention of illness and injury by expanding screening programs for breast and cervical cancer;[86] and addressing the needs of those who already have the disease [type 2 diabetes] to prevent and reduce serious complications.[87] In these examples, the term "prevention" is used to refer to secondary prevention, either explicitly, or implicitly (e.g., reference to screening or early detection), thus suggesting a shift in the term's meaning compared to earlier periods.

Conclusions

All data sources have limitations. Throne speeches, like other government speeches, have purposes ranging from inspiration to information to political marketing. Nevertheless, throne speech content provides a rich source of insight into legislative priorities and concerns, and it enables systematic coding and comparison over time. The data set allows us to see, from the perspective of successive provincial governments, priorities and concerns emerge and fade over the historical sweep of the Province of Alberta. Thus, without denying the value of deeper historical analysis of the episodes we have described in this chapter, the Alberta throne speech data set provides a valuable survey of the public health landscape in Alberta over time.

A key insight emerged from our analysis of the Manning years of the mid-1940s through the mid-1960s. Premier Manning's SC government was very concerned with health and spoke of it frequently in throne speeches during their lengthy time in office. However, we detected a shift in the use of the term "public health" during that time. Prior to the late 1950s, "public health" was used, by governments of Manning and others, to describe a range of activities and services of both a preventive and curative orientation. Starting around 1958, the use of "public health" by Manning's government and others seemed to drift toward an increasing emphasis on treatment, management, diagnostics, and rehabilitation activities within the context of publicly funded medical care. From the current vantage point of widespread confusion about what public health is and does, including a tendency to conflate public health and medical care, it seems that this contemporary confusion may date back to this mid-century shift in usage by Alberta government leadership, which coincided with provincial and national attention to building capacity for hospital and physician services.

Also providing contemporary insight is our analysis of the concept of prevention and how it was used over time in the Alberta throne speech data set. Early in the hundred-year period, prevention was used in the context of efforts to halt the spread of communicable disease and to ensure access to preventive health services for all Albertans, thus conveying a population-wide scope and alignment with primary prevention. Later, we found evidence of declining relative emphasis on prevention, based on its increasing co-occurrence with treatment (which tends to be expensive and appealing to the public) in the same statement, and an apparent drift toward secondary forms of prevention that focused on identifying individuals at risk for the purpose of tailored intervention to prevent further progression of disease.

In terms of the objects of prevention, we saw significant recent focus on certain health concerns, including addictions, especially alcohol and drug dependence, as well as cancer. Although these are important concerns in the Alberta context, it is significant to note that there are many other important health concerns, such as injury and diabetes, that did not receive the same level of explicit attention in the Alberta throne speeches. Health and illness occur in social, economic, political, and moral contexts that shape perceptions of importance and urgency,[88] including whether or the extent to which they may appear in a government throne speech. Perceptions of importance and urgency may or may not be proportionate to the prevalence or incidence of the problem, with certain illnesses and populations seen as more important or deserving than others.

Collectively, the findings of this chapter shed light on contemporary discourse around the "weakening" of public health in Canada. We have identified subtle shifts in how concepts of public health and prevention have been discussed and conceptualized over time by one source — provincial government throne speeches in Alberta. Our analysis suggests that these concepts have, over time, changed in emphasis, and have in many ways become increasingly indistinguishable from downstream medical care, which is focused on treatment and management of illness at the individual level.[89] If we wish to strengthen public health as a policy priority, we must find ways to articulate, defend, and advance its core features in a way that aligns with a broad vision of public health (i.e., upstream or root causes of health equity) even if the context is unfriendly.[90]

NOTES

1   Alberta Public Health Association. "Public Health: Taking It to the Streets." Created in 1993, video, available from the authors; Susan Nall Bales, Andrew Volmert, and Adam Simon, *Overcoming Health Individualism: A FrameWorks Creative Brief on Framing Social Determinants in Alberta* (Washington: FrameWorks Institute, March 2014), http://www.frameworksinstitute.org/pubs/mm/albertahealth/.

2   Robert G. Evans and Gregory L. Stoddart, "Producing Health, Consuming Health Care," in *Why Are some People Healthy and Others Not? The Determinants of Health of Populations*, ed. Robert G. Evans, Morris L. Barer, and Theodore R. Marmor (New York: Aldine de Gruyter, 1994); Daniel J. Dutton, et al., "Effect of Provincial Spending on Social Services and Health Care on Health Outcomes in Canada: An Observational Longitudinal Study," *Canadian Medical Association Journal* 190, no. 1 (2018), https://doi.org/10.1503/cmaj.170132.

3   "About," Comparative Agendas Project, accessed 14 February 2019, https://www.comparativeagendas.net/pages/About.

4   Alberta speeches from the throne can be found in Legislative Assembly of Alberta, *Journals of the Legislative Assembly of the Province of Alberta* (Edmonton, 1963–present, https://www.assembly.ab.ca/assembly-business/assembly-records/journals) and in the Alberta Legislature Library (Edmonton: 1906–present), https://librarysearch.assembly.ab.ca/client/en_CA/public/search/results?qu=u239632&st=TL; speeches from the throne and related data were also extracted from Jack Lucas and Jean-Philippe Gauvin, "Alberta Throne Speeches 1906–2017 (Comparative Agendas Project)," 2019, https://doi.org/10.5683/SP2/0WH5FH, Borealis, V1.

5   Building on original efforts by Frank Baumgartner and Bryan Jones, a master codebook was developed by Shaun Bevan, Senior Lecturer in Quantitative Political Science and Director of Research (Data) for the School of Social and Political Science at the University of Edinburgh (http://www.sbevan.com/index.html). The Canadian arm of the Comparative Agendas Project is led by Jean-Philippe Gauvin at Concordia University (https://www.comparativeagendas.net/canada); Gauvin and a team of other researchers have digitized and coded Canadian federal and provincial throne speeches from 1960–2015. The remaining Alberta Throne Speeches (1906–1959 and 2015–2017) were digitized and coded by Jack Lucas, Associate Professor in the Department of Political Science at the University of Calgary. Data from Lucas and Gauvin, "Alberta Throne Speeches."

6   Legislative Assembly of Alberta, *Journals of the Legislative Assembly of Alberta. Second Sessions of the Third Legislature* (Edmonton: J.W. Jeffery, Government Printer, 1914); Legislative Assembly of Alberta, *Journals of the Legislative Assembly of Alberta. Third Sessions of the Twentieth Legislature* (Edmonton, 1985).

7 . The master codebook (see note #5) was adapted to the Canadian context by Stuart Soroka, Professor of Communication Studies and Political Science at the University of Michigan (formerly of McGill University). Stuart Soroka, *Canadian Policy Agendas Data: Oral Questions* (McGill University, April 2009); Stuart Soroka, *Canadian Policy Agendas Topic Codebook* (McGill University, May 2005). See Stuart Soroka, Erin Penner, and Kelly Blidook, "Constituency Influence in Parliament," *Canadian Journal of Political Science* 42, no. 3 (2009).

8   To convey the breadth of the major topic code, we provide the sub-topic codes from the Canadian version of the master codebook (Soroka, *Canadian Policy Agendas Topic Codebook*, 7): general (includes combinations of multiple subtopics); health care reform, costs, and availability; health care funding arrangements; regulation of prescription drugs, medical devices, and medical procedures; health facilities construction and regulation; mental illness and mental retardation; medical fraud, malpractice, and physician licensing requirements; elderly health issues; infants, children, and immunization; health manpower needs and training programs; military health care; drug and alcohol treatment; alcohol abuse and treatment; tobacco abuse, treatment, and education; illegal drug abuse, treatment, and education; specific diseases; research and development; and other.

9   "Lowess" refers to Locally Weighted Scatterplot Smoothing, which is a regression analysis-based tool to create a smooth line through a timeplot or scatter plot, and is particularly useful in situations with "noisy data values, sparse data points, or weak interrelationships." "Lowess Smothing in Statistics: What is it?," Statistics How To, modified on 6 October 2013, https://www.statisticshowto.datasciencecentral.com/lowess-smoothing/

10 Legislative Assembly of Alberta, *Journals of the Legislative Assembly of Alberta. Third Session of the Tenth Legislature* (Edmonton: A. Shnitka, King's Printer, 1946), 8.

11 Legislative Assembly of Alberta, *Journals of the Legislative Assembly of Alberta. Third Session of the Tenth Legislature*, 8.

12 Legislative Assembly of Alberta, *Journals of the Legislative Assembly of Alberta. Fifth Session of the Tenth Legislature* (Edmonton: A. Shnitka, King's Printer, 1948), 8.

13   Legislative Assembly of Alberta, *Journals of the Legislative Assembly of Alberta. Fourth Session of the Eleventh Legislature* (Edmonton: Printed by A. Shnitka, King's Printer for Alberta, 1951), 8.

14   Legislative Assembly of Alberta, *Journals of the Legislative Assembly of Alberta. Second Session of the Twelfth Legislature* (Edmonton: A. Shnitka, Queen's Printer for Alberta, 1954), 8.

15   Legislative Assembly of Alberta, *Journals of the Legislative Assembly of Alberta. Fourth and Fifth Sessions of the Twenty-Third Legislature* (Edmonton: 1996 and 1997), 3.

16   Legislative Assembly of Alberta, *Journals of the Legislative Assembly of Alberta. Third Session of the Twenty-Fourth Legislature* (Edmonton: 1999), 3.

17   Legislative Assembly of Alberta, *Journals of the Legislative Assembly of Alberta. Fourth and Fifth Sessions of the Twenty-Fourth Legislature* (Edmonton: 2000 and 2001), 9.

18   Legislative Assembly of Alberta, *Journals of the Legislative Assembly of Alberta. Second Session of the Fourth Legislature* (Edmonton: Printed by J.W. Jeffery, King's Printer, 1919), 8.

19   *An Act respecting the Department of Public Health*, S.P.A. 1919, c. 16.

20   *An Act respecting Public Health*, S.P.A. 1910, c. 17; *An Act to amend the Public Health Act*, S.P.A. 1919, c. 46; "Public Health Bills are given First Reading," *Edmonton Bulletin*, 25 February 1919, Alberta Legislature Library, Scrapbook Hansard.

21   Legislative Assembly of Alberta, *Journals of the Legislative Assembly of Alberta. Fifth Session of the Fourteenth Legislature* (Edmonton: Printed by L.S. Wall, Printer to the Queen's Most Excellent Majesty, 1963), 9.

22   Alberta Legislative Assembly, *Report of the Special Legislative and Lay Committee Inquiring into Preventive Health Services in the Province of Alberta* (Edmonton: 1965).

23   For an in-depth discussion of Alberta's transition to medical insurance, see, *Alberta's Medical History: Young and Lusty, and Full of Life* (Red Deer, AB: R. Lompard, 2008), especially "The Roots of Medicare are in Alberta (1927–1946)," 605–630.

24   Legislative Assembly of Alberta, *Journals of the Legislative Assembly of Alberta. Second Session of the Twenty-Fifth Legislature* (Edmonton: 2002), 4.

25   Federal, Provincial and Territorial Advisory Committee on Population Health (ACPH), *Toward a Healthy Future: Second Report on the Health of Canadians* (Ottawa, Health Canada, 1999), http://publications.gc.ca/site/eng/82290/publication.html.

26   Two possible exceptions to Klein's otherwise biomedical/behavioral orientation toward health in his 2002 throne speech are about developing community-based health projects under an Indigenous health strategy and taking steps to enhance the health of vulnerable children. However, efforts vis-à-vis those issues could take many forms, and the mere mention of these topics does not necessarily signal a social determinants of health orientation.

27   Legislative Assembly of Alberta, *Journals of the Legislative Assembly of Alberta. Second Session of the Twenty-Fifth Legislature* (Edmonton: 2002), 5.

28   The sub-topic codes in the original Canadian codebook (Soroka, *Canadian Policy Agendas Topic Codebook*) did not work well for our purposes; in particular, the "general" sub-code (300) was large and diverse, and the existing codes did not distinguish between prevention and treatment/management, which we felt was key for our purposes. We therefore developed our own sub-topic coding through an iterative process wherein two team members undertook multiple independent assessments of batches of throne speech quasi-sentences. Once those two team members were consistent in their coding, the coding was applied by a third team member to ascertain consistency and defensibility of coding.

29   John Church and Neale Smith, "Health Reform in Alberta: The Introduction of Health Regions," *Canadian Public Administration* 51, no. 2 (June 2008).

30   Legislative Assembly of Alberta, *Journals of the Legislative Assembly of Alberta. Second Session of the First Legislature* (Edmonton: Printed by Jas. E. Richards, Government Printer, 1907), 8.

31   Legislative Assembly of Alberta, *Journals of the Legislative Assembly of Alberta. Third Session of the Fourth Legislature* (Edmonton: Printed by J.W. Jeffery, King's Printer, 1920), 9.

32   Legislative Assembly of Alberta, *Journals of the Legislative Assembly of Alberta. First Session of the Sixth Legislature* (Edmonton: W.D. McLean, Acting King's Printer, 1927), 10.

33   Legislative Assembly of Alberta, *Journals of the Legislative Assembly of Alberta. Ninth Session of the Eighth Legislature* (Edmonton: A. Shnitka, King's Printer, 1940), 8.

34   Legislative Assembly of Alberta, *Journals of the Legislative Assembly of Alberta. First Session of the Eleventh Legislature* (Edmonton: A. Shnitka, King's Printer, 1949), 9.

35   Malcolm Ross Bow and F. T. Cook, "The History of the Department of Public Health of Alberta," *Canadian Journal of Public Health* 26, no. 1 (1935).

36 Legislative Assembly of Alberta, *Journals of the Legislative Assembly of Alberta. First Session of the First Legislature* (Edmonton: Jas. E. Richards, Government Printer, 1906), 14; Legislative Assembly of Alberta, *Journals of the Legislative Assembly of Alberta. Second Session of the First Legislature*; *An Act respecting Public Health*, S.P.A. 1907, c. 12; "The Last Legislative Oratory for 1907," *Edmonton Journal*, 15 March 1907, Alberta Legislature Library, Scrapbook Hansard.

37 Legislative Assembly of Alberta, *Journals of the Legislative Assembly of Alberta. Third Session of the Fourth Legislature* (Edmonton: Printed by J.W. Jeffery, King's Printer, 1920), 9.

38 Legislative Assembly of Alberta, *Journals of the Legislative Assembly of Alberta. First Session of the Fifth Legislature* (Edmonton: Printed by J.W. Jeffery, King's Printer, 1922), 12.

39 Legislative Assembly of Alberta, *Journals of the Legislative Assembly of Alberta. Third Session of the Sixth Legislature* (Edmonton: Printed by W.D. McLean, King's Printer, 1929), 8.

40 *An Act to amend The Public Health Act*, S.P.A. 1929, c. 36.

41 Legislative Assembly of Alberta, *Journals of the Legislative Assembly of Alberta. First Sessions of the Eighth Legislature* (Edmonton: A. Shnitka, King's Printer, 1936), 11.

42 Legislative Assembly of Alberta, *Journals of the Legislative Assembly of Alberta. First Session of the Ninth Legislature* (Edmonton: A. Shnitka, King's Printer, 1941), 10.

43 Legislative Assembly of Alberta, *Journals of the Legislative Assembly of Alberta. Second Session of the Ninth Legislature* (Edmonton: A. Shnitka, King's Printer, 1942), 7.

44 Legislative Assembly of Alberta, *Journals of the Legislative Assembly of Alberta. First Sessions of the Tenth Legislature* (Edmonton: A. Shnitka, King's Printer, 1945), 10.

45 Legislative Assembly of Alberta, *Journals of the Legislative Assembly of Alberta. First Sessions of the Tenth Legislature*, 10.

46 Legislative Assembly of Alberta, *Journals of the Legislative Assembly of Alberta. First Sessions of the Eleventh Legislature*, 9.

47 Legislative Assembly of Alberta, *Journals of the Legislative Assembly of Alberta. Third Session of the Tenth Legislature*, 8.

48 Legislative Assembly of Alberta, *Journals of the Legislative Assembly of Alberta. First Session of the Twelfth Legislature* (Edmonton: A. Shnitka, Queen's Printer for Alberta, 1953).

49 Legislative Assembly of Alberta, *Journals of the Legislative Assembly of Alberta. First Sessions of the Eleventh Legislature*, 9.

50 Legislative Assembly of Alberta, *Journals of the Legislative Assembly of Alberta. Second Session of the Thirteenth Legislature* (Edmonton: Printed by A. Shnitka, Printer to the Queen's Most Excellent Majesty, 1956), 7.

51 Legislative Assembly of Alberta, *Journals of the Legislative Assembly of Alberta. Third Session of the Thirteenth Legislature* (Edmonton: Printed by A. Shnitka, Printer to the Queen's Most Excellent Majesty, 1957), 7.

52 Legislative Assembly of Alberta, *Journals of the Legislative Assembly of Alberta. Fourth Session of the Thirteenth Legislature* (Edmonton: Printed by L.S. Wall, Printer to the Queen's Most Excellent Majesty, 1958), 5–6.

53 Legislative Assembly of Alberta, *Journals of the Legislative Assembly of Alberta. Fifth Session of the Thirteenth Legislature* (Edmonton: Printed by L.S. Wall, Printer to the Queen's Most Excellent Majesty, 1959), 6; Legislative Assembly of Alberta, *Journals of the Legislative Assembly of Alberta. Second Session of the Fourteenth Legislature* (Edmonton: Printed by L.S. Wall, Printer to the Queen's Most Excellent Majesty, 1961), 4.

54 Legislative Assembly of Alberta, *Journals of the Legislative Assembly of Alberta. Fourth Sessions of the Fourteenth Legislature* (Edmonton: Printed by L.S. Wall, Printer to the Queen's Most Excellent Majesty, 1962), 4.

55 Legislative Assembly of Alberta, *Journals of the Legislative Assembly of Alberta. Fifth Session of the Fourteenth Legislature*, 3.

56 Legislative Assembly of Alberta, *Journals of the Legislative Assembly of Alberta. First Session of the Fifteenth Legislature* (Edmonton: Printed by L.S. Wall, Printer to the Queen's Most Excellent Majesty, 1964), 6.

57 Legislative Assembly of Alberta, *Journals of the Legislative Assembly of Alberta. Second Session of the Fifteenth Legislature* (Edmonton: Printed by L.S. Wall, Printer to the Queen's Most Excellent Majesty, 1965), 4.

58 Legislative Assembly of Alberta, *Journals of the Legislative Assembly of Alberta. Fourth and Fifth Sessions of the Fifteenth Legislature* (Edmonton: Printed by L.S. Wall, Printer to the Queen's Most Excellent Majesty, 1966), 4.

59   Legislative Assembly of Alberta, *Journals of the Legislative Assembly of Alberta. Fifth Sessions of the Fifteenth Legislature* (Edmonton: Printed by L.S. Wall, Queen's Printer, 1967), 5.

60   Legislative Assembly of Alberta, *Journals of the Legislative Assembly of Alberta. Third Session of the Sixteenth Legislature* (Edmonton: Printed by L.S. Wall, Queen's Printer, 1970), 5.

61   Legislative Assembly of Alberta, *Journals of the Legislative Assembly of Alberta. Second Session of the Seventeenth Legislature* (Edmonton: Printed by the Queen's Printer for the Province of Alberta, 1973), 8.

62   Legislative Assembly of Alberta, *Journals of the Legislative Assembly of Alberta. Second Session of the Seventeenth Legislature*, 8.

63   Legislative Assembly of Alberta, *Journals of the Legislative Assembly of Alberta. Second Session of the Twentieth Legislature* (Edmonton: Printed by the Queen's Printer for the Province of Alberta, 1984), 5.

64   Legislative Assembly of Alberta, *Journals of the Legislative Assembly of Alberta. Second Session of the Twenty- First Legislature* (Edmonton, 1987), 8.

65   Legislative Assembly of Alberta, *Journals of the Legislative Assembly of Alberta. Second Session of the Twenty- Sixth Legislature* (Edmonton, 2006), 7.

66   Legislative Assembly of Alberta, *Journals of the Legislative Assembly of Alberta. Second Session of the Twenty- Sixth Legislature*, 7.

67   Legislative Assembly of Alberta, *Journals of the Legislative Assembly of Alberta. Third Session of the Twenty- Sixth Legislature* (Edmonton, 2007 and 2008), 7.

68   Legislative Assembly of Alberta, *Journals of the Legislative Assembly of Alberta. Third Session of the Twenty- Sixth Legislature*, 7.

69   Legislative Assembly of Alberta, *Journals of the Legislative Assembly of Alberta. Second Session of the Twenty- Seventh Legislature* (Edmonton, 2009), 9.

70   Legislative Assembly of Alberta, *Journals of the Legislative Assembly of Alberta. Fourth Session of the Twenty-Second Legislature* (Edmonton, 1992–1993), 7.

71   Legislative Assembly of Alberta, *Journals of the Legislative Assembly of Alberta. Third Session of the Nineteenth Legislature* (Edmonton: Printed by the Queen's Printer for the Province of Alberta, 1981), 6.

72   Fran Baum, *The New Public Health: An Australian Perspective* (Oxford: Oxford University Press, 1998); Mervyn Susser, "Does Risk Factor Epidemiology Put Epidemiology at Risk? Peering into the Future," *Journal of Epidemiology and Community Health* 52, no. 10 (October 1998); Louise Potvin and Catherine M. Jones, "Twenty-five Years after the Ottawa Charter: The Critical Role of Health Promotion for Public Health," *Canadian Journal of Public Health* 102, no. 4 (August 2011).

73   Legislative Assembly of Alberta, *Journals of the Legislative Assembly of Alberta. First Session of the Sixth Legislature*, 10; Legislative Assembly of Alberta, *Journals of the Legislative Assembly of Alberta. Fourth Session of the Sixth Legislature* (Edmonton: Printed by W.D. McLean, King's Printer, 1930), 8.

74   Legislative Assembly of Alberta, *Journals of the Legislative Assembly of Alberta. Eighth Session of the Eighth Legislature* (Edmonton: A. Shnitka, King's Printer, 1939), 7; Legislative Assembly of Alberta, *Journals of the Legislative Assembly of Alberta. Third Session of the Twelfth Legislature* (Edmonton: Printed by A. Shnitka, Queen's Printer for Alberta, 1955).

75   Many of these references to prevention were in the context of references to public health by the Aberhart government (1940–1943), and the "post-war public health program" by the Manning government (1944–1946 and 1949–1950). Lucas and Gauvin, "Alberta Throne Speeches."

76   Legislative Assembly of Alberta, *Journals of the Legislative Assembly of Alberta. Ninth Session of the Eighth Legislature* (Edmonton: A. Shnitka, King's Printer, 1940), 9.

77   Legislative Assembly of Alberta, *Journals of the Legislative Assembly of Alberta. First Session of the Twentieth Legislature* (Edmonton: Printed by the Queen's Printer for the Province of Alberta, 1983), 7-8.

78   Legislative Assembly of Alberta, *Journals of the Legislative Assembly of Alberta. Second Session of the Twenty- First Legislature* (Edmonton: 1987), 8.

79   Legislative Assembly of Alberta, *Journals of the Legislative Assembly of Alberta. First Session of the Sixth Legislature* (1927); Legislative Assembly of Alberta, *Journals of the Legislative Assembly of Alberta. Second Session of the Sixth Legislature* (1928); Legislative Assembly of Alberta, *Journals of the Legislative Assembly of Alberta. Fourth Session of the Sixth Legislature* (1930); and Legislative Assembly of Alberta, *Journals of the Legislative Assembly of Alberta. Eight Session of the Eighth Legislature* (Edmonton: A. Shnitka, King's Printer, 1939).

80   See note #74.

81   Lucas and Gauvin, "Alberta Throne Speeches."

82   Public Health Agency of Canada. *Glossary of Terms*. https://www.canada.ca/en/public-health/services/public-health-practice/skills-online/glossary-terms.html. Last modified 18 December 2022.

83   Legislative Assembly of Alberta, *Journals of the Legislative Assembly of Alberta. Second Session of the Seventeenth Legislature* (Edmonton: Printed by the Queen's Printer for the Province of Alberta, 1973); Legislative Assembly of Alberta, *Journals of the Legislative Assembly of Alberta. Fourth Session of the Eighteenth Legislature* (Edmonton: Printed by the Queen's Printer for the Province of Alberta, 1978), 4.

84   Legislative Assembly of Alberta, *Journals of the Legislative Assembly of Alberta. Third Sessions of the Twentieth Legislature*, 8.

85   Legislative Assembly of Alberta, *Journals of the Legislative Assembly of Alberta. Third Session of the Twenty-Fourth Legislature* (Edmonton: 1999), 3.

86   Legislative Assembly of Alberta, *Journals of the Legislative Assembly of Alberta. Fourth and Fifth Sessions of the Twenty-Fourth Legislature* (Edmonton: 2000 and 2001), 9.

87   Legislative Assembly of Alberta, *Journals of the Legislative Assembly of Alberta. Second Session of the Twenty-Fifth Legislature* (Edmonton: 2003), 8.

88   Samantha King, *Pink Ribbons, Inc. Breast Cancer and the Politics of Philanthropy* (Minneapolis: University of Minnesota Press, 2006); Kirsten Bell, Darlene McNaughton, and Amy Salmon, "Introduction," in *Alcohol, Tobacco, and Obesity: Morality, Mortality, and the New Public Health*, eds. Kirsten Bell, Darlene McNaughton, and Amy Salmon (New York: Routledge, 2011).

89   Daniel J. Dutton, et al., "Effect of Provincial Spending on Social Services and Health Care on Health Outcomes in Canada: An Observational Longitudinal Study," *Canadian Medical Association Journal* 190, no. 1 (2018); Michael Hayes, et al., "Telling Stories: News Media, Health Literacy and Public Policy in Canada," *Social Science & Medicine* 64, no. 9 (May 1, 2007), https://doi.org/10.1016/j.socscimed.2007.01.015.

90   Lindsay McLaren, "In Defense of a Population-Level Approach to Prevention: Why Public Health Matters Today," *Canadian Journal of Public Health* 110, no. 3 (2019).

3

Albertans' Health over Time: What We Know (and Why We Don't Know What We Don't Know)

Lindsay McLaren and Rogelio Velez Mendoza

Introduction

Our intention with this chapter is to present an overview of the health status of the Alberta population from 1919 to 2019. However, this is not a straightforward task, nor one without controversy.

First, what constitutes "the population" is not always clear, consistent, or inclusive. As seen in Chapter 1 and elsewhere in this volume, there are many examples throughout Alberta's public health history where "the public" or "the population" excluded certain groups, often based on problematic assumptions about Indigeneity, ethnicity, gender, socio-economic circumstances, or other social dimensions. Second, what constitutes "health" can be debated, and how health is understood and experienced, versus measured, is not always concordant. In their 1946 constitution, the World Health Organization famously defined health as "a state of complete physical, mental and social well-being and not merely the absence of disease or infirmity."[1] In contrast to this broad definition, much of what we know about the "health" of Albertans is based more narrowly on sickness and death. We encourage the reader to keep in mind that what we know about population health and illness over time reflects social processes and power dynamics pertaining to what aspects of health are counted, among whom, to what end, and who gets to decide.

This chapter presents one version of Albertans' health over time, which draws on quantitative data — namely, leading causes of death as recorded in Alberta's vital statistics, which were published in provincial annual reports across our one hundred-year period of interest,[2] supplemented by other quantitative information that is likewise available over a long period of time, such as historical statistics on notifiable diseases, diseases which, by law, must be reported to government authorities.[3] Notwithstanding the challenges noted above, we believe that compiling information that is available over a long time period provides an important, albeit partial, opportunity to better understand our history as it pertains to health and illness including societal efforts to address health problems.

The chapter proceeds as follows. First, continuing with the question of how we know what we know, we briefly introduce some of the key sources consulted. Then, using those sources, we present trends over time, beginning with a broad overview of the period of interest, approximately 1919 to 2019, followed by a more detailed analysis of discrete time periods. We contextualize the statistics with contemporary events and discourse gleaned from debates in the Alberta legislature, changes in the administrative structure of the provincial Department of Public Health, and news media. We take the liberty of going into some depth for topics that do not appear elsewhere in this volume, such as motor vehicle accidents and seat belts.

How Do We Know What We Know? Disease and Death Statistics, 1919–2019

Vital statistics, or "systematically tabulated information concerning births, marriages, divorces, separations, and deaths based on registrations of these vital events," constitute the earliest and longest-standing source of formally recorded, quantitative information about the health of the Alberta population and indeed across Canada.[4] Following the passing of census and vital statistics legislation for Upper and Lower Canada in 1847 and then the Dominion of Canada in 1879,[5] provincial legislation was passed throughout the late nineteenth and early twentieth centuries, with Alberta passing its first Vital Statistics Act (An Act respecting the Registration of Births, Marriages and Deaths) in 1907.[6] To improve upon processes under the former Northwest Territories Ordinances, Alberta's 1907 act provided for the appointment of postmasters throughout the province to serve as registrars, which reportedly permitted "much fuller and more accurate returns of births, marriages and deaths."[7]

Speaking to long-standing administrative connections between vital statistics and public health, a new provincial Vital Statistics Act, passed in 1916, created the positions of Registrar General of Vital Statistics, which was held by the minister of agriculture (the government department responsible for public health at the time), and Deputy Registrar General of Vital Statistics, which fell to the provincial medical officer of health.[8] The act remained with the Department of Agriculture until 1919, when it was transferred to the newly established Department of Public Health.[9] Vital Statistics remained under the Department of Public Health (or the Department of Health as it was sometimes called) until 1994, when the act was transferred to the Department of Municipal Affairs and then later, around 1998, to the Department of Government Services (called Service Alberta at the time of writing).[10]

Another important and long-standing source of health (illness) statistics in Alberta is notifiable diseases, defined as "a disease that, by statutory requirements, must be reported to the public health authority in the pertinent jurisdiction when the diagnosis is made [because it is] deemed of sufficient importance to the public health to require that its occurrence be reported to health authorities."[11] Notifiable disease reporting is part of a broader set of activities in public health surveillance (i.e., the ongoing, systematic collection, analysis, and interpretation of data and its timely dissemination to decision makers to inform action).[12] Retaining content from prior territorial ordinances,[13] Alberta's inaugural Public Health Act retained legislated responsibilities for notifiable disease reporting, authorizing regulation by the Provincial Board of Health.[14] At the time of writing, the list of notifiable diseases is found in the Communicable Diseases Regulation of the provincial Public Health Act.[15]

Historical news media sheds some light on social perceptions around designating a disease as notifiable. For example, designating venereal diseases as notifiable permitted public reporting of important trends over time, such as a decline in syphilis in Alberta between the 1940s and 1960s (see also below).[16] The practice, moreover, permitted clarification of the number of cases of food poisoning (salmonella; 65) versus measles (1,968) in Edmonton in 1967, when public concern seemed disproportionately focused on the rarer problem.[17] Designating a condition as notifiable can be controversial. This was the case with HIV: when the Alberta Hospital Association passed a resolution in 1988 recommending that HIV be reported under the notifiable diseases regulations of the Public Health Act, Dr. John Gill, chair of the Provincial Advisory Committee on AIDS argued that the resolution shows "a disappointing lack of understanding" in that such an action would discourage people from getting tested.[18] HIV became a notifiable disease in Alberta in 1998.[19]

A final example of an important and long-standing source of health (illness) statistics in Alberta —for non-communicable disease — is the provincial cancer registry, which began in the early 1940s amid recognition of cancer as a growing problem in Alberta and across the country; the registry continues today.[20]

The Health of the Alberta Population, 1919–2019

Some important caveats apply to the statistics presented below. First, what one might call reporting infrastructure has changed over time, such that accuracy and completeness of records may be imperfect in any given year, and the degree of inaccuracy and incompleteness changes over time. As one illustration, the 1921 *Report of the Provincial Board of Health*, prepared by Dr. W.C. Laidlaw, stated that "in most of the infectious diseases there has been an increase over the year 1920, and this increase can be explained by the fact that infectious diseases are being more fully reported. It is not considered that the incidence of disease was any higher this year than in previous years, as judging by the death-rate the incidence must have been practically the same."[21] We accordingly encourage readers to focus more on trends over time than on specific numbers.

Second, the ways in which diseases and causes of death are classified has changed over time. This presents a particular challenge to the trends presented in Table 3.1 and Figure 3.1, which we attempt to mitigate by extracting more or less exactly what was presented in the provincial annual reports for the purpose of year-to-year comparison, with details provided in Appendix B on page 430. For the rest of the chapter, readers are directed to the endnotes in which we provide additional details about the statistics presented.

The Health of the Alberta Population Since 1915: Broad Overview

Table 3.1 shows the three most common causes of death from 1920 to 2010 at ten-year intervals.[22]

TABLE 3.1: Leading causes of death (number of deaths), all ages, Alberta, 1920 to 2010, 10-year intervals. Ranking based on absolute number of deaths for Selected Causes, all ages.[23]

Year	Rank 1 (# of deaths)	Rank 2 (# of deaths)	Rank 3 (# of deaths)
1920	Influenza (603)	Pneumonia (all forms) (398)	Violent causes (excl. suicide) (365)
1930	Diseases of the heart (564)	Malignant tumors (482)	Pneumonia (all forms) (468)
1940	Diseases of the heart (1,086)	Malignant tumors (759)	Diseases of the arteries (517)
1950	Diseases of the heart (2,046)	Malignant tumors (997)	Cerebral haemorrhage (693)
1960	Diseases of the heart (2,800)	Malignant tumors (1,439)	Cerebral haemorrhage (934)
1970	Diseases of the heart (3,171)	Malignant tumors (1,827)	Violent causes (excl. suicide) (981)
1980	Diseases of the heart	Malignant tumors (2,627)	Cerebrovascular diseases (1,057)
1990	Diseases of the heart (3,777)	Malignant tumors (3,607)	Violent causes (excl. suicide) (1,066)
2000	Malignant tumors (4,775)	Diseases of the heart (4,548)	Cerebrovascular diseases (1,271)
2010	Malignant tumors (5,649)	Diseases of the heart (4,785)	Violent causes (excl. suicide) (1,390)

For those causes of death listed in Table 3.1, the rates of death, from 1915 to 2015, are shown in Figure 3.1. For this and subsequent figures, rates refer to the number of deaths per 100,000 population during a one-year period in Alberta.[24]

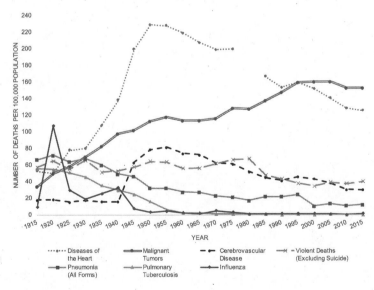

Fig. 3.1: Select leading causes of death, 1915 to 2015 (5-year intervals). Rate per 100,000 population.[25]

Overall, Table 3.1 and Figure 3.1 show that communicable diseases, and specifically influenza, were the most important causes of death around 1920 but were soon overtaken by non-communicable diseases — first heart disease, which dominated from the 1930s to the 1980s, and then cancer, which surpassed heart disease in the 1990s. These latter groups of diseases dwarfed influenza and other communicable diseases in terms of their absolute (number) and relative (rate) impacts on mortality across the Alberta population.

We structure the remainder of the chapter by presenting statistics on somewhat more specific causes of death within discrete time periods (1910–1922, 1923–1940, 1941–1959, 1960–1977, 1985–2015), defined based on the classification system, generally the International Classification of Diseases system, used to classify and tabulate the vital statistics in Alberta's annual reports.[26] Figures 3.2a to 3.2i include the top five causes of death in the first year of the time period in question; in some cases we included additional causes of death that otherwise seemed important or interesting due to, for example, a major increase or decrease. For each time period, we also consider elements of the public health context and activities aligning with one or more of the prominent causes of morbidity or mortality in more detail.

1910–1922: Communicable Diseases

Figure 3.2a presents leading causes of death for Albertans from 1910 to 1922. During this early period in Alberta's history, the leading causes of death were communicable in nature. Diarrhea and enteritis, specific to Albertans under two years of age, and typhoid fever figured prominently in 1910 but decreased fairly rapidly thereafter in terms of both incidence and mortality, in part reflecting early public health efforts relating to waterworks, sewerage, and immunization.

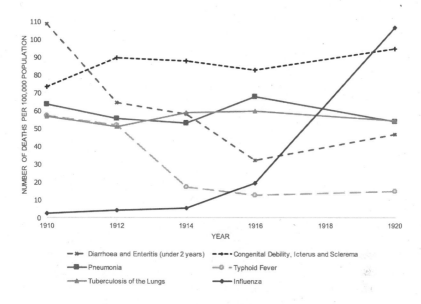

Fig. 3.2a: Leading causes of death (individual codes), 1910 to 1920. Rate per 100,000 population.[27]

Although reported deaths from influenza were relatively uncommon in Alberta early in this period, they increased significantly late in the decade reflecting the 1918/19 influenza pandemic, which was described in the inaugural provincial Department of Public Health's annual report in 1919.

> The influenza epidemic which late in the year 1918 swept the province with such disastrous results had by the beginning of 1919 materially declined, and while there were one or two waves, they had not the virulence of the first wave, and declined more rapidly. 7,185 cases were reported during the year [1919], the last cases being reported in the month of May. 31,051 cases were reported in 1918, thus making a total of 38,236 for the epidemic.[28]

Table 3.2 shows cases and deaths due to influenza in Alberta during those pandemic years and, by contrast, years on either side. During the pandemic, there were 38,236 cases and over 4,300 deaths[29] in a population of just over 500,000.[30]

TABLE 3.2: Reported annual number of cases of, and deaths from, influenza in Alberta, 1916–1923.[31]

Year	Reported cases (#)	Reported deaths (#)
1916	(not reported)	97
1917	(not reported)	75
1918	31,051	3,315
1919	7,185	1,049
1920	2,753	603
1921	3	75
1923	(not reported)	272

The illnesses noted in Figure 3.2a were the biggest contributors to mortality at the time. There were others that — while not necessarily causing large numbers of deaths — raised concern because of rising incidence, rapid spread, and impact on health and well-being. One example was venereal diseases which, in the context of World War I, were prevalent among Canadian soldiers[32] and extended to the civilian population. Venereal disease was described in the Alberta legislature in 1917 as "the scourge [that] was increasing at a tremendous rate, through the ignorance of the people" by Dr. George D. Stanley, MLA for High River; his comment provides insight into views on the causes of those diseases.[33] In 1920 a venereal disease division was established within the provincial Department of Public Health, which was responsible for treatment (i.e., every person with a venereal disease must place himself under treatment by a qualified practitioner); education (i.e., all persons attending treatment are informed about precautions to prevent spread of infection; as well, two films on the subject were shown across the province, and booklets were distributed); and reporting of cases.[34] Gonorrhea and syphilis became notifiable diseases in Alberta in 1919 and 1921, respectively.[35]

1923–1940: Communicable Diseases Persist, and an Epidemiological Transition Begins, in a Context of Economic Depression

Figures 3.2b and 3.2c present, respectively, leading causes of death in Alberta from 1923 to 1929 and from 1931 to 1939. Communicable diseases, including pneumonia, tuberculosis, and influenza persisted as important causes of death during the 1920s and 1930s in Alberta. The persistence of communicable disease deaths underpinned the 1924 creation of an infectious disease branch within the provincial Department of Public Health. Deaths from influenza continued to show periodic spikes. In 1937, for example influenza caused 472 deaths in Alberta, compared to 340 the year before. Based on news media coverage, there was concern, which did not materialize, that the 1937 outbreak might rival the 1918/19 pandemic.[36]

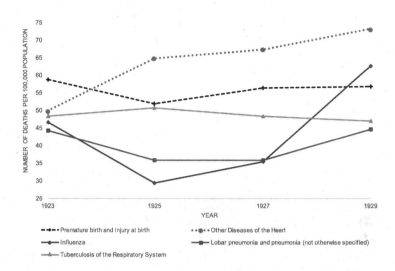

Fig. 3.2b: Leading causes of death (individual codes), 1923 to 1929. Rate per 100,000 population.[37]

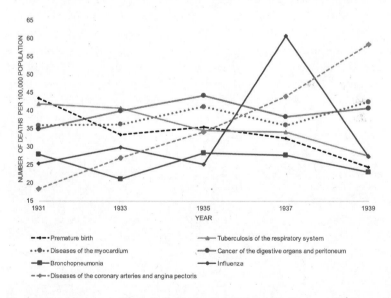

Fig. 3.2c: Leading causes of death (individual codes), 1931 to 1939. Rate per 100,000 population.[38]

Epidemics of polio struck the province in 1927 — with 353 cases, including fifty-three deaths — and in 1930, when there were 150 cases and thirty-two deaths. However, as we shall soon see, Alberta's most significant polio outbreak was yet to come.[39] The 1927 outbreak occurred mostly in and around Edmonton, while the 1930 outbreak largely affected areas south of Red Deer, including Calgary, suggesting that those in the Edmonton area had developed some immunity that protected them later.[40] Although 1937 was a significant polio year for Canada, Alberta was less affected than provinces such as Ontario.[41] Approximately half of Alberta's 169 reported cases that year occurred in and around Medicine Hat; the incidence of polio in Medicine Hat at the time was the highest ever experienced by any Alberta municipality. As described by historian Christopher Rutty and colleagues, polio sparked frustration and fear throughout the first half of the twentieth century due to a lack of understanding of its cause, the unpredictability of outbreaks, and the fact that it primarily affected middle-class children and families,[42] who have relatively high political voice (see Chapter 1). In this context, the Alberta government passed the Poliomyelitis Sufferers Act in 1938, which provided free treatment for polio patients.[43]

Alongside the persistence of communicable diseases, non-communicable diseases began to appear among the leading causes of death during the 1920s and 1930s. Deaths from diseases of the circulatory system (e.g., heart, myocardium, coronary arteries), for example, increased during the 1920s and 1930s. In the 1930s, cancer appeared for the first time in the top five causes of death, causing considerable public and professional concern,[44] including a discussion in 1931 by the Edmonton Board of Health to make cancer a notifiable disease (this did not materialize).[45] This transition from communicable to non-communicable diseases as primary causes of death led Deputy Minister of Health, Dr. Malcolm Bow to lament in 1937 that "we have done relatively little for those over forty years of age [who are more likely to suffer from] [c]ancer, diabetes, diseases of the heart and arteries, accidents."[46]

Insight into other health concerns of this period may be gleaned from the content and structure of the provincial Department of Public Health, including dental health in the 1920s. In 1930, a division of mental health was created within the provincial department. However, contrary to its name, the mental health division focused entirely on provincial institutions for patients with mental illnesses, including those considered "refractory or disturbed" and "idiots, imbeciles . . . and defectives." It also focused on mental hygiene clinics, which dealt with "problem cases referred by schools, courts, police, physicians, health departments, hospitals, charities, homes, parents and the Department of Neglected Children;"

perhaps not surprisingly, the director of mental health, Dr. C. A. Baragar, worked closely with the provincial Eugenics Board (see also Chapter 1).[47]

1941–1959: Cancer, Nutrition, and a Resurgence of Polio

Leading causes of death in Alberta during the 1940s and 1950s are shown in Figure 3.2d (1941–1949) and Figure 3.2e (1951–1959). The context for these statistics is the period during and after World War II, which included wartime restrictions such as food rationing, followed by post-war economic growth and development of the welfare state. The 1940s represented the last period that any communicable disease, in particular tuberculosis (Figure 3.2d), appeared among the top five causes of death for Albertans according to the statistics presented here.

With funding from provincial and federal governments, the Central Alberta Sanatorium (later renamed the Baker Sanatorium) in the Calgary area opened in 1920 to serve civilians and World War I veterans.[48] The provincial Tuberculosis Act, passed in 1936, authorized free tuberculosis treatment, and allowed for significant increases in institutional beds and diagnostic services.[49] The so-called rest cure provided in sanatoriums was the most common treatment for tuberculosis until the 1940s, when the antibiotic streptomycin was discovered, widespread use of which has been credited with contributing importantly to the continued decline in deaths from tuberculosis.[50] As discussed in Chapter 1, the framing and deployment of tuberculosis control efforts in Alberta effectively excluded, on racist grounds, Indigenous patients. These dynamics moreover cast doubt on the reliability of the estimates of the number of Indigenous tuberculosis patients in Alberta.

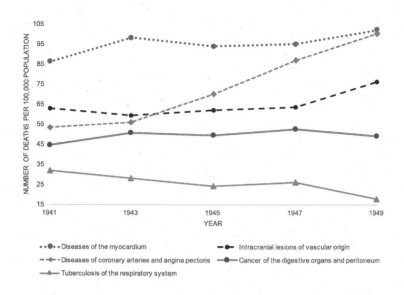

Fig. 3.2d: Leading causes of death (individual codes), 1941 to 1949. Rate per 100,000 population.[51]

By the 1950s, despite an emerging sense of having largely combated communicable disease, illnesses persisted.[52] A notable spike in gonorrhea incidence in the province occurred during the 1940s (see Figure 3.4 on page 80),[53] once again influenced by wartime circumstances and high rates of infection among returning WWII soldiers. Although penicillin had been discovered in the late 1920s, it was in the 1940s that research efforts intensified to permit producing the antibiotic on a larger scale.[54] In 1945 in Alberta, penicillin was added to the list of drugs to be distributed for free by the provincial Department of Public Health for the treatment of gonorrhea.[55]

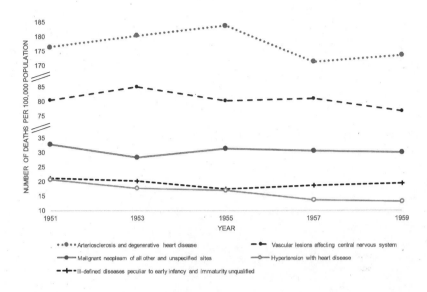

Fig. 3.2e: Leading causes of death (individual codes), 1951 to 1959. Rate per 100,000 population.[56]

In the 1950s, attention shifted again to polio. Alberta's largest polio out-break occurred in 1952/1953, with a total of 2,232 cases and 192 deaths.[57] During August and September of 1953, polio appeared in the local news almost daily, including frequent advertisements for polio insurance (Figure 3.3). The Salk vac-cine was the focus of a large-scale field trial in 1954 led by the U.S. National Foundation for Infantile Paralysis with materials provided by the Toronto-based Connaught Laboratories.[58] Alberta — having been badly affected by the 1953 out-break — was one of a few Canadian jurisdictions to participate in the trial, and over 16,000 Alberta children were enrolled. The trial established that the Salk vaccine was 60 to 90 percent effective depending on the type of poliovirus, and Alberta and other provinces began widespread funding and distribution of the vaccine to school-aged children.[59] Immunization has eliminated polio in Alberta and across Canada. In Alberta, there have been only three cases of symptomatic polio since 1968, with the last one reported in 1979.[60]

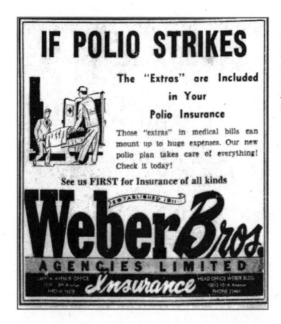

IF POLIO STRIKES

The "Extras" are Included
in Your
Polio Insurance

Those "extras" in medical bills can
mount up to huge expenses. Our new
polio plan takes care of everything!
Check it today!

See us FIRST for Insurance of all kinds

Weber Bros.
AGENCIES LIMITED
Insurance

Fig. 3.3: Advertisement for polio insurance. Originally published in *the Edmonton Journal*, a Division of Postmedia Network Inc. *Edmonton Journal*, 8 August 1953, 34 (one of many examples).

Heart disease was the leading cause of death during the 1940s and 1950s,[61] but cancer was a growing concern. Under the 1940 Cancer Treatment and Prevention Act, the provincial government assumed responsibility for funding procedures related to cancer diagnosis, treatment, and prevention.[62] The Alberta Cancer Registry evolved from a need for a system to support the administration of that new payment model under the 1940 act.[63] Starting out as a file-card data collection system, the registry expanded and evolved over time; in 1953, registration of patients with government-administered cancer clinics — at that time in Edmonton, Calgary, and Lethbridge — became a prerequisite for physicians to be paid for treating cancer patients. In 1968, it became mandatory for medical laboratories in Alberta to send pathology reports concerning cancer to the registry, and in 1974, physicians became legally required to register cancer patients.

In line with the shift toward non-communicable diseases as major causes of death, the 1940s saw growing interest in nutrition on the part of the provincial Department of Public Health.[64] In 1947, a nutrition division was created within the provincial department, with Public Health Nutritionist, Elva M. Perdue BSc, appointed as director. From the outset, the division's efforts focused on nutrition education, thus illustrating an assumption that lack of knowledge, rather than lack of money and its intersection with other social identities such as ethnicity, was at the root of poor nutrition.[65] The division also participated in dietary surveys to assess nutrition among the Alberta population.[66]

1960–1977: A Focus on Motor Vehicle Accidents

Diseases of the circulatory system and cancer continued to be leading causes of death during the 1960s (Figure 3.2f) and 1970s (Figure 3.2g). A new entry among the leading causes of death starting in the 1960s was motor vehicle accidents. This was a period of considerable provincial and national discussion around traffic safety, including the role of seat belts.[67]

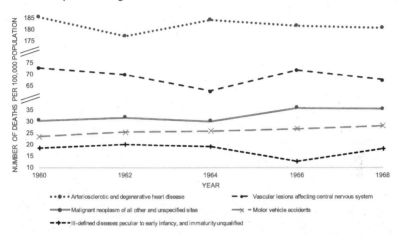

Fig. 3.2f: Leading causes of death (individual codes), 1960 to 1968. Rate per 100,000 population.[68]

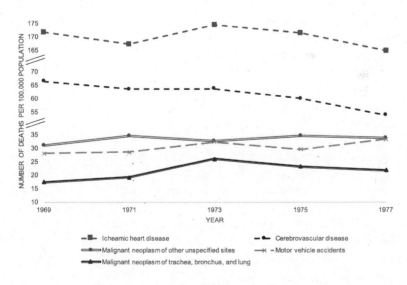

Fig. 3.2g: Leading causes of death (individual codes), 1969 to 1977. Rate per 100,000 population.[69]

There had been a few references to seat belts in Alberta news media as early as the 1950s. In 1954, the Farm Women's Union of Alberta passed a resolution recommending that all manufacturers of motor cars provide safety belts as standard equipment in cars,[70] one of several examples of involvement by women's groups in advocating for seat belts.[71] In 1955 and 1956, members of the Alberta Safety Council,[72] including safety director Paul Lawrence, attended meetings of the National Safety Council in Chicago, where seat belts were major topics of discussion.[73] Awareness of the safety benefits of seat belts[74] manifested in their mandatory use in stock car racing, including in Edmonton,[75] and their adoption in other limited circumstances.[76] In 1955, the Chrysler Corporation announced from Detroit that seat belts would be made available as "dealer-installed optional equipment" in its 1955 cars; the initiative would come to Canada soon after.[77]

Discussion about seat belts grew in frequency and intensity during the 1960s. Alongside a growing chorus of pro-seat belt voices by medical professionals and others,[78] automobile industry standards slowly advanced, beginning with seat belt attachments to permit their installation in vehicles.[79] Uptake of seat belt certification in Alberta was hastened in 1963 when the cabinet of the governing SC party passed an order-in-council stipulating that seat belts sold in the province must meet specific safety standards.[80] However, it was still up to consumers to decide whether or not to purchase and install seat belts in their vehicles. Although other jurisdictions passed legislation requiring all new cars sold to be equipped with seatbelts, Alberta preferred to wait.[81] In 1962, Premier Ernest Manning stated that the provincial government had "no intention of requiring car owners to have them installed."[82] He then predicted that seat belts would become standard equipment in all cars, in time.[83] In fact, he was largely correct: by early 1964 three major car manufacturers — American Motors (Canada), Chrysler Canada, and General Motors — had announced that all new cars, including those purchased in Alberta, would have seat belts pre-installed, to the delight of long-standing Highways Minister Gordon Taylor.[84]

With seat belts physically in place, for the most part, the discussion in the late 1960s shifted to use which, at the time, was low.[85] In Alberta, there was a very strong sentiment, which endured well into the 1970s and 1980s, that seat belt use should not be legislated and that education was the best approach.[86] The Alberta Safety Council, with Mr. Paul Lawrence as safety director and later general manager, continued to be a vocal proponent for seat belts and was frequently in the news,[87] publicizing the benefits of seat belt use and answering common questions, such as whether seat belts are necessary for short trips in town at a slower speed limit (yes; a large proportion of traffic deaths occur within 25 miles [around 40 kilometres] of home, and at speeds of less than 40 miles per hour [around 65 kilometres per hour]), and whether the potential risk of being belted in if a vehicle is burning or submerged outweighs the benefit (no; even in such circumstances, chances of remaining conscious to free oneself are increased when wearing a seat belt).[88] A 1969 survey by the council estimated that, even though approximately three-quarters of cars had seat belts installed, fewer than one in four individuals surveyed said that they used them on a regular basis.[89]

During the 1970s, in the face of persistently low seat belt use, attention began to shift to the idea of making it compulsory to wear seat belts, building on precedents elsewhere, including Australia.[90] In Canada, Minister of National Health and Welfare, Marc Lalonde, in the 1974 context of his newly released *A New Perspective on the Health of Canadians Report*, urged provincial governments to consider compulsory seat belt legislation.[91] Although some Canadian provinces advanced such legislation,[92] Alberta resisted, despite efforts, including by Mr. George Ho Lem, Social Credit MLA for Calgary McCall. In the mid-1970s Mr. Ho Lem made two attempts to introduce legislation in the form of private members bills to amend the provincial Highway Traffic Act to mandate seatbelt use.[93] There was very little discussion and no apparent support for the proposed amendment in the legislature, and the bill did not progress.

In 1975, Mr. Ho Lem was back with Bill 213, to amend the Highway Traffic Act such that seat belt use would be required but only on public highways where the prescribed speed limit was 50 mph (around 80 km/h) or more.[94] This time, the bill underwent second reading, with Mr. Ho Lem delivering an impassioned description and rationale, including the benefits of seat belts for reducing suffering, deaths, and hospital costs; the success of compulsory seat belt legislation elsewhere; analogies with other legislation such as for helmet use on motorcycles; and his perspective about public perceptions shifting to be more supportive of seat belt legislation. Considerable discussion followed, nearly all of which was opposed, and the bill timed out.[95] In these and subsequent debates, the points of opposition raised in the legislature were similar and may be summarized into several themes, which are listed along with illustrative examples in Table 3.3. Overall, these wide-reaching points of opposition led to strong reluctance to embrace compulsory seat belt legislation in Alberta, even when other Canadian jurisdictions were beginning to move in that direction.[96] We continue the seat belt story below.

TABLE 3.3: Points of opposition to compulsory seatbelt legislation (thematic groupings), along with illustrative examples, from the Alberta legislature, 1970s.[97]

Point of opposition	Illustrative examples (quotations)
Uncertainty about the benefits of seat belts / it's not just about seat belts.	" . . . it has not been proven that wearing seat belts is a complete safety factor [. . .] I would hope, before we pass legislation [. . .] that we make every effort to study, research, and bring back the report to the Legislature whether the research proves that wearing seat belts is an effective way of saving people from being injured or killed." —Rudolph Zander (PC), MLA for Drayton Valley, *Alberta Hansard*, 13 February 1975.
	"I should point out, though, that the statistics on morbidity and mortality relative to automobile accidents have been coming down across the country without regard to whether that particular jurisdiction has mandatory seat belt legislation." —Hugh Horner (PC), MLA for Barrhead, *Alberta Hansard*, 25 March 1977.
Harms of seat belts ("I know someone . . . ")	"Out of dozens of examples in my own constituency [. . .] There was one incident where a man and a lady were travelling and at an intersection they piled in with a gravel truck [. . .] The man, a person [of] 180 pounds, was in a seat belt. He couldn't loosen the seat belt [. . .] By that time, the car exploded and the person burned." —John Batiuk (PC), MLA for Lamont, *Alberta Hansard*, 13 February 1975.
Seat belt use can't be enforced	"One is the problem of enforcement. How does a policeman see somebody who's only wearing a lap belt and not a shoulder belt? How does he obtain a conviction if an apprehended person says he has just snapped loose his seat belt at the moment his vehicle is stopped?" —Roy Farran (PC), MLA for Calgary-North Hill, *Alberta Hansard*, 20 November 1975.
I believe in seat belts, just not in being forced to wear them.	"No one will deny the wearing of seat belts is of some help in reducing the extent of injury in highway accidents [. . .] However, we must be aware that encouraging people to use seat belts and making sure the car has seat belts are very different from enforcing people to use seat belts. It is to this latter element of coercion [. . .] that I take exception [. . .] By requiring that seatbelts be used, the freedom of choice is lost." —Clifford Doan (PC), MLA for Innisfail, *Alberta Hansard*, 13 February 1975.

1985–2015: Some Key Successes, and New Challenges

Continuing among the top causes of death in the 1980s, 1990s, and early 2000s was cancer (Figure 3.2h and 3.2i). Priorities for cancer prevention were reducing the prevalence of cigarette smoking (see also Chapter 9), research into the influence of diet, and the development of programs for early diagnosis, especially for colorectal, breast, and cervical cancer.[98] Also in the mid-1980s, and against the backdrop of an international wave of enthusiasm around community-based health promotion and disease prevention activities,[99] was the Steve Fonyo Cancer Prevention Program, a community-based education demonstration project focused on cancer risk reduction and early detection.[100]

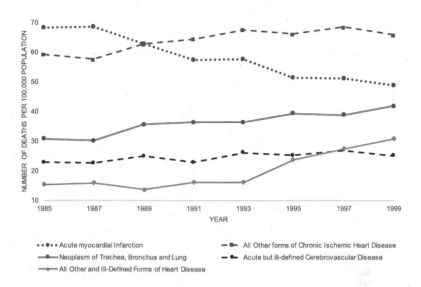

Fig. 3.2h: Leading causes of death (individual codes), 1985 to 1999. Rate per 100,000 population.[101]

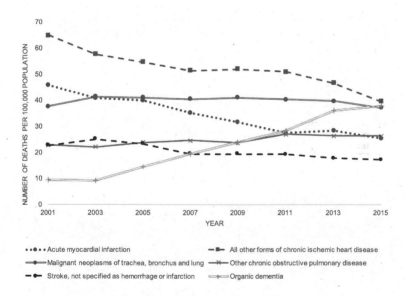

Fig. 3.2i: Leading causes of death (individual codes), 2000 to 2015. Rate per 100,000 population.[102]

A notable health trend in Alberta during this most recent period (1980s–present) was a peak, followed by a steep decline, in the incidence of gonorrhea (Figure 3.4). In the 1980/81 period, Alberta had the highest incidence of gonorrhea in Canada, which was believed to reflect a variety of factors including "a buoyant economic climate" that resulted in a proportionally larger number of individuals considered high risk (e.g., young, single workers, and visitors), greater awareness of sexually transmitted disease among members of the public and health professionals, and improvements in reporting processes.[103] An increasingly comprehensive program for the control of sexually transmitted infections was developed, including the establishment of diagnostic and treatment clinics in Calgary, Edmonton, and Lethbridge;[104] contact tracing; consulting and referral services to physicians; data monitoring and surveillance; free medication; counselling by professional social workers; and education, including efforts to present venereal disease as a public health problem rather than a moral one.[105] Starting in the early 1980s, incidence in Alberta started to show a significant decline,[106] which has been attributed in part to changes in sexual practices stemming from increased awareness of HIV-AIDS.[107]

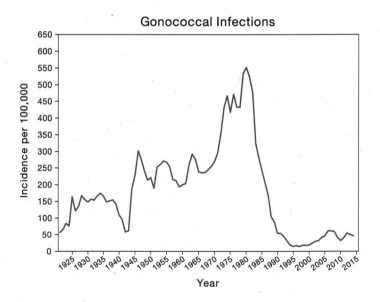

Fig. 3.4: Incidence of Gonococcal Infections (Gonorrhea), Alberta, 1919 to 2014. Figure reproduced from Alberta Health, Surveillance and Assessment Branch and Office of the chief medical officer of health, *Alberta Notifiable Disease Incidence: A Historical Record, 1919–2014* (Government of Alberta, 2015), 8.

Returning to seat belts, government deliberations continued into the 1980s, including repeated attempts to introduce mandatory legislation. In 1980, Mr. Dennis L. Anderson (PC), MLA for Calgary-Currie, introduced private member Bill 204: An Act to Amend the Highway Traffic Act, which would require "that each individual *under the age of 18* travelling in a motor vehicle wear a seat belt or be held by a child restraint device" (italics added), with a penalty for drivers who did not comply.[108] Following discussion at second reading, including presentation of statistics from other provinces showing that seat belt use increased following the introduction of mandatory legislation, the bill was left to die on the Order Paper.[109] Somewhat frustratingly, some members took issue with the arbitrariness of age eighteen as a cut-off. Mr. John B. Zaozirny QC (PC), MLA for Calgary Forest-Lawn, for example, argued that using eighteen years as a cut-off for mandatory seat belt use, but sixteen years as legal driving age would amount to encouraging the seventeen-year-old to break the law.[110]

Aside from occasional questions,[111] the next time seat belts appeared prominently in the legislature was in 1983–1984, in the context of discussions around ways to reduce health care expenditures, including the possible implementation of hospital user fees.[112] Leader of the Official Opposition, W. Grant Notley (NDP), was vehemently opposed to user fees on the basis that they are contrary to the concept of equality in treatment.[113] He, along with Dr. Walter A. Buck (Independent, MLA for Clover Bar), argued that the Lougheed government could not introduce a user fee without first considering all other alternatives — including preventive measures such as mandatory seat belt legislation, which could save lives and money.[114]

In the context of a 1983 legislative discussion, Janet Koper (PC, MLA for Calgary-Foothills) suggested that "seat belt" in previous bills be substituted with "mandatory use of *child restraint devices* in motor vehicles for *children from birth to five years of age*" (italics added).[115] Koper's suggestion was formalized as government Bill 83: Child Transportation Safety Act, introduced by Minister of Transportation, Marvin E. Moore (PC) in October 1984.[116] The rationale for the bill, presented at second reading, focused on the large number of deaths due to automobile accidents among children and the inability of young children to make decisions for themselves. Likely in anticipation of pushback, Moore was explicit that the proposed legislation was "not in any way associated with seat belts for all adults, and [he did not] intend to expand it in that way or to introduce legislation in that regard."[117] Although some members expressed disappointment that the bill did not go further,[118] it received broad support and passed third reading in November 1984.[119]

With the election of Don Getty's Progressive Conservative government in 1985, the door opened to revisit the issue of mandatory seat belt legislation for everyone, with indications that the mood in the legislature was shifting.[120] During the Speech from the Throne on 5 March 1987, the Getty administration announced that "based on extensive consultation with Albertans through their elected representatives, my government will introduce legislation requiring the use of seat belts in automobiles in a further effort to reduce the number of people injured in automobile accidents."[121] Several members of the legislature expressed enthusiastic support, while others were resigned, maintaining that although they were personally opposed to mandatory seat belts, they were compelled to accept the views of their constituents and Albertans more generally.[122]

Bill 9, which made seat belt use compulsory for all in Alberta, passed and took effect on 1 July 1987.[123] The new legislation was accompanied by regulations outlining exceptions to the new rules.[124] Nonetheless, and notwithstanding a hiatus in implementation and enforcement due to a legal challenge, the benefits of mandatory seat belt legislation in Alberta soon became apparent:[125] five months after the legislation was introduced, it was reported that use averaged about 80 percent, which was the highest of any province in Canada,[126] and the number of fatalities in 1990 had decreased by 16 percent from 1989. Perhaps emblematic of Alberta's cultural shift, Kenneth R. Kowalski (PC, MLA for Barrhead) commented a year later that "I was one of those who opposed the idea of mandatory seat belt legislation because I thought the invasion of individual rights was paramount and more important, but as I stand here on this particular day in May of 1991, I have to come clean on this matter and basically say without a moment of hesitation in my mind that seat belts do save lives."[127]

Conclusions

This chapter presents an overview of the health of the Alberta population over a hundred-year period, using statistics that were available over the full period of interest. We are not aware of other efforts to compile and present this historical information for Alberta. The basic storyline of this chapter, which includes shifts over time in predominant health problems (e.g., communicable to non-communicable diseases and injuries); approaches (e.g., education, legislation, and health service delivery); and tensions (e.g., urban versus rural infrastructure, benefits and drawbacks of disease reporting, the balance between government intervention and individual liberties) is not unique to Alberta, yet we aimed to tell the story in a way that showcased local responses and personalities within that common story.[128]

We began — and now end — the chapter with the important, yet fraught, question, "how do we know what we know?" While the answer to that question certainly includes elements of a technical nature, such as statistical data and reporting infrastructure, it also embodies elements of power and privilege that determine what information is gathered, by and from whom, to what end, what is to be done about it, and who gets to decide. We encourage anyone who is interested in the public's health to keep these considerations in mind.

NOTES

1   World Health Organization, "Constitution of the World Health Organization: Principles," About WHO, accessed on 4 November 2018, http://www.who.int/about/mission/en/.

2   Vital statistics were published in the annual report of the Department of Agriculture from 1905 to 1917. In 1919, they were transferred to the newly established Department of Public Health.

3   Alberta Health, Surveillance and Assessment Branch, and Office of the Chief Medical Officer of Health, *Alberta Notifiable Disease Incidence: A Historical Record, 1919–2014* (Government of Alberta, 2015). https://open.alberta.ca/dataset/09ff0f40-1cfc-48fd-b888-4357104c3c32/resource/c5ceca04-ccda-4811-9ed0-03a3cbe8c0fb/download/7019844-notifiable-disease-incidence-1919-2014.pdf. This report presents a compilation of historical data from 1919 to 2014 on select notifiable communicable diseases. The data were gathered from sources including the source files from the Government of Alberta (1919–1924), the *Annual Report of Notifiable Diseases of the Dominion of Canada* (1925–1978), the *Cumulative Annual Notifiable Disease List* from Alberta Health and Wellness (1979–1984), and Alberta's Communicable Disease Reporting System (1985–2014). For several diseases, incidence rates are available as early as 1919, corresponding to when these diseases were designated as reportable.

4   *A Dictionary of Epidemiology*, 4th ed., Ed. John M. Last (Oxford: Oxford University Press, 2001), 187 "vital statistics".

5   Statistics Canada "History of Vital Statistics" (Government of Canada, modified 8 April 2020), https://www.statcan.gc.ca/eng/health/vital/2012001/hvs; Statistics Canada, "A 100 Years and More of Statistics Acts" (*The Daily*, Government of Canada, modified 3 December 2018), https://www150.statcan.gc.ca/n1/daily-quotidien/181203/dq181203h-eng.htm; Kelsey Lucyk, Mingshan Lu, Tolulope Sajobi, and Hude Quan, "Administrative Health Data in Canada: Lessons from History," BMC Medical Informatics and Decision Making 69, no. 15 (2015). Statistics Canada, "A 100 Years and More of Statistics Acts.

6   Statistics Canada "History of Vital Statistics"; *An Act respecting the Registration of Births, Marriages and Deaths*, Statutes of the Province of Alberta (S.P.A.), 1907, c. 13.

7   "The Legislature on the Weed Question," *Edmonton Journal*, 2 March 1907, 1.

8   An Act respecting Vital Statistics, S.P.A. 1916, c. 22.

9   *An Act to amend the Vital Statistics Act*, S.P.A. 1919, c. 45, assented 17 April 1919.

10   Provincial Archives of Alberta, An Administrative History of the Government of Alberta, 1905–2005 (Edmonton: The Provincial Archives of Alberta, 2006), 286; Service Alberta, "Alberta Vital Statistics Annual Review," Open Government Publications (Edmonton, AB: Alberta Government, 2006), https://open.alberta.ca/publications/1485-3809.

11   Last, *A Dictionary of Epidemiology*, 125.

12   Alberta Health Services "Public Health Surveillance," (Government of Alberta, accessed 18 May 2020, https://www.albertahealthservices.ca/services/Page13513.aspx. See also Last, *A Dictionary of Epidemiology*, 174.

13   *An Ordinance respecting Public Health*, Ordinances of the Northwest Territories 1902, c. 4.

14   *An Act respecting Public Health*, 1907.

15   *Communicable Diseases Regulation*, 238/1985, https://open.alberta.ca/publications/1985_238#summary

16   This is notwithstanding some of the implementation challenges to notifiable disease reporting, which may lead to under-reporting. For example, in commenting on the 1967 Edmonton Board of Health annual report, city Medical Officer of Health, Dr. G.H. Ball, "said that he believes there are at least twice as many actual cases of salmonella poisoning in Edmonton as are reported." "City Will Step Up Food Poison Study," *Edmonton Journal*, 12 September 1967, 13; "Venereal Disease Still Major Health

Problem," *Edmonton Journal*, 17 September 1966, 23. In her address to the Alberta Association of Medical Record Librarians, J.D. Hanna, Division of Social Hygiene, Department of Public Health, supervisor, reported on trends in venereal diseases including syphilis, for which the number and incidence of cases in Alberta was quite a bit lower in 1965 (171 cases, 11.2 per 100,000) than in 1946 (246 cases, 30.6 per 100,000).

17   "City Will Step Up Food Poison Study," *Edmonton Journal*, 12 September 1967, 13.

18   "AIDS Proposal Opposed," *Edmonton Journal*, 27 November 1988, 27.

19   Alberta Health and Wellness, *Public Health Notifiable Disease Management Guidelines, Human Immunodeficiency Virus (HIV)* (Government of Alberta, January 2011, superseded 2021 and 2022), https://open.alberta.ca/dataset/78566f8e-622e-448d-b579-4a838b642689/resource/dbc68c10-7fff-41c3-8063-2ec6a3872f9d/download/guidelines-human-immunodeficiency-virus-2011.pdf

20   In his presidential address at the Canadian Public Health Association's 26th annual meeting in 1937, Malcolm Bow identified cancer as one of "eight major health problems facing us to-day irrespective of the particular section of Canada in which we live" due to the "tremendous toll of life levied by this disease." Malcolm R. Bow, "Public Health Yesterday, To-Day, and To-Morrow," *Canadian Journal of Public Health* 28, no. 7 (July 1937).

21   Alberta Department of Public Health, *Annual Report of the Department of Public Health of the Province of Alberta 1921*, 11-12 (all Alberta Department of Public Health reports are printed in Edmonton, by: J.W. Jeffery, King's Printer, for report years 1919-1923; W.D. McLean, King's Printer, for report years 1924-1933; A. Shnitka, King's Printer, for report years 1934-1949; A. Shnitka, Queen's Printer, for report years 1950-1955; and L.S. Wall, Queen's Printer, for report years 1956-1968).

22   These cause of death categories represent major headings contained within the annual vital statistics reports. Although the categories are broad, they are perhaps the ones most amenable to comparisons over time. They are compiled by statistics officers for the purpose of identifying leading causes of death in the report summaries and to making comparisons over time. See for example, the summaries in the Alberta Department of Public Health, Annual Report *1924*, 77–78; Alberta Department of Public Health, *Annual Report of the Vital Statistics Branch 1937*, 7–8; Alberta Department of Public Health, *Annual Report of the Vital Statistics Branch 1947*, 6–7, 119; Alberta Department of Public Health, *Annual Report of the Bureau of Vital Statistics*, 2–3, 63. The five- and ten-year intervals used in Table 3.1 and Figure 3.1 result in the omission of peak periods of certain causes of death, such as the 1918/19 influenza epidemic.

23   The number of deaths from "diseases of the heart" in 1980 is not reported because it is noted to be "understated" in the 1980 annual report (1980 Vital Statistics Report, province of Alberta). Brief contemporary definitions of each cause of death are as follows: *Influenza*: an acute respiratory infection caused by the influenza virus; includes seasonal and other forms of influenza; *pneumonia*: a form of acute respiratory infection that affects the lungs; *tuberculosis*: a disease caused by bacteria that most often affects the lungs; *violent causes (excluding suicide)*: includes transport accidents, poisoning, self-harm, falls, homicides, war, drowning, etc.; *diseases of the heart*: includes rheumatic heart disease, coronary heart disease, congenital heart disease, and heart attacks; *cancer or malignant tumors*: a large group of diseases that can affect any part of the body and are characterized by the rapid creation of abnormal cells that grow beyond their usual boundaries and can invade or spread to other parts of the body; *diseases of the arteries*: generalized and localized diseases that affect arteries, including those that result in arterial occlusion (blockage) and those that do not; *cerebral haemorrage*: an escape of blood from a ruptured vessel in the brain; rupture can occur for different reasons; *cerebrovascular disease*: disease of blood vessels supplying the brain. Sources: "Fact Sheets", World Health Organization, https://www.who.int/news-room/fact-sheets; "Cerebral hemorrhage," Mosby's Medical Dictionary, https://medical-dictionary.thefreedictionary.com/Cerebral+hemhorrage; "Cardiovascular disease," Encyclopaedia Britannica, https://www.britannica.com/science/cardiovascular-disease/Diseases-of-the-arteries

24   Sometimes the rates presented in this chapter pertain to particular age groups, and this is specified as it occurs. In general, the rates presented were drawn directly from the annual reports of the provincial department responsible for public health and vital statistics at the time.

25   Sources: Alberta Vital Statistics Reports, Alberta Vital Statistics Reviews, Statistics Canada, 1915 to 2015. Data were extracted from the Vital Statistics Reports summary sections and tables labelled *Certain Causes of Death, Selected Causes of Death*, or *Leading Causes of Death* for the years 1915–1995 (See Appendix A for sources). Data for "Diseases of the heart" are missing in 1980 because they are reported to be unreliable that year. Starting in 2000, data were taken from Statistics Canada. This is because the province's summary classification of Leading Causes changed in 2000 with the adoption of ICD-10. Population figures were extracted from: Population from 1905 to 1970 taken from: "Table 32: Population, Birth, Marriages, Death and Rates for the years 1905 – 1970," in Alberta Department of

Health, *Annual Report of the Division of Vital Statistics 1970* (Edmonton: Printed by L.S. Wall, Printer to the Queen Most Excellent Majesty, 1972), 121. Population from 1975 to 1995 taken from: Respective Vital Statistics Annual Reports for each corresponding year. Population from 2000 to 2015 taken from: Statistics Canada "Population estimates on July 1st, by age and sex" Frequency: Annual Table: 17-10-0005-01 (formerly CANSIM 051-0001).

26   The process to classify causes of death is complex and has changed significantly over time. The most common system for classification of diseases internationally is the International Classification of Diseases (ICD), which was adopted by the International Statistical Institute in 1899. In 1905, when the Department of Agriculture first reported statistics on causes of death for the province of Alberta, diseases were classified using a list of fourteen main categories with a total of 101 individual codes or causes. Starting in 1910, the province seems to have adopted the ICD system, using ICD-2, and thereafter adopted each iteration of the ICD.

27   Classification system is not named but cause numbers match ICD-2 codes. Includes deaths at all ages. Sources: Alberta Department of Agriculture, *Annual Report 1910* (Edmonton, 1911), 217–218; Alberta Department of Agriculture, *Annual Report 1912* (Edmonton, 1913), 80–81; Alberta Department of Agriculture, *Annual Report 1914* (Edmonton: Printed by J.W. Jeffrey, Government Printer, 1915), 24–25; "Deaths during the Year 1916, by ages and sexes," Alberta Department of Agriculture, *Annual Report 1916* (Edmonton: Printed by J.W. Jeffrey, King's Printer, 1917), 198–201; For the year 1918, the value for "Diarrhoea and Enteritis (Under 2 years)" is not given; and "Influenza" includes the sum of the "Influenza" and "Influenza (Epidemic)" categories. "Causes of Death during the Year 1918, by Ages and Sexes (for the Whole province)," Alberta, *Annual Report of the Vital Statistics Branch 1918* (Edmonton), 67–73; "Causes of Death during the Year 1920, by ages and sexes (for the whole province)," Alberta Department of Public Health, *Annual Report of the Vital Statistics Branch 1920* (Edmonton: Printed by J.W. Jeffery, King's Printer, 1921), 28–43. Population source: "Table 32: Population, Birth, Marriages, Death and Rates for the years 1905 – 1970," in Alberta Department of Health, *Annual Report of the Division of Vital Statistics 1970* (Edmonton: Printed by L.S. Wall, Printer to the Queen Most Excellent Majesty, 1972), 121.

28   Alberta Department of Public Health, *Annual Report 1919*, 9.

29   Alberta, *Annual Report of the Vital Statistics Branch 1918* (Edmonton), 67; Alberta Department of Public Health, *Annual Report 1919*, 45.

30   The population of Alberta was 495,351 in 1916; "Census of the Prairie Provinces, 1916," Library and Archives Canada, modified 29 November 2019, https://www.bac-lac.gc.ca/eng/census/1916/Pages/about-census.aspx). Alberta's population was 588,454 in 1921 ("Census of Canada, 1921," Library and Archives Canada, modified 21 February 2019, https://www.bac-lac.gc.ca/eng/census/1921/Pages/introduction.aspx).

31   Sources: Alberta Department of Agriculture, *Annual Report 1916*, 178 and 196; Alberta Department of Agriculture, *Annual Report 1917* (Edmonton: Printed by J.W. Jeffery, King's Printer, 1918), 165 and 184; Alberta, *Annual Report of the Vital Statistics Branch 1918* (Edmonton), 67; Alberta Department of Public Health, *Annual Report 1919*, 9 and 45; Alberta Department of Public Health, *Annual Report 1920*, 9 and 47; Alberta Department of Public Health, *Annual Report 1921* (Edmonton: Printed by J.W. Jeffery, King's Printer, 1922), 12 and 101; Alberta Department of Public Health, *Annual Report 1923* (Edmonton: Printed by J.W. Jeffery, King's Printer, 1924), 7 and 92. "Not reported" (which refers to number of cases) means that influenza was not included in the Statistical Table that often accompanied the provincial medical officer's report, because it did not figure amongst the most common diseases that year. Data on the number of deaths comes from the vital statistics on causes of death.

32   A.F.W. Peart, "The Venereal Disease Problem in Canada," *Canadian Journal of Public Health* 44, no. 5 (May 1953).

33   "Education and Agriculture Estimates in Legislature," *Edmonton Bulletin*, 20 March 1917, Alberta Legislature Library, Scrapbook Hansard, https://librarysearch.assembly.ab.ca/client/en_CA/search/asset/141864/0. The Scrapbook Hansard (https://librarysearch.assembly.ab.ca/client/en_CA/scrapbookhansard) provided insight into legislative debates prior to the establishment of the Alberta Hansard in 1972.

34   "Report of the Director of the Division of Venereal Diseases," in Alberta Department of Public Health, *Annual Report 1920*, 21–2.

35   Alberta Health, *Alberta Notifiable Disease Incidence*. The idea of designating venereal diseases as notifiable diseases was discussed at least as early as 1916: at a meeting of the Alberta congress of Social Service, held 25 November 1916 in Calgary, a resolution was passed "asking government for legislation to include venereal diseases in the list of notifiable diseases, and to undertake to provide Wasserman Test and the Salverson treatment free of charge to every physician who will register a patient." "Social Service Congress Asks for Dower Law," *Edmonton Journal*, 25 November 1916, 9.

36   "'1918 Type' 'Flu Epidemic Feared," *Edmonton Journal*, 7 January 1937, 9.

37   Classification system is not named but cause numbers match ICD-3 codes. For the years 1923 and 1925, the causes of deaths for Indigenous ("Indian") and non-Indigenous people were published in two separate tables. We added the numbers from the two tables to present a total sum for the province. This was to be consistent with other years, where a single table presents causes of death for Indigenous and non-Indigenous peoples. Note that statistics for Indigenous peoples are incomplete at best. Includes deaths at all ages. Sources: "Deaths during the Year 1923—by Ages and Sexes for the Whole Province (Indians Excepted)" and "Death during the Year 1923, by ages and sexes, of Indians Living on Reserves," Alberta Department of Public Health, *Annual Report 1923* (Edmonton: Printed by W.D. McLean, King's Printer, 1924), 96–107 and 164–165; "Deaths during the Year 1925—by Ages and Sexes for the Whole Province (Indians Excepted)," and "Death during the Year 1925, by ages and sexes, of Indians Living on Reserves," Alberta Department of Public Health, *Annual Report 1925* (Edmonton: Printed by W.D. McLean, King's Printer, 1926), 96–109 and 142–144; "Table 9: Causes of Death by Sex and Ages—for the Whole Province," Alberta Department of Public Health, *Annual Report 1927* (Edmonton: Printed by W.D. McLean, King's Printer, 1928), 70–83; "Table 13: Causes of Death by Sex and Ages, 1929, for the Whole Province," Alberta Department of Public Health, *Annual Report 1929* (Edmonton: Printed by W.D. McLean, King's Printer, 1931), 106–119. Population source: "Table 32: Population, Birth, Marriages, Death and Rates for the years 1905 – 1970," in Alberta Department of Health, *Annual Report of the Division of Vital Statistics 1970* (Edmonton: Printed by L.S. Wall, Printer to the Queen Most Excellent Majesty, 1972), 121.

38   Classification system is not named but cause numbers match ICD-4 codes. Includes deaths at all ages. Sources: "Table 17: Causes of Death by Sex and Age, for the Whole Province, 1931," Alberta Department of Public Health, *Annual Report of the Vital Statistics Branch 1931* (Edmonton: Printed by W.D. McLean, King's Printer, 1932), 47–63; "Table 17: Causes of Death by Sex and Age, for the Whole Province, 1933," Alberta Department of Public Health, *Annual Report of the Vital Statistics Branch 1933* (Edmonton: Printed by W.D. McLean, King's Printer, 1934), 48–65; "Table 17. Causes of Death by Sex and Age for the Whole Province, 1935," Alberta Department of Public Health, *Annual Report of the Vital Statistics Branch 1935* (Edmonton: Printed by A. Shnitka King's Printer, 1936), 48–65; "Table 17. Causes of Death by Sex and Age for the Whole Province, 1937," Alberta Department of Public Health, *Annual Report of the Vital Statistics Branch 1937* (Edmonton: Printed by A. Shnitka, King's Printer, 1938), 48–65; "Table 17. Causes of Death by Sex and Age for the Whole Province, 1939," Alberta Department of Public Health, *Annual Report of the Vital Statistics Branch 1939* (Edmonton: Printed by A. Shnitka, King's Printer, 1940), 48–65. Population source: "Table 32: Population, Birth, Marriages, Death and Rates for the years 1905 – 1970," in Alberta Department of Health, *Annual Report of the Division of Vital Statistics 1970* (Edmonton: Printed by L.S. Wall, Printer to the Queen Most Excellent Majesty, 1972), 121.

39   Alberta Department of Public Health, *Annual Report 1927*; Alberta Department of Public Health, *Annual Report 1930*.

40   R. B. Jenkins, "Some Findings in the Epidemic of Poliomyelitis in Alberta, 1927," *Canadian Public Health Journal* 20, no. 5 (May 1929); A. C. McGugan, "Anterior Poliomyelitis in Alberta in 1930," *Canadian Public Health Journal* 22, no. 12 (December 1931).

41   According to Rutty et al., the 1937 outbreak included almost 4,000 reported cases of polio across the country, of which over 2,500 were in Ontario. Christopher J. Rutty, Luis Barreto, Rob Van Exan, Shawn Gilchrist, "Conquering the Crippler: Canada and the Eradication of Polio," *Canadian Journal of Public Health* 96, no. 2 (Mar–Apr 2005): I7.

42   Rutty et al., "Conquering the Crippler," I4. See also Geraldine Huynh, "University of Alberta Hospital Acute and Convalescent Polio Care and the Reintegration of Polio Patients into Albertan Communities, 1953--80," *Canadian Bulletin of Medical History* 36, no. 1 (Spring 2019).

43   Alberta Department of Public Health, *Annual Report 1938*, 13.

44   "City May Start Active Campaign to Check Cancer," *Edmonton Journal*, 28 March 1930, 17.

45   "Health Inspectors Asking Higher Pay; May Be Granted," *Edmonton Journal*, 15 October 1931, 13.

46   Malcolm R. Bow and F. Thomas Cook, "History of the Department of Public Health of Alberta," Canadian Public Health Journal 28, no. 1 (1937).

47   C. A. Baragar, M.D., Commissioner of Mental Institutions and Director of Mental Health, "Mental Health Division," in Alberta Department of Public Health, *Annual Report 1930*, 58.

48   Alberta Department of Public Health, *Annual Report 1920*. The WWI veterans had reportedly been transferred from the military hospital in Frank, Alberta, of which Dr. A.H. Baker was in charge. Baker served as medical superintendent for the new Central Alberta Sanatorium and was the inaugural director of the provincial Division of Tuberculosis Control upon its establishment in 1936. The Central Alberta Sanatorium also reportedly treated Japanese evacuees during WWII. "Baker Memorial

Sanatorium," Asylum Projects, https://www.asylumprojects.org/index.php/Baker_Memorial_
Sanatorium.

49   Alberta Department of Public Health, *Annual Report 1936*, 7–8. Hospitalization or treatment was
      provided at no charge to "persons who have been residents of the Province for twelve successive
      months out of the twenty-four months immediately preceding admission." *An Act Respecting the
      Prevention and Treatment of Tuberculosis*, S.P.A. 1936, c. 50. See also George Jasper Wherrett, *The
      Miracle of the Empty Beds: A History of Tuberculosis in Canada* (Toronto: University of Toronto Press,
      1977), 182.

50   Canadian Public Health Association "History of Tuberculosis." During the early 2000s, an important
      new concern has emerged: multidrug-resistant Mycobacterium tuberculosis. Public Health Agency
      of Canada, *The Chief Public Health Officer's Report on the State of Public Health in Canada 2013 –
      Tuberculosis – past and present*.

51   Classification system is labelled "Int. List No.," which corresponds to ICD-5 codes. Includes deaths at
      all ages. Sources: "Table 17. Causes of Death by Sex and Age for the Whole Province, 1941," Alberta
      Department of Public Health, *Annual Report 1941* (Edmonton: Printed by A. Shnitka, King's Printer,
      1942), 48–67; "Table 17. Causes of Death by Sex and Age for the Whole Province, 1943," Alberta
      Department of Public Health, *Annual Report 1943* (Edmonton: Printed by A. Shnitka, King's Printer,
      1945), 48–67; "Table 16. Causes of Death by Sex, Age and Residence for the Whole Province, 1945,"
      Alberta Department of Public Health, *Annual Report of the Vital Statistics Branch 1945* (Edmonton:
      Printed by A. Shnitka King's Printer, 1947), 33–53; "Table 17. Causes of Death by Sex and Age in
      Alberta, by Place of Residence, 1947," Alberta Department of Public Health, *Annual Report of the Vital
      Statistics Branch 1947* (Edmonton: Printed by A. Shnitka King's Printer, 1948), 35–57; "Table 17. Causes
      of Death by Sex and Age in Alberta, by Place of Residence, 1949," Alberta Department of Public Health,
      Annual Report of the Vital Statistics Branch 1949 (Edmonton: Printed by A. Shnitka King's Printer,
      1951), 35–57. Population source: "Table 32: Population, Birth, Marriages, Death and Rates for the years
      1905 – 1970," in Alberta Department of Health, *Annual Report of the Division of Vital Statistics 1970*
      (Edmonton: Printed by L.S. Wall, Printer to the Queen Most Excellent Majesty, 1972), 121.

52   "Alberta Has Lowest Death Rate," *Calgary Herald*, 9 March 1960, Alberta Legislature Library,
      Scrapbook Hansard, https://librarysearch.assembly.ab.ca/client/en_CA/search/asset/165143/0.

53   See Alberta Department of Public Health annual reports for the following years on indicated pages:
      1941: 763 cases (21), 1942: 577 cases (20), 1943: 602 cases (21), 1944: 902 cases (22), 1945: 1,039 cases
      (26), 1946: 1,479 cases (22), 1947: 1,476 cases (22), 1948: 1,903 cases (23), 1949: 1,113 cases (24), 1950:
      951 cases (24).

54   Christopher Rutty and Sue C. Sullivan, *This is Public Health: A Canadian History* (Ottawa: Canadian
      Public Health Association, 2010).

55   Alberta Department of Public Health, *Annual Report 1945*, 94; Alberta Department of Public Health,
      Annual Report *1947*, 22.

56   Classification system is the "Intermediate List" of ICD-6 (also known as List A). Includes deaths at
      all ages. Please note broken y-axis. Sources: "Table 17. Causes of Death (Intermediate List) by Sex and
      Age in Alberta, by Place of Residence, 1951," Alberta Department of Public Health, *Annual Report
      of the Vital Statistics Branch 1951* (Edmonton: Printed by A. Shnitka Queen's Printer for Alberta,
      1953), 30–38; "Table 8. Deaths by Cause and Sex, by Age, in Alberta, 1953," Alberta Department of
      Public Health, *Annual Report of the Vital Statistics Branch 1953* (Edmonton: Printed by A. Shnitka
      Queen's Printer, 1955), 30–37; "Table 8: Deaths, by Cause and Sex, by Age, Alberta 1955," Alberta
      Department of Public Health, *Annual Report of the Bureau of Vital Statistics 1955* (Edmonton: Printed
      by A. Shnitka, Queen's Printer, 1956), Part III, 22–29; "Table 8: Deaths, by Cause and Sex, by Age,
      Alberta 1957," Alberta Department of Public Health, *Annual Report 1957* (Edmonton: Printed by A.
      L.S. Wall, Queen's Printer, 1959), Part III, 21–28; "Table 8: Deaths, by Cause and Sex, by Age, Alberta
      1959," Alberta Department of Public Health, *Annual Report 1959* (Edmonton: Printed by A. L.S. Wall,
      Queen's Printer, 1961), Part III, 32–40. Population source: "Table 32: Population, Birth, Marriages,
      Death and Rates for the years 1905 – 1970," in Alberta Department of Health, *Annual Report of the
      Division of Vital Statistics 1970* (Edmonton: Printed by L.S. Wall, Printer to the Queen Most Excellent
      Majesty, 1972), 121.

57   Alberta Department of Public Health, *Annual Report 1952*, 17 (774 cases, 81 deaths); Alberta
      Department of Public Health, *Annual Report 1953*, 20 (1458 cases, 111 deaths).

58   This sentence belies a much longer and more complex history, for which the reader is directed to work
      by Rutty et al., "Conquering the Crippler."

59   Rutty et al., "Conquering the Crippler;" Albert Department of Public Health, *Annual Report 1955*.

60   Alberta Health, *Alberta Notifiable Disease Incidence*, 14.

61   "Alberta Has Lowest Death Rate," Scrapbook Hansard.

62   *An Act relating to the Treatment and Prevention of Cancer*, S.A. 1940, 49. ("The Cancer Treatment and Prevention Act").

63   Alberta Health Services, Alberta Cancer Registry, https://www.albertahealthservices.ca/cancer/Page17367.aspx

64   Alberta Department of Public Health, *Annual Report 1947*, 21 and 54–56; Alberta Department of Public Health, *Annual Report 1948*, 22 and 47–48; Alberta Department of Public Health, *Annual Report 1949*, 22 and 55–56; Alberta Department of Public Health, *Annual Report 1950*, 22 and 56–61.

65   Alberta Department of Public Health, *Annual Report 1947*, 54–6; Alberta Department of Public Health, *Annual Report 1948*, 47–8; Alberta Department of Public Health, *Annual Report 1949*, 55–6; Alberta Department of Public Health, *Annual Report 1950*, 56–61.

66   For example, during 1947 and 1948, a family dietary survey was carried out in the Foothills Health Unit (specifically, in the areas of High River, Milo and Queenstown, Royalties, and Okotoks). This survey was a collaborative effort involving the Nutrition Services division of the provincial Department of Public Health, the Foothills Health Unit nursing staff, the nutrition specialist of the provincial Department of Agriculture, and the Nutrition Division of the federal Department of National Health and Welfare. Beginning in 1947, 236 families were invited by Foothills Health Unit staff to participate in the survey, of which 122 families (450 people) agreed. August 1947 and January 1948 dietary records were completed, and for 239 of the individuals, a medical examination, including physical and dental examinations and blood tests, was done in May 1948. Survey participants received a report on recommended dietary changes, a pamphlet summarizing the findings was distributed more broadly throughout the health unit, and "vitamin capsules and other medications were made available to those requiring them." From the point of view of the provincial Department of Public Health, this was a positive experience — the 1948 annual report comments on the "splendid co-operation" by the people residing in the foothills district and the staff at the health unit. Alberta Department of Public Health, *Annual Report 1947*, 54–56; Alberta Department of Public·Health, *Annual Report 1948*, 47–48.

67   An article about life expectancy in Canada in the *Calgary Herald* in 1972 identified traffic deaths as "the biggest killer" but "also the simplest to tackle," including via seat belt use. "Canadians May Get the Life Expectancy They Deserve," *Calgary Herald*, 11 September 1972, 18.

68   Classification system is the "Intermediate List" of ICD-7 (also known as List A). Includes deaths at all ages. Please note broken y-axis. Sources: "Table 8: Deaths, by Cause and Sex, by Age, Alberta 1960," Alberta Department of Public Health, *Annual Report of the Division of Vital Statistics 1960* (Edmonton: Printed by A. L.S. Wall, Queen's Printer, 1962), 27–35; "Table 8: Deaths, by Cause and Sex, by Age, Alberta 1962," Alberta Department of Public Health, *Annual Report 1962* (Edmonton: Printed by A. L.S. Wall, Printer to the Queen's Most Excellent Majesty, 1964), Part II, 29–37; "Table 8: Deaths, by Cause and Sex, by Age, Alberta 1964," Alberta Department of Public Health, *Annual Report 1964* (Edmonton: Printed by A. L.S. Wall, Printer to the Queen's Most Excellent Majesty, 1966), Part II, 29–37; "Table 6: Deaths, by Cause and Sex, by Age, Alberta, 1966," Alberta Department of Public Health, *Annual Report 1966* (Edmonton: Printed by A. L.S. Wall, Printer to the Queen's Most Excellent Majesty, 1968), Part II, 32–49; "Table 6: Deaths by Cause and Sex, by Age, Alberta, 1968," Alberta Department of Health, *Annual Report 1968* (Edmonton: Printed by A. L.S. Wall, Printer to the Queen's Most Excellent Majesty, 1970), Part II, 41–45. Population source: "Table 32: Population, Birth, Marriages, Death and Rates for the years 1905 – 1970," in Alberta Department of Health, *Annual Report of the Division of Vital Statistics 1970* (Edmonton: Printed by L.S. Wall, Printer to the Queen Most Excellent Majesty, 1972), 121.

69   Classification system is the "Intermediate List A" of ICD-8 (also known as List A). Data from 1971 and 1973 was extracted from the list of causes of death for each province contained in the *Vital Statistics Annual publication, Volume II, Deaths* by Statistics Canada (Alberta Vital Statistics reports for those years are not available). Includes deaths at all ages for residents and non-residents. Please note broken y-axis. Sources: "Table 6: Deaths by Cause and Sex, by Age, Alberta, 1969," Alberta Department of Health, *Annual Report 1969* (Edmonton: Printed by A. L.S. Wall, Printer to the Queen's Most Excellent Majesty, 1971), Part II, 45–54; "Table 21. Deaths and Rates by Cause and Sex, Canada and Provinces, 1971," Statistics Canada, *Vital Statistics: Volume III - Deaths 1971* (Ottawa: The Minister of Industry, Trade and Commerce, 1974), 132–151; "Table 21. Deaths and Rates (per 100,000 population) by Cause and Sex, Canada and Provinces, 1973," Statistics Canada, *Vital Statistics: Volume III – Deaths 1973* (Ottawa: The Minister of Industry, Trade and Commerce, 1975), 132–151; "Table 11b: Deaths Occurring in Alberta, Cause by Sex, 1975," Alberta Social Services and Community Heath, *Vital Statistics Annual Review 1975 and 1976* (Edmonton: 1978), 37–47; "Table 11b: Deaths Occurring in Alberta, Cause by Sex, 1977," Alberta Social Services and Community Heath, *Vital Statistics Annual Review 1977* (Edmonton: 1978), 36–46. Population sources: "Table 32: Population, Birth, Marriages, Death and Rates for the years 1905 – 1970," in Alberta Department of Health, *Annual Report of the Division of Vital Statistics 1970* (Edmonton: Printed by L.S. Wall, Printer to the Queen Most

Excellent Majesty, 1972), 121; Alberta, Social Services and Community Health, *Annual Report 1971–72* (Edmonton, 1972), 33; Alberta, Social Services and Community Health, *Annual Report 1973–74* (Edmonton, 1974), 16; and Alberta, Social Services and Community Health, *Annual Report 1975–76* (Edmonton, 1977), 37.

70 "District Personals, Morinville" *Edmonton Journal*, 4 December 1954, 37. The Farm Women's Union of Alberta began in 1915–16 as the United Farm Women of Alberta, which was the first provincial organization of farm women in Alberta. They became the Farm Women's Union of Alberta in 1949 (Nanci Langford, "United Farm Women of Alberta," in *The Canadian Encyclopedia. Historica Canada*, last edited 16 December 2013, https://www.thecanadianencyclopedia.ca/en/article/united-farm-women-of-alberta). Farm women in Alberta continued to be supportive of seat belts; for example, at the sixth annual Western Canada Farm Safety Conference, it was reported that "The women have . . . been active in selling seat belts for cars." "Women Contribute to Farm Safety," *Edmonton Journal*, 13 February 1963, 17).

71 For example, at a 1962 meeting, the National Council of Women announced that they would work with the Canadian Highway Safety Conference to sponsor a campaign focused on the installation and use of seat belts in vehicles ("Bilingualism, immigration on Council agenda," *Edmonton Journal*, 7 February 1962, 21; "Women Promote Seat Belt Use," *Edmonton Journal*, 3 May 1962, 19); also that year, District Two of the Alberta Women's Institute announced their upcoming conference which would feature a talk on seat belts by William J. Perkins of the Alberta Safety Council ("WI District Two to Confer Here," *Edmonton Journal*, 10 March 1962, 20). The intersection of women and seat belts revealed strong gender stereotypes of the time; for example, an *Edmonton Journal* article from 10 January 1962 featured Nell Siemens, "a bit of a traffic stopper herself," who had launched a country-wide campaign to make Canadian women more conscious of traffic safety "through the women, she hopes to make more careful drivers out of Canada's men . . . [and to] get their husbands and children to take safety precautions, such as wearing safety belts . . . but 'they shouldn't nag.'" ("Rules for Safety in Traffic World," *Edmonton Journal*, 10 January 1962, 26). Furthermore, the co-ordinator of women's activities with the Alberta Safety Council, Mrs. L.R. Betts of Edmonton, asserted that "the woman's hand in traffic safety" is to teach safety to her children ("Women Steer Safety Drive," *Edmonton Journal*, 9 May 1962, 17).

72 The Alberta Safety Council is a non-government, not-for-profit organization that was established in approximately the early 1950s and remains active at the time of writing (https://www.safetycouncil.ab.ca/). In its early years the organization was primarily focused on farm and rural safety, but grew to encompass transportation and children's safety by the 1960s, and workplace health and safety in the 1970s.

73 "Use of Seat Belts in Autos Topic at Safety Convention," *Edmonton Journal*, 27 October 1955, 13; "Plan Inventory Traffic Mishaps," *Edmonton Journal*, 1 November 1956, 6.

74 For example, in 1954, the Ontario Medical Association recommended that safety belts be made compulsory equipment in automobiles. "Doctors Recommend Car Safety Belts," *Edmonton Journal*, 27 August 1954, 26.

75 For example, "20 Cars Enter Stock Car Races," *Edmonton Journal*, 14 May 1953, 19.

76 "Belt for 'Suicide Seat,'" *Edmonton Journal*, 9 February 1954, 4.

77 "Plan Safety Belts for Automobiles," *Edmonton Journal*, 26 April 1955, 23.

78 For example, in 1960 the Canadian Medical Association recommended installation and use of seat belts by all car occupants ("Doctors Caution Ambulance Drivers," *Edmonton Journal*, 15 June 1960, 74); and throughout the 1960s Alberta physicians spoke up in favour of seatbelts, often based on their experiences with accident victims in hospital ("Automobile Safety Campaign Gains City Police Approval," *Edmonton Journal*, 11 September 1964, 1 [Dr. F.M. Christie, Lethbridge]; "No Seat Belt No Sympathy," *Edmonton Journal*, 11 June 1965, 60 [Dr. M.T. Carpendale, Edmonton]; and "Quiet Ones Concern Doctors Most When Injured are Brought to Emergency Ward," *Edmonton Journal*, 22 August 1968, 29.

79 "CSA Preparing Basis for Car Safety Belts," *Edmonton Journal*, 25 May 1962, 26; "Standards Set," *Edmonton Journal*, 9 October 1962, 9. "Auto Seat Belts Standards Met," *Edmonton Journal*, 14 December 1962, 23.

80 The safety standards could be those of the Canadian Standards Association or the U.S. Society of Automotive Engineers. "Cabinet Would Set New Speed Limits," *Edmonton Journal*, 20 March 1963, 3; "Seat Belts Will Need Approval," *Edmonton Journal*, 26 June 1963, 38.

81 "New York Cars Must Have Seat Belts," *Edmonton Journal*, 28 April 1962, 55; "BC Enacts Seat Belts for '64," *Edmonton Journal*, 7 March 1963, 2; "Safety Belts Made a Must," (New Zealand), *Edmonton Journal*, 14 September 1964, 20. In 1965, New York became the first U.S. State to require safety belts in

the rear as well as in the front seats of passenger vehicles ("World Notes," *Edmonton Journal*, 21 July 1965, 6).

82   "Seat Belts Predicted in All Cars," *Edmonton Journal*, 8 February 1962, 21; see also "No Seat Belts in this Car," *Edmonton Journal*, 15 January 1964, 1.

83   "Seat Belts Predicted in All Cars," *Edmonton Journal*.

84   "3 Firms to Include Seat Belts," *Edmonton Journal*, 28 January 1964, 23.

85   "Motorists Ignoring Shoulder Harnesses," *Edmonton Journal*, 25 June 1968, 3.

86   "No Law for Seat Belt Use," *Edmonton Journal*, 1 March 1966, 22; "Seat Belt Use May Be Enforced," *Edmonton Journal*, 30 March 1968, 1. Alongside seatbelt discussions was growing attention to drinking and driving, as illustrated by the creation of a Division of Alcoholism in the provincial Department of Public Health in 1965 with the major aim "to prevent alcoholism by means of treatment, education and research" ("Division of Alcoholism," in Alberta Department of Public Health, *Annual Report 1965*, 122–126) and a new 1966 law stipulating that the license of a driver who refused to take a breath test would be subject to suspension. ("Canada Looks at Auto Safety," *Edmonton Journal*, 17 June 1966, 14).

87   The Alberta Motor Association was also involved in efforts to promote seat belt use and road safety; one example was their "Bring 'em back alive" (BEBA) campaign, which involve broad publicizing of the BEBA campaign (e.g., car decals, highway overpass signs, schools, roadside restaurants) during holiday long weekends ("Province-wide Safety Drive will 'Bring 'em Back Alive," *Edmonton Journal*, 8 May 1968, 60; "Drivers Get Message – Bring 'em Back Alive", *Calgary Herald*, 1 May 1969, 32).

88   "Seat Belts can Cut Deaths in Alberta by Third — if Used," *Edmonton Journal*, 6 May 1963, 47.

89   For example, "Plan Inventory Traffic Mishaps," *Edmonton Journal*, 1 November 1956, 6; "126 Die on Roads; Death Toll up 24%," *Edmonton Journal*, 27 July 1960, 3; "Safety Official Urges Use of Seat Belts," *Edmonton Journal*, 1 February 1962, 22; "Road Death Figures are Growing Worry," *Edmonton Journal*, 23 June 1964, 8; "No Law for Seat Belt Use," *Edmonton Journal*, 1 March 1966, 22; "Photograph Urged on Driving License," *Calgary Herald*, 9 June 1969, 30.

90   For example, at the 1972 Ontario Traffic Conference, representatives from the auto industry, police, and teaching, legal and medical professions reportedly agreed that the wearing of seat belts in autos should be made compulsory. "Mandatory Seat Belt Use Proposed at OTC," *Calgary Herald*, 16 May 1972, 6. "Buckle up or Else," *Calgary Herald*, 15 July 1971, 6; "In the Driver's Seat," *Calgary Herald*, 24 September 1971, 71. "Mandatory Use of Seat Belts Cuts Australia Deaths," *Calgary Herald*, 30 May 1972, 6. "Australia Requires Use of Seat Belts," *Calgary Herald*, 28 February 1972, 20.

91   Provincial Minister of Health and Social Development, Neil Crawford (PC), attended the provincial health ministers' meeting in February of 1974, where federal minister Marc Lalonde urged provincial governments to consider compulsory seatbelt legislation. When questioned about this in the Alberta Legislature, Mr. Crawford responded, "as desirable as that proposal was . . . my feeling was that it would be an extremely difficult matter to enforce" Alberta. Legislative Assembly of Alberta, 18 March 1974 (Neil Crawford, PC) (Alberta Hansard transcripts are available at https://www.assembly.ab.ca/assembly-business/transcripts/transcripts-by-type). See also: The Honourable Marc Lalonde, "Beyond a New Perspective," Fourth annual Matthew B. Rosenhaus Lecture, 104th Annual Meeting of the American Public Health Association, 18 October 1976, Miami Beach, Florida, in *American Journal of Public Health* 67, no. 4 (April 1977).

92   Ontario and Quebec passed compulsory seat belt legislation in 1976, followed by Saskatchewan and British Columbia in 1977.

93   Alberta. Legislative Assembly of Alberta, 2 May 1974 (George Ho Lem, SC).

94   Alberta. Legislative Assembly of Alberta, 29 January 1975 (George Ho Lem, SC).

95   Alberta. Legislative Assembly of Alberta, 13 February 1975 (George Ho Lem, SC).

96   For example, provinces of Ontario, Saskatchewan, and British Columbia implemented mandatory seat belt legislation in 1976, 1977, and 1977 respectively, with Newfoundland and Labrador (1982), New Brunswick (1983), Nova Scotia (1984), and Manitoba (1984) following in the early 1980s. Canadian Council of Motor Transport Administrators (CCMTA), *CCMTA Road Safety Report Series: National Occupant Restraint Program 2010 - Annual Monitoring Report 2009*, prepared for the Canadian Council of Motor Transport Administrators Standing Committee on Road Safety Research and Policies (Ottawa: CCMTA, 2010), http://ccmta.ca/images/publications/pdf/norp_report09.pdf

97   It is interesting and important, from the point of view of public health more broadly, to note the similarities between the points of opposition to compulsory seat belt legislation, and the points of opposition to other public health interventions, such as community water fluoridation (see Chapter 9: *Mobilizing Preventive Policy*).

98   Alberta Cancer Board, Taking Stock.

99   For example: Caroline Schooler, John W. Farquhar, Stephen P. Fortmann, and June A. Flora, "Synthesis of Findings and Issues from Community Prevention Trials," *Annals of Epidemiology* 7, no. 7 (1997); S. Leonard Syme, "Social Determinants of Health: the Community as an Empowered Partner," *Preventing Chronic Disease* 1, no. 1 (2004):A02 (epub); Louise Potvin and David McQueen (editors), *Health Promotion Evaluation Practices in the Americas: Values and Research* (New York: Springer, 2008).

100 The community members were invited from, for example, health care agencies, educational institutions, service clubs, voluntary agencies, media, and civic governments. Judy M. Birdsell, H. Sharon Campbell, S. Elizabeth McGregor, Gerry B. Hill, "Steve Fonyo Cancer Prevention Program: Description of an Innovative Program," *Canadian Journal of Public Health* 83, no. 3 (May/June 1992).

101 Classification system is reported to be ICD-9 ("ICD-9 282 Selected Causes of Death"); however, the numbers do not match ICD-9 codes. Includes deaths at all ages for residents and non-residents. Sources: "Table 11: Deaths, Cause by Sex and Age, 1985," Alberta Community and Occupational Health, *Vital Statistics Annual Review 1985* (Edmonton: 1986), 18–49; "Table 11: Deaths, Cause by Sex and Age, 1987," Alberta Community and Occupational Health, *Vital Statistics Annual Review 1987* (Edmonton: 1988), 25–55; "Table 11: Deaths, Cause by Sex and Age, 1989," Alberta Health, *Vital Statistics Annual Review 1989* (Edmonton: 1990), 28–50; "Table 11: Cause of Death by Age and Sex, 1991," Alberta Health, *Vital Statistics Annual Review 1991* (Edmonton: 1992), 22–44; "Table 11: Deaths, Cause by Gender and Age, 1993," Alberta Municipal Affairs, *Vital Statistics Annual Report 1993* (Edmonton: 1994), 20–46; "Table 11: Deaths, Cause by Gender and Age, 1995," Alberta Municipal Affairs, *Vital Statistics Annual Review 1995* (Edmonton: 1996), 18–40; "Table 11: Deaths, Cause by Gender and Age, 1997," Alberta Municipal Affairs, *Vital Statistics Annual Review 1997* (Edmonton: 1998), 18–40; "Table 11: Deaths, Cause by Gender and Age, 1999," Alberta Government Services, *Vital Statistics Annual Review 1999* (Edmonton: 2000), 18–40. Population source: Respective Vital Statistics Annual Report for each corresponding year.

102 Classification system is reported to be ICD-10: "Causes of death are bases [sic] on the International Classification of Diseases 10th Edition" and uses 358 Selected Causes of Death; however, the numbers do not match ICD-10 codes. Sources: "Table 15: Deaths, Cause by Gender and Age, 2001," Alberta Government Services, *Alberta Vital Statistics Annual Review 2001* (Edmonton: 2002), 25–54; "Table 15: Deaths, Cause by Gender and Age, 2003," Alberta Government Services, *Alberta Vital Statistics Annual Review 2003* (Edmonton: 2004), 25–54; "Table 18: Deaths, Cause by Gender and Age, 2005," Alberta Government Services, *Alberta Vital Statistics Annual Review 2005* (Edmonton: 2006), 28–57; "Table 18: Deaths, Cause by Gender and Age, 2007," Service Alberta, *Alberta Vital Statistics Annual Review 2007* (Edmonton: 2008), 28–57; "Table 20: Deaths, Cause by Gender and Age, 2009," Service Alberta, *Alberta Vital Statistics Annual Review 2009* (Edmonton: 2010), 30–59; "Table 20: Deaths, Cause by Gender and Age, 2011," Service Alberta, *Alberta Vital Statistics Annual Review 2011* (Edmonton: 2012), 30–59; "Table 20: Deaths, Cause by Gender and Age, 2013," Alberta Government, Service Alberta, *Alberta Vital Statistics Annual Review 2013* (Edmonton: 2014), 36–61; "Top 10 Leading Causes of Death in Alberta in 2015," Service Alberta, *Alberta Vital Statistics: Annual Review 2015* (Edmonton: 2017), 15. Population source: Statistics Canada "Population estimates on July 1st, by age and sex" Frequency: Annual Table: 17-10-0005-01 (formerly CANSIM 051-0001).

103 Alberta Department of Social Services and Community Health, *Annual Report 1979–80*, 28; Alberta Department of Social Services and Community Health, *Annual Report 1980–81* (Edmonton: 1984), 28. For Alberta Department of Social Services and Community Health Reports (1974/75-1984/85), no printer information is listed.

104 In addition to the clinics in Calgary, Edmonton, and Lethbridge, a mobile clinic permitted contact tracing and treatment across the province (Alberta Department of Social Services and Community Health, Annual Report, 1977–78 (Edmonton: 1979), 14; Alberta Department of Social Services and Community Health, *Annual Report 1979–80*, 28), and a clinic in Fort McMurray provided the same diagnostic and treatment services under the auspices of the Fort McMurray Health Unit (Alberta Department of Social Services and Community Health, *Annual Report 1980–81*, 28).

105 See the Alberta Department of Health and Social Development and Department of Social Services and Community Health Annual reports, 1973–74 to 1985–86; "VD Increasing, Grade 8 Told," *Calgary Herald*, 19 March 1975, 26.

106 Alberta Department of Social Services and Community Health, *Annual Report 1983–84* (Edmonton: 1984), 8; Alberta Department of Social Services and Community Health, Annual Report, 1985–86 (Edmonton, 1986), 10.

107 Alberta Health, *Alberta Notifiable Disease Incidence*.

108 Alberta. Legislative Assembly of Alberta, 26 March 1980 (Dennis Anderson, PC).

109   Alberta. Legislative Assembly of Alberta, 15 May 1980 (Dennis Anderson, PC). Discussion timed out, and the Bill was "left to die on the Order Paper" as described in: Alberta. Legislative Assembly of Alberta, 1 May 1984 (Janet Koper, PC), 609.

110   We say "frustratingly" because, as stated by Mr. Anderson who introduced the bill, seat belts are beneficial for all ages, yet the concession was made to address concerns about undue coercion of adults. Alberta: Legislative Assembly of Alberta, 15 May 1980 (Dennis Anderson, PC).

111   For example, questions to the minister of transportation as to why there has been no action on seat belts (Alberta. Legislative Assembly of Alberta, 27 April 1981 (John S. Batiuk, PC; Henry Kroeger, PC); Alberta. Legislative Assembly of Alberta, 19 May 1981 (R. Speaker, SC; Henry Kroeger, PC); and as one small part of broader Motion 202: that the Assembly urge the government, through the Department of Transportation, to initiate a multimedia campaign to increase public awareness regarding traffic safety, which also timed out: Alberta. Legislative Assemby of Alberta, 16 March 1982; 23 March 1982; and 1 April 1982.

112   For example, Bill 28 *Appropriation (Interim Supply) Act* of 1983. Alberta. Legislative Assembly of Alberta, 25 March 1983, first reading; 28 March 1983, second reading; 29 March 1983, Committee of the Whole; and 30 March 1983, third reading – when Mr. Notley attempted but failed to intervene.

113   Alberta. Legislative Assembly of Alberta, 30 March 1983.

114   Alberta. Legislative Assembly of Alberta, 30 March 1983.

115   Alberta. Legislative Assembly of Alberta, 24 November 1983 (Janet Koper, PC).

116   Alberta. Legislative Assembly of Alberta, 26 October 1984 (Marvin Moore, PC), Bill 83 first reading.

117   Alberta. Legislative Assembly of Alberta, 2 November 1984, Bill 83 second reading.

118   For example, Mr. Martin expressed that "I am a little disappointed that the government hasn't screwed up its political courage" and Mr. Anderson commented "Of course . . . I would have preferred that we would have gone to legislation for those under 18. Alberta. Legislative Assembly of Alberta, 2 November 1984.

119   Alberta. Legislative Assembly of Alberta, 13 November 1984, Bill 83, third reading [passed].

120   Alberta. Legislative Assembly of Alberta, 12 August 1986.

121   Alberta. Legislative Assembly of Alberta, 5 March 1987.

122   Alberta. Legislative Assembly of Alberta, 20 March 1987; 25 March 1987.

123   Bill 9 *Highway Traffic Amendment Act*, 1987: Alberta. Legislative Assembly of Alberta, 12 March 1987, first reading; 13 April 1987, second reading; 9 June 1987, Committee of the Whole; 10 June 1987, third reading.

124   For example, you don't need a seatbelt if you are driving in reverse, John Zazula "June 22, 1987: Albertans Prepare for Seatbelt Law," *CBC Edmonton*, last updated: 23 June 2016, https://www.cbc.ca/news/canada/edmonton/june-22-1987-albertans-prepare-for-seatbelt-law-1.3649730

125   See, for example, David L. Ryan and Guy A. Bridgeman "Judging the Roles of Legislation, Education and Offsetting Behaviour in Seat Belt Use: a Survey and New Evidence from Alberta," *Canadian Public Policy* 18, no. 1 (March 1992). See also Alberta. Legislative Assembly of Alberta, 3 May 1990.

126   Alberta. Legislative Assembly of Alberta, 9 December 1987 (Stanley Schumacher, PC).

127   Alberta. Legislative Assembly of Alberta, 2 May 1991 (Kenneth Kowalski, PC).

128   Rutty and Sullivan, *This is Public Health*.

4

Public Health Governance: A Journey of Expansion and Tension

Lindsay McLaren, Rogelio Velez Mendoza, and Donald W.M. Juzwishin

Introduction

Public health, by definition, involves multiple societal sectors and the tensions between them; these include the public sector (government), the private sector, and civil society. Although all are important, public health's reliance on "the organized efforts of society" to promote and protect the health of the population means that the public sector has always been prominent.[1] In this chapter, we consider legislative and institutional dimensions of Alberta's public health governance throughout the province's history. Specifically, this chapter focuses on settler-colonial public health administration. The federal structure that has provided some colonial public health services for First Nation and Inuit communities — and how those communities have revamped it to their benefit — is considered in Chapter 7.

There are at least two reasons why a historical study of public health governance is of value. First, law provides, at least in theory, a powerful mechanism for action. But that mechanism is not necessarily straightforward and cannot be assumed to be positive, thus shedding light on important nuances of public health. For instance, as outlined in Alberta's current provincial Public Health Act, when a communicable disease has been confirmed, a medical officer of health is authorized to "take whatever steps [they] consider necessary" to protect public health.[2] As seen clearly during the COVID-19 pandemic, these legal authorities and the politics that surround them can contribute to key tensions and contested dialogue around lines of authority.[3] A second reason why the historical study of public health governance is useful is that legislative and institutional dimensions contribute to shaping the contours of public health by providing parameters around its scope. The broad vision of public health embraced in this volume requires collaboration across sectors and departments (e.g., those focused on housing, social services, environment, labour, social services, education, finance, etc., as well as health care), which governance arrangements, such as where public health is administratively situated and mechanisms for coordination with other departments or sectors, may facilitate or impede.

The objective of this chapter is to chart key legislative and institutional aspects of public health governance in Alberta, in a way that illustrates how these dimensions contribute to shaping its scope and boundaries over time. Our chapter narrative is built around two key pieces of information: the administrative structure of the provincial department responsible for public health, and the provincial Public Health Act. Although there are many pieces of legislation at multiple levels of government that are pertinent to public health, Alberta's *Public Health Act* is central and has existed for nearly as long as the province itself, thus providing a consistent source of information to consider change over time. Key sources include: 1) *An Administrative History of the Government of Alberta, 1905–2005*, which is a historical compilation of Alberta public administration created by the Provincial Archives of Alberta; 2) the legislation itself, that is, the various iterations of Alberta's Public Health Act and amendments; 3) the annual reports of the provincial Department of Public Health and other departments historically responsible for public health in Alberta; 4) provincial task force reports and commissions; and finally, 5) discussion and debates within the legislature, as recorded in the *Alberta Hansard* and Scrapbook Hansard.[4]

Setting the Stage: The Broad Context of Alberta's Public Health Governance History

To organize this chapter, we have divided it into six chronological sections corresponding to what we considered to be meaningful periods or eras of Alberta's public health governance history. As a backdrop for those sections, we provide several tables and figures. First, Table 4.1 presents a chronological overview of formal public health governance in Alberta, including the provincial department or ministry responsible for public health, along with the minister, deputy minister, and provincial medical officer of health.

TABLE 4.1: Government of Alberta: Departments responsible for public health and the provincial minister, deputy minister, and provincial medical officer of health (or similar position), 1905–present.

Year	Department	Minister	Deputy Minister	Provincial MOH (or similar)
1905	Agriculture	William Findlay (Liberal)	George Harcourt	*N/A*
1906	Agriculture	William Findlay (Liberal)	George Harcourt	Dr. A.E. Clendennan
1907	Agriculture	William Findlay (Liberal)	George Harcourt	L.E.W. Irving
1908	Agriculture	William Findlay (Liberal)	George Harcourt	L.E.W. Irving
1909	Agriculture	William Findlay (Liberal) Duncan Marshall (Liberal)	George Harcourt	L.E.W. Irving
1910	Agriculture	Duncan Marshall (Liberal)	George Harcourt	L.E.W. Irving
1911	Agriculture	Duncan Marshall (Liberal)	George Harcourt	L.E.W. Irving
1912	Agriculture	Duncan Marshall (Liberal)	George Harcourt	Dr. W.C. Laidlaw
1913	Agriculture	Duncan Marshall (Liberal)	George Harcourt	Dr. W.C. Laidlaw
1914	Agriculture	Duncan Marshall (Liberal)	George Harcourt	Dr. T.J. Norman, pro tem.
1915	Agriculture	Duncan Marshall (Liberal)	George Harcourt, Horace A. Craig	Dr. T.J. Norman, pro tem.
1916	Agriculture	Duncan Marshall (Liberal)	Horace A. Craig	Dr. T.J. Norman, pro tem.
1917	Agriculture	Duncan Marshall (Liberal) George Peter Smith (Liberal)	Horace A. Craig	Dr. T.J. Norman
1918	Provincial Secretary (Jan – July)	George Peter Smith (Liberal)	Edmund Trowbridge	Dr. T.J. Norman
	Municipal Affairs (Aug – Dec)	Wilfrid Gariépy (Liberal)	John Perrie	
1919	Municipal Affairs (Jan – March)	Alexander G. MacKay (Liberal)	Judson H. Lamb	Dr. W.C. Laidlaw
	Public Health (April -)	Alexander G. MacKay (Liberal)	John Perrie, Dr. Telfer Joshua (T.J.) Norman	
1920	Public Health	Alexander G. MacKay (Liberal) Charles R. Mitchell (Liberal)	Dr. T.J. Norman	Dr. W.C. Laidlaw

TABLE 4.1: *(continued)*

Year	Department	Minister	Deputy Minister	Provincial MOH (or similar)
1921	Public Health	Charles R. Mitchell (Liberal)	Dr. W.C. Laidlaw	Dr. W.C. Laidlaw
		Richard G. Reid (UFA)		
1922	Public Health	Richard G. Reid (UFA)	Dr. W.C. Laidlaw	Dr. W.C. Laidlaw
1923	Public Health	Richard G. Reid (UFA)	Dr. W.C. Laidlaw	Dr. W.C. Laidlaw
		George Hoadley (UFA)		
1924	Public Health	George Hoadley (UFA)	Dr. W.C. Laidlaw	Dr. W.C. Laidlaw
1925	Public Health	George Hoadley (UFA)	Dr. W.C. Laidlaw	Dr. W.C. Laidlaw
1926	Public Health	George Hoadley (UFA)	Dr. W.C. Laidlaw	Dr. R.B. Jenkins
			R.B. Owens (Acting)	
1927	Public Health	George Hoadley (UFA)	Dr. Malcolm Ross Bow	Dr. R.B. Jenkins
1928	Public Health	George Hoadley (UFA)	Dr. Malcolm Ross Bow	Dr. R.B. Jenkins
1929	Public Health	George Hoadley (UFA)	Dr. Malcolm Ross Bow	Dr. A.C. McGugan
1930	Public Health	George Hoadley (UFA)	Dr. Malcolm Ross Bow	Dr. A.C. McGugan or Dr. M.R. Bow[1]
1931	Public Health	George Hoadley (UFA)	Dr. Malcolm Ross Bow	Dr. A.C. McGugan or Dr. M.R. Bow
1932	Public Health	George Hoadley (UFA)	Dr. Malcolm Ross Bow	Dr. A.C. McGugan or Dr. M.R. Bow
1933	Public Health	George Hoadley (UFA)	Dr. Malcolm Ross Bow	Dr. A.C. McGugan or Dr. M.R. Bow
1934	Public Health	George Hoadley (UFA)	Dr. Malcolm Ross Bow	Dr. A.C. McGugan or Dr. M.R. Bow
1935	Public Health	George Hoadley (UFA)	Dr. Malcolm Ross Bow	Dr. A.C. McGugan or Dr. M.R. Bow
		Wallace W. Cross (SC)		
1936	Public Health	Wallace W. Cross (SC)	Dr. Malcolm Ross Bow	Dr. A.C. McGugan or Dr. M.R. Bow
1937	Public Health	Wallace W. Cross (SC)	Dr. Malcolm Ross Bow	Dr. A.C. McGugan or Dr. M.R. Bow
1938	Public Health	Wallace W. Cross (SC)	Dr. Malcolm Ross Bow	Dr. A.C. McGugan or Dr. M.R. Bow
1939	Public Health	Wallace W. Cross (SC)	Dr. Malcolm Ross Bow	Dr. A.C. McGugan or Dr. M.R. Bow
1940	Public Health	Wallace W. Cross (SC)	Dr. Malcolm Ross Bow	Dr. A.C. McGugan or Dr. M.R. Bow
1941	Public Health	Wallace W. Cross (SC)	Dr. Malcolm Ross Bow	Dr. A.C. McGugan or Dr. M.R. Bow

Year	Department	Minister	Deputy Minister	Provincial MOH (or similar)
1942	Public Health	Wallace W. Cross (SC)	Dr. Malcolm Ross Bow	Dr. A.C. McGugan or Dr. M.R. Bow
1943	Public Health	Wallace W. Cross (SC)	Dr. Malcolm Ross Bow	Dr. A.C. McGugan or Dr. M.R. Bow
1944	Public Health	Wallace W. Cross (SC)	Dr. Malcolm Ross Bow	Dr. A.C. McGugan or Dr. M.R. Bow
1945	Public Health	Wallace W. Cross (SC)	Dr. Malcolm Ross Bow	Dr. A.C. McGugan or Dr. M.R. Bow
1946	Public Health	Wallace W. Cross (SC)	Dr. Malcolm Ross Bow	Dr. A.C. McGugan or Dr. M.R. Bow
1947	Public Health	Wallace W. Cross (SC)	Dr. Malcolm Ross Bow	Dr. A.C. McGugan or Dr. M.R. Bow
1948	Public Health	Wallace W. Cross (SC)	Dr. Malcolm Ross Bow	Dr. A.C. McGugan or Dr. M.R. Bow
1949	Public Health	Wallace W. Cross (SC)	Dr. Malcolm Ross Bow	Dr. A.C. McGugan or Dr. M.R. Bow
1950	Public Health	Wallace W. Cross (SC)	Dr. Malcolm Ross Bow	Dr. A.C. McGugan or Dr. M.R. Bow
1951	Public Health	Wallace W. Cross (SC)	Dr. Malcolm Ross Bow	Dr. A.C. McGugan or Dr. M.R. Bow
1952	Public Health	Wallace W. Cross (SC)	Dr. Malcolm Ross Bow Dr. Ashbury Somerville (Acting)	Dr. A.C. McGugan or Dr. M.R. Bow
1953	Public Health	Wallace W. Cross (SC)	Dr. Ashbury Somerville	Dr. Ashbury Somerville
1954	Public Health	Wallace W. Cross (SC)	Dr. Ashbury Somerville	Dr. Ashbury Somerville[2]
1955	Public Health	Wallace W. Cross (SC)	Dr. Ashbury Somerville	Dr. Ashbury Somerville[3]
1956	Public Health	Wallace W. Cross (SC)	Dr. Ashbury Somerville	Dr. Ashbury Somerville[4]
1957	Public Health	Wallace W. Cross (SC) Joseph D. Ross (SC)	Dr. Ashbury Somerville	Dr. Ashbury Somerville[5]
1958	Public Health	Joseph D. Ross (SC)	Dr. Ashbury Somerville	Dr. Ashbury Somerville[6]
1959	Public Health	Joseph D. Ross (SC)	Dr. Ashbury Somerville	Dr. Ashbury Somerville[7]
1960	Public Health	Joseph D. Ross (SC)	Dr. Ashbury Somerville	Dr. Ashbury Somerville[8]

Year	Department	Minister	Deputy Minister	Provincial MOH (or similar)
1961	Public Health	Joseph D. Ross (SC)	Dr. Ashbury Somerville Dr. Malcolm G. McCallum	Dr. Ashbury Somerville[9]
1962	Public Health	Joseph D. Ross (SC)	Dr. Malcolm G. McCallum	Dr. Malcolm G. McCallum[10]
1963	Public Health	Joseph D. Ross (SC)	Dr. Malcolm G. McCallum	Dr. Malcolm G. McCallum[11]
1964	Public Health	Joseph D. Ross (SC)	Dr. Malcolm G. McCallum	Dr. Malcolm G. McCallum[12]
1965	Public Health	Joseph D. Ross (SC)	Dr. Malcolm G. McCallum	Dr. Malcolm G. McCallum
1966	Public Health	Joseph D. Ross (SC)	Dr. Malcolm G. McCallum	Dr. Malcolm G. McCallum
1967	Public Health	Joseph D. Ross (SC)	Dr. Malcolm G. McCallum	Dr. Malcolm G. McCallum
	Health		Dr. Patrick Blair Rose	Dr. Patrick Blair Rose
1968	Health	Joseph D. Ross (SC)	Dr. Patrick Blair Rose	Dr. Patrick Blair Rose
1969	Health	Joseph D. Ross (SC) James Henderson (SC)	Dr. Patrick Blair Rose	Dr. Patrick Blair Rose
1970	Health	James Henderson (SC)	Dr. Patrick Blair Rose	Dr. Patrick Blair Rose
1971	Health	James Henderson (SC)	Dr. Patrick Blair Rose	N/A[13]
	Health & Social Development	Neil Crawford (PC)	Bruce Strathearn Rawson	
1972	Health & Social Development	Neil Crawford (PC)	Bruce Strathearn Rawson	N/A
1973	Health & Social Development	Neil Crawford (PC)	Bruce Strathearn Rawson	N/A
1974	Health & Social Development	Neil Crawford (PC)	Bruce Strathearn Rawson	N/A
1975	Health & Social Development	Neil Crawford (PC)	Bruce Strathearn Rawson	N/A
	Social Services & Community Health	Helen Hunley (PC)	Bruce Strathearn Rawson, Stanley H. Mansbridge[14] Dr. Jean Nelson[15]	

Year	Department	Minister	Deputy Minister	Provincial MOH (or similar)
1976	Social Services & Community Health	Helen Hunley (PC)	Stanley H. Mansbridge, Dr. Jean Nelson[16]	N/A
1977	Social Services & Community Health	Helen Hunley (PC)	Stanley H. Mansbridge Dr. Jean Nelson	N/A
1978	Social Services & Community Health	Helen Hunley (PC)	Stanley H. Mansbridge Dr. Jean Nelson	N/A
1979	Social Services & Community Health	Helen Hunley (PC) Robert Bogle (PC)	Stanley H. Mansbridge, David M. Stolee (Acting)[17] Sheila Durkin[18]	N/A
1980	Social Services & Community Health	Robert Bogle (PC)	Stanley H. Mansbridge,[19] David M. Stolee (Acting) Sheila Durkin[20]	Dr. John Waters[21]
1981	Social Services & Community Health	Robert Bogle (PC)	Stanley H. Mansbridge[22] David M. Stolee (Acting)[23] Sheila Durkin[24]	Dr. John Waters
1982	Social Services & Community Health	Robert Bogle (PC) Neil Webber (PC)	Sheila Durkin[25]	Dr. John Waters
1983	Social Services & Community Health	Neil Webber (PC)	Sheila Durkin[26]	Dr. John Waters
1984	Social Services & Community Health	Neil Webber (PC)	Sheila Durkin[27] David S. Kelly (Acting)[28]	Dr. John Waters
1985	Social Services & Community Health	Neil Webber (PC) Connie Ostermann (PC)	Robert R. Orford[29]	Dr. John Waters
1986	Social Services & Community Health	Connie Ostermann (PC)	Robert R. Orford[30]	Dr. John Waters
	Community & Occupational Health	Bill Diachuk (PC) Jim Dinning (PC)		

TABLE 4.1: (*continued*)

Year	Department	Minister	Deputy Minister	Provincial MOH (or similar)
1987	Community & Occupational Health	Jim Dinning (PC)	Robert R. Orford	Dr. John Waters
1988	Community & Occupational Health	Jim Dinning (PC)	Robert R. Orford, Jan D. Skirrow	Dr. John Waters
		Nancy J. Betkowski (PC)	Rheal Joseph LeBlanc	
1989	Community & Occupational Health	Nancy J. Betkowski (PC)	Rheal Joseph LeBlanc	Dr. John Waters
	Health			
1990	Health	Nancy J. Betkowski (PC)	Rheal Joseph LeBlanc	Dr. John Waters
1991	Health	Nancy J. Betkowski (PC)	Rheal Joseph LeBlanc	Dr. John Waters
1992	Health	Nancy J. Betkowski (PC)	Rheal Joseph LeBlanc	Dr. John Waters
		Shirley A.M. McClellan (PC)		
1993	Health	Shirley A.M. McClellan (PC)	Rheal Joseph LeBlanc, Donald J. Philippon	Dr. John Waters
1994	Health	Shirley A.M. McClellan (PC)	Donald J. Philippon	Dr. John Waters
1995	Health	Shirley A.M. McClellan (PC)	Bernard J. Doyle (Acting), Jane Fulton	Dr. John Waters
1996	Health	Shirley A.M. McClellan (PC)	Jane Fulton	Dr. John Waters
		Halvar C. Jonson (PC)		
1997	Health	Halvar C. Jonson (PC)	Donald M. Ford (Acting)	Dr. John Waters / Dr. Karen Grimsrud (Deputy MOH)[31]
1998	Health	Halvar C. Jonson (PC)	Donald M. Ford	Dr. John Waters / Dr. Karen Grimsrud (Deputy MOH)
1999	Health	Halvar C. Jonson (PC)	Donald M. Ford, Gilmer Lynne Duncan	Dr. John Waters / Dr. Karen Grimsrud (Deputy MOH)

Year	Department	Minister	Deputy Minister	Provincial MOH (or similar)
2000	Health	Halvar C. Jonson (PC)	Gilmer Lynne Duncan	Dr. John Waters
	Health & Wellness	Gary Mar (PC)	Gilmer Lynne Duncan,	Dr. Nicholas Bayliss[32]
			Shelley Ewart-Johnson	Dr. Karen Grimsrud (Deputy MOH)
2001	Health & Wellness	Gary Mar (PC)	Shelley Ewart-Johnson	Dr. Nicholas Bayliss
				Dr. Karen Grimsrud (Deputy MOH)
2002	Health & Wellness	Gary Mar (PC)	Shelley Ewart-Johnson,	Dr. Nicholas Bayliss
			Roger F. Palmer	Dr. Karen Grimsrud (Acting)[33]
2003	Health & Wellness	Gary Mar (PC)	Roger F. Palmer	Dr. Nicholas Bayliss
				Dr. Karen Grimsrud (Deputy MOH)
2004	Health & Wellness	Gary Mar (PC)	Roger F. Palmer,	Dr. Nicholas Bayliss
		Iris Evans (PC)	Patricia Meade	Dr. Karen Grimsrud (Deputy MOH)
2005	Health & Wellness	Iris Evans (PC)	Patricia Meade	Dr. Nicholas Bayliss
				Dr. Karen Grimsrud (Deputy MOH)
2006	Health & Wellness	Iris Evans (PC)	Patricia Meade	Dr. Nicholas Bayliss
		Dave Hancock (PC)		Dr. Karen Grimsrud (Deputy MOH)
2007	Health & Wellness	Dave Hancock (PC)	Patricia Meade	Dr. Nicholas Bayliss
				Dr. Karen Grimsrud (Acting MOH)[34]
2008	Health & Wellness	Dave Hancock (PC)	Linda Miller (Acting)	Dr. Karen Grimsrud (Acting MOH)
		Ron Liepert (PC)		
2009	Health & Wellness	Ron Liepert (PC)	Linda Miller	Dr. Andre Corriveau
2010	Health & Wellness	Ron Liepert (PC)	Jay G. Ramotar	Dr. Andre Corriveau
		Gene Zwozdesky (PC)		
2011	Health & Wellness	Gene Zwozdesky (PC)	Jay G. Ramotar	Dr. Andre Corriveau
		Fred Horne (PC)	Marcia Nelson	
2012	Health & Wellness	Fred Horne (PC)	Marcia Nelson	Dr. Andre Corriveau
	Health			Dr. James Talbott

Year	Department	Minister	Deputy Minister	Provincial MOH (or similar)
2013	Health	Fred Horne (PC)	Marcia Nelson	Dr. James Talbott
			Janet Davidson	
2014	Health	Fred Horne (PC)	Janet Davidson	Dr. James Talbott
		Stephen Mandel (PC)		
2015	Health & Seniors	Stephen Mandel (PC)	Janet Davidson	Dr. James Talbott
		Sarah Hoffman (NDP)	Carl G. Amrhein	
2016	Health & Seniors	Sarah Hoffman (NDP)	Brandy Payne[35]	Dr. Karen Grimsrud
	Health		Carl G. Amrhein	
2017	Health	Sarah Hoffman (NDP)	Brandy Payne[36]	Dr. Karen Grimsrud
			Carl G. Amrhein	
			Milton Sussman	
2018	Health	Sarah Hoffman (NDP)	Brandy Payne[37]	Dr. Karen Grimsrud
			Milton Sussman	
2019	Health	Sarah Hoffman (NDP)	Milton Sussman	Dr. Deena Hinshaw
		Tyler Shandro (UCP)	Lorna Rosen	

Gender and ethnic diversity in these leadership positions has been rather limited; this is a legacy with which public health, with its emphasis on social justice, must continue to contend. Moreover, Alberta's provincial government has been characterized by long periods of time with the same government. These include the thirty-six-year period of Social Credit leadership (1935–1971), which saw the transition from the Department of Public Health to the Department of Health; and the forty-four-year period of Progressive Conservative leadership (1971–2015), during which time there were several iterations of the provincial department responsible for public health.

Next, Figures 4.1 presents the divisions and branches that constitute the department responsible for public health, from 1919 to 1993.

	1919	1920	1921	1922	1923	1924	1925	1926	1927	1928	1929	1930	1931	1932	1933	1934	1935
Department of Public Health																	
Mental Health												- - - - - - - - - - - - - -»					
Eugenics Board[2]										- -»							
Public Health Education										- -»							
Hospital Inspection and Coroner's Supervision of Operations / Hospital Inspection								- - - - - - - - - - - / - - - - - - - - - - - - - -»									
Provincial Dentist / Dental Hygiene								- - - - - - - - - - - / - - - - - - - - - - - - - -»									
Infectious Diseases / Communicable Diseases						- - / -»											
Institutions[1]							- -»									
Venereal Diseases / Social Hygiene			- - - - - - - - - - - - - / -»													
Municipal Hospitals / Hospitals / Charity and Relief / Hospital, Charity, and Relief / Municipal Hospitals, Charity and Relief / Municipal Hospitals		- - - - - - - / - - - - - - - - - - - - - / - - / - - - - - - - - / - - - - - / - - - - - - - -»															
Provincial Laboratories		- -»															
Public Health Nursing		- -»															
Provincial Sanitary Engineer / Sanitary Engineering and Sanitation		- - - - - - - - - - - - - - - - / - - - - - - - - - - - - - -»															
Medical Officer of Health / Provincial Board of Health		- - - - - / -»															
Vital Statistics		- -»															

[1] Institutions: Central Alberta Sanatorium; Mental Hospital, Ponoka; Mental Institute, Oliver; Training School, Red Deer were previously reported individually

[2] Later included as part of the Mental Health Division.

Legend	
- -|	End
|- -	Start
-/-	Name change
- -»	Continues

Fig. 4.1: Provincial higher-level divisions and branches under the ministries and departments responsible for public health in Alberta, 1919–1993.

Note: This figure includes all divisions/branches at higher levels in the organizational structure. In some cases, the highest level was not illustrative of the organization; in that case, the next level was used. The table also excludes administrative or support divisions. Some reports are not clear about structure.

	1936	1937	1938	1939	1940	1941	1942	1943	1944	1945	1946	1947	1948	1949	1950	1951	1952
Cerebral Palsy Clinics													- - - - - - -»				
Nutrition										- - - - - - - - - - - - -»							
Entomology						- -»											
Cancer Control / Cancer Services					- - / -»												
Child Welfare and Mothers' Allowance / Child Welfare		- - - - - - - / - - - - - - - - - -															
Tuberculosis Control	»- -»																
Mental Health	»- -»																
Eugenics Board	»- -»																
Public Health Education	»- -»																
Municipal Hospitals / Hospital and Medical Services	»- / - - - - - - - - - - -»																
Hospital Inspection	»- -																
Dental Hygiene	»- -																
Communicable Diseases	»- -»																
Institutions[3]	»- -																
Social Hygiene	»- -»																
Provincial Laboratories	»- -»																
Public Health Nursing	»- -»																
Sanitary Engineering and Sanitation	»- -»																
Provincial Board of Health	»- -»																
Vital Statistics	»- -»																

[3] Transferred to Mental Health

Legend	
- -|	End
|- -	Start
-/-	Name change
- -»	Continues

Fig. 4.1 (*continued*)

Fig. 4.1 (*continued*)

	Department of Public Health													Department of Health				
	1953	1954	1955	1956	1957	1958	1959	1960	1961	1962	1963	1964	1965	1966	1967	1968	1969	1970
Epidemiology														Start	-	-	-	Continues »
Alberta Health Plan														Start	-	End		
Alcoholism Services											Start	-	-	-	-	-	End	
Industrial Health									Start	-	-	-	-	-	-	-	-	Continues »
Medical Services[4]			Start	-	-	-	-	-	-	-	-	-	-	-	-	-	-	Continues »
Local Health Services		Start	-	-	-	-	-	-	-	-	-	-	-	-	-	-	-	Continues »
Civil Service Nurse[6]	Start	-	-	-	-	-	-	-	-	-	-	-	-	-	-	End		
Nursing Aides School	Start	-	-	-	-	End												
Health Units[5]	Start	-	-	-	End													
Arthritis Services	Start	-	-	-	-	-	-	-	-	-	-	-	-	-	-	-	End	
Cerebral Palsy Clinics[6]	»	-	-	-	-	-	-	-	-	-	-	-	End					
Nutrition[5]	»	-	-	-	End													
Entomology[5]	»	-	-	End														
Cancer Services	»	-	-	-	-	-	-	-	-	-	-	-	-	-	-	End		
Tuberculosis Control	»	-	-	-	-	-	-	-	-	-	-	-	-	-	-	-	-	Continues »
Mental Health	»	-	-	-	-	-	-	-	-	-	-	-	-	-	-	-	-	Continues »
Eugenics Board	»	-	-	-	-	-	-	-	-	-	-	-	-	-	-	-	-	Continues »
Public Health Education[5]	»	-	-	-	End													
Hospital and Medical Services / Hospitals	»	-	-	-	-	Name change	-	-	-	-	-	-	-	-	-	-	End	
Communicable Diseases[5]	»	-	-	-	End													
Social Hygiene	»	-	-	-	-	-	-	-	-	-	-	-	-	-	-	-	-	Continues »
Provincial Laboratories	»	-	-	-	-	-	-	-	-	-	-	-	-	-	-	-	-	Continues »
Public Health Nursing / Municipal Nursing[6]	» Name change	-	-	-	End													
Sanitary Engineering and Sanitation / Environmental Health Division[7]	»	-	-	-	-	-	-	-	-	-	-	-	-	Name change	-	-	-	Continues »
Provincial Board of Health	»	-	-	-	-	-	-	-	-	-	-	-	-	-	-	-	-	Continues »
Vital Statistics	»	-	-	-	-	-	-	-	-	-	-	-	-	-	-	-	-	Continues »

[4] Split from Hospitals. Includes: School for Nursing Aides
[5] Transferred to Local Health Services Division
[6] Transferred to Medical Services
[7] Transferred to new Environment Department after 1971

Legend
- -| End
- |- - Start
- -/- Name change
- - -» Continues

	Dept. of Health and Social Development / Social Services and Community Health																	Department of Health			
	1971	1972	1973	1974	1975	1976	1977	1978	1979	1980	1981	1982	1983	1984	1985	1986	1987	1990	1991	1992	1993
Special Health Projects (Services)					- - - - - - - - - - - - - - -																
Misc. Health Services				- - - -																	
Research and Planning				- - - - - - - - - - - - - - - - -															
Services for the Handicapped / Rehabilitation Services[13]		- -																			
Emergency Welfare Services[8]		- - - - - - - -																			
Public Assistance[8]		- - - - - - - - - - - - - - - -																
Metis Rehabilitation (Development)[8]		- - - - - - - - - - - - - - - - - - -															
Maintenance and Recovery[8]		- - - - - - - - - - - - - - - - - - - -														
Homes and Institutions[9]		- - - - - - - - - - - - - -																
Preventive Social Services / Community Social Services		- - - - - - - - - - - - - - - - - / - - - - - - - - - -														
Epidemiology	»- - - - - -																			
Industrial Health	»- - - - - - - - -																		
Medical Services	»- - - - - - - - -																		
Local Health Services / Community Health Services	»- - - - - - - - - - - - - - - - - - - / - - - - - - - - - -														
Child Welfare		- -																
Tuberculosis Control	»- - - - - - - - - - - - - - -																	
Mental Health	»- -																				
Income Support / Income Security[13]				- -							- - - - - - - - - - -									
Eugenics Board	»-																			
Social Hygiene[10]	»- - - - - - - - - - - - - - - - - -																
Provincial Laboratories	»- - - - - - - - - - - - - - - - - -				- - - - - - - - - - - -						
Provincial Board of Health[11]	»- -				- - - - - - -						
Vital Statistics[12]	»- -																

Missing Reports

[8] Transferred to Social Services at one point.
[9] Included in Social Services Delivery
[10] Transferred to Communicable Diseases Control And Epidemiology
[11] Temporarily under Community Health Services
[12] Transferred to Finance Information and Support Services
[13] Transferred to Policy and Program Development

Legend
- -| End
|- - Start
-/- Name change
- -» Continues

Fig. 4.1 (*continued*)

	Dept. of Health and Social Development / Social Services and Community Health																	Department of Health			
	1971	1972	1973	1974	1975	1976	1977	1978	1979	1980	1981	1982	1983	1984	1985	1986	1987	1990	1991	1992	1993
Acute and Long term Care																		|------		--|
Provincial Nursing Consultant																		.....	.. --|		
Provincial Medical Consultant																		.....	.. --|		
Policy and Planning Services / Health Strategy and Evaluation																		- - --	- - -	- -	--|
Occupational Health and Safety																-----					
Public Health Services													|------	---		---	---	- --	---	--|
Policy and Program Development													----								
Children Services Program / Family and Children Services												----- /-----									
Division Support Branch												------ --- --									
Associate Deputy Minister (Service Delivery)												------ --- --									
Family and Community Support Services[14]												----- --- --- --- ---							
Residencial Services												----- --- --									
Finance information and Support Services / Program Support												----- --- --- --- ---							
Health Promotion and Protection[14]												----- --- --- --								
Rehabilitative Programs[14]												----- --- --									
Aids to Daily Living										----											
Family Maintenance and Court Services / Family Relations										----- /-----										
Day Care										----- --										
Office of the Public Guardian								----- --- --- --- --- --- --								
Social Services Delivery					----- --- --- --												
Services to Special Groups				----															
Communicable Diseases Control And Epidemiology[14]									----- --- --- --- --- --								

[14] Included in Public Health Services

Missing Reports

Legend	
- -|	End
|- -	Start
-/-	Name change
- -»	Continues

Fig. 4.1 (*continued*)

The figure illustrates that the number and breadth of divisions and branches within the Department of Public Health have changed significantly over time. It also provides a glimpse into the changing nature of how public health was understood and organized within government, as we discuss further below and in Chapter 2.

Finally, Table 4.2 identifies several health-related commissions, committees, and reports of the Alberta government, from the 1920s to the 2010s.

TABLE 4.2: Overview of select public health-related commissions, task forces and reports in Alberta, 1919–2019.

Year	Title / Chair	Purpose	Response or Outcome
1928–29	*Report of the Inquiry into Systems of State Medicine* / Chris Pattison and Fred White[1]	In response to recognition of a disparity in health care between rural and urban citizens and the cost to patients, the report explored the feasibility of introducing state medicine.	The report determined that state medicine would be feasible but the cost would be high.[2] The report recommended two plans, one for rural health care and another for urban populations. In February 1930 a motion to consider instituting a system of state medicine as described in the report was entertained but defeated.[3] The provincial government opted to emphasize preventive health services, child and maternal hygiene, sanitary inspections, control of communicable disease and public health education.[4]
1929– (unknown)	Advisory Committee of Health *(Ministerial Committee)* / Malcolm R. Bow[5]	The purpose of this Committee was to advise the government on matters which were of concern to the health of the Alberta public, for example, public health by-laws, hospital bylaws, and emergency methods for epidemics.[6] The Committee met once a year and was composed of representatives from: the College of Physicians and Surgeons; the Faculty of Medicine, University of Alberta; physicians at large; the city medical officers of health; the nursing profession; city hospitals; municipal hospitals; urban laymen; rural laymen; urban women; and rural women.[7]	Following committee recommendation, provincial legislative authority was granted to establish health units,[8] and two full-time health units (in Red Deer and Okotoks-High River) were established with a cost-sharing arrangement between the province (50%), municipality (25%), and the Rockefeller Foundation (25%). The health units would concentrate on preventive medicine and public health functions, including prevention of epidemics, sanitary inspections of food and water, medical inspections of pre-school and school children, educational activities, and vital statistics. The committee also recommended that the provincial government should provide financial support to municipalities to permit caring for patients and creating "isolation hospitals" during contagious diseases outbreaks. Finally, the committee recommended compulsory medical inspections for all school children in the province.[9] The next year, recommendations concerning provincial hospital regulations, and physical examinations of rural school children by qualified physicians, were adopted.[10] In 1932, the committee recommended an inquiry into the issue of maternal mortality, and the maintenance of budgetary appropriations related to prevention services during the years of the depression.[11] From 1933 to 1937 no meetings of this committee were held; after 1937, there is no information about the committee in the annual reports.[12]

TABLE 4.2: *(continued)*

Year	*Title* / Chair	Purpose	Response or Outcome
1933–34	The Final Report of the *Legislative Commission on Medical Health Services* / George Hoadley[13]	Prompted by ongoing concerns about inadequate and inequitable access to health care across Alberta, this report – like others before it – considered the feasibility of making adequate health services available to all Albertans at an affordable cost. A similar report had been produced in British Columbia, which foresaw no added expense to the province or to employers and thus recommended state medicine.[14]	This report's recommendations were written into Alberta's Health Insurance Act of 1935. Legislation to provide health insurance for Albertans (a five-year plan under which powers of boards of health would be extended to provide "state medicine" on a modified scale[15]) was passed but not proclaimed because the UFA lost the 1935 election and the new Social Credit government was not prepared to fund the program. The commission was convinced that any system of medical administration that did not make provision for prevention could not function in the best interests of the insured. "Prevention lies at the very base of any efficient health structure."[16] For provision of public health services in rural Alberta, the commission recommended new full-time health units like the ones in existence. It also recommended further expansion of public health programs, such as tuberculosis control and public health nursing services, and the re-establishment of a travelling clinic service for those parts of the Province where a similar service did not exist.[17]
1965	*Report of the Special Legislative and Lay Committee Inquiring into Preventive Health Services in the Province of Alberta* / A. Somerville[18]	This report was prompted by recognition that preventive and public health services in Alberta were fragmented and uncoordinated.[19]	The report's 247 recommendations constituted the foundational structures and functions of preventive health services in the province. The report recommended the establishment of nine health regions with a single board, with the purpose of equalizing preventive health services across the province. Although proposed legislation to establish health regions was discussed in 1968, it did not pass because critics said the plan would mean the loss of autonomy at the provincial level.[20] Also, Edmonton and Calgary municipal governments were opposed, arguing that although they would be responsible for most the taxes required for financing the regions, the proposed infrastructure would benefit rural areas more.[21] This report contributed to legislation that permitted the creation of an amalgamated provincial department of Health and Social Development in 1971.[22]

Year	Title / Chair	Purpose	Response or Outcome
1989	*The Rainbow report:* Our Vision for Health, by the Premier's Commission on Future Health Care for Albertans / L. Hyndman[23]	The purpose of the report was to examine: 1) health care services and costs in the province, 2) future health requirements as they relate to population trends, and 3) incentives and mechanisms to maintain the quality and accessibility of health services.	The report recommended a "phased-in budgetary shift to prevention" that would involve: regionalization of health services delivery infrastructure to ensure focus on local needs; greater attention to human resources planning; better health data collection; and "some private financing to increase choice and competition and redefinition of insured services."[24] The phased in approach to prevention did not materialize, and our research leads us to believe that this was the inflection point at which financial support for the public health enterprise began to substantively erode. The financial appetite of medical procedures and hospital infrastructure in the health care system became insatiable, and issues such as waiting lists and access dominated the daily news. Premier Getty (PC) did not act on the regionalization suggestion; however, his successor, Premier Klein (PC) used the Rainbow Report as the foundation for 'regionalization' in 1994, which included uniting 128 acute care hospital boards, 25 public health boards and 40 long-term care boards into 17 health regions.[25]
1991	*Partners in Health:* the government of Alberta's response to the Premier's Commission on the Future Health Care of Albertans / Nancy Betkowski[26]	Following the release of the Rainbow report, Premier Don Getty (PC) formed a Cabinet Task Force to review the report's findings and recommendations, which it found to be unsatisfactory. It was argued that improving the health system is not a matter of more money but rather a matter of better management. The Rainbow report cost $4.2 million, but its proposals were felt to be too vague[27] The Partners in Health report was to be the next step to implement the recommendations.	The Getty (PC) government only accepted 16 of the 21 recommendations from the Rainbow report.[28] Regarding public health, the government agreed with the Rainbow report that additional funds should be provided for health promotion and illness/injury prevention. The government increased the promotion and prevention budget by $1 million in 1991/2 with incremental increases expected thereafter.

Year	*Title* / Chair	Purpose	Response or Outcome
2000–01	*Framework for Reform:* Report of the Premier's Advisory Council on Health / D. Mazankowski[29]	This advisory council was formed for the purpose of providing strategic advice to Premier Klein (PC) on the preservation and future enhancement of quality health services for Albertans and on the continuing sustainability of the publicly funded health system.[30]	Recommendations included: encouraging support for the determinants of health; focusing on customers; redefining comprehensiveness; investing in technology and electronic health records; reconfiguring health system governance; encouraging choice, competition and accountably; diversifying revenue sources; incentivizing health care providers; pursuing quality; mobilizing the health sector as an asset in creating wealth; and establishing a transition plan to drive change. The 17 regional health boards were reduced to nine, and in 2008 those nine were collapsed to one – Alberta Health Services.
			The Report mentioned that, compared with the 'big ticket' items like hospital care and diagnostic tests, very little is spent on health promotion and disease and injury prevention. The report states that the health of all Albertans should be promoted and improved by taking a global view of all the factors that determine and affect people's health, including basic public health measures, economic well-being, early childhood development, education, housing, nutrition, employment status, quality of the environment, lifestyle choices and healthy behaviours.
			The report urged the government to permit private enterprises to compete in the health field, while keeping the system largely publicly funded, which was interpreted by critics as opening the door to privatization.[31] It has been argued that the focus of reforms on the institutional part of the health system in Canada has been at the expense of the public health.[32]

We have omitted some potentially important recent reports, such as the 2019 ten-year review of Alberta Health Services commissioned by the United Conservative Party government, which require more time to pass before their historical significance becomes clear.[5]

1) Public Health Governance Prior to 1905: Early Foundations of Public Health

Public health activities in Alberta predated the formal establishment of the province in 1905. Indeed, collective efforts to promote the well-being of communities date back millenniums, to long-standing practices of Indigenous Peoples. One example from Treaty 7 territory is the Kainai Nation's Kainayssini or guiding principles for protecting and preserving their culture and community, including traditional ways of using the land, language, and spirituality, all of which are fundamental dimensions of health and well-being (see Chapter 7).

In terms of settler-colonial society, organized public health efforts are different, and much more recent, dating to the late nineteenth century. They illustrate public health's firm origins in communicable disease control with physicians in leadership roles — an enduring and challenging legacy. Under the territorial Public Health Ordinance that was in place between 1870 and 1905, public health activities were governed locally. In 1871, for example, a territorial board of health was established at Fort Edmonton, the Hudson's Bay trading post, in response to a smallpox outbreak.[6] In one of many illustrations of the colonial orientation of early formal public health practice, although reports suggest that most of the local residents were Cree or Métis, the board, which was named the Saskatchewan Board of Health, after the river Edmonton sits on, was comprised of non-Indigenous Hudson's Bay officials and local missionaries[7] who were unlikely to fully reflect local interests. The board was temporary; it ceased when the outbreak abated and was re-established when smallpox re-appeared in the area in 1876. The intermittent and reactive nature of early formal public health infrastructure was not unique to Alberta.[8]

In 1892, the incorporation of the Town of Edmonton permitted the creation of a more permanent local board of health at that location. Once again prompted by a smallpox outbreak, the council for the new town promptly passed a bylaw to establish a board of health, which was made up of the mayor, Matt McCauley, and four councillors.[9] Although the town of Calgary was incorporated in 1894, it did not establish a formal board of health until 1909. However, it did have a precursor: a Market and Health Committee, which council established in 1884 and which was responsible for sanitation, public scales, and the removal of dead animals from the streets.[10]

The Town of Edmonton's first medical officer of health, appointed upon the establishment of the board, was Dr. Edward Braithwaite, who also served as surgeon to the Royal North-West Mounted Police, coroner, and medical officer to the Canadian National Railways and the lumber industry.[11] Although a breadth of roles in this context is not surprising, from the point of view of a broad vision of public health concerned with upstream determinants of health equity, public health's early connections with colonial and extractive sectors and industries that are harmful to health equity are important to note. Within the context of rapid population growth (for example, between 1896 and 1913, the "wheat boom" drew over 60,000 people to Edmonton), conditions were challenging. A historical article by medical officer of health for the Edmonton Board of Health James Howell described living conditions during the 1890s in the new town: "Many lived in tents on the riverbank and drank river water. Mud houses were common, water and sewage systems almost non-existent. Unwanted garbage, impure food and milk, overcrowded living conditions and smelly slaughterhouses continued to dominate the list of problems."[12] In that context, Dr. Braithwaite had a considerable range of responsibilities including inspection of public and private premises, placing quarantines, and ensuring that the "poor and indigent" were looked after; the latter signalling some downstream recognition of connections between social conditions and health.[13]

2) 1905–1918: Navigating the Challenges of an Emergent State

Alberta's Public Health Act: Key Content and Changes, 1905–1918
• Alberta passed its first Public Health Act as a province in 1907. It provided for the appointment of a provincial health officer and a provincial board of health and included a long list of their duties and powers. Under the new act, local boards of health became mandatory. Outside of municipalities, areas could be defined as health districts and could create a local board of health under the supervision of the Provincial Board of Health.
• In 1910, a new Public Health Act was passed that extended the Provincial Board of Health's powers. The new act also reduced the provincial board to three permanent members (this structure would last until 1970): a medical officer of health,[14] sanitary engineer, and bacteriologist.

Upon establishment of the province of Alberta in 1905, provincial authority for public health activities was assigned to the Department of Agriculture, where it remained until 1918.[15]

There were only six government departments in the early years of Alberta public administration — Agriculture, Attorney General, Public Works, Provincial Secretary, Treasury, and Education.[16] Accordingly, the activities and functions of each were in some cases not obvious from the department name. The Department of Agriculture was a case in point, with its initial purview including "all that part of the administration of the Government of the Province which relates to agriculture, statistics and the public health, including hospitals."[17]

In 1906, a Public Health Branch was established within the Department of Agriculture, and the Minister of Agriculture, Hon. W.T. Findlay, appointed Dr. A.E. Clendennan as the province's first public health officer.[18] In the 1906 annual report of the new branch, limitations of the territorial ordinances were identified, including that they assigned jurisdiction to the Dominion government in certain domains. These limitations prompted Alberta's first Public Health Act, which was passed in 1907.[19] Also under the territorial ordinance, a bacteriological laboratory had been established in Regina, which Alberta continued to use via arrangements with the new Saskatchewan government (also established in 1905). However, long delays before results were received led to a desire for a laboratory in Alberta. A provincial laboratory was established in 1907 as a branch of Alberta's Department of Agriculture, with Dr. D.G. Revell, provincial bacteriologist and professor of anatomy at the University of Alberta serving as the inaugural (1907–1911) director.[20] ProvLab, as it came to be known, was transferred to the University of Alberta in 1911[21] and fell under the joint jurisdiction of the provincial government and the University of Alberta, thus initiating an enduring relationship between the two institutions.[22]

The 1907 Public Health Act provided for the formal creation of a provincial medical officer of health and a provincial board of health, a structure that would remain largely unchanged until 1970.[23] The general duties and functions of the board[24] included to "take cognizance of the interests of health and life among the people of the province" and to make investigations and inquiries concerning "the effects of localities, employments, conditions, habits and other circumstances upon the health of the people."[25] This early wording appears to align with a broad view of health and its determinants, albeit focused in practice on communicable disease control.[26] The provincial board's purview included studying and making use of vital statistics; making inquiries and investigations about the causes of disease; and making and implementing strategies to prevent, limit, and suppress disease. These latter activities were enshrined in the provincial board's authorization to make and issue regulations for a wide range of scenarios and purposes.

The provincial board's extent and scope of authority subsequently expanded. For example, the inaugural (1907) Public Health Act authorized the provincial board to "make and issue such rules and regulations, *not conflicting with any law in force in the province*" (italics added).[27] The 1910 act did not contain this stipulation, and instead clarified the legal supremacy of the Public Health Act: "should any Act in force within the province conflict with this Act, then, *and in every such case this Act shall prevail*" (italics added).[28] Also, whereas the 1907 act provided an itemized list of issues and circumstances for which the provincial board could create regulations,[29] the 1910 act and subsequent iterations clarified that the list should not be taken as comprehensive; that is, it "shall not be taken to curtail or limit the general power to make orders, rules, and regulations."[30]

Alberta's early provincial legislation also contributed to strengthening local public health governance, which in some areas such as Edmonton already existed. Local boards of health were established in Lethbridge and in Calgary between 1908 and 1909.[31] Membership of local boards, under the provincial legislation, was to consist of the mayor (or commissioner), the clerk of the municipal council, the city engineer, and the medical health officer.[32] This arrangement, which was most apparent in the cities where public health governance advanced most quickly, illustrates formalized overlap between public health governance and city governance more generally,[33] which continued in Alberta until approximately the 1980s.

On 1 January 1918, provincial authority for public health in Alberta shifted to the Department of the Provincial Secretary.[34] Under the leadership of Hon. George P. Smith, a public health nursing branch was added, sanitary inspectors were hired and acts were drafted, including the Venereal Diseases Prevention Act and the Municipal Hospitals Act.[35] Only a few months later, in August 1918, the administrative home for public health once again changed, to the provincial Department of Municipal Affairs.[36] Although situating public health within Municipal Affairs would appear to be a good fit with public health's local orientation at the time, there is little to be gleaned from this relationship from the department's 1918 annual report.[37]

A serious outbreak of influenza reached Alberta in 1918: over 38,000 people in Alberta got ill and over 4,300 hundred died. A need for stronger public health infrastructure was identified by government and public health leaders, which set the stage for the passing of Alberta's Department of Public Health Act in 1919.[38]

3) 1919–1929: Prioritizing the Public Health: Establishing a Provincial Department

Alberta's Public Health Act: Key Content and Changes, 1919–1929
• A 1919 amendment extended the list of communicable diseases to include influenza among others.
• Four amendments during the 1920s signalled continued expansions to the scope and authority of the Provincial Board of Health. These included extensions to the list of who could perform vaccinations (1921) and the extension of the board's inspection and enforcement powers (1922).
• A 1929 amendment created full-time health districts, consisting of several rural and outlying municipalities, through which various departmental programs and services could be delivered. Full-time health districts were to appoint a district board of health with authority to enforce the provisions of the act.

The need for a provincial public health department in Alberta had been discussed at least as early as 1917. At a South Edmonton Conservatives rally held on 25 May of that year, one of the speakers, Mrs. Clyde Macdonald, quipped that the minister of agriculture, to whom responsibility for public health fell, "value[d] noxious weeds more than human life, as proven by his expenditures," advocating for a separate department for public health.[39] A separate department was also supported by "medical men" including the Alberta Medical Association, the Edmonton Academy of Medicine, and the Edmonton Dental Society.[40] At least some Alberta doctors were more concerned with leadership than with departmental structure: according to a 28 November 1917 article in the *Edmonton Journal*, "it is suggested by the doctors that there should be a competent deputy minister, presumably a trained medical man, at the head of the health department, which might be attached to any one of the existing government departments so long as it had a separate official at its head."[41] However, in an early illustration of tensions that persist today, others were opposed to the idea that leadership would be best served by a doctor because "medical men are concerned only with curing the ills which beset us from day to day, and are not interested in preventive measures such as it is the business of a public health department to establish."[42]

Following an address delivered at the January 1919 United Farm Women of Alberta Convention,[43] Hon. A.G. MacKay introduced Bill 19 to establish a department of public health to the legislature on 18 February 1919; second and third readings took place later that month.[44] On 17 April 1919, An Act

Respecting the Department of Public Health received royal assent under the provincial Liberal government, making Alberta the second province in Canada, after New Brunswick, to establish such a department. MacKay became Alberta's first Minister of Health, Dr. T.J. Norman was appointed deputy minister; and Dr. W.C. Laidlaw was appointed provincial medical officer of health under this new arrangement.[45] The new department was responsible for "all that part of the administration of the government of the province, which relates to public health," which included matters falling under the following legislation: the Public Health Act, the Public Health Nurses Act, the Registered Nurses Act, the Municipal Hospitals Act, the Hospitals Ordinance, the Venereal Diseases Act, the Medical Profession Act, the Alberta Pharmaceutical Association Act, the Dental Association Act, the Marriage Ordinance, and the Vital Statistics Act.[46] Responsibilities were wide ranging and included control and monitoring of infectious diseases, inspections, approval of plans for waterworks and sewage, education about public health matters, vital statistics, and the provincial laboratory.[47]

Not surprisingly, the next decade was an active one in terms of infrastructure, legislation, and program development. In the 1920s, several new branches and divisions were added, including for venereal diseases, infectious diseases, social hygiene, dental public health, and public health education.[48] By the mid-1920s, only the cities of Calgary and Edmonton had full-time medical officers of health; accordingly, the early activities of the new infectious disease branch included helping smaller communities across the province to implement efforts to control the spread of communicable diseases.[49] In 1928, the newly established Eugenics Board, and newly-passed Sexual Sterilization Act fell under the authority of the new department (see Chapter 1).

4) 1930–1970: Public Health in Alberta: Expansion and Compromise

---

Alberta's Public Health Act: Key Content and Changes, 1930–1970

- Over thirty amendments to the Public Health Act were passed, speaking to a period of significant public health activity in the province.

- The scope of the Public Health Act continued to include new or expanded regulations pertaining to, for example, dairy products (1933, 1935); air and water pollution (1945, 1946, 1957); waterworks, including sewage systems (1944); and processes for municipalities to pass public health legislation, such as milk pasteurization (1945, 1962) and water fluoridation (1952, 1956, 1958, 1964, 1966).

- With respect to local/regional public health infrastructure, a 1934 amendment authorized city local boards of health to i) supply medical, dental, and surgical services; ii) employ physicians, dentists, and nurses; and iii) deliver services to school districts. For areas outside of cities, several amendments expanded or clarified parameters around the organization of health districts, and, starting in 1947, health units.

- In 1970, the provincial medical officer of health position was struck from the act and was replaced by a deputy minister of health.

The 1930s saw the continued evolution of local public health infrastructure in rural areas. A 1929 amendment to the provincial Public Health Act had allowed the minister of health to establish full-time health districts, the precursor to health units[50] that consisted of several municipalities, which made possible the organization and delivery of a range of programs and services in communities that were too small to support specialized services on their own.[51] Although the legislation was in place, the Great Depression of the early 1930s meant that the ambitious plans had to be put on hold. Under an initiative by the private, philanthropic Rockefeller Foundation to support health units in rural areas across North America, two health units in Alberta were created on a pilot basis in 1931: Red Deer, and Okotoks-High River, which was later named Foothills.[52] Writer Bill Carney describes this innocuously as a return to an earlier tradition of seeking charitable assistance to support health services.[53] In fact, this significant contribution of the Rockefeller Foundation to early public health infrastructure should be viewed critically as an early example of philanthro-capitalism and the depoliticized views about the causes of ill health that usually come with it.[54]

Meanwhile, in the larger cities, strong local public health governance continued.[55] A 1934 amendment to the provincial Public Health Act enhanced the capacity of city boards of health, by authorizing them to provide medical and dental services to schoolchildren, including to enter into agreements with school districts to do so. With respect to intersectoral dimensions of public health, there are several examples of connections between local public health and schools around this time. In Edmonton, for example, the membership parameters for the local board of health during the 1930s included representatives from the Edmonton public and separate school boards, along with previous members such as the mayor and local physicians.[56] In Calgary, a relationship between local public health authorities and school boards materialized around health record-keeping, led by the city's Medical Officer of Health, Dr. W.H. Hill, and which Hill later credited with increasing immunization uptake by enabling public health practitioners to be in closer contact with children.[57]

Efforts to strengthen public health services in the late 1920s and early 1930s became connected with attempts to establish universal health care insurance. In 1928, the legislature formed a committee to examine the feasibility of introducing "state medicine" in Alberta (see Table 4.2).[58] A state medicine motion was introduced in the legislature but was defeated, with legislators instead opting to emphasize preventive health services, child and maternal hygiene, sanitary inspections, and public health education.[59] The issue of provincial health insurance was raised again in 1933, and Alberta's Health Insurance Act of 1935 described a five-year plan to provide health insurance.[60] The act was passed but not proclaimed because the new Social Credit government was not prepared to implement the plan. Although universal health care insurance was not yet forthcoming, interest and support for the public health component of the 1928/29 state medicine report remained, perhaps underscored by the report's statement that prevention lies "at the very base of any efficient health structure."[61]

Social assistance at municipal, provincial, and federal levels evolved during and following the Depression (see also Chapter 12). To accompany programs provided by municipalities, Alberta's provincial Department of Public Health had a Charity and Relief Branch that, from 1926 to 1932, provided accommodation, food, clothing, and medical services to residents outside of municipalities and to "transients."[62] In 1936, perhaps in recognition of the significant health implications of economic destitution, provincial responsibility for the Child Welfare and Mothers' Allowance Branch was moved to the Ministry of Health from the attorney general.[63] Administration of provincial public relief functions followed suit in 1937; these social welfare functions remained in the Department of Public Health until 1944 when the provincial Department of Public Welfare was created.[64] Federal social programs were also created around this time; for example, in 1930 the federal government introduced a means-tested pension program for those over age 70 with an annual income of less than $125 with matching contributions from Alberta.[65] National unemployment insurance was introduced in 1940, but it initially excluded over half of the workforce; exclusions included, for example, farm workers, domestic workers, fishers, forestry workers, other seasonal workers, and married women.[66] Speaking to weaknesses in efforts to address social determinants of health, there were no universal social programs in Canada prior to the Second World War.

The Rockefeller Foundation funding for the experimental health units ran out in 1936. With the support of most involved areas, legislation to continue this organizational structure was created and passed throughout the 1930s and 1940s, culminating in the Health Unit Act of 1951.[67] The number of health units grew rapidly, and by 1960 there were twenty-four health units across the province, serving approximately 93 percent of Alberta's population outside of Edmonton and Calgary.[68] Their purview continued to emphasize prevention of mostly physical health concerns; key activities included physical examinations, education in child and maternal hygiene, and control of communicable diseases including via immunizations.

Reflecting the health concerns of the time, various new branches and divisions were created within Alberta's Department of Public Health during this period (Figure 4.1), including those focused on mental health (1930), tuberculosis control (1936), cancer control (1941), entomology (1944), nutrition (1947), industrial health (1963), and alcoholism services (1965). Existing divisions, such as Sanitation, adapted to new demands, including those presented by growing infrastructure in towns and cities.[69] Federally, following important civil society activism, the targeted pension program for seniors became universal in 1951. Seniors thus became, and continue to be, among the groups best served by social programs in Alberta and across the country, with demonstrable benefits for population well-being and health equity.[70] In 1966, the federal Pearson government implemented the Canada Assistance Plan, which supported provinces, territories, and municipalities in providing social programs, including income supports. The Canadian Assistance Plan was significant in that it embodied — to a greater extent than programs that came before — society's responsibility for well-being and its social determinants.[71]

5) 1970s to 1980s: Individualism and Efficiency

> **Alberta's Public Health Act: Key Content and Changes, 1970s–1980s**
>
> - In the mid-1980s, Alberta's Public Health Act was completely rewritten. The new act, passed in 1984, amalgamated six existing acts, changed the role of the Provincial Board of Health to that of an advisory and appeal body, updated the provisions for communicable disease control, and presented fewer stipulations around the membership of local boards of health.

The 1970s marked the beginning of the Progressive Conservative reign in Alberta government, which lasted over forty years (Table 4.1). As articulated by Edward LeSage, professor emeritus of government studies at the University of Alberta, Premier Peter Lougheed (1971–1985) brought in "sweeping modernizing reforms to the provincial public administration" that represented a "pronounced break from the Social Credit administration and policy ambitions."[72] For public health, changes that occurred in this context signalled an inflection point.

The nature of local boards of health seemed to be shifting. While local boards in 1973 consisted of the mayor, the medical officer of health, the municipal engineer, and three appointed taxpayers, by 1977 they required simply a representative from city council, who could be the mayor or a city councillor, the medical officer of health and eight members from the community. In Calgary, where city council had been serving as the de facto board of health since its 1922 city charter, these changes may have been particularly significant.[73] Furthermore, while local boards of health continued throughout the 1970s to include public health professionals, there were important changes: in 1977, the position of medical officer of health became non-voting, and the position of municipal engineer had been eliminated.[74]

On a national and international scale, important social trends were occurring, including the health promotion movement (see also Chapter 10), signalled federally by the 1974 report, *A New Perspective on the Health of Canadians* by then federal Health Minister Marc Lalonde, and the 1986 *Ottawa Charter for Health Promotion*, which presented "new" ways of thinking about public health.[75] It explicitly embraced a holistic vision of health (encompassing physical, mental, and social well-being), to be supported via a range of actions at individual, community, health services, and broader societal levels.[76] Further, foreshadowing the later prominence of the social determinants of health, the Ottawa Charter identified "prerequisites for health" including peace, shelter, education, food, income, a stable ecosystem, sustainable resources, social justice, and equity.[77]

Against that backdrop, an amendment to Alberta's Public Health Act in the early 1970s revised the preamble to Section 7, General Duties of the Provincial Board of Health, to read "the . . . Board may . . . make and issue orders, rules and regulations for *the protection and improvement of health and* the prevention, mitigation and suppression of disease" (italicized wording was not included in the previous act).[78] This change hints at some alignment with health promotion's emphasis on improving health to accompany the existing focus on preventing illness. Aside from this, however, the collective and upstream spirit of health promotion seemed to be largely thwarted by a prominent and rapidly growing sentiment of individualism and a focus on efficiency in all government departments including health.

The new Public Health Act of 1984 provides an illustration of this shift. The new act was to be a "total rewrite"; it was Alberta's first entirely new Public Health Act since 1910, and was intended to replace the previous act, which was described as "archaic and overlapping." The new act would be streamlined by a redrafting of the "tremendous number of regulations," as well as consolidation of existing public health legislation. From the outset, the language used to describe the new act, for example, "greater flexibility," "restructuring," "in the spirit of deregulation," "increased financial autonomy," betrayed a pervasive government concern with rationalization and systematization,[79] suggesting a concern with system efficiencies more so than peoples' well-being. Although health promotion was discussed, its framing did not align with how the concept was intended to be used —as a lens or approach to create supportive environments for all. Rather, content such as an emphasis on health campaigns to support the financial autonomy of local boards suggests that it was more accurately a vehicle for the individualized "lifestyle drift" that has come to characterize health promotion in the neoliberal era.[80]

There were several other features of the proposed act, which was introduced to the legislature on 6 April 1984 by PC MLA Janet Koper. For example, the Provincial Board of Health, which had existed since 1907 with the broad mandate to understand and take action to prevent or limit disease, was eliminated. The mandate of its replacement, the Public Health Advisory and Appeal Board, was to advise the minister, and to hear appeals of decisions by local boards. It also had a new membership: whereas the provincial board had specified membership from certain public health roles, the membership of the new board was open ended, consisting of seven to eleven members appointed by the lieutenant governor in council; there were no requirements for public health specialists.[81]

Despite the breadth of revisions and their potentially significant implications for the role and substance of public health, the ensuing legislative debate focused almost entirely on one item in the act: a new section on "recalcitrant

patients." While the act had always bestowed considerable authority on medical officers of health to act as they deemed necessary to prevent or limit disease
spread, the proposed 1984 act articulated powers to "apprehend" and "detain"
people in circumstances where they refused to comply with a public health order
(e.g., an isolation order). Considering the context of George Orwell's *1984*,[82] it is
perhaps unsurprising that these sections of the proposed act preoccupied discussion and debate including in the media. For example, one article published in the
Edmonton Journal described the act as giving "sweeping powers to medical officers of health, allowing them to enter premises without a warrant." An editorial
in the same newspaper likened the new act to "arbitrary arrest and incarceration"
that would permit doctors to "short-circuit the legal process . . . to detain patients, with or without their consent" to address communicable diseases.[83]

Although resistance to language like "detainment" is not surprising, one
must recognize that this debate was occurring in the context of advances in human rights legislation. The Canadian Charter of Rights and Freedoms, which
purports to "protect the rights of all Canadians from infringements by laws, policies or actions of governments" became part of Canada's Constitution in 1982,
and Alberta passed a Bill of Rights in 1980.[84] From 1910 to 1980, Alberta's Public
Health Act had paramountcy; starting in 1984 that clause was revised to state
that "this Act prevails over any enactment with which it conflicts, other than
the Alberta Bill of Rights." Furthermore, the creation with the 1984 act of an
Advisory and Appeals Board led to a lengthy new section detailing the appeals
process that appears near the beginning of the 1984 act, speaking to its prominence in that legislation.

Considering this broader context, the fixation on the new section on recalcitrant patients thus seems somewhat disproportionate and may have crowded
out discussion and debate on other potentially significant changes such as the
elimination of the provincial medical officer of health and the Provincial Board
of Health. The fixation also seems rather narrow when considered alongside
other government activities at the time that brought massive implications for
population well-being and health equity, such as significant cuts to public sector
activities including public education, where problematic narratives of "parental
choice," underpinned by an incorrect assumption that marketplace competition
is appropriate for public sector services, opened the door to public funding for
private schools[85] (high-quality public education is a key social determinant of
health). With respect to other content in the Public Health Act, there was some
limited discussion around the proposed movement of milk pasteurization legislation from the Public Health Act to the Dairy Industry Act. The Health Unit
Association of Alberta publicly expressed concern about this proposed change,

suggesting that it would weaken public health considerations by municipalities around this issue. However, the issue was largely dismissed on the basis that the legislation would be transferred intact to the new act, arguing that it would thus not constitute a change in procedures.[86]

Ultimately, the discussion and debate, which largely focused on the "new" powers of public health officials, subsided, and Bill 25, The Public Health Act 1984, passed third reading on 30 May 1984, receiving royal assent the following day.[87]

6) 1990s-Present: The Neoliberal Legacy and Self-Critical State

Alberta's Public Health Act: Key Content and Changes, 1990s–present
• A 1996 amendment reflected the 1994 Regional Health Authorities Act, which entailed a total restructuring of health service delivery, including public health services, in Alberta.
• A 1998 amendment replaced the Public Health Advisory and Appeal Board with the Public Health Appeal Board, with the sole mandate to hear appeals. This amendment also created two new positions — chief medical officer and deputy chief medical officer — responsible for monitoring the health of Albertans and making recommendations to the minister of health.
• A 2016 amendment authorized the minister of health to require the minister of education to provide student enrolment data to permit cross-referencing with immunization records, and it strengthened reporting requirements for immunizations and adverse events.

Considering the significance of the changes to the Public Health Act in 1984, it is perhaps not surprising that some subsequent amendments represented a return to the pre-1984 structure. In 1998, for example, an amendment added the provincial positions of chief (and deputy chief) medical officers of health, whose duties included monitoring the health of Albertans and making recommendations to the minister and to regional health authorities on measures to protect and promote health and prevent disease and injury.[88] These positions appear reminiscent of the provincial medical officer of health position that existed for much of Alberta's history (1907 to 1970), although they now functioned in a different socio-political and epidemiologic context.

Starting in the 1990s, several additional significant changes to public health administration in Alberta occurred, within the broader context of neoliberalism, which arrived with vigour in Canadian federal and provincial politics in the 1990s. A hallmark of neoliberalism is a scaling back of government intervention in regulatory processes and public services, in favour of private and corporate responsibility for well-being, underpinned by a dominant ethos of individualism and overarching concern with economic growth. Neoliberal economic and social policies, whose manifestations include public sector funding cuts and restructuring, have demonstrably negative effects on population well-being and health equity.[89] An important federal example was the 1996 demise, under the Chretien Liberals, of the Canada Assistance Plan. Its replacement, the Canada Health and Social Transfer, combined federal transfers for health care and social programs and reduced the total budget by $7 billion over three years. In contrast to Canada Assistance Plan, where transfers were conditional upon provinces and territories agreeing to provide aid to all in need without exception, the Canada Health and Social Transfer gave provincial governments more discretion over how to spend the funds, which is highly problematic in a neoliberal context where government cost-cutting becomes an orchestrated imperative.[90]

Public sector cuts and restructuring were dramatic in Alberta under PC Premier Ralph Klein, whose 1992 election victory, as described by Professor of Political Science, John Church, "signalled a shift from a moderate, urban-based conservative agenda to a more radical and rural-based right-wing agenda."[91] Despite the fact that significant privatization and public sector cuts had already occurred under the prior PC government of Don Getty,[92] Klein effectively created a narrative of "out of control spending" by government, which he used to justify a series of ideologically driven actions that further gutted the public sector with massive implications for health care, health determinants, and social and health equity.[93] For example, one of the first initiatives, described as "a clear harbinger of things to come," was to drastically reduce the number of people on social assistance by introducing "workfare," a highly punitive and stigmatizing initiative where persons receiving social assistance must work for their benefits.[94] Under regionalization of Alberta's health care system, about which much has been written, in 1995 seventeen regional health authorities replaced the previous 148 health facility and health unit boards; in the process, local boards of health, including in Calgary and Edmonton, were dissolved.[95] More restructuring followed: in April 2003, the regional authorities were further consolidated into nine health regions.[96] The process of regionalization was experienced by some as fracturing the public health community in the province by making it more difficult for people to connect, and significant efforts — such as the Alberta Public Health Association's Millennium Project — were made to try to mend that fracture.[97]

Beyond the formal public health system, that is, the narrow version of public health, Klein's neoliberal activities eroded social determinants of health through drastic cuts to public services, programs, and workers. This was aptly described by author and former provincial politician Kevin Taft in his scathing critique of Klein, *Shredding the Public Interest*, who gave a sense of the magnitude of the cuts and how they were experienced.

> In the first year [1993], they cut more than $800 million from public spending. Public sector job reductions were immense, including in the first year alone 778 teachers and 2300 hospital staff. They reduced or eliminated various benefits and programs, usually with sharpest effect on seniors, families with young children, and the poor (though some benefits were actually increased to very low-income seniors). They imposed a 5 percent pay cut on MLAs and public sector workers, including civil servants, teachers, nurses, and university staff. They raised health care insurance premiums substantially while de-insuring many services.
>
> The cuts continued the following year. By the end of 1995, public spending had fallen $1.9 billion since the Klein government came into office, and more than 4500 civil service jobs had been eliminated. Many hundreds more were cut in 1996. Direct fees and premiums for public services continued to climb. In Calgary the Grace Hospital, the Colonel Belcher Hospital, and the Holy Cross Hospital were closed, and the Calgary General/Bow Valley Centre was slated for closure. In Edmonton . . . hospital-bed numbers were cut by 44% from 1994 to 1996.
>
> Under Ralph Klein's government, public programs in Alberta became the most poorly supported in Canada. . . . The cuts occurred so quickly and in such confusion that they became hard to follow. By fiscal year 1995/96, per student funding for schools dropped to 14% below the Canadian average. From 1992 to 1995 the Calgary Regional Health Authority lost about 1400 staff, and the Capital Health Authority about 4000. From 1992 to 1995, the total province-wide loss of employed registered nurses was estimated at almost 8275, or a staggering 43% of all employed nurses in Alberta. . . .
>
> Under the [previous] Getty government, support for Alberta's public programs went from the highest in Canada to below average; under the Klein government it hit rock bottom. [98]

In short, it would be a considerable understatement to say that the Klein administration and its ideological underpinnings had a negative impact on public health, understood broadly as the science and art of preventing disease and promoting health through organized societal efforts, in which social determinants of health figure prominently. On a constructive note, emblematic of the damage of the Klein government was the 1996 founding, in response, of the Parkland Institute, a non-partisan research centre whose vision of "research and education for the common good" aimed to provide an antidote to the dominant narratives of privatization and austerity and provide a space and community for alternative perspectives and policies; it continues to serve this role.[99]

In May 2008, in the context of public discontent with the regional health system structure, Premier Ed Stelmach (PC) announced another significant episode of health system restructuring, in which the health regions were consolidated into a single, provincial authority. Alberta Health Services became the largest health care delivery organization in Canada; analysis of this change is available from many sources.[100]

With respect to the broad vision of public health that anchors this volume, we conclude with brief reference to the historic 2015 provincial election that led to a majority NDP government under Premier Rachel Notley, thus ending over 40 years of Progressive Conservative rule in Alberta. As described by reporter Graham Thompson,

> After years as a social justice champion, Notley became a social justice premier. Her government raised the minimum wage to $15 an hour, instituted an Alberta Child Benefit, reduced school fees, protected gay-straight alliances in schools and introduced workplace protections for farm workers.[101]

The NDP reign was ultimately short-lived, as the 2019 provincial election resulted in a majority United Conservative Party government under Premier Jason Kenney, once again to the detriment of Albertans' health and well-being.[102] We will eagerly await what light is shed on these most recent governments, with respect to population well-being and health equity, by the next 100-year history of public health in Alberta.

Conclusion

Although we focused on Alberta in this chapter, there are broad similarities with public health governance in other Canadian provinces.[103] The work of political scientist Jack Lucas is illustrative.[104] In his work on historical urban governance in five policy domains — policing, public health, public schools, public transit, and water — across six Canadian cities in three provinces, Lucas showed that, rather than city- or province-specific histories, there was evidence for domain-specific histories (e.g., history of public health governance) that transcend geographies.[105] Such cross-jurisdictional patterning reminds us that the public health governance story in Alberta is part of a larger trajectory of governance across Canada, although certain periods — such as Klein's austerity and restructuring measures of the 1990s — continue to stand out.

Our chapter omits many significant aspects of governance such as how institutional arrangements were experienced and the nuance of how governance activities played out "on the ground." Indeed, any number of points made in this chapter could benefit from more in-depth analysis. Nonetheless, we draw attention in closing to an apparent thread where the incoherent and misunderstood version of public health seen today has roots in: the likely non-innocuous financial contributions of the Rockefeller Foundation in the 1930s, the growing separation of public health from peoples' daily lives through weakened connections with local governments in the 1970s, and the destruction of social determinants of health under the ideological tentacles of neoliberalism in the 1980s and 1990s.

NOTES

1   Christopher Rutty and Sue Sullivan, *This Is Public Health: A Canadian History* (Ottawa: Canadian Public Health Association, 2010), https://cpha.ca/sites/default/files/assets/history/book/history-book-print_all_e.pdf.

2   *Public Health Act*, R.S.A. 2000, c. P-37.

3   Marjorie MacDonald, "Introduction to Public Health Ethics 1: Background," in *Briefing Notes*, edited by National Collaborating Centre for Healthy Public Policy (Montréal: National Collaborating Centre for Healthy Public Policy, 2014), accessed 2 November 2018, http://www.ncchpp.ca/docs/2014_Ethics_Intro1_En.pdf/; Sammy Hudes, "Following weeks of pressure, Kenney declares state of emergency, closes high schools," *Calgary Herald*, November 25, 2020, https://calgaryherald.com/news/local-news/live-at-430-kenney-to-unveil-new-covid-19-restrictions-following-weeks-of-pressure.

4   Provincial Archives of Alberta, *An Administrative History of the Government of Alberta, 1905–2005* (2006), https://open.alberta.ca/publications/0778547140. Alberta's Public Health Acts and Amendment Acts were accessed via the HeinOnline database of historical government documents, available through the University of Calgary library system; many of these documents are also available through the Government of Alberta's open source database, https://open.alberta.ca/dataset. The annual reports of provincial departments were available in electronic or hard copy from the University of Calgary library or Alberta's Legislative Library in Edmonton. The *Alberta Hansard* (https://www.assembly.ab.ca/assembly-business/transcripts/transcripts-by-type) is the official record of the Legislative Assembly, starting with the 1st session of the 17th Legislature in 1972. Prior to 1972, insight into legislative debates is available from the Scrapbook Hansard (https://librarysearch.assembly.ab.ca/client/en_CA/scrapbookhansard).

5   Ministry of Health, "Alberta Health Services Review" (Government of Alberta, last updated April 16, 2020), https://www.alberta.ca/alberta-health-services-review.aspx.

6   Gerald Predy, "A Brief History of Public Health in Alberta," *Canadian Journal of Public Health* 75, no. 5 (1984); Bill Carney, *Public Health: People Caring for People* (Edmonton: Health Unit Association of Alberta, 1994); James M. Howell, "Edmonton Board of Health Celebrates 100 Years — or More," *Canadian Journal of Public Health* 83, no. 4 (July/August 1992).

7   Howell, "Edmonton Board of Health," 306.

8   Howell, "Edmonton Board of Health," 306; Rutty and Sullivan, *This is Public Health*.

9   Predy, "A Brief History of Public Health in Alberta"; Howell, "Edmonton Board of Health," 306; Jack Lucas, "Historical Overview: Public Health Governance in Calgary" and "Historical Overview: Public Health Governance in Edmonton," in *Canadian Urban Policy Governance Backgrounders*, ed. Jack Lucas, (Calgary: Canadian Urban Policy Governance Backgrounders, 2015), https://doi.org/10.5683/SP/HLKDPK. As described by Lucas, the bylaw to establish Edmonton's Board of Health was created by a Civic Health and Relief Committee that existed prior to 1892, and then approved by the Council of the new town.

10   Lucas, "Historical Overview: Calgary."

11   Howell, "Edmonton Board of Health," 306–07.

12   Howell, "Edmonton Board of Health," 306.

13   Carney, *Public Health.*

14   "Provincial Health Officer" in the 1907 Public Health Act became "Provincial Medical Officer of Health" in the 1910 Act.

15   Bow and Cook, "The Department of Public Health"; John J. Heagerty, "Provincial Department of Health, Alberta," in *Four Centuries of Medical History in Canada and a Sketch of the Medical History of Newfoundland* (Toronto: The MacMillan Company of Canada Ltd, at St. Martin's House, 1928), 372–75.

16   Provincial Archives of Alberta, *An Administrative History.*

17   *Act respecting the Department of Agriculture*, S.P.A. 1906, c. 8; Provincial Archives of Alberta, *An Administrative History*, 517.

18   Heagerty, "Provincial Department of Health," 372–75; Alberta Department of Agriculture, *Annual Report 1905–6*, 162.

19   Alberta Department of Agriculture, *Annual Report 1905–6*; *An Act respecting Public Health*, S.P.A. 1907, c. 12; Heagerty, "Provincial Department of Health," 372–75.

20   Alberta Health Services, "History: ProvLab, Laboratory Services," accessed 1 June 2020, https://www.albertahealthservices.ca/lab/Page14604.aspx/.

21   Alberta Health Services "History: ProvLab."

22   Alberta Health Services "History: ProvLab"; Doug Wilson, interview by Rogelio Velez Mendoza, 12 December 2019.

23   *An Act respecting Public Health*, S.P.A. 1907; Heagerty, "Provincial Department of Health," 372–75.

24   The provincial medical officer of health was a key member of the provincial board of health, serving as secretary (as per the 1907 Public Health Act) and then as chair (1910–1970). See *An Act respecting Public Health*, S.P.A. 1907; *An Act respecting Public Health*, S.P.A. 1910, c. 17; *An Act respecting Public Health*, R.S.A. 1922, c. 58; *An Act respecting Public Health*, R.S.A. 1942, c. 183; *An Act respecting Public Health*, R.S.A. 1955, c. 255; and *Public Health Act*, R.S.A. 1970, c. 294.

25   This wording first appeared in the Public Health Act in 1907 and remained there until the early 1980s.

26   Canadian Public Health Association (CPHA), *Public Health: A Conceptual Framework*, Canadian Public Health Association Working Paper, Second Edition (Ottawa: CPHA, 2017), https://www.cpha.ca/sites/default/files/uploads/policy/ph-framework/phcf_e.pdf

27   *An Act respecting Public Health*, S.P.A. 1907.

28   *An Act respecting Public Health*, S.P.A. 1910.

29   Amongst the list of circumstances for which the provincial board could make and issue regulations, the 1907 Public Health Act did contain a clause accommodating "generally, all such matters, acts and things as may be necessary for the protection of the public health and for ensuring the full and complete enforcement of every provision of this Act." Nonetheless, the new explicit statement in 1910 seems illustrative of the growing scope of authority of the provincial board.

30   *An Act respecting Public Health*, S.P.A. 1910. A similar sentiment was conveyed in subsequent acts (see 1922 R.S.A.; 1942 R.S.A.; 1955 R.S.A.; 1970 R.S.A.; 1980 R.S.A.)

31   Heagerty, "Provincial Department of Health;"; Lucas, "Historical Overview: Calgary."

32   Provincial legislation concerning the membership of local boards of health changed in 1908, to the mayor, the medical health officer, the city / municipal engineer (if there was one), and three ratepayers appointed by municipal council. In 1921, this changed again, to clarify that appointed ratepayers serving on local boards of health were not allowed to be members of local council; this latter stipulation was removed in 1923. Lucas, "Historical Overview: Calgary."

33   In Calgary, the 1922 City Charter stated that the city's board of health and the city council would be one and the same, and that "the city council had all the powers and duties of a local board of health under the Public Health Act." Lucas, "Historical Overview: Calgary."

34   For example, the *Report of the Provincial Medical Officer of Health and Deputy Registrar General*, within the 1917 Department of Agriculture annual report, noted that "the Public Health Branch was, late in the year, transferred to the Provincial Secretary's department, and in future, reports will be issued under that department." Alberta Department of Agriculture, *Annual Report 1917* (Edmonton: Printed by J.W. Jeffery, King's Printer, 1918), 165.

35   Heagerty, "Provincial Department of Health;"; *An Act for the Prevention of Venereal Disease*, S.P.A 1918, c. 50, assented to 13 April 1918; *The Municipal Hospitals Act*, S.P.A 1918, c. 15.

36   Bow and Cook, "Department of Public Health"; Heagerty, "Provincial Department of Health."

37   Alberta Department of Municipal Affairs, *Report 1918* (Edmonton: Printed by J.W. Jeffery, King's Printer, 1919), 6.

38   Predy, "A Brief History of Public Health," 366.

39   "Temperance Workers Stormed Sifton and Thus Forced Him to Grant People Their Rights," *Edmonton Journal*, 26 May 1917, 9.

40   "To Ask Premier for a Separate Health Branch: Delegation of City Doctors Will Present Request to Government Officials," *Edmonton Journal*, 28 November 1917, 3. See also "Care of School Children Outlined in Report to Public by Medical Men," *Edmonton Journal*, 8 September 1917, 5 and "Alberta Doctors Want Department of Public Health," *Edmonton Journal*, 29 September 1917, 5.

41   "To Ask Premier for a Separate Health Branch," *Edmonton Journal*.

42   "As I Was Saying Today," *Edmonton Journal*, 4 January 1919, 9; "As I Was Saying Today," *Edmonton Journal*, 18 January 1919, 7.

43   "United Farm Women of Alberta Convention Program," *Edmonton Journal*, 21 January 1919, 17.

44   Bill No. 19, *An Act respecting the Department of Public Health* (Edmonton; J.W. Jeffery, King's Printer, A.D. 1919); "Separate Health Department, Public Hospital Changes Bill Introduced in Legislature," *Edmonton Journal*, 19 February 1919; "Loans Dangerous Remarks MacKay Over Seed Bills," *Edmonton Journal*, 27 February 1919, 16.

45   MacKay continued to serve as minister of municipal affairs during the initial stages of the Department of Public Health, thus holding two ministerial roles. Laidlaw began his term as provincial medical officer of health in 1912 and remained until 1914 when he was granted leave of absence to serve overseas. Upon return, Laidlaw served again as provincial medical officer of health and deputy minister. Bow and Cook, "Department of Public Health." Alberta Department of Public Health, *Annual Report 1919*. "Bill Regarding Establishment of Employment Agencies among Important Measures Taken Up," *Edmonton Bulletin*, 25 February 1919, 36.

46   *An Act respecting the Department of Public Health*, S.P.A. 1919, c. 16, assented to 17 April 1919.

47   *An Act respecting the Department of Public Health*, S.P.A. 1919.

48   Alberta Department of Public Health, *Annual Report 1920* (Edmonton: Printed by J.W. Jeffery, King's Printer, 1921); Alberta Department of Public Health, *Annual Report 1924* (Edmonton: Printed by W.D. McLean, Acting King's Printer, 1926); Alberta Department of Public Health, *Annual Report 1925* (Edmonton: Printed by W.D. McLean, Acting King's Printer, 1926); Alberta Department of Public Health, *Annual Report 1926* (Edmonton: Printed by W.D. McLean, Acting King's Printer, 1927); Alberta Department of Public Health, *Annual Report 1928–29* (Edmonton: Printed by W.D. McLean, King's Printer, 1930).

49   Other than Edmonton and Calgary, local boards of health at the time had medical practitioners who served the medical officer of health role in a part-time capacity, which was not always effective for several reasons: "The medical practitioner [of local boards in outlying areas] does not make a competent health officer for the reason that he has not the special training, and further, he is dependent upon the goodwill of the people for his livelihood, and any measures such as quarantine, prosecution for maintaining insanitary conditions and matters of this description, tend to injure his local practice." "Infectious Diseases Branch," Alberta Department of Public Health, *Annual Report 1924*, 7.

50   For a detailed analysis of the health units, see Adelaide Schartner, *Health Units of Alberta* (Edmonton: Health Unit Association of Alberta Co-Op Press, 1982).

51   *An Act to amend the Public Health Act*, P.S.A. 1929, c. 36, assented to March 20, 1929. Bow and Cook, "The Department of Public Health."

52   Carney, *Public Health*; Alberta Department of Public Health, *Annual Report 1931* (Edmonton: Printed by W.D. McLean, King's Printer, 1932).

53   Carney, *Public Health*, 23. By "earlier tradition," Carney was referring to the charitable support of the Grey Nuns who tended to the ill as part of their missionary work starting around 1860 in what was to become the province of Alberta.

54   Anne-Emanuelle Birn and Elizabeth Fee, "The Rockefeller Foundation and the International Health Agenda," *The Lancet* 381, Issue 9878 (2013); Anne-Emanuelle Birn, "Philanthrocapitalism, Past and

Present: The Rockefeller Foundation, the Gates Foundation, and the Setting(s) of the International/ global Health Agenda," *Hypothesis* 12, no. 1.

55   For example, the 1924 *Annual Report* of the Department of Public Health notes that only Edmonton and Calgary had full-time local medical officers of health at the time; "all other local boards employ[ed] a part-time man." Alberta Department of Public Health, *Annual Report 1924*, 7.

56   Specifically, as summarized by Lucas, the Edmonton Board of Health consisted in 1930 of "the mayor, medical officer of health, city engineer, and a member of the board of trustees from the Edmonton School Board and one from the Separate School Board, along with two aldermen and two medical practitioners qualified under Alberta law," and in 1936 of "the mayor, one member of the public school board, one member of the separate school board, two aldermen and two doctors." Lucas, "Historical Overview: Edmonton."

57   W.H. Hill, "Recording Child Hygiene Activities in Calgary," *Canadian Journal of Public Health* 36, no. 7 (July 1945). Dr. W.H. Hill was also the inaugural president of the Alberta Public Health Association.

58   Alberta Legislative Assembly, *Report of the Inquiry into Systems of State Medicine*, Sessional Paper No. 43, 1929 (Edmonton: W.D. McLean, King's Printer, 1929).

59   "Alberta Not Ready to Start Scheme of Health Insurance," *Edmonton Journal*, 25 February 1930, 11; "Cost Is Stumbling Block in State Medicine Scheme," *Edmonton Journal*, 28 February 1929, 13; T.B. Windross, "More Than One Thousand Lives Saved Annually by Alberta Health Services," *Calgary Herald*, 21 July 1934.

60   Alberta Legislative Assembly, Commission on State Medicine and Health Insurance, *Final Report of the Legislative Commission Appointed to Consider and Make Recommendations to the Next Session of the Legislature as to the Best Method of Making Adequate Medical and Health Services Available to All the People of Alberta* (Legislative Assembly of Alberta, 1934); "Contend 'State Medicine' Real Need in Province," *Edmonton Journal*, 4 March 1932; David Naylor, *Private Practice, Public Payment: Canadian Medicine and the Politics of Health Insurance, 1911–1966* (Kingston and Montreal: McGill-Queen's Press – MQUP, 1986), 54–6; "'State Medicine' Bill Introduced," *Edmonton Journal*, 19 March 1934.

61   Alberta Legislative Assembly, *Final Report of the Legislative Commission*, 10–11.

62   "Charity and Relief Branch," in Alberta Department of Public Health, *Annual Report 1926*, 25; Provincial Archives of Alberta, *Administrative History*, 285, 289.

63   Provincial Archives of Alberta, *Administrative History*, 285.

64   Provincial Archives of Alberta, *Administrative History*, 285.

65   James Muir, "Alberta Labour and Working-Class Life, 1940–1959," in *Working People in Alberta: a History*, Alvin Finkel et al. (Edmonton: AU Press, 2011).

66   Alvin Finkel, *Social Policy and Practice in Canada: A History* (Waterloo, ON: Wilfrid Laurier Press, 2006).

67   Several amendments to the *Public Health Act* during the 1930s and 1940s served to clarify and strengthen the legislative parameters of health districts and then health units (e.g., 1929, 1932, 1937, 1938, 1942, 1944, 1945, 1947, and 1949). These details were largely transferred to the Health Unit Act upon its creation in 1951 (An Act to provide for the Constitution and Establishment of Health Units ("The Health Unit Act"), S.P.A. 1951, c. 38). The Health Unit Act was repealed upon proclamation of the 1984 Public Health Act, which once again included a lengthy section on health units. *Public Health Act*, S.A. 1984, c. P-27.1, assented to 31 May 1984.

68   Predy, "A Brief History of Public Health in Alberta," 367; Alberta Department of Public Health, *Annual Report 1960* (Edmonton: Printed by L.S. Wall, Queen's Printer, 1962), 27.

69   Provincial Archives of Alberta, *Administrative History*, 285.

70   Muir, "Alberta Labour and Working-Class Life." See also J.C. Herbert Emery and Jesse A. Matheson, "Should Income Transfers be Targeted or Universal? Insights from Public Pension Influences on Elderly Mortality in Canada, 1921–1966," *The Canadian Journal of Economics* 45, no. 1 (2012).

71   Finkel, *Social Policy and Practice in Canada*.

72   Edward C. LeSage, "Introduction," in Provincial Archives of Alberta, *Administrative History, 1905–2005*.

73   Lucas, "Historical Overview: Calgary."

74   Lucas, "Historical Overview: Calgary."

75   Minister of Health and Welfare, *A New Perspective on the Health of Canadians — A Working Document* (Ottawa, ON: Minister of Health and Welfare, 1981); World Health Organization, "The Ottawa Charter for Health Promotion. First International Conference on Health Promotion, Ottawa, 21 November 1986," in *Health Promotion*, ed. World Health Organization (New York City: World Health

Organization, 1986), https://www.who.int/teams/health-promotion/enhanced-wellbeing/first-global-conference.

76   World Health Organization, "The Ottawa Charter for Health Promotion."

77   World Health Organization, "The Ottawa Charter for Health Promotion."

78   *An Act to Amend the Public Health Act*, S.A. 1971 (Bill 64), c. 87, assented to 27 April 1971.

79   Alberta. Legislative Assembly of Alberta, 6 April 1982; 23 April 1982; 19 March 1984; 6 April 1984. Note that versions of the proposed changes were discussed in the legislature in 1982, when Hon. Robert Bogle (PC), minister of social services and community health, introduced Bill 30: "The Public Health Amendment Act," which ultimately "was left to die on the Order Paper" (Alberta. Legislative Assembly of Alberta, 28 May 1984), only to be revived in 1984.

80   Alberta. Legislative Assembly of Alberta, 28 May 1984; "Lifestyle drift" describes a tendency for policy initiatives to tackle the social determinants of health to drift downstream towards individual lifestyle factors; it is a general trend of investing in individual behavioral interventions. See, for example, Gemma Carey at al., "Can the Sociology of Social Problems Help Us to Understand and Manage 'Lifestyle Drift'?" *Health Promotion International* 32, no. 4 (2017).

81   From 1910 until 1970, the legislated membership of the provincial board of health included the provincial medical officer of health (Chair), the provincial sanitary engineer, and the provincial bacteriologist. The membership shifted with a 1970 Public Health Act amendment to include the deputy minister as chair (the position of provincial medical officer of health was struck from the act in 1970); along with the Director of the Division of Environmental Health and the Director of the Provincial Laboratory. With the 1984 Act, there were no specified parameters of membership on the new provincial board.

82   References to the iconic book, *1984*, written in 1949 by English novelist George Orwell appeared in popular discourse, including David J. Lowe, "New law like '1984,'" letter, *Edmonton Journal*, 9 April 1984, and in the legislature; for example, Alberta. Legislative Assembly of Alberta, 8 May 1984 (John Gogo, PC).

83   Janet Vlieg, "Act Would Force Treatment," *Edmonton Journal*, 7 April 1984, 8; Roy Cook, "Should Doctors be Above the Law?" *Edmonton Journal*, 31 May 1984, 6.

84   Alberta's Bill of Rights followed the creation of various provincial offices during the 1960s and 1970s focused on fiduciary and human rights matters, such as the Office of the Ombudsman (est. 1967), the Office of the Auditor General (est. 1978) and the Office of the Chief Electoral Officer (est. 1977). Provincial Archives of Alberta, *Administrative History of Alberta, 1905–2005*. The Canadian "Bill of Rights" as a federal statute was passed in 1960 and twenty-two years later was enshrined in the Constitution.

85   Winston Gereluk, "Alberta Labour in the 1980s," in *Working People in Alberta: a History*, Alvin Finkel et al. (Edmonton: AU Press, 2011).

86   Rick Pedersen, "Public Health Act Criticized," *Edmonton Journal*, 15 May 1984, 12; Alberta. Legislative Assembly of Alberta, 29 May 1984 (Janet Koper, PC).

87   Alberta. Legislative Assembly of Alberta, 30 May 1984; 31 May 1984.

88   *Public Health Amendment Act*, S.A. 1998, c. 38; *Public Health Act*, R.S.A. 2000, c. P-37; *Public Health Amendment Act*, S.A. 2002, c. 38; *Public Health Amendment Act*, S.A. 2009, c. 13; *Public Health Amendment Act*, S.A. 2016, c. 25.

89   Ted Schrecker and Clare Bambra, *How Politics Makes Us Sick: Neoliberal Epidemics* (Basingstoke: Palgrave Macmillan, 2015); David Stuckler and Sanjay Basu, *The Body Economic: Why Austerity Kills* (Toronto: HarperCollins, 2013); Ronald Labonté and David Stuckler, "The Rise of Neoliberalism: How Bad Economics Imperils Health and What to Do about It," *Journal of Epidemiology and Community Health* 70 (2016).

90   Finkel, *Social Policy and Practice in Canada*.

91   John Church and Neale Smith, "Health Reform in Alberta: the Introduction of Health Regions," *Canadian Public Administration* 51, no. 2 (2008).

92   Gereluk, "Alberta Labour in the 1980s."

93   See for example Lee Parsons, "Canada: Alberta Premier Berates Homeless in Visit to Shelter," *World Socialist Web Site*, 22 December 2001, https://www.wsws.org/en/articles/2001/12/can-d22.html.

94   Jason Foster, "Revolution, Retrenchment, and the New Normal: The 1990s and Beyond," in *Working People in Alberta: a History*, Alvin Finkel et al. (Edmonton: AU Press, 2011).

95   Regionalization is not unique to Alberta. As stated by Karen Born et al, "Regionalization took place across Canada during the 1990s, transforming the way health care was governed and operated." Karen Born, Terrance Sullivan, and Robert Bear, "Restructuring Alberta's Health System," *Healthydebate*, 10 October 2013, http://healthydebate.ca/2013/10/topic/politics-of-health-care/restructuring-alberta-

health; John Church and Neale Smith, "Health Reform in Alberta: Fiscal Crisis, Political Leadership, and Institutional Change within a Single-party Democratic State," in *Paradigm Freeze: Why it Is so Hard to Reform Health-care Policy in Canada*, eds. Harvey Lazar et al. (Montreal & Kingston: McGill-Queen's University Press, 2013); Paul Barker and John Church, "Revisiting Health Regionalization in Canada: More Bark than Bite?" *International Journal of Health Services* 47, no. 2 (2016); Born, Sullivan, and Bear, "Restructuring Alberta's Health System;" Gregory P. Marchildon, *Health Systems in Transition: Canada*, 2nd ed. (Toronto: University of Toronto Press, 2013). *Regional Health Authorities Act*, S.A. 1994, c. R-9.07; Lucas, "Historical Overview: Calgary."

96   Lucas, "Historical Overview: Calgary."

97   See Rogelio Velez Mendoza, Kelsey Lucyk, Isabel Ciok, Lindsay McLaren, Frank Stahnisch, "The History of the Alberta Public Health Association" (narrative report produced for the Alberta Public Health Association) (Calgary, AB: Alberta Public Health Association, 2017), www.apha.ab.ca.

98   Kevin Taft, *Shredding the Public Interest: Ralph Klein and 25 Years of One-Party Government* (Edmonton: The University of Alberta Press and the Parkland Institute, 1997), 28–31.

99   "Home," Parkland Institute, accessed 4 May 2023, https://www.parklandinstitute.ca; Sarah Pratt, *Parkland Institute. 25 Years of Research and Education for the Common Good* (Edmonton: Parkland Institute, 2021), https://assets.nationbuilder.com/parklandinstitute/pages/1/attachments/original/1645306782/parkland-institute-25-years-research-and-education-for-the-common-good.pdf?1645306782.

100 Lucas, "Historical Overview: Calgary." For example: Born, Sullivan, and Bear, "Restructuring Alberta's Health System."

101 Graham Thomson, "Rachel Notley," *The Canadian Encyclopedia*, Historica Canada, last edited 6 September 2019, https://www.thecanadianencyclopedia.ca/en/article/rachel-notley.

102 Cristina Santamaria-Plaza, "Public Policy and Health: A Critical Public Health Analysis of Alberta's UCP Government Policy Agenda" (unpublished honour's thesis, Bachelor of Health Sciences Program, University of Calgary, 2020).

103 See for example Rutty and Sullivan, *This is Public Health.*

104 Jack Lucas, *Fields of Authority: Special Purpose Governance in Ontario, 1815-2015* (Toronto: University of Toronto Press, 2016); Jack Lucas, "Patterns of Urban Governance: a Sequence Analysis of Long-term Institutional Change in Six Canadian Cities," *Journal of Urban Affairs* 39, no. 1 (2017).

105 Lucas, "Patterns of Urban Governance".

NOTES TO TABLE 4.1

1   From 1930 to 1952, the Provincial Medical Officer is not specifically listed in the annual report; it is our best guest that either Dr. M.R. Bow (Deputy Minister) or Dr. A.C. McGugan (Director, Communicable Diseases Division), held or acted in this role during these years.

2   Alberta Department of Public Health, *Annual Report 1954* (Edmonton: Printed by A, Shnitka, Queen's Printer 1956), 10.

3   Albert Department of Public Health, *Annual Report 1955* (Edmonton: Printed by A. Shnitka, Queen's Printer, 1956), 2.

4   Albert Department of Public Health, *Annual Report 1956* (Edmonton: Printed by A. Shnitka, Queen's Printer, 1958), 2.

5   Albert Department of Public Health, *Annual Report 1957* (Edmonton: Printed by L.S. Wall, Queen's Printer, 1959), 2.

6   Albert Department of Public Health, *Annual Report 1958* (Edmonton: Printed by L.S. Wall, Queen's Printer, 1960), 2.

7   Albert Department of Public Health, *Annual Report 1959* (Edmonton: Printed by L.S. Wall, Queen's Printer, 1961), 2.

8   Alberta Department of Public Health, *Annual Report 1960* (Edmonton: Printed by L.S. Wall, Queen's Printer, 1962), 2.

9   Alberta Department of Public Health, *Annual Report 1961* (Edmonton: Printed by L.S. Wall, Printer to the Queen's Most Excellent Majesty, 1963), 2.

10   Alberta Department of Public Health, *Annual Report 1962* (Edmonton: Printed by L.S. Wall, Printer to the Queen's Most Excellent Majesty, 1964), 2.

11   Alberta Department of Public Health, *Annual Report 1963* (Edmonton: Printed by L.S. Wall, Printer to the Queen's Most Excellent Majesty, 1965), 2.

12   Alberta Department of Public Health, Annual Report 1964 (Edmonton: Printed by L.S. Wall, Printer to the Queen's Most Excellent Majesty, 1966), 2.

13   'N/A' – this was during the period when "Provincial Medical Officer of Health" was struck from the *Public Health Act*, and the Deputy Minister was to serve the role of Chair of the Provincial Board of Health. The 1984 amendment to the *Public Health Act* stated that the Minister may designate a physician employed by the Department to serve as a medical officer of health for the purpose of Part 4 of the Act (communicable diseases).

14   Chief Deputy Ministers of Social Services and Community Health. Stanley Mansbridge had the title of "Chief Deputy Minister," and the Deputy Ministers of Public Health (Dr. Jean Nelson and then Dr. Sheila Durkin) and of Social Services (David Stolee) both reported to him. Don Junk (ret'd), former Assistant Deputy Minister: Department of Social Services and Community Health, Policy and Planning (mid-October 1977 to 1 April 1981); Department of Social Services and Community Health, Rehabilitation Services (mid 1981); Department of Hospitals and Medical Care (late 1981 to 1988); Department of Health (approximately 1989 to June 1991), in discussion with the authors.

15   Dr. Jean Nelson was appointed acting deputy minister of Community Health and Social Development in 1974 and as deputy minister in 1975, making her the first woman to hold a deputy minister's appointment in Alberta. Dr. Nelson died on January 15, 1979. Lloyd C. Grisdale, "Concern for Children," *Canadian Medical Association Journal* 120, no. 10 (May 1979): 1276 and W. Helen Hunley "Dr. Jean Nelson: Courage and Spirit," *Canadian Medical Association Journal* 120, no. 10 (May 1979): 1276.

16   "Two Ontario Men Ill after Flue Shots," *Edmonton Journal*, 22 December 1976, 6.

17   David Stolee was the Deputy Minister of Social Services, within the Department of Social Services and Community Health. Don Junk, in discussion with the authors.

18   Deputy Ministers of Health Services

19   Don Junk, in discussion with the authors.

20   Deputy Ministers of Health Services

21   Dr. John Waters' obituary (Date of passing: 6 July 2001) stated "For the past 21 years he has been employed as the Provincial Health Officer, Alberta Health and Wellness." "John Robert Waters M.D. FRCP(C)," *Winnipeg Free Press*, 8 July 2001, https://passages.winnipegfreepress.com/passage-details/id-62201/John_Waters

22   Stanley H. Mansbridge, until approx. Feb 1981. Don Junk, in discussing with the authors.

23   David Stolee was Acting ADM until approximately July 1981. Don Junk, in discussing with the authors.

24   Deputy Ministers of Health Services

25   Deputy Ministers of Health Services

26   Deputy Ministers of Health Services

27   Deputy Ministers of Health Services

28   Deputy Ministers of Health Services

29   Deputy Minister of Community Health

30   Deputy Minister of Community Health

31   Keith Gerein, "Familiar Face Hired as Alberta's New Chief Medical Officer of Health," *Edmonton Journal*, updated 11 March 2016. According to this article, Dr. Grimsrud "served as the province's deputy medical officer of health for around a decade before being appointed as the acting chief in 2007. Her stint in that role lasted until the summer of 2008, when she and three other public health officials were told their contracts were not being renewed by Ed Stelmach's Progressive Conservative government."

32   Darcy Henton, "Looking for a New Top Health Officer: Dr. Nicholas Bayliss Steps Down," *Edmonton Sun*, 8 December 2006. According to this article, Dr. Bayliss "took the province's top health officer job in 2000" and "will be stepping down from his post March 31 [of 2007]."

33   "10 Calgarians Report Food Poisoning," *Calgary Herald*, 23 January 2002, 17.

34   "Mumps Vaccine Campaign on Hold," *Edmonton Journal*, 12 December 2007, 1

35   Associate Minister of Health

36   Associate Minister of Health

37   Associate Minister of Health

NOTES TO TABLE 4.2

1   Alberta Legislative Assembly, *Report of the Inquiry into Systems of State Medicine* (Edmonton: W.D. McLean, King's Printer, 1929), Sessional Paper No. 43, 1929.

2   Alberta Legislative Assembly, *Report of the Inquiry into Systems of State Medicine*, Abstract. Robert Lampard, *Alberta's Medical History: Young and Lusty, and Full of Life*. (Robert Lampard, 2008).

3   "Alberta Not Ready to Start Scheme of Health Insurance," *Edmonton Journal*, 25 February 1930, 11.

4   "Cost Is Stumbling Block in State Medicine Scheme," *Edmonton Journal*, 28 February 1929, 13; "More Than One Thousand Lives Saved Annually by Alberta Health Services," *Calgary Herald*, 21 July 1934.

5   Alberta Department of Public Health, *Annual Report 1930* (Edmonton: Printed by W.D. McLean, King's Printer, 1931); Alberta Department of Public Health, *Annual Report 1931* (Edmonton: Printed by W.D. McLean, King's Printer, 1932).

6   "Hon. George Hoadley Defends Policy of Importing British Women Doctors into Alberta," *Edmonton Journal*, 15 February 1929.

7   Malcolm R. Bow and F. T. Cook, "The History of the Department of Public Health of Alberta," *Canadian Public Health Journal*, 26, no. 8 (August 1935): 384–396.

8   *Special Legislative and Lay Committee Inquiring into Preventive Health Services in the Province of Alberta*. Report (Edmonton: The Committee, 1965).

9   The Committee met on March 6, 1930, Alberta Department of Public Health, *Annual Report 1930*, 7–8, https://librarysearch.assembly.ab.ca/client/en_CA/search/asset/47192/0

10   Alberta Department of Public Health, *Annual Report 1931*, 8.

11   Alberta Department of Public Health, *Annual Report 1932* (Edmonton: Printed by W.D. McLean, King's Printer, 1933), 8.

12   Alberta Department of Public Health, *Annual Report 1937* (Edmonton: Printed by A. Shnitka, King's Printer, 1938); Alberta Department of Public Health, *Annual Report 1938* (Edmonton: Printed by A. Shnitka, King's Printer, 1939).

13   Alberta Legislative Assembly, Commission on State Medicine and Health Insurance, *Final Report of the Legislative Commission Appointed to Consider and Make Recommendations to the Next Session of the Legislature as to the Best Method of Making Adequate Medical and Health Services Available to All the People of Alberta* (Legislative Assembly of Alberta, 1934).

14   "Contend 'State Medicine' Real Need in Province," *Edmonton Journal*, 4 March 1932); David Naylor, *Private Practice, Public Payment: Canadian Medicine and the Politics of Health Insurance, 1911–1966* (Kingston and Montreal: McGill-Queen's Press - MQUP, 1986), 54–56.

15   "'State Medicine' Bill Introduced," *Edmonton Journal*, 19 March, 1934, 1.

16   Alberta Legislative Assembly, *Final Report of the Legislative Commission*, 10–11.

17   Alberta Legislative Assembly, *Final Report of the Legislative Commission*, 24.

18   *Special Legislative and Lay Committee Inquiring into Preventive Health Services* (Edmonton, 1965)

19   *Special Legislative and Lay Committee Inquiring into Preventive Health Services*, xii.

20   "Committee Blasts Health Region Act," *Edmonton Journal*, 8 November 1968, 53; "A Bad Act," *Calgary Herald*, 11 November 1968, 4.

21   "Health Regions Plan Scrapped," *Calgary Herald*, 25 September 1969, 37.

22   Suggested in *Special Legislative and Lay Committee Inquiring into Preventive Health Services*, 69.

23   Premier's Commission on Future Health Care for Albertans, and Louis D. Hyndman, *The Rainbow Report: Our Vision for Health* (The Commission, 1989), accessed 3 June 2020, https://ia800309.us.archive.org/33/items/rainbowreportourprem/rainbowreportourprem.pdf

24   Gregory P. Marchildon, *Health Systems in Transition: Canada* (Toronto: University of Toronto Press, 2006), 109.

25   "Rainbow Report — Our Vision for Health," Making Medicare: The History of Medicare in Canada, 1914–2017, *Canadian Museum of History*, accessed 3 June 2020, www.historymuseum.ca/cmc/exhibitions/hist/medicare/medic-8g02e.html

26   Alberta Government, *Partners in Health: The Government of Alberta's response to the Premier's Commission on Future Health Care for Albertans*, November 1991, accessed 3 June 2020, https://archive.org/details/partnersinhealth00albe/page/n9

27   "B.C.'s Doctors' Medicine," *Edmonton Journal*, 15 November 15, A14.

28   "Health-care Report Skirts Funding: MD," *Red Deer Advocate*, 6 December 1991, A2.

29   *A Framework for Reform: Report of the Premier's Advisory Council on Health*, December 2001, http://www.assembly.ab.ca/lao/library/egovdocs/2001/alpm/132279.pdf

30   Open Government description of *A Framework for Reform: Report of the Premier's Advisory Council on Health*, accessed 3 June 2020, https://open.alberta.ca/publications/0778515478

31   "Critics Misrepresenting Report, Says Mazankowski," *Edmonton Journal*, 14 March 2002, 7.

32   Ak'ingabe Guyon, Trevor Hancock, Megan Kirk, Marjorie MacDonald, Cory Neudorf, Penny Sutcliffe, G. Watson-Creed, "The Weakening of Public Health: A Threat to Population Health and Health Care System," *Canadian Journal of Public Health* 108 no. 1 (2017): E1–E6.

5

The Non-Profit Sector: Trials and Tribulations of the Alberta Public Health Association

Rogelio Velez Mendoza and Lindsay McLaren

Introduction

Although substantive provincial legislation offering protection from second-hand tobacco smoke early 2000s, there were pressures from non-governmental organizations in the province as early as the 1970s. In 1978, one such organization — the Alberta Public Health Association — passed a resolution to urge the Government of Alberta to prohibit smoking in schools and in public places. This would be the first of more than twenty tobacco-related resolutions from the Alberta Public Health Association. In its role as a non-profit public health advocacy association, the Alberta Public Health Association has worked for decades to strengthen public health in Alberta. These efforts were almost always an exercise in persistence, they were sometimes to no avail, and they have been significantly eroded in recent years.

Public health, by definition, engages multiple societal sectors, including public/government; private; and civil, such as non-governmental organizations. In this chapter, the focus is non-governmental organizations, or the non-profit sector, in Alberta. The non-profit sector is characterized by its community-based and charitable approach to caring for problems facing society.[1] It can play a role in society by identifying and addressing issues that are not directly or adequately addressed by the private sector or the government. However, problems arise when essential services and supports, such as the provision of basic social and material resources, fall to this sector when it is not equipped to address them.[2]

The chapter begins by introducing the non-profit sector and its history in Alberta. Then, to illustrate the role and activities of that sector in public health, we examine one association in detail: the Alberta Public Health Association. We draw on findings from a study of the history of this organization for which we scanned the private archives as well as the Provincial Archives of Alberta for information on the activities of the Alberta Public Health Association since its foundation in 1943.[3] Our analysis focuses on resolutions passed by membership since its establishment, which present a consistently available marker of priorities and concerns. Although many groups and associations within the Alberta non-profit sector are relevant to advancing public health goals,[4] we focus on this organization for two main reasons: first, of the large number of non-profit associations in Alberta, this is the only one explicitly focused on public health. Second, the Alberta Public Health Association was established in 1943 and thus, compared to more recently established associations, permits some historical analysis.[5]

The Alberta Public Health Association has a history of active involvement in advocating for solutions to diverse public health concerns in Alberta. Showing some consistency with public sector activities, early Alberta Public Health Association priorities, such as protecting the interests of the public health workforce and advocating for regulation of food service establishments during the 1950s and 1960s, gave way to a focus on non-communicable disease prevention activities, such as smoking regulations, and on public policy to address social determinants of health. The organization's presence and level of activity ebbed and flowed in response to the broader economic, political, and health system contexts. This ebb and flow is informative for understanding the Alberta Public Health Association specifically, and the non-profit sector in Alberta more generally. This is especially true from a contemporary point of view when the organization, and some other public health associations across the country, appear to be at a historical low point in terms of capacity and impact.[6]

The Non-Profit Sector in Canada and Alberta

The non-profit sector in Canada is substantial. Measured by the size of its workforce (paid staff and volunteers) relative to the size of the country's economy, Canada's non-profit sector is proportionately second only to that of the Netherlands.[7] In 2015, Canada's non-profit sector consisted of over 161,000 organizations employing more than two million people.[8] Organizations range from small groups to larger institutions; examples are sports and recreation organizations, social service organizations, universities, and museums. To be considered part of the non-profit sector, an organization's functions must, to some extent, occur voluntarily; that is, the organization's membership is voluntary rather than required by law or as a condition of citizenship or profession, and some of the work is performed by individuals without pay.[9]

The size and nature of the contemporary non-profit sector is a product of a long tradition of charity and charitable organizations in Canada that must be situated within socio-political and colonial contexts. Since before Canadian confederation in 1867, major religious organizations have been involved in providing services such as education, health care, and recreation to their constituencies through their charitable organizations.[10] One example originated with the so-called three Grey Nuns who in 1863 established an orphanage in what is now the City of St. Albert, Alberta and they continue to be involved in health care.[11] More broadly, charitable associations started appearing in Canada in and around the late nineteenth and early twentieth century. Examples include the Red Cross, the Canadian Mental Health Association, and the Canadian National Institute for the Blind.[12] Following the creation of the province of Alberta in 1905, some national and international associations opened local branches; for example, the YWCA started providing shelter and support to women informally in 1907 and was incorporated in Calgary in 1910.[13]

The legal history of the non-profit sector in Alberta can be argued to have started in 1922 with the ascension of the Act respecting Benevolent and Other Societies ("The Benevolent Societies Act").[14] Under this act, a group of five or more persons could become incorporated for any benevolent, philanthropic, or charitable purpose but not for carrying on a trade or business. The act was expanded in 1924 as The Societies Act,[15] when being incorporated under the Societies Act became the first step for many Alberta organizations to secure formal non-profit status. These acts were designed to allow organizations incorporated as societies to receive donations and have members; at the same time, the act was intended to protect the public against false or illegitimate societies.[16] The Alberta Public Health Association registered under this act in 1955.[17]

In the context of population growth in Canada and Alberta at the beginning of the twentieth century, governments were increasingly pressured to strengthen state infrastructure to address circumstances such as poverty and unemployment, and to support citizens who were affected by the issues. Early examples of the latter in Alberta included the Children's Protection Act (1909), the Workmen's Compensation Act (1908) and the Mothers' Allowance Act (1919).[18] The First World War and the Great Depression of the 1930s provided further impetus for government to play a more active role in providing for the well-being of its citizens with legislation such as the Welfare of Children Act (1925), which among other things encouraged the formation of child welfare associations and aid societies; an Act to establish the Alberta Women's Bureau (1928), which aimed to improve social and educational conditions in communities; and an Act to create a Bureau of Relief and Public Welfare (1936) which was created to look after "transient indigents"[19] and to manage their treatment when sick.[20] Eventually, a provincial health care system was proposed by the Hoadley Commission in 1934; the proposal led to the Alberta Health Insurance Act of 1935,[21] which was the precursor of Alberta's participation in national Medicare beginning in 1969.[22]

Despite an evolving public sector, delivery of some services remained in the hands of non-profit organizations, although this changed over time with shifting economic and political climates. One early example in the health care context is the Victorian Order of Nurses, which established chapters in Edmonton and Calgary in 1909 and provided nursing to those otherwise unable to obtain those services.[23] From the early 1910s, the order delivered nursing services and baby clinics in Calgary to care for new babies and mothers. The Edmonton Branch of the order continued to provide nursing services for decades, working separately from but alongside public sector nurses, and later focusing their efforts on home nursing services.[24]

In later decades, government austerity led to situations where services that were previously partially or fully in the public sector, shifted to the non-profit sector. Two time periods illustrate this shift. The first is the economic downturn of the early 1980s. The decline in oil prices, prompted by international oil crises of the 1970s, had significant implications for Alberta's economy, which was — and is — heavily dependent on oil and gas. Alberta's Progressive Conservative Party governments, led by Peter Lougheed (1971–1985) and then Don Getty (1985–1992) increasingly relied on the non-profit sector to fill gaps in public infrastructure.[25] For example, in the late 1970s, non-profit food banks opened across Alberta, first in major cities and later in smaller communities. Food banks were not intended to replace or supplement public sector programs such as income supports, but in light of gaps in those supports, demand for and reliance on food banks grew.[26] Social worker and historian Baldwin Reichwein noted that gradually, "well-intentioned voluntary responses to poverty conditions led to a volunteer-driven and quasi-public welfare system as a supplementation of governments' public welfare programs."[27] This is an example of a subtle shift in sectoral responsibility that would have significant, and enduring, implications for Albertans' health and well-being.

A second example occurred during the 1990s. Between 1992 and 1999, there were significant and ideologically driven reductions in government program spending across Canada.[28] In Alberta, these cuts took place under conservative Premier Ralph Klein, whose term began in 1992 following a political campaign focused heavily on reducing public debt that had accumulated since 1986.[29] Klein misleadingly framed Alberta's dire economic situation as a problem emanating from too much government spending, particularly on health care.[30] In a strong embodiment of neoliberalism, his government's remedy included significant spending cuts to public services and bureaucratic reforms under the guise of increasing administrative efficiency and accountability. Between the 1992/93 and 1995/96 fiscal years, the Klein government reduced the real per capita funding to provincial ministries by approximately 13 percent for education, 16 percent for health care, and 28 percent for family and social services.[31] At the same time, they lowered corporate taxes, thus reducing revenue for public services, and they privatized services; for example, the 1995 Action Plan for Social Services allowed Child and Family Services regional authorities to contract with private providers for service delivery.[32]

This "Klein Revolution" strongly impacted the non-profit sector and its place in Alberta society. With cuts to public services, unmet social needs increasingly fell to non-profit organizations and individuals and families, which in turn faced new challenges and less support. New contracts between government and the non-profit sector, previously designed to support the day-to-day operation and activities of organizations, now included complex and time-consuming accountability requirements, which were not always feasible, especially for small organizations. Further, provincial funding was contained to short-term projects, which hindered the long-term planning capacity of such organizations. According to Harrison and Weber, "the non-profit sector through this time lacked sustainable and long-term funding — an unfortunate legacy that survives today."[33]

Collectively, these circumstances set the stage for a contemporary non-profit sector in Alberta characterized by a very large number of organizations working to provide important public functions but with restricted capacity. Additionally, their activities are often poorly, or not at all, coordinated, thus contributing to duplication of efforts and competition for limited funds. As of 2015, there were 24,800 non-profit organizations in Alberta, and the number appears to be increasing.[34] Only 43 percent of non-profit organizations in Alberta employed staff in 2015, while the remainder were run entirely by volunteers, which itself presents considerable constraints around achieving objectives.[35] The largest category of non-profit organizations in Alberta in 2011, representing 38 percent of all non-profit organizations in the province, were those classified as "social services," including child welfare, child services and day care, youth services and youth welfare, family services, services for handicapped and elderly persons, temporary shelters, and disaster/emergency prevention and control, among others.[36] It was the provincial Ministry of Family and Social Services that experienced the largest proportionate funding cuts during the 1990s. The proliferation of non-profit organizations in family and social service domains is no coincidence: it speaks to a negative legacy of those cuts, and of a shift from public to non-profit sector responsibility more generally.

Following "social service," the second largest non-profit sector category in Alberta is arts and culture (12 percent), followed by religious organizations (8 percent), and then health (6 percent),[37] which includes our focal example of the Alberta Public Health Association.[38]

Spotlight: The Alberta Public Health Association

The Alberta Public Health Association was established in 1943, when the province was shifting from economically depressed conditions toward an increasingly urbanized and industrialized society. Several health professional associations came together with the aim to help coordinate health services and strengthen public health.[39] Upon its creation, the Alberta Public Health Association was, and continues to be, primarily a professional organization governed by a voluntary board that is elected by the membership. Regular board meetings and the Annual General Meetings included presentation of reports from the organization's sections or subcommittees, which changed over time but included, at one point or another, sections focused on public health professional groups, including nurses and sanitary inspectors, and topics, including environmental health, epidemiology, family health, and health promotion.[40]

Methods

One way to depict the activities of the organization over time is to examine the association's resolutions. Resolutions constitute an explicit marker of members' priorities and concerns, and they are available for the association's entire history.[41] As mechanisms of association action, resolutions may also provide insight into the presence and impact of one non-profit association in a broader public health context.

Here we present the findings from our analysis of the collection of the Alberta Public Health Association's resolutions, from 1944 to 2017 (n=443 in total), which we coded and organized based on their alignment with core public health functions as described by the Public Health Agency of Canada.[42] Public health functions include health promotion, health protection, disease and injury prevention, health surveillance, and emergency preparedness. To fully capture the breadth of the resolutions, we added four categories: social determinants of health; public health workforce; association-related (e.g., resolutions related to board governance) and other. Our coding category definitions, which we established and finalized through an iterative process,[43] are shown in Table 5.1 (See page 155).

Findings

The trends over time in the content of member resolutions provide an indication of shifts in their attention to and levels of activity in the categories. We first present broad trends from 1944 to 2017, and then we consider and historically contextualize each decade in more detail.

Figure 5.1 shows the content of the Alberta Public Health Association's resolutions from 1944 to 2017.

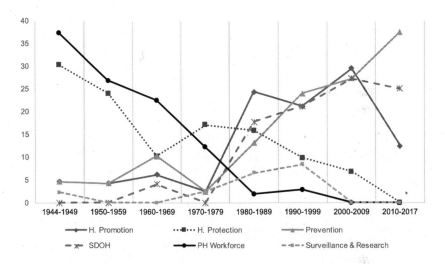

Fig. 5.1: Resolutions carried by the Alberta Public Health Association, 1944–2017, organized according to their alignment with key public health domains (described in Table 5.1), expressed as a percent of total resolutions by decade. Note: two time periods (1944–1949, and 2010–2017) are partial decades.

As seen in Figure 5.1, resolutions related to the public health workforce (solid black line, circle marker) were prevalent early in the Alberta Public Health Association's history, especially the 1940s, but declined steadily thereafter, ultimately almost disappearing. Resolutions focused on health protection activities (dotted line, square marker) also featured prominently during the organization's earliest years, and likewise declined over the course of the association's history, albeit more gradually. In contrast, resolutions focused on disease and injury prevention (grey solid line, triangle marker), health promotion (dark grey line, diamond marker) and social determinants of health (grey dashed line, X marker) were relatively scarce during the 1940s–1970s but showed a notable increase during the 1980s. Overall, and consistent with trends in public health observed elsewhere,[44] a growing focus on resolutions with a focus on root causes of health problems is apparent over time.[45]

1940s: The Alberta Public Health Association – An Association for the Public Health Workforce

Nursing and medical services in Alberta expanded rapidly during the 1940s, with the creation of health units, mental institutions, sanatoriums, and hospitals, and other infrastructure, especially as part of the post-WWII infrastructure expansions.[46] Of particular importance to public health, rural nursing expanded during the 1940s and 1950s. Rural nurses were responsible for providing many public health services to Albertans, such as physical examinations and vaccinations.[47]

In its first year, the Alberta Public Health Association included members who worked in health-related settings, including provincial and municipal departments, divisions, and boards of health.[48] W.H. Hill, a physician, was elected the first president of the organization in 1943, followed by public health nurse, Ms. Helen G. McArthur in 1944 (see Chapter 13).[49] The resolutions show that proposals and requests were made to the provincial government to improve working conditions for the public health workforce; almost 40 percent of the resolutions passed during the 1940s were related to the workforce. These resolutions included, for example, requests to improve salaries and pensions for public health professionals, increase the number of staff in health units, and provide education for public health workers.[50]

The second main preoccupation of the Alberta Public Health Association during the 1940s, was processes and legislation to improve sanitary conditions for Albertans. These resolutions covered issues like milk packaging, regulations on commercial activities, and food handling and service establishment practices.[51] For example, in a 1946 resolution, the organization expressed concern that there were not limits on who could open a restaurant or bakeshop and advocated for a provincial regulation stipulating that the opening of such an establishment would require written permission from the local board of health.[52]

During the 1940s, two long-serving leaders in the provincial Department of Public Health — Dr. Wallace Warren Cross, minister of public health from 1935 to 1957, and Dr. Malcolm Ross Bow, deputy minister of public health from 1927 to 1952 (see Chapter 13) — were active members of the Alberta Public Health Association. Bow, for example, delivered a presentation at the inaugural annual general meeting, titled "Hopes for the Future of Public Health in Alberta,"[53] and was listed as a working member of the organization in a 1945 association directory.[54] In 1948, Bow once again presented at the annual general meeting, this time about provincial trends in polio incidence and the new Dominion Health Grants, which provided support for professional public health training and provincial public health initiatives, such as efforts to prevent and control tuberculosis, venereal disease, and cancer.[55] Also in 1948, the organization passed a resolution to consider setting up a mental health section, and in so doing, to seek support and approval of such a section from Bow, then deputy minister of health, along with the director of the Mental Health Division of the Department of Public Health, Dr. R.R. MacLean.[56] Overall, the Alberta Public Health Association seemed to have a presence in, and a good working relationship with, provincial governmental public health during the 1940s.

1950s: Continued Emphasis on the Workforce and Health Protection

The organization continued to maintain a relationship with the provincial Department of Public Health in the 1950s; for example, Health Minister Cross attended and delivered greetings at the association's annual meeting in 1954, and he spoke about the importance of health education and public relations in 1956.[57] However, there are indications that the Alberta Public Health Association desired a greater voice in provincial public health matters. In a 1950 resolution, they expressed disappointment at not having been invited by the provincial government "to express their group opinion in convention regarding important public health matters as distribution of federal health grants, proposed changes in the size of Rural Health Units, etc."[58] In this resolution, which was intended to be forwarded to Premier Manning and to Dr. Cross, the members lamented that "not only is this exclusion [of the Alberta Public Health Association] from such useful cooperation discouraging to the public health workers of the province, but also that the government is failing to take advantage of the aggregate opinion of the group whose intimate proximity to the public health problems of our people best equip them to interpret such problems to the Provincial Government."[59] To the extent that the organization was left out of discussions concerning health matters in the province, perhaps this is one illustration of the shift toward an increasingly downstream and diffuse meaning of "public health" in the 1950s, discussed in Chapter 2.

The two main concerns of the 1940s — the public health workforce and health protection — continued to be prominent during the 1950s (Figure 5.1). Of the forty-eight non-association-related resolutions passed during the 1950s, thirty-six (75 percent) focused on those two issues. Concerning workforce issues, the Alberta Public Health Association advocated for issues affecting nurses, such as the need for training and uniforms, and access to educational materials.[60] These ongoing preoccupations were reflected in the content of the *Alberta Health Worker* — a publication created in 1941 by public health workers in Alberta, which became the official publication of the organization in 1949 — consisting of articles written by and targeted to nurses, sanitary inspectors, and other public health professionals in the province.[61] Early issues of the *Worker* included articles on the organization and legislation of public health in Alberta, the topic of undulant fever in the province's cattle industry, provincial dairy regulations, methods of dealing with bedbugs in rural areas, and removing the high mineral content in water in Edmonton.[62]

1960s: New Social Concerns

Beginning in the 1960s, Alberta experienced a period of economic growth, facilitated by booms in the energy and construction industries.[63] The populations of Alberta's cities grew. While Alberta remained politically conservative throughout the 1960s, 1970s, and 1980s, social change movements that were occurring across North America and western Europe influenced the younger generations of Albertans who now comprised the workforce and voting majority.[64] Social movements in support of feminism, environmentalism, anti-racism, LGBTQ2S+ rights, and human rights took hold in the province throughout the 1960s and 1970s.[65]

As early as 1964, and reflecting changing social attitudes, the Alberta Public Health Association held a panel on sex education at its annual convention.[66] The 1967 convention in Edmonton featured a panel presentation on abortions and abortion law reform in recognition and support of women's reproductive rights.[67] Environmental concerns also began to permeate the organization's priorities starting in the 1960s; for example, in 1965 there was a panel on air and water pollution.[68]

The administrative relationship between social welfare and health that was in place in government during this period (see Chapter 12) is apparent in the Alberta Public Health Association activities,[69] which makes sense considering that many members — such as public health nurses, physicians, and dentists working in health units in rural areas — worked directly with communities and would have observed the importance of social factors, such as income and housing, for health and well-being. In 1964, in what may be an illustration of "health imperialism" (top-down directive by the health sector), the members passed a resolution to advocate to the provincial Department of Welfare for the boundaries of welfare officers' jurisdictions to align with the health unit boundaries and for the offices of the two agencies to be located in the same building to facilitate greater collaboration.[70] However, a 1967 resolution highlighted encroachment of the Department of Welfare into the responsibilities of the Department of Health, and suggested that a committee be formed to "investigate this problem."[71] That resolution, however, was defeated.[72]

1970s: Growing Focus on Advocacy

In 1971, the Alberta Public Health Association declared that "the objects of the Association shall be to promote community health in all its aspects and to maintain an affiliation with the Canadian Public Health Association."[73] With this, the organization appears to have formalized a shift from a professional association primarily focused on serving the needs of public health workforce members, to an advocacy association that voiced a broader array of concerns in the interest of the public's health. This shift is implicitly represented in the meeting minutes of the association throughout the 1970s and is also conveyed through the shifting nature of resolutions: the 1970s is the decade during which, for the first time, resolutions focused on the public health workforce were not the most common.[74]

During the 1970s, the organization embraced a partnership approach, aiming to bring together multiple organizations around shared concerns. At the 1979 annual general meeting, for example, psychologist and later president, Helen Simmons, recommended "that [the Alberta Public Health Association] take a proactive stand on identifying significant health issues and elicit other voluntary health organizations and address them from a position of taking concerted action."[75] This constitutes an early example of a coalition or collective impact approach, which involves "bring[ing] people together, in a structured way, to achieve social change."[76]

Alberta Public Health Association priorities evolved alongside important evolutions in public health more broadly, specifically a shift toward health promotion. Resolutions about health promotion, that is, the process of enabling people to increase their control over and to improve their health,[77] started to increase in number during the 1970s, likely prompted in part by the introduction of the *Lalonde Report* in 1974, which drew explicit attention to determinants of health beyond human biology and the health care system.[78] However, although health promotion encompassed a broad range of actions, including building healthy public policy, creating supportive environments, strengthening community actions, developing personal skills, and reorienting health services, our analysis suggests that some of these actions were given more attention than others.[79]

Specifically, an emphasis on promoting healthy lifestyles was prominent at the organization's annual conventions in the late 1970s. One example is the 1977 convention in Calgary, for which the conference theme was "Lifestyles."[80] The next year, in Red Deer, presentations included health promotion-inspired topics such as, "The Health Service's Main Motives for Prevention," "A Cost-Benefit Approach to Investing in Occupational Health Programs," and "Improvement to Employee Fitness."[81] This tendency of the organization to privilege certain elements of health promotion, that is, those focused on lifestyles and health services, over others such as empowering communities and advocating for health-promoting policy, is consistent with critical scholarship on how health promotion has been taken up in the Canadian context.[82]

Alongside an increasing focus of the Alberta Public Health Association resolutions on health promotion during the 1970s was a decreasing focus on traditional health protection strategies. One important exception, however, was milk pasteurization, which continued to be a focus of their resolutions. According to the provincial Public Health Act at the time, a plebiscite was required for municipalities to enact pasteurization bylaws.[83] In a 1971 resolution, members entertained a proposal to remove the plebiscite requirement, which would facilitate the local implementation of pasteurization.[84] The resolution did not pass the first time but was later carried on 6 April 1973.[85] Illustrative of their presence in provincial public health matters, the resolution was referenced in the Alberta legislature on April 10 of that year,[86] and in May 1973 the Public Health Act was amended to permit municipal councils to pass a pasteurization bylaw without a plebiscite.[87]

Despite some growing attention to social determinants elsewhere in the country, including a federally funded field experiment of a guaranteed annual income in Dauphin, Manitoba (1974– 1979),[88] the Alberta Public Health Association resolutions around poverty and income inequality were limited and were, in fact, absent during the 1970s, perhaps reflecting challenges both specific to Alberta (e.g., politically conservative context) and general to public health (e.g., lifestyle drift, as it was later named[89]). Attention to social determinants of health in the Alberta Public Health Association re-appeared during the late 1980s and figured prominently in the association's concerns during the early 2000s.

1980s: Health Promotion and New Interest in Social Determinants of Health

The 1980s was by far the most active decade in the Alberta Public Health Association's history, as indicated by the size of the membership and the number of resolutions passed. During the 1980s, 107 resolutions were carried, and in 1985, membership reached the highest point in its history with approximately 450 members.

At the beginning of the decade, the organization put forward its goals in a 1981 document that outlined their intentions, which included to develop a unifying vision of health, to be an acknowledged representative of the health interests of Albertans, to monitor social, political, economic and environmental circumstances, and to be an effective liaison with government and other groups.[90] This decade also appears to have been a period where partnerships and engagement with members were strong, as evident in the pages of the newsletter, *The Promoter*, which was published three or four times a year.[91]

This active decade coincided with challenging economic circumstances, including high unemployment rates in the province. When assuming the organization's presidency in 1982, Gerry Predy pointed out how rising unemployment, high interest rates and inflation were detrimental to public health practice (if not quite yet drawing the connection between those factors and the public's health), remarking that "health and social programs [had to] struggle to compete for scarce financial resources."[92] For the organization to be effective in its role, it needed to link "professional and technical competence to political and social action."[93] Predy later proposed a change in the organization's statement of philosophy, with the new version asserting that health be considered "an integral part of the social, political, economic, ecologic whole." For that reason, according to Predy, the Alberta Public Health Association should be an association that worked within that complexity, using a variety of approaches.[94]

This change in philosophy was reflected in the number and breadth of resolutions passed during the 1980s. While the largest proportion of resolutions during the 1980s was coded as health promotion (n=24, 22 percent of all resolutions during the 1980s), other categories were not far behind. The association's earlier focus on health protection continued to be a priority with seventeen resolutions (16 percent of all 1980s resolutions), but by this time health protection resolutions had expanded beyond food and beverage safety to include issues such as the regulation of landfills, transportation of dangerous goods, indoor air quality, and herbicide and pesticide containers, among others.[95]

The number of resolutions concerned with the social determinants of health also increased, totalling nineteen (18 percent of all resolutions during the 1980s). These resolutions were broad in scope, and included poverty, working conditions, child care, language and cultural barriers to health, and nuclear missile testing.[96] For example, in a 1988 resolution, the organization sought "public health action on inequities," based on knowledge of links between poverty and health, and identified a need for an inequities working group to support and inform 1989 conference planning.[97] The number of resolutions focused on disease and injury prevention also started to increase during the 1980s, with topics such as immunization, automatic daytime vehicle headlights, and mandatory seatbelts.

Although the organization's first resolution regarding tobacco was carried in 1978, the 1980s was the decade during which the association accelerated its involvement in tobacco control activities. Anti-tobacco efforts in Alberta strengthened during the 1980s with the formation of coalitions, such as the Alberta Interagency Council on Smoking and Health, of which the Alberta Public Health Association was a member.[98] The Alberta Public Health Association also participated as one of many members in the provincial Tobacco Reduction Alliance. Embracing the multi-pronged approach adopted by its partners, the organization carried resolutions that addressed various aspects of tobacco control including prohibiting advertising, promotion, and tobacco company sponsorship; banning smoking from indoor public places; and restrictions on the sale of tobacco products to minors.[99] As discussed in Chapter 9, these activities ultimately led to important, albeit not uncontroversial, advances in tobacco control in Alberta.

1990s: Partnerships, Tobacco, and Declining Membership

The 1990s opened with a convention in Calgary that prompted the organization to review its mission and plan for the next year. A membership survey confirmed members' views that the most important function of the organization was to advocate for public health.[100] A theme that permeates the Alberta Public Health Association's archival materials from the 1990s was the need to expand the membership to permit the organization to be a more effective voice in the province. In 1991, the number of members totalled 344, which was lower than the association's peak of 450 in 1985, but still high relative to its history overall (see Figure 5.2). Of the 344 members in 1991, approximately half were health unit employees, while the rest included university and government employees, and some students. The most represented profession was nurses, including community health nurses. Despite many efforts, the organization did not meet their stated goal of having 500 members by 1993, the fiftieth anniversary of the association; in fact, by March of that year, membership had declined to 289.[101]

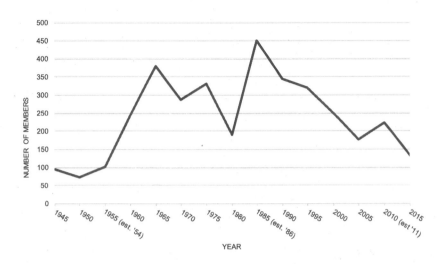

Fig. 5.2: Size of the Alberta Public Health Association membership, 1945–2015. Sources: Minutes from the Alberta Public Health Association's Annual General Meetings and annual reports.

Considering that members were largely public health workers within the health care system, it is not surprising that health care system reform — specifically regionalization of the provincial health care system — was a preoccupation of the organization during the 1990s; archival materials indicate that core committees even reduced their other work to concentrate on regionalization. In August of 1992, in the context of discussions around reforms, Alberta's Minister of Health, Nancy J. Betkowski, approached the organization to request that they outline what they saw as priorities and challenges to public health. The association's response was threefold: i) the need for continued action including the achievement of provincial health goals, objectives and actions; ii) the need to position public health within the reform process, along with education of politicians and the public to understand the contributions and key role public health plays in the health system; and iii) the need for sustained funding to carry out the organization's work, which included a request for a sustaining grant.

In the 1993/94 annual report, President Pearl Upshall stated that members could be proud of the association's input into the provincial government report, *Health Goals for Alberta: A Progress Report*. Speaking about the report, which was a compilation of all suggestions from community workshops and roundtables held by the Ministry of Health around the province, Upshall commented that, "the content of this and other health reform documents are full of public health."[102] However, Alberta's health system reforms in the 1990s, including the Klein government's 1994 passing of the Regional Health Authorities Act, entailed major structural changes. For the Alberta Public Health Association, it meant rethinking its previous ways of gaining members because the health units, abolished with the 1994 Health Authorities Act, were previously a main source of membership. The organization also lost an important partner with the abolishment of the Health Unit Association of Alberta.[103]

In 1995, the organization was distinguished as one of the few provincial organizations funded by the National Literacy Secretariat to discover how health could improve when literacy levels were strengthened. An important outcome of the organization's Partnership Project on Literacy and Health was an increase in awareness of intersectoral connections between literacy and health among various organizations.[104] A booklet on the relationship between literacy and health, titled *Health for All Albertans*, which was designed to serve as both a fact sheet and a discussion paper, was produced and distributed to partner organizations and to MLAs. Illustrative of the organization's governmental presence at the time, the booklet elicited fifteen responses from MLAs, one of whom tabled the booklet as a report submitted to the Legislative Assembly of Alberta, as noted in the *Hansard*.[105]

Within the context of the "Klein Revolution" and its damaging effects on the public sector and thus the public's health, the 1990s was characterized by a multi-pronged approach by the Alberta Public Health Association. Among resolutions carried during that decade, those focused on health promotion, disease and injury prevention, and social determinants of health were most common (Figure 5.1). Regarding disease and injury prevention, resolutions focused on tobacco reduction efforts continued, and nearing the end of the decade, resolutions revealed additional important partnerships with organizations such as Action on Smoking and Health (see Chapter 13).[106]

2000–Present: Loss of Funding, Struggling to Survive

The new millennium started with comprehensive efforts by the Alberta Public Health Association to examine strengths and weaknesses in public health in general, and of the organization in particular. The Millennium Project was undertaken; as outlined in the project's final report, *Public Health in Alberta: Showcasing our Past; Creating our Future*, this project featured public health initiatives selected from submissions solicited from health authorities across the province. The association expected that this initiative, which concluded in fall of 2001, would raise the profile of public health and offer an opportunity to re-establish connections around the province, which were felt to have been severed by regionalization. As part of phase two of the project, over two hundred people from around the province were involved in discussions through focus groups, interviews, meetings, and at the organization's 2001 annual convention. The result was *Public Health in Alberta: A Proposal for Action*, a publication targeted to both lay audiences and policy-makers that aimed to strengthen public health moving forward. According to the 2001 annual report, the Minister of Health & Wellness, Gary Mar, commended the report and noted that his ministry was committed to working closely with the Alberta Public Health Association.[107]

The Ministry of Health & Wellness contributed annual funding to the organization, including $75,000 in 2004,[108] $75,000 in 2007, and $79,000 in 2008.[109] This Ministry funding was essential to stabilizing the association.[110] Then, however, the funds were cut suddenly. In January 2009, the Alberta Public Health Association had understood that their annual ministry funding would be frozen at $100,000 for 2009/10. Yet, in February 2009, the organization learned that this funding would be cut completely, effective that year.[111] Not surprisingly, the loss put the association in a difficult situation with respect to maintaining existing operations, which was further compounded by discontinued website support from a neighbouring public health association.[112] Once the funding notice was received, the organization undertook efforts to evaluate their financial situation and future direction. They also reached out to other sources of funding, with little success.[113]

Alberta Public Health Association continued its work to the extent possible, relying entirely on volunteer time and capacity. Some key recent achievements have been possible through collaborations coupled with in-kind support from board members' workplaces and external sources of funding. Examples include the Alberta Public Health Association History Project, which was funded by a grant from the Alberta Historical Resources Foundation;[114] and two events that were co-hosted by the Alberta Public Health Association and the O'Brien Institute for Public Health at the University of Calgary: a 2018 provincial forum on the theme of "In Defense of Public Health,"[115] in recognition of the Alberta Public Health Association's seventy-fifth anniversary; and a 2019 all-candidates forum on public health, held in advance of the provincial election that year and intended in part to strengthen the organization's role as an advocacy association for public health in the province.[116] Although the number of resolutions per year decreased during the first decades of the twenty-first century, the organization has continued to carry resolutions and otherwise engage in key issues, many of which are related to the social determinants of health, including resolutions on provincial income support programs, food security, and affordable housing, including — in collaboration with First Nation organizations — housing for Indigenous communities.[117]

Conclusion

As highlighted here, the Alberta Public Health Association has a noteworthy history when one considers the scope and tenacity of its efforts. Alberta Public Health Association has been one key player in Alberta's public health history, both reflecting and shaping — often in partnership — the provincial public health landscape. It has done so largely by convening professionals, with relatively fewer examples of engaging with communities ("the public" in public health). The association's voice was not always heard, and in recent years it has struggled to maintain its membership and capacity. Indeed, when considered relative to its history, the organization's capacity and impact has declined considerably in a relatively short period of time. As such, it stands as one example of challenges facing organizations in the non-profit sector more generally.

Non-profit associations in general, and public health associations in particular,[118] are uniquely positioned to serve as a hub to unite public health communities, including diverse professionals and members of publics, in mobilizing as a collective toward strengthening population well-being and health equity, via various forms of advocacy including representational (e.g., strategies for "selling" public health goals to decision makers and to the broader public) and facilitational (e.g., a more democratic approach to advocacy that centres on listening to and working with communities whose voices are under-represented in research and policy debates) forms.[119] From that perspective, the formidable challenges facing the Alberta Public Health Association and some other public health associations across the country are unfortunate. The challenge remains for public health associations to attract and engage members and to build capacity — including via alignment with partners, allies, and communities — to realize the role and vision that they are so well positioned to hold.

TABLE 5.1: Categories used to code the Alberta Public Health Association resolutions based on core public health functions and adapted to cover the breadth of their resolutions.

Code	Description	Examples
Health Promotion	Health promotion contributes to and shades into disease prevention (see below) by catalyzing healthier and safer behaviours. Comprehensive approaches to health promotion may involve community development or policy advocacy and action regarding environmental and socioeconomic determinants of health and illness.	Intersectoral community partnerships to solve health problems; advocacy for healthy public policies; health education; catalyzing the creation of physical and social environments to support health (e.g., bike paths, promoting access to social networks for institutionalized seniors).
Health Protection	Efforts to ensure safe food and water, including the regulatory framework for control of infectious diseases and protection from environmental threats. Health protection efforts often aim to protect others; for example, breathalyzer laws.	Restaurant inspections; institutional facility inspections (e.g., Foster Home Training & Home Investigation); water treatment monitoring; air quality monitoring/enforcement; quarantine. Also includes provision of expert advice to national regulators of food and drug safety.
Disease & Injury Prevention	Measures to prevent the occurrence of disease and injury, and to arrest the progress and reduce the consequences of disease or injury once established. It overlaps with health promotion, especially as regards educational programs targeting safer and healthier lifestyles.	Immunization; investigation and outbreak control; efforts to prevent behaviors deemed unhealthy or unsafe (e.g., not wearing a bicycle helmet); screening and early detection of cancer; availability of prophylactic drugs; warning labels on products.
Health Surveillance & Academic research*	Surveillance: "information for action" – gathering of information to permit early recognition of outbreaks, disease trends, and health factors which in turn inform policy and program intervention. Academic research is defined as organized and methodic efforts to produce knowledge related to people's health.	Periodic health surveys; Cancer and other disease registries; Communicable disease reporting; Ongoing analysis of data to identify trends or emerging problems, (e.g., recognition of increasing syphilis cases); Report to practitioners of increasing threat, what they need to look for, and intervention required.
Emergency Preparedness and Response	Activities that provide the capacity to respond to acute harmful events that range from natural disasters to infectious disease outbreaks and chemical spills. Often inter-jurisdictional.	Responses to environmental disasters such as floods, avalanches, or biological events like disease outbreaks, etc.

TABLE 5.1: *(continued)*

Code	Description	Examples
Social Determinants of Health	The social determinants of health and health inequities are conditions in which people are born, grow, live, and work, which are shaped by the distribution of money, power and resources. Include but are not limited to: income, education, gender and other axes of social stratification such as race/ethnicity and disability (and associated forms of exclusion e.g., racism, sexism), physical environment, social environment, and healthy childhood development (including child care)	Advocacy for guaranteed income; literacy and health; relations between culture and health; efforts to reduce poverty and inequality.
Public Health Workforce	Related to availability of jobs, training, creation of new positions, workplace conditions and compensation.	Public health workforce salaries negotiation; improving working conditions and availability of supplies
Association-Related	Related to APHA internal work and management, including the role/function of the organization.	Change of bylaws, change of name of purpose. Administrative changes (e.g. hiring new staff)
Other Aspects of Public Health	Other, non-specific aspects of public health.	

* Recognizing that they are distinct, resolutions are coded related to academic research along with health surveillance because i) both concepts contribute to understanding the impacts of efforts to improve health and reduce the impact of disease in a systematic manner, and ii) the number of resolutions in both categories was relatively small.

NOTES

1   Trevor Harrison and Barret Weber, *Neoliberalism and the Non-Profit Social Services Sector in Alberta* (Edmonton: Parkland Institute, 2015), 6.

2   Harrison and Weber, *Neoliberalism*, 13, 16, 36–37.

3   Alberta Historical Resources Foundation - Heritage Preservation Partnership Program research grant, 2015-2018, "Public health advocacy: lessons learned from the history of the Alberta Public Health Association," (McLaren L, Lucyk K, Stahnisch F). Results from this project include a narrative history of the association (Rogelio Velez Mendoza et al., *The History of the Alberta Public Health Association*, Calgary: APHA, 2017), a complete list of association presidents, and a complete list of resolutions. These are available on the APHA website: https://www.apha.ab.ca/public-health-resources

4   Two of many examples are the Alberta Policy Coalition for Chronic Disease Prevention (https://abpolicycoalitionforprevention.ca), of which APHA is a member and Vibrant Communities Calgary, which advocates for long-term strategies that address root causes of poverty in Calgary (http://vibrantcalgary.com).

5   Although APHA marks its year of establishment in 1943, there are a few mentions of the organization in local newspapers in 1942. The organization has its origins in the Alberta Public Health Officials Association, which preceded it. APHA archival materials indicate that its first president was Dr. W.H. Hill, but the newspaper articles mention a prior president named Dr. H. Siemans, from the Lamont Public Health District. See *Edmonton Journal*, 2 October 1942, 15 (announcement); "Wives Feed Husbands Better than Selves," *Calgary Herald*, 2 October 1942, 13; "Public Health Officials Elect Dr. H. Siemans," *Calgary Herald*, 2 October 1942.

6   The Canadian Network of Public Health Associations (CNPHA), "A Collective Voice for Advancing Public Health: Why Public Health Associations Matter Today," *Canadian Journal of Public Health* 110, no. 3 (2019).

7   Michael H. Hall et al., *The Canadian Nonprofit and Voluntary Sector in Comparative Perspective* (Toronto: Imagine Canada, 2005), 9.

8   Nilima Sonpal-Valias, "Paradoxes in Paradise: Neoliberalism in Alberta's Developmental Disability Field" (PhD diss., University of Calgary, 2016), 5, Prism Database, https://prism.ucalgary.ca/items/8d945d1e-5344-4e31-83b6-275198cf7e0f; Statistics Canada, *Cornerstones of Community: Highlights of the National Survey of Nonprofit and Voluntary Organizations* (2003, 2005), https://www150.statcan.gc.ca/n1/pub/61-533-s/61-533-s2005001-eng.htm.

9   Sonpal-Valias, *Paradoxes in Paradise*, 5.

10   Hall et al., *The Canadian Nonprofit*, 22.

11   Pauline Paul, "A History of the Edmonton General Hospital: 1895–1970, 'be faithful to the duties of your calling,'" (Ph.D. diss., University of Alberta, 1994, ERA [Education & Research Archives] database, https://era.library.ualberta.ca/items/da01f69f-e833-402f-b9a4-d0764687920f).

12   Carl A. Meilicke and Janet L. Storch, *Perspective on Canadian Health and Social Policy: History and Emerging Trends* (Ann Harbor, Michigan: University of Michigan, Health Administration Press, 1980), 4.

13   For a history of the YWCA in Calgary, see YW Calgary, "Our History", https://www.ywcalgary.ca/about-us/our-history/; and Antonella Fanella, Pernille Jakobsen, Lee Tunstall, and Young Women's Christian Association, *Creating Cornerstones: A History of the YWCA of Calgary* (Calgary: YWCA of Calgary, 2011).

14   *An Act respecting Benevolent and other Societies Act* ("The Benevolent Societies Act"), R.S.A. 1922, c. 159. This act was a provincial revision of the Northwest Territories' Ordinance respecting Benevolent and other Societies Act, O.N.T. 1891-1892, no. 19.

15   *Act respecting Benevolent and Other Societies* ("The Societies Act"), S.P.A., 1924, c. 11.

16   "Davidson Will Ask Questions about Quarrel," *Edmonton Journal*, 27 March 1924, Alberta Legislature Library, Scrapbook Hansard, https://librarysearch.assembly.ab.ca/client/en_CA/search/asset/143249/0; "Summary of Legislation Passed at Session," *Edmonton Journal*, 12 April 1924, 16; An Act respecting Benevolent and other Societies Act, 1924.

17   *Act respecting Benevolent and Other Societies*, 1924; "Alberta Non-Profit Listing," Open Government Program, Government of Alberta, https://open.alberta.ca/opendata/alberta-non-profit-listing; APHA, Minutes of the Annual General Meeting, 6 September 1955, Provincial Archives of Alberta (PAA).

18   *Act for the Protection of Neglected and Dependent Children*, S.P.A. 1909, c. 12; *Act with Respect to Compensation to Workmen for Injuries Suffered in the Course of Their Employment*, S.P.A. 1908, c. 12; *Act Granting Assistance to Widowed Mothers Supporting Children*, S.P.A. 1919 c. 6.

19   *Act to Establish a Bureau of Relief and Public Welfare and to Provide for the Administration of Unemployment Relief*, S.P.A. 1936, c. 34. According to the act, "'indigent' means a person who is actually destitute of means from his own resources of obtaining the food, clothing and shelter necessary for his immediate wants;" and "'transient indigent' means any indigent within the Province in respect of whose maintenance or partial maintenance there is no liability upon any municipality in the Province."

20   *Act respecting the Welfare of Children*, S.P.A. 1925, c. 4; *Act respecting the Alberta Women's Bureau*, S.P.A. 1928, c. 13; *Act to Establish a Bureau of Relief and Public Welfare and to Provide for the Administration of Unemployment Relief*, S.P.A. 1936, c. 4.

21   *An Act respecting Health Insurance*, S.P.A. 1935, c. 49 (assented to 23 April 1935); Robert Lampard, *Alberta's Medical History: Young and Lusty, and Full of Life* (Red Deer: R. Lompard, 2008), 605–609.

22   *An Act respecting the Alberta Health Care Insurance Plan*, S.A. 1969, c. 43.

23   Victorian Order of Nurses (Edmonton Branch) fonds, History/Biographical Sketch, Provincial Archives of Alberta; Donald Smith, *Calgary's Grand Story* (Calgary: University of Calgary Press, 2005), 50.

24   Some argued this was a product of the not-for-profit groups being under pressure from government funding cuts. See "Victorian Order of Nurses to Shut Down Alberta Operations," *CBC Calgary*, 25 November 2015, https://www.cbc.ca/news/canada/calgary/von-victorian-order-nurses-closing-alberta-1.3336643; "Victorian Order of Nurses Shutting Down Operations in 6 Provinces," *The Canadian Press and Global News*, 25 November 2015, https://globalnews.ca/news/2361476/victorian-order-of-nurses-shutting-down-operations-in-six-provinces/.

25   Harrison and Weber, *Neoliberalism*, 26.

26   Baldwin Reichwein, *Benchmarks in Alberta's Public Welfare Services: History Rooted in Benevolence, Harshness, Punitiveness and Stinginess* (Edmonton: Alberta College of Social Workers, 2003), 26.

27   Reichwein, *Benchmarks*, 26. See also Valerie Tarasuk et al., "A Survey of Food Bank Operations in Five Canadian Cities," *BMC Public Health* 14 (28 November 2014), https://doi.org/10.1186/1471-2458-14-1234.

28   Hall et al., *The Canadian Nonprofit*, 25.

29   Sonpal-Valias, *Paradoxes in Paradise*, 151–2.

30   Sonpal-Valias, *Paradoxes in Paradise*, 152.

31   Sonpal-Valias, *Paradoxes in Paradise*, 154.

32   Harrison and Weber, *Neoliberalism*, 28–29.

33   Harrison and Weber, *Neoliberalism*, 29–30.

34   Harrison and Weber, *Neoliberalism*, 3; Calgary Chamber of Voluntary Organizations (CCVO), *Points of Light: The State of the Alberta Non-profit Sector* (Calgary, 2011), 2. In May 2020, there were 26,201 non-profit organizations registered as "Active" in Alberta. "Alberta Non-Profit Listing," Open Data, Alberta Government, updated 1 May 2020, https://open.alberta.ca/opendata/alberta-non-profit-listing

35   Harrison and Weber, *Neoliberalism*, 3.

36   CCVO, *Points of Light*, 11, 38. The International Classification of Non-profit Organizations system groups organizations into twelve major activity groups, see: Lester Salamon and Helmut K. Anheier, *Defining the Nonprofit Sector: A Cross-national Analysis* (Manchester: Manchester University Press, 1997). For more information on each category see: https://unstats.un.org/unsd/publication/seriesf/seriesf_91e.pdf.

37   CCVO, *Points of Light*, 11.

38   CCVO, *Points of Light*, 11.

39   These associations included health inspectors, medical officers, and public health nurses. Velez Mendoza et al. *The History of the Alberta Public Health Association*.

40   The reader can consult the archival holdings related to the APHA, which are housed at the Provincial Archives of Alberta (archival processing was in progress at the time of writing). These include annual reports, conference programs, newsletters, and other documents.

41   The complete list of resolutions can be found on the APHA website: https://www.apha.ab.ca/resources/Documents/APHA%20Resolutions%20-%20Master%20Document%20-%20FINAL%20for%20website%20(Dec%2030%202017).docx (hereafter cited as Historical APHA Resolutions).

42   Public Health Agency of Canada, *Core Competencies for Public Health in Canada: Release 1.0* (Public Health Agency of Canada, September 2007), https://www.phac-aspc.gc.ca/php-psp/ccph-cesp/pdfs/cc-manual-eng090407.pdf; Historical APHA Resolutions.

43   This iterative process consisted in three instances of inter-coder verifications, where two individuals independently coded a sample of the total resolutions to compare the proposed categories and make further adjustments. A third individual coder was brought in for the third instance to check the accuracy of categories. The categories were extracted from Canadian Public Health Association (CPHA), *Public Health: A Conceptual Framework*, Canadian Public Health Association Working Paper, Second Edition (Ottawa: CPHA, 2017), https://www.cpha.ca/sites/default/files/uploads/policy/ph-framework/phcf_e.pdf; Christopher David Naylor, *Learning from SARS: Renewal of Public Health in Canada* —Report of the National Advisory Committee on SARS and Public Health. National Advisory Committee, 2003); Public Health Agency of Canada, *Core Competencies*; Atlantic Provinces Public Health Collaboration, *Public Health 101: An Introduction to Public Health* (Nova Scotia Health Promotion and Protection and the Public Health Agency of Canada, November 2007), https://novascotia.ca/dhw/publications/Public-Health-Education/Public-Health-101-An%20Introduction-to-Public-Health.pdf.

44   CPHA, *Public Health, A Conceptual Framework*, 5.

45   National Collaborating Centre for Determinants of Health, *Let's Talk: Moving Upstream* (Antigonish, NS: National Collaborating Centre for Determinants of Health, St. Francis Xavier University, 2014), http://nccdh.ca/images/uploads/Moving_Upstream_Final_En.pdf.

46   Paul Boothe and Heather Edwards, *Eric J. Hanson's Financial History of Alberta, 1905–1950* (Calgary: University of Calgary Press, 2003), 21.

47   Boothe and Edwards, *Eric J. Hanson's Financial History of Alberta*, 100.

48   "Public Health Officials Elect Dr. H. Siemans," *Calgary Herald;* Minutes of the Annual Meeting, Alberta Public Health Association, 2 and 3 October, 1944, PAA.

49   Alberta Public Health Association, *Annual Report 1993–94* (1994).

50   See Historical APHA Resolutions.

51   See Historical APHA Resolutions.

52   APHA, Minutes of the Annual General Meeting, 16 and 17 September 1946, PAA.

53   APHA, Minutes of the Annual General Meeting, 2 and 3 October 1944, PAA.

54   John H. Brown, Jean Clark J, and C. Ellinger, "A Classified Directory of Alberta Public Health Workers Association." *Alberta Health Worker* 5, no. 1 (February 1945).

55   APHA, Minutes of the Annual General Meeting, 7 and 8 September 1948, PAA.

56   APHA, Minutes of the Annual General Meeting, 7 and 8 September 1948, PAA.

57   APHA, Minutes of the Annual General Meeting, 1–3 September 1954 and 29–31 August 1956.

58   Christopher Rutty and Sue C. Sullivan, *This Is Public Health: A Canadian History* (Ottawa: Canadian Public Health Association, 2010); APHA, Minutes of the Annual General Meeting, 4–6 September 1950, PAA.

59   APHA, Minutes of the Annual General Meeting, 4–6 September 1950, 2, 3. The association was also concerned by both the financing of public health services and practice, which in Alberta was thought to be at a standstill. APHA, Minutes of the Annual General Meeting, 10 and 12 September 1952, PAA.

60   See Historical APHA Resolutions.

61   See *Alberta Health Worker* 1, no. 1 (April 1946) and *Alberta Health Worker* 9, no. 1 (November 1949).

62   *Alberta Health Worker* 1, no. 1 (April 1946).

63   Alvin Finkel et al., *Working People in Alberta: A History* (Edmonton: Athabasca University Press, 2012).

64   Finkel et al., *Working People in Alberta*.

65   Finkel et al., *Working People in Alberta*, 142.

66   Program, APHA Annual Convention 1964, Calgary. APHA convention programs and annual reports are available in the APHA Archives, PAA.

67   Program, APHA Annual Convention 1967, Edmonton.

68   "Sanitary Landfill Practices — A Panel Discussion," a panel discussion presented at the Sectional Meeting of Sanitary Inspectors, chaired by W. Boulton. Program, APHA Annual Convention 1960, Edmonton; "Air and Water Pollution Control Programs in Alberta," Program, APHA Annual Convention 1965, Edmonton. The latter session was a panel featuring: G.H. Ball, Medical Officer of Health, Edmonton; S.L. Dobko, Air and Water Pollution Control Section, Alberta Department of Public Health; J.H. Broomhall, Provincial Public Health Inspector, Alberta Department of Public Health; and R. Ferguson, Water Pollution Control Engineer, Alberta Department of Public Health.

69 Specifically, the formation of the Department of Health and Social Development, which replaced the previous Department of Health and Department of Social Development in 1971 (see Chapter 4); also, Legislative Assembly of Alberta, *Report of the Special Legislative and Lay Committee Inquiring into Preventive Health Services in the Province of Alberta* (Edmonton: 1965).

70 CPHA, Minutes of the Annual General Meeting (Alberta Division), 2 and 3 April 1964, PAA.

71 Sean A. Valles, *Philosophy of Population Health: Philosophy for a New Public Health Era* (London: Routledge, 2018).

72 CPHA, Minutes of the Annual General Meeting, (Alberta Division), 7 April 1967, PAA.

73 APHA, Minutes of the Annual General Meeting, 16 April 1971, PAA.

74 For example, in 1974, the sections of the association, which were previously based on professions (e.g., public health nurses, public health inspectors) were replaced by five function-oriented sections, namely Health Services Administration, Environmental Health, Epidemiology and Disease Control, Health Promotion, and Family Health. See APHA, Minutes of the Annual General Business Meeting, 16 April 1971; APHA, Minutes of the General Business Meeting, 18 April 1974. This decade also brought other changes; for example, in 1971, it changed its name back to Alberta Public Health Association from Canadian Public Health Association (Alberta Division).

75 APHA, Minutes of Executive Meeting, 17-18 April 1979 April, PAA.

76 National Collaborating Centre for Determinants of Health, *Collective Impact and Public Health: An Old/New Approach — Stories of two Canadian Initiatives* (Antigonish, NS: National Collaborating Centre for Determinants of Health, St. Francis Xavier University, 2007), 2, http://nccdh.ca/images/uploads/comments/Collective_impact_and_public_health_An_old_new_approach_Two_Canadian_initiatives_EN_FV.pdf.

77 "Health Promotion," World Health Organization, last updated 2024, https://www.who.int/topics/health_promotion/en/.

78 Marc Lalonde, *A New Perspective on the Health of Canadians: A Working Document* (Ottawa: Queen's Printer, 1974). Heather Macdougall, "Reinventing Public Health: A New Perspective on the Health of Canadians and Its International Impact," *Journal of Epidemiology and Community Health* 61, no. 11 (2007).

79 "The Ottawa Charter for Health Promotion," World Health Organization, accessed 1 March 2019, https://www.who.int/healthpromotion/conferences/previous/ottawa/en/.

80 Program, APHA Annual Convention 1977, Calgary.

81 Program, APHA Annual Convention 1978, Red Deer.

82 Katherine L. Frohlich and Louise Potvin, "Health Promotion through the Lens of Population Health: Toward a Salutogenic Setting," *Critical Public Health* 9, no. 3 (1 September 1999).

83 *Public Health Act*, R.S.A. 1970, c. 294, 4479–4480.

84 APHA, Minutes of the Annual General Business Meeting, 16 April 1971, PAA.

85 APHA, Minutes of the Annual General Business Meeting, 5 April 1973, PAA.

86 APHA, Minutes of the Annual General Meeting, 5–6 April 1973; Alberta. Legislative Assembly of Alberta, 10 April 1973 (Mr. Ashley Cooper, SC). https://docs.assembly.ab.ca/LADDAR_files/docs/hansards/han/legislature_17/session_2/19730410_1430_01_han.pdf

87 *Act respecting Public Health*, S.A., 1973 c. 47 (specifically the change to section 10). See also, Alberta. Legislative Assembly of Alberta, 10 May 1973, 57-3112. https://docs.assembly.ab.ca/LADDAR_files/docs/hansards/han/legislature_17/session_2/19730510_2000_01_han.pdf

88 Evelyn L. Forget, "The Town with No Poverty: The Health Effects of a Canadian Guaranteed Annual Income Field Experiment," *Canadian Public Policy* 37, no. 3 (2011); David A. Croll, *Poverty in Canada. Report of the Special Senate Committee on Poverty* (Ottawa: King's Printer, 1971).

89 Fran Baum and Matthew Fisher, "Why Behavioural Health Promotion Endures Despite its Failure to Reduce Health Inequities," *Sociology of Health & Illness* 36, no. 2 (2014).

90 Helen Simmons, "Annual Report of the President" (1981–82). APHA Archives, PAA.

91 APHA started publishing a newsletter for its members in 1968. The newsletter was renamed *The Promoter* in 1992 and was published up until at least 2008.

92 "Dr. Gerry Predy Accepts Office of President," *APHA Newsletter* (June 1982).

93 "Dr. Gerry Predy Accepts Office of President."

94 Supplement to the *APHA Newsletter*, January 1983.

95 See Historical APHA Resolutions.

96 Other related resolutions included nuclear disarmament and cruise missile testing; for the members were "cognizant of the negative effect such a nuclear disaster would have on the health of populations in terms of extremely high mentality, morbidity, environmental, ecological and health services,

disruption, social disorganization and long-term far-reaching effects on any surviving population." See *Historical APHA Resolutions.*

97 See Historical APHA Resolutions.

98 APHA, "Second Vice-president Report" for 13 March 1979 and 17 April 1979, in APHA, *Annual Report 1979–80* (1980), PAA. APHA was represented at steering committee meetings that led to the establishment of this Council in 1979.

99 Program, APHA Annual Convention 1981, Edmonton.

100 APHA, *Annual Report 1990–1991* (1991).

101 APHA, *Annual Report 1991–92* (1992); APHA, *Annual Report, 1992–93* (1993). The low membership led APHA to consider offering direct membership in addition to the CPHA co-membership. The idea materialized in 1993. It seems to be working at first, with thirty new direct members in the first year of implementation, but they could not make the goal of the anniversary. By the end of the decade, the membership committee conceived a plan to emphasize a targeted and personalized approach. Approximately two hundred recruitment packages were distributed, but only fifteen new memberships were received.

102 APHA, *Annual Report 1993–94*; Alberta Ministry of Health, *Health Goals for Alberta: Progress Report* (Edmonton: Alberta Health, 1993); Donald J. Philippon and Sheila A. Wasylyshyn, "Health-care reform in Alberta," *Canadian Public Administration* 39 (1996).

103 APHA, *Annual Report 1999–2000* (2000), 9; APHA, *Annual Report 2000-2001* (2001), 3.

104 APHA, *Annual Report 1995–96* (1996).

105 APHA, *Partnership Project on Literacy and Health Final Report*, March 1997; Alberta. Alberta Legislative Assembly of Alberta, 20 August 1996 (Mr. Zwozdesky, Lib). https://docs.assembly.ab.ca/ LADDAR_files/docs/hansards/han/legislature_23/session_4/19960820_1330_01_han.pdf

106 APHA used the numbers from Canadian Centre for Substance Abuse, 1994.

107 APHA, *Annual Report 2001–2002*, 12.

108 Of that amount, $50,000 was for the Alberta Healthy Living Network project. APHA Commitment to Collaborate with AHLN on Healthy Living. APHA, Minutes of the Annual General Meeting, 2005.

109 APHA, *Annual Report 2007–08* (2008).

110 APHA, *Annual Report 2006–07* (2007), 5 and 7.

111 APHA, *Annual Report 2008/09* (2009), 9–10.

112 Namely, the Public Health Association of British Columbia. APHA, *Annual Report 2008/09*, 9.

113 APHA, *Annual Report 2008/09*, 10.

114 Results from this project include a narrative history of the association (Velez Mendoza et al., *The History of the Alberta Public Health Association*), a complete list of association presidents, and a complete list of resolutions. These are available on the APHA website: https://www.apha.ab.ca/public-health-resources

115 This event was held in conjunction with annual Campus Alberta conference, "Campus Alberta Health Outcomes and Public Health Annual Forum," O'Brien Institute for Public Health, accessed 8 July 2020, https://events.ucalgary.ca/obrien/#!view/event/event_id/101855.

116 APHA and the O'Brien Institute for Public Health at the University of Calgary, "All Party Candidate Forum: A Healthy Alberta Through Healthier Policies," O'Brien Institute for Public Health, accessed 8 July 2020, https://events.ucalgary.ca/obrien/#!view/event/event_id/101777.

117 APHA, "Support for a comprehensive poverty reduction among persons with disabilities," Minutes of the Annual General Meeting, 4 March 2005; "Increased food security for low-income Albertans," APHA, Minutes of the Annual General Meeting, 6 June 2006; "Support for Guaranteed Annual Income for Albertans," APHA, Minutes of the Annual General Meeting, 16 May 2014; "Support for advocacy efforts to improve access to affordable housing," APHA, Minutes of the Annual General Meeting, 2017.

118 CNPHA, "A Collective Voice."

119 Katherine E. Smith and Ellen A. Stewart, "Academic Advocacy in Public Health: Disciplinary 'Duty' or Political 'Propaganda'?" *Social Science & Medicine* 189 (2017).

6

Public Health Education: Power and Politics in Alberta Universities

Lindsay McLaren, Rogelio Velez Mendoza, and Frank W. Stahnisch

Introduction

This volume was prompted, in part, by concerns expressed in recent discourse about the weakening of public health and about its identity in the contemporary context.[1] These concerns manifest in, among other things, a strong tendency to conflate public health with publicly funded medical care, which has the effect of diluting public health's unique contributions including its focus on population well-being and health equity via emphasis on prevention, health promotion, and upstream thinking about root causes of health problems.[2]

Public health education figures prominently in these concerns. Robust programs of public health education are essential foundations of a strong and effective public health community.[3] Our aim in this chapter is to consider how public health education programs in Alberta have evolved, collectively and independently, and how they have shaped the capacity, visibility, and impact of public health in the province. We focus on programs at the University of Alberta, the University of Calgary, and the University of Lethbridge (see Table 6.1 on page 179), which are a subset of all relevant programs and education opportunities in the province.[4]

We situate our discussion within the broader Albertan and Canadian context, in which relatively recent national developments in public health figure prominently, starting in the 2000s.[5] A timeline of some of the key events is shown in Table 6.2 on page 180.

Twentieth-Century Public Health Education in Canada and Alberta

In what may be considered both a necessity and a perpetual challenge for the field, public health education across Canada and in Alberta is historically closely tied to medicine, as well as to nursing, albeit in different ways. One example in Alberta is the close relationship, beginning early in the province's history, between the Faculty of Medicine at the University of Alberta and the provincial public health laboratory. Another example is the training courses in public health nursing offered by the University of Alberta that were prompted in part by the 1918 influenza pandemic.[6]

1905–1970s: Public Health Education and its Tethers to Medicine

In terms of a stand-alone program of study for public health in Canada, one must historically look beyond Alberta to Ontario, where in 1927 a School of Hygiene was established at the University of Toronto that was separate from the university's School of Medicine.[7] This occurred in a context of significant discussion in the United States around the need for specialized public health education, including a 1913 conference sponsored by the Rockefeller Foundation whose contributions, as noted in Chapter 4, must be placed in critical context. As described by public health historian Elizabeth Fee, "[Rockefeller] Foundation officials were convinced that a new profession of public health was needed. It would be allied to medicine but also distinct, with its own identity and educational institutions."[8] The conference led to the Welch-Rose Report of 1915,[9] which envisioned an "Institute of Hygiene" that would "train public health leaders and advance knowledge of the sciences of hygiene."[10] Several such institutes or schools were created with financial support from the Foundation, including at the University of Toronto, the only public health school in Canada until 1945.[11] According to Fee, the authors of the Welch-Rose Report had different perspectives on the appropriate balance of public health science and practice;[12] this is a tension that persists in public health, including public health education, today.[13]

In 1945, a French-language stand-alone program of study for public health was established at Université de Montréal.[14] There were then two institutions in Canada at that time offering graduate diplomas in public health, primarily to physicians. However, this first era of stand-alone public health education in Canada was temporary, and by the 1970s, both schools were absorbed into the universities' faculties of medicine.[15] Perhaps there was a perception at that time that public health was no longer relevant in the face of the apparent conquest of infectious diseases, advances in biomedical science and the development of new technologies for the treatment of disease, and the introduction and evolution of public medical insurance.[16]

In Alberta, the early, medically anchored version of public health education expanded when the University of Alberta established a Department of Preventive Medicine within its Faculty of Medicine around 1949. That department is described in hindsight as providing medical students with a perspective that situates health and illness in broader context.[17] The 1960s was a period of important social and political change in Alberta that had implications for public health education: The province became increasingly urbanized as the population of its major cities doubled, and there was a significant political and administrative transition from Social Credit leadership, largely under Ernest Manning, to the lengthy Progressive Conservative reign of Peter Lougheed starting in 1971.[18] The introduction of Medicare in Canada in the late 1960s prompted further diversification of medical and nursing facilities[19] and, in that context, the creation of the University of Calgary in 1966 laid the foundation for its new Faculty of Medicine.[20] In a legacy that presents significant challenges to a broad version of public health — and which persists today —, that faculty would become home to the division (later Department) of Community Health Sciences, which was established in 1970 with John H. Read as the inaugural head.

The University of Lethbridge was founded one year after the University of Calgary and soon offered undergraduate programs in nursing.[21] In the 1970s, the specialty of community medicine was recognized by Canada's Royal College of Physicians, and medical officers of health in Alberta, including Gerry Predy, were involved in launching a residency program in Alberta.[22] However, according to public health physicians Richard Massé and Brent Moloughney, in those early days of the specialty, some of the trainees had to leave Canada to pursue their academic training in the basic public health sciences, suggesting that options for specialized public health training in Canada in the 1970s were still limited.[23] At the University of Alberta, a Master of Health Services Administration program was established in the Faculty of Medicine in 1968, under the directorship of Carl Meilicke, which aimed to fill an educational gap in western Canada.[24]

> "Either a foundation or an annoying legacy, depending on where you sit" — Ruth Wolfe, speaking of some of these early programs from the perspective of public health education today.[25]

Overall, this period up until the early 1970s may be considered a first era in public health education in Alberta and Canada.[26] Although nationally it included Canada's first stand-alone public health programs, under the name "hygiene," public health education programs during this era, especially in Alberta, retained close ties with medicine and health care. If the goals of public health are around preventing disease and injury and promoting health, well-being, and health equity, then these ties — as illustrated by the quote from Ruth Wolfe — present a conundrum of being both a historical reality and an enduring challenge.

1970s–2000: The Influx of Health Promotion

The 1970s to approximately the year 2000 may be viewed as a second era in public health education in Alberta and elsewhere. A precursor to the University of Lethbridge's Faculty of Health Sciences was founded in 1980,[27] and in 1981 the University of Calgary's Division of Community Health Sciences, within the Faculty of Medicine, became a department, with Ed Love as head.[28] Under Love's headship, the community medicine residency program, later to become the Public Health And Preventive Medicine residency program, was founded in 1982, as western Canada's youngest program. Initially, however, intake was exclusively through re-entry positions for already practicing physicians; direct entry was not available until the late 1990s.[29]

At the University of Alberta, a centre focused on injury prevention was established in 1989 within the University of Alberta Hospitals' Department of Surgery, under the leadership of Louis Francescutti (see Chapter 13).[30] Also at the University of Alberta, in 1996 a Department of Public Health Sciences was created within the Faculty of Medicine and Dentistry, with Tom Noseworthy as chair. That department hosted the province's first master of public health program. The initial cohort included fifteen students who specialized in health care policy and management; other specialties were added later, including occupational and environmental health, clinical epidemiology, and global health.[31]

Public health education in Alberta during this second era was influenced by significant national and international developments in prevention and health promotion, including the 1974 federal Lalonde Report, the 1986 Ottawa Charter for Health Promotion (briefly, an international agreement toward the goal of "Health for All," see Chapter 10),[32] and enduring international signposts in the understanding of population health and the social determinants of health, including the historical work of British scholar Thomas McKeown.[33] McKeown's work questioned the role of "active human intervention," particularly in the form of curative medical practice, in driving nineteenth and early twentieth-century improvements in population health status (e.g., life expectancy), as compared to improved levels and distribution of social, political, and economic resources.[34] These events significantly influenced members of public health communities in

Alberta, and contributed to important cross-institution collaboration in research and education, specifically around health promotion.[35]

At the University of Alberta, the creation of infrastructure for health promotion research and education is widely attributed to the leadership of Doug Wilson (see Chapter 13) who, during his tenure as dean of the Faculty of Medicine (1984–1994) began to see the importance of prevention and health promotion.[36] The Health Sciences Council, of which he was a member, agreed that a cross-faculty health promotion entity would be preferable to one situated in the Faculty of Medicine, where it would likely be overwhelmed by other focuses such as acute care.[37] After successfully securing provincial government funding, the University of Alberta's Centre for Health Promotion Studies was formally launched in 1996 as a freestanding, interdisciplinary academic unit. The centre had both a research and an education mandate, and that same year it launched a master of science degree program and a postgraduate diploma program, which were unique in the country at the time.[38] Wilson served as the centre's initial director, followed by Miriam Stewart (1997–2001) and then Kim Raine (2002–2008) (see Chapter 13).[39]

Health promotion research and education in the province was not limited to the University of Alberta, however. In the mid-1990s, in the wake of the Ottawa Charter, a significant federal grant opportunity allowed for the creation of several health promotion centres across the country, including two in Alberta. In addition to the Centre for Health Promotion at the University of Alberta, the Regional Centre for Health Promotion Studies at the University of Lethbridge was funded under this program.[40] The Lethbridge centre was affiliated with nursing within the Faculty of Health Sciences, under the leadership of Judith Kulig. The University of Calgary also had the multi-faculty (kinesiology, sociology, nursing, social work, and community health sciences) Health Promotion Research Centre, led by Billie Thurston and later by Ardene Robinson Vollman which, although not funded under the national program, was considered to be a valued partner in the province.[41] The three centres, along with the Alberta Centre for Well-Being, now the Alberta Centre for Active Living, and an Indigenous research group, formed the Alberta Consortium for Health Promotion Research, which supported collaborative research and education in health promotion, including distance education classes offered collaboratively between the Universities of Alberta and Calgary. [42]

Overall, a number of developments in public health education in Alberta occurred during the 1970s, 1980s, and especially the 1990s, many of which set the stage for the acceleration of events in the early 2000s.

The 2000s: An Inflection Point for Public Health and Public Health Education in Canada and Alberta

The global Severe Acute Respiratory Syndrome pandemic, which occurred in 2003,[43] heightened national attention to public health, and it can be considered to have ushered in a third era in public health education. The pandemic prompted the realization that Canada did not have sufficient public health human resource capacity, and the report of a national task force chaired by former University of Toronto president David Naylor strongly recommended greater investment to create more human resources in public health.[44] Significant outcomes of the Naylor Report, as it came to be known, included the creation of the Public Health Agency of Canada in 2004 and the National Collaborating Centres for Public Health in 2005,[45] the release of a Pan-Canadian framework for public health human resources planning in 2005, and the subsequent development of core competencies for public health practice including both cross-cutting and discipline-specific competencies.[46]

Collectively, the circumstances around the pandemic led to a surge in education and training opportunities for public health in Canada, including master of public health programs, schools of public health, and undergraduate public health programs. Writing in 2011, Massé and Moloughney identified that the number of such programs had increased from around five in 1990s to fifteen in September 2011.[47] Notably, that latter number included early adopters in Alberta; namely, the University of Alberta's School of Public Health, which was the only public health school in the process of pursuing accreditation at the time; and the University of Lethbridge, which was named as one of "a limited number" of institutions in Canada offering undergraduate programs focused on public health at that time.[48]

Also occurring on the national (and international) stage were important advancements in public health research. The formation of the Canadian Institutes of Health Research in 2000 signified a symbolically and substantively important transition from the former entity, the Medical Research Council.[49] With respect to our focus here, the Canadian Institute for Health Information's Institute of Population and Public Health was important. One of the Canadian Institutes of Health Research institute's flagship initiatives was the Applied Public Health Chairs program, which, in partnership with the Public Health Agency of Canada and other partners, funded midcareer scholars pursuing innovative, applied research in population and public health and health equity. This program, which was part of post-pandemic efforts to strengthen public health research capacity, included two Alberta researchers (of thirteen nationally) in the first cohort (2008–2013, Kim Raine, University of Alberta and Alan Shiell, University of Calgary), and two (of fourteen nationally) in the second cohort (2014–2019, Candace Nykiforuk, University of Alberta and Lindsay McLaren, University of Calgary).[50]

Growth and Expansion of Public Health Education Programs, and the Rise and Fall of a Pan-provincial School of Public Health

Members of the University of Alberta, University of Calgary, and University of Lethbridge public health communities all credit these national events as significantly influencing their respective public health education developments in the new millennium.[51] It is worth noting that these developments occurred in the context of a politically disruptive Alberta environment of the '90s and '00s, including the ideologically driven public sector cuts of the Ralph Klein government that spanned more than a decade starting in 1992 (see Chapter 4), regionalization of the health care system in the neoliberal context of the mid-1990s, and — coinciding with the global financial crisis — the subsequent creation of Alberta Health Services, a single provincial health services authority, in 2008.[52] As described below, public health education programs in Alberta during this period evolved independently and inter-dependently of one another, and they illustrate dimensions of power and politics as they play out in post-secondary education.

THE UNIVERSITY OF ALBERTA

In the post-pandemic context, Doug Wilson and others at the University of Alberta began to realize that they already had many ingredients for a stand-alone School of Public Health. In addition to the Department of Public Health Sciences, the Centre for Health Promotion Studies, and the Injury Prevention Centre, they had existing expertise in other key areas of public health, including environmental health, occupational health, and health administration, thus rounding out many of the areas required for accreditation by the U.S. based Council on Education for Public Health.[53]

> "It seemed to me that we didn't have to come up with a whole lot of money, we just had to come up with the will to do it" — Doug Wilson[54]

Then-provost Carl Amrhein agreed that the idea of a School of Public Health was an exciting one, and in early 2005 he formed a task force, chaired by Wilson, to investigate the idea further.[55] Wilson concedes that some competitive spirit, stemming from the University of Calgary's recent creation of a new Faculty of Veterinary Medicine, factored into the decision to work toward the new school.

Broad support was sought and secured from across the University of Alberta campus, including from the dean of the Faculty of Medicine, Tom Marrie, which was somewhat noteworthy because the new initiative meant that the Faculty of Medicine would lose their public health sciences department to the new School of Public Health.[56]

The report of the task force was accepted by Amrhein, and in March of 2006, the board of governors of the University of Alberta approved the creation of a School of Public Health, making it Canada's first stand-alone school in the modern era.[57] Former Alberta Deputy Minister of both Health and Wellness and of Education, Roger Palmer, was appointed interim dean to get the faculty up and running; he was succeeded in that position by Sylvie Stachenko (2009–2011), Lory Laing (interim 2011–2013), Kue Young (2013–2019), and Shanthi Johnson (2019–present).[58] The approval of the establishment of the school by the university's board of governors had stipulated that it must be accredited by the Council on Education for Public Health; the school achieved this accreditation in 2012, making it the first in Canada to achieve that milestone.[59] From an initial departmental structure, the school shifted to a non-departmental structure in 2013, in part to avoid the school being dominated by larger departments.[60] The school brought many pockets of public health together, with one main exception being the community medicine (now called public health and preventive medicine) residency program, which remained within the Faculty of Medicine and Dentistry.[61]

The School of Public Health offers several graduate programs (see Table 6.1 on page 179) including a master of public health professional degree as well as research-intensive, thesis-based MSc and PhD degrees. It also offers graduate embedded certificates, and professional development in the form of a fellowship in health system improvement. A core curriculum redesign of the master of public health program, completed in 2017, produced a curriculum shaped by the conventional five bodies of knowledge — epidemiology, biostatistics, psychosocial determinants of health, environmental determinants of health, and health policy & management — but it "departs radically from the former conventional siloed approach" by integrating those bodies of knowledge into team-taught, interdisciplinary core courses.[62]

As the first of its contemporary kind in Canada, the School of Public Health at the University of Alberta ushered in a new era in public health education. Other Canadian universities soon followed suit, such as the University of Saskatchewan and the University of Toronto, which established their schools of public health in 2007 and 2008 respectively.[63] However, while it was certainly a significant achievement for the province and for Canada, and worthy of celebration, the announcement of the School of Public Health at the University of Alberta was not met with quite the same degree of enthusiasm elsewhere in Alberta.

THE UNIVERSITY OF CALGARY[64]

Following the establishment of the Department of Community Health Sciences and the community medicine residency program in the '80s, and the shift to direct entry into the residency program in the '90s, developments in public health research and education accelerated at the University of Calgary in the early 2000s, largely anchored in the Faculty of Medicine.[65] The developments in Calgary were somewhat complex, with many things going on at once.

Early developments occurred in the undergraduate realm with the Bachelor of Health Sciences (BHSc) program,[66] and notably the health and society major,[67] which is affiliated with the Department of Community Health Sciences. Development of a program proposal began in late 2001, and the new BHSc program formally began with the first class of students in fall of 2003.[68] In 2005, consistent with a theme of philanthropically funded programs in Calgary to which a critical lens must be applied,[69] it became the O'Brien Centre for the Bachelor of Health Sciences Program. Within the BHSc program, the unique health and society major focuses on health equity and public health, and students have to select a social science concentration.[70] The first class of BHSc students graduated from the four-year program in 2007, one year before the University of Lethbridge launched its Bachelor of Health Sciences in Public Health.

Around 2004, within the context of growing national support for population and public health research, there was a significant philanthropic donation to the University of Calgary to support research in that domain. International population and public health scholars Penny Hawe, who held the university's Markin Chair in Health and Society, and Alan Shiell had been recruited to the University of Calgary to advance their work and were situated within the Department of Community Health Sciences.[71] A small but growing group of faculty members[72] made it possible to create a new population and public health specialization within the graduate program (MSc and PhD), which aligned with the Canadian Institutes of Health Research's Institute of Population and Public Health.[73] Meanwhile, the community medicine residency program (the name of the specialty changed to Public Health & Preventive Medicine in 2012) grew in size during the early 2000s, although its integration with other education programs in the department remained limited.

In 2005, Harvey Weingarten, the university president at the time, announced the position of adviser to the president on health and wellness, which was initially held by Ron Zernicke, former dean of Kinesiology at Calgary, and then by David Low (2005–2007), who was recruited from Texas where he had served as president of the University of Texas Health Science Center at Houston.[74] Public health nurse and academic administrator Ardene Robinson Vollman was hired to support this new position. Robinson Vollman worked with Zernicke and then Low, along with Richard Musto and Bretta Maloff from the Calgary Health Region, as it was called at the time, to engage with and secure support from faculties across campus for a university-wide research and education initiative in public health, including the possibility of a cross-faculty master of public health program. Unfortunately, despite securing broad support, the dean of medicine at the time, Grant Gall, was not supportive and that university-wide initiative came to a halt.[75]

Meanwhile, the national post-pandemic sense of urgency around public health had prompted inter-institution discussions between the Universities of Alberta, Calgary, and Lethbridge. The involvement of Lethbridge was facilitated in part by the fact that David Low, the University of Calgary's president's adviser on health and wellness, was originally from Lethbridge.[76] A tripartite committee was formed, which envisioned a pan-Alberta public health coalition, including the idea of a cross-institution School of Public Health. With Alberta being a small province, it was felt that no one university had the capacity to develop their own School of Public Health, but by working together they could meet the accreditation standards. The institutions collectively hired Bob O'Reilly, former associate dean of the University of Calgary's Faculty of Education, to advise and coordinate the activities. For one of the tripartite meetings in early 2006, the committee hosted Harrison Spencer, president of the U.S.-based Association of Schools of Public Health,[77] to discuss accreditation possibilities for the cross-institution school, or at least that was the understanding of Calgary and Lethbridge members.[78] The tripartite committee meetings ultimately led to a memorandum of understanding (see summary points in Figure 6.1 on page 182) which was ceremoniously signed by the presidents of the three universities, with the Premier of Alberta in attendance, in May of 2006.[79] However, the enthusiasm for the memorandum of understanding had been dampened when, to the surprise of some, the University of Alberta announced its School of Public Health in March of that year.[80]

> "We have the battle of Alberta with hockey, and we have the battle
> of Alberta with universities too." — Ardene Robinson Vollman[81]

Feeling that the tripartite discussions had fallen apart, the University of Calgary members turned their attention back to strengthening public health research and education internally. David Low was succeeded as adviser on health and wellness by Wayne Giles, dean of kinesiology, and then by Tom Noseworthy, head of the Department of Community Health Sciences, with a name change from adviser to the president to adviser to the provost. Robinson Vollman worked with Giles and Noseworthy to develop a proposal for a multi-faculty research program in public health, and for a master of public health program, and once again secured considerable support from faculties across campus. The proposal for the MPH program was approved by the Faculty of Medicine, but it was rejected by members of the Department of Community Health Sciences, who preferred a thesis-based option. With that decision, which occurred around 2007, the idea of an MPH program at the University of Calgary dissipated, which in Robinson Vollman's view "took the University of Calgary out of the national presence of university schools of public health."[82]

Although the MPH goal was abandoned, efforts toward a public health research institute at the University of Calgary continued. Starting in 2004, the Faculty of Medicine had started to develop research institutes, which were intended to cut across the faculty's departmental organization and to connect the university with the broader community including Alberta Health Services. After the first six institutes had been formed, a final "Institute 7" was envisioned that would focus on health services research.[83] Within the national context of support for population and public health research, coupled with the significant efforts of Robinson Vollman, Noseworthy, Musto, and others to build and strengthen public health at the University of Calgary over the course after the Severe Acute Respiratory Syndrome period, "Institute 7" became the Calgary Institute for Population and Public Health; in 2010 it was renamed the O'Brien Institute for Public Health with Bill Ghali as Director.[84] Although the institute is not an educational entity per se, it forms an important part of the context of public health-related education at the University of Calgary, and it continues a historical legacy of emphasis on health services research, to the detriment of a broad vision of public health.

THE UNIVERSITY OF LETHBRIDGE

When Chris Hosgood began his tenure as dean of health sciences in the summer of 2005, one of the first things the academic historian experienced was the growing sense of urgency about public health capacity in the post-pandemic period.[85] The University of Lethbridge was poised to respond: an undergraduate program in public health had been partly developed, and Hosgood had a mandate to work with expert colleagues to complete the program's development and secure funding to deliver it.[86]

It was in this context that the University of Lethbridge enthusiastically entered the tripartite discussions with the University of Alberta and the University of Calgary. As a smaller, primarily undergraduate institution at the time, Lethbridge would arguably benefit the most from such an arrangement. Hosgood participated in the tripartite committee meetings, including the one with Harrison Spencer, which he likewise understood to be about accreditation of an Alberta-wide School of Public Health. It was surprising and disappointing to the University of Lethbridge when the University of Alberta announced their School of Public Health in March 2006.[87]

Nonetheless, with the notion of a province-wide school off the table, the University of Lethbridge continued with its efforts to develop what would become a successful program of public health education in southern Alberta. The efforts to develop the BHSc in Public Health degree aligned with Hosgood's mandate to expand health sciences from a school into a faculty (which was achieved in May of 2009) and coincided with the institution's transition from an undergraduate to a comprehensive university, which occurred around 2006–2007. Hosgood could see an opportunity for developments in public health to contribute to these broader goals by strengthening education, research, and community engagement.

> "The purpose of education within the University [isn't] just to train the next generation of health professionals, it [is] also to educate the next generation of health professionals." — Chris Hosgood[88]

Health Sciences at the University of Lethbridge at that time was described by Hosgood as somewhat peripheral to the academy. Many of the faculty members, in addition to being new to the university and faculty, had health professional backgrounds and lived and worked in a practice-oriented culture that was different from the academic orientation of the university. For Hosgood, part of building a foundation for public health education was helping people to understand that education and training are not the same thing. While the program needed to meet professional and practice needs, it also had to meet the degree requirements of a university.

Under Hosgood's leadership, provincial funding for a four-year BHSc in Public Health degree program was secured, and the first students enrolled in the fall of 2008. A view of public health as "art and science" underpinned collaboration with the Faculty of Arts and Science, to help ensure that graduates would emerge as critical thinkers with a broad, multidisciplinary view of health.[89] And, consistent with some of the concerns that prompted this volume as a whole, Sharon Yanicki, Assistant Professor and former Program Coordinator for the

BHSc in Public Health degree program, commented that "although the field of public health isn't new, it's an area that isn't all that well known or understood. The program aims to change that."[90]

The BHSc public health program at Lethbridge initially had three specializations and a practicum.[91] Although the economic recession of 2008–2009 resulted in a loss of funding and consequently a scaling back of ambitions, the program continued to grow and evolve. From a handful of students in 2008, the program increased to fifty-five in 2012 and to around 175 in 2019.[92] In contrast to the initial sense of the program as peripheral, by 2011 Yanicki described it as having "definitely found its niche within the faculty and within the fabric of the University as well," with one illustration being high enrolment in public health courses by students in other programs.[93]

A significant boost came from the program's successful external review in 2014, where some reviewers who had perhaps anticipated what Hosgood described as a "mickey mouse" program, came away impressed.[94] Fuelled by their successes, the University of Lethbridge continued to build their public health education offerings (Table 6.1), to include a combined Bachelor of Health Sciences / Bachelor of Management degree program, launched in fall of 2012; a Post-Diploma Bachelor of Health Sciences (public health major, health leadership minor), launched in fall 2016; as well as graduate programs including an MSc major in public health and a PhD program in population studies in health.[95]

Conclusions

There is no hard-and-fast rule as to the minimum number of years needed before an event can be called historical.[96] For this chapter, our attention was drawn to a relatively recent period when a great deal of activity in public health education occurred in Alberta and across Canada. A caveat with this recent focus, of course, is that we continue to live this history, and there will continue to be more of it, even by the time this volume is published. Nonetheless, this recent story, which considers how different levels (undergraduate, graduate) and types (research, practice) of public health education programs have evolved in Alberta, is important and should be told. With respect to our chapter objective, which included a consideration of how public health education programs in Alberta have shaped the capacity, visibility, and impact of public health in the province, we conclude with a few comments and observations.

Independence and Inter-dependence

The idea of a pan-Alberta School of Public Health as envisioned in the original tripartite committee agreement did not materialize, which "knocked the wind out of the sails"[97] for some of those involved. This outcome illustrates issues of power and politics in post-secondary education, with the University of Alberta having the size, prestige, and capacity to pursue its own goals. This somewhat uncomfortable interpretation has implications for understanding tensions in the province, between and within particularly the larger institutions, as well as between urban and rural settings.[98]

Despite that outcome, one must recognize the success of many of the individual programs as judged by metrics such as student demand and enrolment, faculty recruitment, and external review and accreditation. Furthermore, the current programs, when viewed collectively (Table 6.1), would appear to be complementary. Alongside the independent developments, efforts to work together have continued,[99] with the Campus Alberta Health Outcomes and Public Health framework representing one mechanism.[100] Pertinent to our focus here, the Campus Alberta Health Outcomes and Public Health meeting grants initiative permitted meetings to be held with public health education representatives from the three institutions in 2019, which suggested that there is appetite to "work toward unity of purpose in public health education" in Alberta.[101]

A Critical Perspective on Public Health Education

We began this chapter by acknowledging some challenges to public health's identity and impact, including the strong tendency to conflate it with publicly funded health care and its perpetually challenging connection with medicine,[102] and the problematic phenomenon of lifestyle drift: the tendency for policy to acknowledge the need for action on upstream social determinants of health inequalities but then to drift downstream to focus on individual lifestyle factors and access to biomedical solutions to health problems.[103]

Critical scholarship sheds light on the implications of these challenges in the context of public health education. In an editorial accompanying a series of papers on public health education in the journal *Critical Public Health*, American scholar Daniel Skinner said that "we must guard against some of our most important concepts — diversity, wellness, equity — being reduced to buzzwords that lose their critical edge and radicality."[104] There is a risk in public health education of these core concepts being diluted or depoliticized, depending on what is taught and how. A study by American scholars Michael Harvey and Margaret McGladrey tackled this issue via an analysis of the theories taught in MPH programming in the U.S.[105] They argue:

> The specific theories employed within public health to explain
> the origins and distribution of health, morbidity, and mortality

profoundly shape subsequent approaches to public health research and practice. For instance, if they are theorized as arising from the summation of individual behaviors, then the task of public health is to better understand and change health-related behaviors, particularly among so-called high-risk individuals, groups, and populations. Alternatively, if such distributions are theorized as arising from unequal distributions of economic resources, then the task of public health is to understand the drivers of economic inequality and pursue reductions in economic inequality. . . . The theories provided to MPH students . . . will shape their understanding of health disparities and subsequent public health practice.[106]

Focusing on theories taught in the social and behavioural sciences competency area (which applies to all accredited programs of public health), and based on an analysis of course syllabi, these authors identified that behavioural health theory represented over 90 percent of the most commonly taught theories, to the relative exclusion of theories that engage with structural determinants of health. This suggests that MPH students may graduate with "an insufficient theoretical toolbox that leaves them poorly equipped to address health inequalities with socio-structural etiology."[107] In Alberta, although recognition of this concern has prompted efforts in some programs to ensure an interdisciplinary approach to public health education that emphasizes critical thinking, it remains a formidable challenge.[108]

In a Canadian study of seventy-six graduate-level programs in public health listed by the Public Health Agency of Canada, Yassi and colleagues found that while 65 percent of programs required at least one quantitative methods course, only 26 percent required qualitative methods.[109] While quantitative methods are certainly important, this asymmetry — which exists in some programs in Alberta[110] — illustrates a persistent methodological hegemony that presents a barrier to appreciating the historical, socio-economic, cultural, colonial, and political context and processes that produce and perpetuate poor health and health inequities.[111] Furthermore, just one-quarter (25 percent) of programs considered in Yassi et al.'s study had at least one required course related to social theory or social determinants of health, thus supporting the findings of Harvey and McGladrey above, in the Canadian context, and only 3 percent required a course in ecological determinants of health. These authors conclude with this observation: "our examination suggests that the majority of schools of public health may still be frozen in old paradigms wherein interdisciplinary inquiry and the development of skills to work with communities to implement and evaluate interventions to promote and protect collective health are still only peripheral considerations."[112] If a goal of public health is to engage with and work to illuminate, communicate, and demonstrate leadership in redressing broader structural determinants of health, well-being, and health equity, then these findings encapsulate some significant challenges facing public health education in Alberta.

Layered upon this challenge is a political economic context that underpins a focus on lucrative but substantively void markers of program quality such as "job readiness"[113] and relatedly, as particularly evident in Calgary, a dominant and increasing trend of private philanthropy.[114] A recent study in the United States considered the increasing trend of accredited public health schools being renamed for private donors, and argued that this trend has unique implications for public health; namely, that it can "implicitly redefine the 'public' in public health, promoting the perception that public health should... serve and celebrate private profit."[115]Although this phenomenon is not new,[116] it takes on renewed importance in the contemporary political economic context, which is highly unfriendly to post-secondary education in Alberta and demands scrutiny.[117]

In our opinion, finding ways to effectively address these challenges would ignite an exciting, critical, and more reflexive fourth era of public health education, in Alberta and beyond.

TABLE 6.1: Summary of public health education programs offered at the Universities of Lethbridge, Calgary, and Alberta (current as of February 2019).

	University of Lethbridge Faculty of Health Sciences	University of Calgary Department of Community Health Sciences, Cumming School of Medicine	University of Alberta School of Public Health
Undergraduate	Bachelor of Health Sciences, Major: Public Health Bachelor of Health Sciences / Bachelor of Management Combined Degree program, Health Sciences Major: Public Health[1]	Bachelor of Health Sciences (Major: Health & Society)	N/A
Graduate (MSc, PhD)	MSc Health Sciences – Public Health specialization PhD in Population Studies in Health, 6 concentrations[2]	MSc and PhD programs, 7 specializations[3]	MSc program, 7 specializations[4] PhD program, 4 specializations[5]
Graduate (MPH)	N/A	N/A	Master of Public Health, 7 specializations[6]
Medical residency	N/A	Public Health and Preventive Medicine Residency program	Public Health and Preventive Medicine Residency program (*Note*: situated in the Faculty of Medicine and Dentistry)
Other	Post-diploma Bachelor of Health Sciences, Major: Public Health; Minor: Health Leadership (2 years)	N/A	Embedded certificates, which can be laddered into a degree University of Alberta North initiative (MPH students recruited from the North with Indigenous knowledge holders or elders acting as mentors) Fellowship in Health Systems Improvement

TABLE 6.2: Timeline of some key events pertinent to the history of public health education in Alberta. "First era" of schools of public health in Canada (approx. 1920–1970); "second era" (1970s–early 2000s); "third era" (early 2000s–present). Compiled from various sources referenced elsewhere in this chapter.

Year	Event
1915	The American *Welch-Rose Report* was published. This report described the poor state of public health in the United States and lack of appropriate training for public health officers, and it recommended the creation of stand-alone "Schools of Hygiene" that were separate from, but connected to, schools of medicine.
1927	The School of Hygiene at the University of Toronto was established (First stand-alone school of public health in Canada)
1945	Second school of public health established in Canada, at l'Université de Montréal
1949	The Department of Preventive Medicine was created within the Faculty of Medicine at the University of Alberta (around 1949).
1968	The Master of Health Services Administration (MHSA) program was launched at the University of Alberta, within the Division of Health Services Administration
1970s	The schools of public health in Toronto and Montreal were absorbed into faculties of medicine
	The Division of Community Health Sciences was created within the Faculty of Medicine at the University of Calgary
	The Community Medicine specialty was recognized by the Royal College of Physicians of Canada
1974	Release by the federal government of *A New Perspective on the Health of Canadians* (Lalonde Report)
1980	The faculty of Health Sciences was established at the University of Lethbridge
1981	The Division of Community Health Sciences became the Department of Community Health Sciences, in the Faculty of Medicine at the University of Calgary
1986	Release of the *Ottawa Charter for Health Promotion*, stemming from the First International Conference on Health Promotion held in Ottawa
1995	The Master of Health Services Administration (MHSA) program at the University of Alberta was discontinued
1996	The Centre for Health Promotion Studies was formally launched at the University of Alberta. That same year, the Centre launched a thesis-based Master of Science degree program and a postgraduate degree program.
	The Department of Public Health Sciences was created in the Faculty of Medicine and Dentistry at the University of Alberta, and offered a Master of Public Health program
2000	The Canadian Institutes of Health Research (CIHR) was created, replacing its predecessor the Medical Research Council, which was established in 1960. One of the new institutes was the Institute of Population and Public Health
2002	The Alberta Government established the Campus Alberta initiative, as a framework comprised of principles to support educational institutions to work together in providing learning opportunities for Albertans
2003	Global pandemic of SARS

TABLE 6.2: *(continued)*

Year	Event
2003	Release of federal report, *Learning from SARS: Renewal of Public Health in Canada*. A report of the National Advisory Committee on SARS and Public Health (the Naylor Report).
	The University of Calgary launched its Bachelor of Health Sciences degree program (Fall 2003)
2004	Establishment of the Public Health Agency of Canada (was confirmed as a legal entity in 2006)
2005	Release of the National Framework on Public Health Human Resources Development, Joint Task Group on Public Health Human Resources
2005	The BHSc program at the University of Calgary became the O'Brien Centre for the Bachelor of Health Sciences Program
2006	The University of Alberta created its School of Public Health (March 2006)
	Memorandum of Understanding between the Universities of Alberta, Calgary, and Lethbridge was signed (May 2006)
2008	The Public Health Agency of Canada released Core Competencies for Public Health
2008	The University of Lethbridge launched its Bachelor of Health Sciences in Public Health Degree (Fall 2008)
2009	The School of Health Sciences at the University of Lethbridge became the Faculty of Health Sciences (1 May 2009)
2012	The University of Lethbridge launched its Bachelor of Health Sciences – Public Health / Bachelor of Management combined degrees program (Fall 2012)
	The School of Public Health at the University of Alberta received Accreditation from the U.S.-based Council on Education for Public Health, making it the first accredited school in Canada.
2016	The University of Lethbridge launched its Post-Diploma Bachelor of Health Sciences (Public Health major, Health Leadership minor) program (Fall 2016)
	The University of Alberta added an MPH in Food Safety, in collaboration with the Faculty of Agriculture, Life & Environmental Sciences
2018	Accreditation of the University of Alberta's School of Public Health was renewed for 7 years.

- All of the major causes of death and disability are either preventable or can be substantially reduced through appropriately designed and implemented public health interventions at the population level, including public policy.
  - References the 2001 provincial report, *A Framework for Reform: Report of the Premier's Advisory Council on Health* (the Mazankowski Report), which identifies that a significant element of health care reform is efforts to keep people healthy in the first place.
- Research has become a powerful tool for discovering opportunities to improve health by taking action on broad determinants of health such as education, socioeconomic status, supportive physical and social environments, healthy child development, gender, culture and various lifestyle and personal health factors and coping skills.
- The three universities have worked hard within their respective capacities to meet Alberta's needs for new knowledge and trained manpower (sic), but more must be done, and continuing to work independently of each other will not be enough.
- We will develop a pan-Alberta coalition to synchronize efforts in ways that will help to develop Alberta's capacity to promote health and security across the entire province, contributing to the sustainability of our health care system.
- Together we will integrate our respective programming and specialized facilities in order to offer well-defined career paths and a greater choice of options to students [. . .] Focusing on the broad spectrum of learning in the field of public health and the social determinants of health, we have made a commitment to align, integrate and strengthen our institutions.
- Our commitment to collaboration [. . .] capitalizes on the different mandates and different roles and responsibilities we have within the provincial post-secondary system.
- We will work toward the following public health research and education objectives: (examples: meet regularly to share information and to develop and support collaborative and complementary programs; share physical and human resources; jointly seek alliances and advocates; jointly promote the combined public health and strength and expertise of the three institutions locally, nationally, and internationally).
- In collaboration with our respective regional health authorities, the Universities of Lethbridge, Calgary and Alberta will build and present to government, a demonstrable case for substantial increase in provincial investment dedicated to public health education, research and practice and that will support a pan-provincial, comprehensive School of Public Health.
- The MOU is only an expression of intent and does not, except for the provision dealing with confidentiality and issuance of press releases, create any binding obligations between parties.
  - Accompanying email correspondence from the University of Alberta requested wording that conveyed an agreement to cooperate, rather than a legally binding contract.

To be signed by William Cade, President and Vice Chancellor, University of Lethbridge; Harvey Weingarten, President, University of Calgary; and Indira Samarasekera, President and Vice Chancellor, University of Alberta.

Fig. 6.1: Summary points from the penultimate version (dated February 2006) of the memorandum of understanding for the pan-Alberta public health coalition.[118]

NOTES

1   Louise Potvin, "Canadian Public Health under Siege," *Canadian Journal of Public Health* 105, no. 6 (2014); Ak'ingabe Guyon et al., "The Weakening of Public Health: A Threat to Population Health and Health Care System Sustainability," *Canadian Journal of Public Health* 108, no. 1 (2017).

2   Commission on Social Determinants of Health, *Closing the Gap in a Generation: Health Equity Through Action on the Social Determinants of Health. Final Report of the Commission on Social Determinants of Health* (Geneva: World Health Organization, 2008).

3   The Canadian Network of Public Health Associations, "A Collective Voice for Advancing Public Health: Why Public Health Associations Matter Today," *Canadian Journal of Public Health* 110, no. 3 (2019); Ali Walker and Patricia Doyle-Baker, "Promoting and Strengthening Public Health through Undergraduate Education," *Canadian Journal of Public Health* 110, no. 3 (2019).

4   A potentially large number of education programs could be considered relevant to public health, spanning the natural sciences, social sciences, and humanities, as well as numerous professional programs, all of which may or may not talk explicitly about 'health' or 'public health.' In addition are the many faculty research programs in which students of different levels are nested. Indeed, trying to define or identify the contours of 'public health education' is one illustration of the conundrum presented by a perennial question for public health: how broad is the mandate? See Michael M. Rachlis, "Moving Forward with Public Health in Canada," *Canadian Journal of Public Health* 95, no. 6 (2004). We have focused primarily on a subset of named programs.

5   "Relatively recent" takes on new meaning with the Covid-19 pandemic, ongoing at the time of writing, which, like SARS nearly two decades earlier, has once again brought public health, or at least some aspects of it, to the forefront.

6   Walter H. Johns, *A History of the University of Alberta, 1908–1969* (Edmonton: University of Alberta Press, 1981), 3, 20; Alberta Health Services, "History: Public Health Laboratory (ProvLab)," accessed 6 July 2020, https://www.albertahealthservices.ca/lab/Page14604.aspx.

7   University of Toronto, "Origin Story: How the Dalla Lana School of Public Health Began," Dalla Lana School of Public Health, accessed 6 July 2020, https://www.utoronto.ca/news/origin-story-how-dalla-lana-school-public-health-began.

8   Elizabeth Fee and Liping Bu, "Models of Public Health Education: Choices for the Future?" *Bulletin of the World Health Organization* 85, no. 12 (December 2007).

9   Fee and Bu, "Models of Public Health Education." Karen Kruse Thomas, "Cultivating Hygiene as a Science: The Welch–Rose Report's Influence at Johns Hopkins and Beyond," *American Journal of Epidemiology* 183, no. 5 (2016); William H. Welch and Wickliffe Rose, *Institute of Hygiene: Being a Report Submitted by Dr. William H Welch and Wickliffe Rose to the General Education Board, Rockefeller Foundation.* 27 May 1915. RG 1.1, Series 200L (Sleepy Hollow, NY: Rockefeller Foundation Archives; 1916).

10   According to Elizabeth Fee, the term "hygiene" was sometimes used in North America to convey the scientific basis of public health, as taught in German institutes of hygiene, rather than the British term "public health," which conveyed more of an administrative focus. Fee and Bu, "Models of Public Health Education."

11   Darwin H. Stapleton, "Internationalism and Nationalism: The Rockefeller Foundation, Public Health and Malaria in Italy," *Parasitologia* 42, no. 1 (2000).

12   Fee and Bu, "Models of Public Health Education."

13   Lindsay McLaren and Trevor Hancock, "Public Health Matters — but We Need to Make the Case," *Canadian Journal of Public Health* 110 no. 3 (2019).

14   Richard Massé and Brent Moloughney, "New Era for Schools and Programs of Public Health in Canada," *Public Health Reviews* 33, no. 1 (2011).

15   Massé and Moloughney, "New Era for Schools and Programs"; Christopher Rutty and Sue C. Sullivan, *This Is Public Health: A Canadian History* (Ottawa: Canadian Public Health Association, 2010), 8.9. See also University of Toronto, "Origin Story: Dalla Lana School of Public Health."

16   Rutty and Sullivan, *This is Public Health,* 8.9–8.10; Kue Young and Faith Davis, "Opinion: Public Health Education Under Threats from Provincial Cuts," *Edmonton Journal,* 16 May 2020, https://edmontonjournal.com/opinion/columnists/opinion-public-health-education-under-threat-from-provincial-cuts/wcm/08da6037-1dd0-4bcd-b706-9c257dd5865e/.

17   Donna Richardson, School of Public Health, University of Alberta, *It Begins Here, 2006–2016: Report to the Community* (Edmonton: School of Public Health, University of Alberta, 2016), https://issuu.com/sphuofa/docs/it_begins_here_report_final_websm.

18   Provincial Archives of Alberta, *An Administrative History of the Government of Alberta, 1905–2005* (Edmonton: The Provincial Archives of Alberta, 2006).

19   Jim Connor, "Bookmarks: Making Medicare: New Perspectives on the History of Medicare in Canada," *Canadian Medical Association Journal* 186, no. 12 (2014): E66.

20   Anthony W. Rasporich, *Make No Small Plans: The University of Calgary at Forty* (Calgary: University of Calgary, 2007), 3. For a history of the parallel degree program in nursing, see Geertje Boschma, *Faculty of Nursing on the Move: Nursing at the University of Calgary, 1969–2004* (Calgary: University of Calgary, 2005), 31.

21   Owen G. Holmes, *Come Hell or High Water — A History of the University of Lethbridge* (Lethbridge: Lethbridge Herald, 1972).

22   Doug Wilson, interview by Rogelio Velez Mendoza, 12 December 2019.

23   Massé and Moloughney, "New Era for Schools and Programs."

24   Richardson, School of Public Health, University of Alberta, *It Begins Here*.

25   Ruth Wolfe (Associate Dean, Professional Programs, University of Alberta), personal communication, 21 October 2019.

26   Edward Shorter, *Partnership for Excellence: Medicine at the University of Toronto and Academic Hospitals* (Toronto: University of Toronto Press, 2016), 120–125.

27   "About the Faculty," Faculty of Health Sciences, University of Lethbridge, accessed 7 July 2020, https://www.uleth.ca/healthsciences/content/about-faculty.

28   Department of Community Health Sciences fonds, University of Calgary Archives. CA ACU ARC F0069.

29   *Working towards unity of purpose in public health education: Starting a conversation across three Alberta post-secondary institutions,* Final report from Campus Alberta Health Outcomes and Public Health-funded meeting, 11 February 2019, Calgary (unpublished report).

30   The centre was originally called the Injury Awareness on Prevention Centre; in 1997 it became the Alberta Centre for Injury Control and Research and subsequently the Injury Prevention Centre. Louis Francescutti, interview by Rogelio Velez Mendoza, Edmonton, 30 August 2018. Since 2008, professor and researcher Donald Voaklander has served as the Centre's Director. "Injury Prevention Centre Staff, Injury Prevention Centre, accessed 7 July 2020, https://injurypreventioncentre.ca/about/staff.

31   Richardson, School of Public Health, University of Alberta, *It Begins Here*.

32   Marc Lalonde, *A New Perspective on the Health of Canadians (Lalonde Report)* (Ottawa: Department of National Health and Welfare, 1974), https://www.canada.ca/en/health-canada/services/health-care-system/commissions-inquiries/federal-commissions-health-care/new-perspective-health-canadians-lalonde-report.html.; World Health Organization, "Ottawa Charter for Health Promotion" (Ottawa: World Health Organization, 1986), https://www.who.int/healthpromotion/conferences/previous/ottawa/en/.

33   James Colgrove, "The McKeown Thesis: A Historical Controversy and its Enduring Influence," *American Journal of Public Health* 92, no. 5 (2002). Perhaps emblematic of the population health movement in Canada was the 1994 book *Why are Some People Healthy and Others Not? The Determinants of Health of Populations*, which was a product of the Population Health Program of the Canadian Institute for Advanced Research (eds. Theodore R. Marmor, Morris L. Barer, and Robert G. Evans. New York: A. de Gruyter).

34   Colgrove, "The McKeown Thesis." Although various aspects of McKeown's original thesis were criticized, his work endures because — as described by Colgrove — of i) the importance of the questions he tackled around what are the primary drivers of population health and ii) the attention he drew to social and economic conditions and their influence on health.

35   Doug Wilson, interview; Kim Raine, interview by Rogelio Velez Mendoza, 25 September 2018; Ardene Robinson Vollman, interview by Rogelio Velez Mendoza, 11 February 2020.

36   Kim Raine, interview.

37   Doug Wilson, interview. The University of Alberta's Health Sciences Faculty Council includes several faculties: Medicine & Dentistry; Agriculture, Life and Environmental Sciences; Pharmacy and Pharmaceutical Sciences; Nursing; Rehabilitation Medicine; Kinesiology, Sport & Recreation; and now Public Health. University of Alberta, "Health Sciences Council," accessed 7 July 2020, https://www.ualberta.ca/health-sciences-council/about-us/members.html.

38   The post graduate diploma initiative was later suspended and ultimately abolished. Ruth Wolfe, personal communication.

39   Kim Raine, interview; Doug Wilson, interview; Ruth Wolfe, personal communication; Richardson, School of Public Health, University of Alberta, *It Begins Here*; University of Alberta, "Miriam Stewart,"

Faculty of Nursing, accessed 7 July 2020, https://www.ualberta.ca/nursing/about/contact-us-and-people/professors-emeritae/stewart.html.

40 Ardene Robinson Vollman, interview; Ontario Health Promotion, "The Canadian Consortium for Health Promotion Research," Ontario Health Promotion E-Bulletin, accessed 7 July 2020, http://www.ohpe.ca/node/4620.

41 Kim Raine, interview; Doug Wilson, interview; Ardene Robinson Vollman, interview.

42 Kim Raine, interview; Doug Wilson, interview; Ardene Robinson Vollman, interview; Ontario Health Promotion, "The Canadian Consortium."

43 Rowena Rae and Anda Zeng, "SARS in Canada," in *The Canadian Encyclopedia. Historica Canada*, last updated 25 March 2020, https://www.thecanadianencyclopedia.ca/en/article/sars-severe-acute-respiratory-syndrome. SARS was one of several events that drew attention to public health capacity (or lack thereof) in Canada early in the new millennium. Another event was the *E. coli* outbreak in Walkerton, Ontario in 2000. See Larry W. Chambers et al., "Health Surveillance: An Essential Tool to Protect and Promote the Health of the Public," *Canadian Journal of Public Health* 97, no. 3 (2006): suppl.

44 Christopher David Naylor, National Advisory Committee, *Learning from SARS: Renewal of Public Health in Canada: A Report of the National Advisory Committee on SARS and Public Health* (Ottawa: National Advisory Committee, 2003), https://www.canada.ca/en/public-health/services/reports-publications/learning-sars-renewal-public-health-canada.html.

45 Public Health Agency of Canada, "History," About the Agency, accessed 8 July 2020, https://www.canada.ca/en/public-health/corporate/mandate/about-agency/history.html.; "About Us," National Collaborating Centres for Public Health, accessed 8 July 2020, https://nccph.ca/about-us/.

46 Joint Task Group on Public Health Human Resources, Public Health Agency of Canada, *Building the Public Health Workforce for the 21 Century: A Pan-Canadian Framework for Public Health Human Resources* (Ottawa: Ministry of Health, 2005), http://publications.gc.ca/collections/collection_2008/phac-aspc/HP5-12-2005E.pdf; Public Health Agency of Canada, *Core Competencies for Public Health in Canada: Release 1.0* (Ottawa: Ministry of Health, 2008), http://www.phac-aspc.gc.ca/php-psp/ccph-cesp/pdfs/cc-manual-eng090407.pdf.

47 Massé and Moloughney, "New Era for Schools and Programs."

48 Massé and Moloughney, "New Era for Schools and Programs."

49 Canadian Institutes of Health Research (CIHR), "Milestones in Canadian Health Research," About Us,, accessed 8 July 2020, https://cihr-irsc.gc.ca/e/35216.html.

50 CIHR, "Applied Public Health Chairs [2008–2013 cohort]," Population and Public Health, accessed 11 July 2020, https://cihr-irsc.gc.ca/e/42160.html.; CIHR, "2014 Applied Public Health Chairs [2014–2019 cohort]," Population and Public Health, accessed 11 July 2020, https://cihr-irsc.gc.ca/e/48898.html. A more recent initiative, for which CIHR's Institute of Population and Public Health is a partner, is the Health System Impact Fellowship for senior (postdoctoral and doctoral) trainees. See Cynthia Weijs et al., "Strengthening the Health System through Novel Population and Public Health Fellowships in Canada," *Canadian Journal of Public Health* 110, no. 3 (2019).

51 Doug Wilson, interview; Ardene Robinson Vollman, interview; Chris Hosgood, interview; *Working towards unity of purpose in public health education: Starting a conversation across three Alberta post-secondary institutions*, Final report from Campus Alberta Health Outcomes.

52 See also Geertje Boschma, "Community Mental Health Nursing in Alberta," *Canadian Journal of Gastroenterology* 23, no. 6 (2009): 404; Robert J. Baley, "A Tribute to Grant Gall," *Canadian Journal of Gastroenterology* 23, no. 6 (2009): 404.

53 Doug Wilson, interview; Richardson, School of Public Health, University of Alberta, *It Begins Here*.

54 Doug Wilson, interview.

55 Doug Wilson, interview; Richardson, School of Public Health, University of Alberta, *It Begins Here*.

56 Doug Wilson, interview.

57 Richardson, School of Public Health, University of Alberta, *It Begins Here*; University of Alberta, "Dean's Corner," School of Public Health, accessed 11 July 2020, https://www.ualberta.ca/public-health/about/deans-corner/index.html; "Public Health School at U of A," *Edmonton Journal*, 18 March 2006, 25; Stephen J. Corber, "The History of Public Health in Canada," *Canadian Journal of Public Health* 85, no. 6 (1994).

58 Richardson, School of Public Health, University of Alberta, *It Begins Here*; University of Alberta, "Dean's Corner."

59 Doug Wilson, interview; Richardson, University of Alberta, School of Public Health, *It Begins Here*.

60 Richardson, University of Alberta, School of Public Health, *It Begins Here*; Kim Raine, interview.

61 Ruth Wolfe, personal communication; University of Alberta, "Public Health & Preventive Medicine Residency Program," Department of Medicine, accessed 11 July 2020, https://www.ualberta.ca/department-of-medicine/education/residency-programs/public-health-preventive-medicine/index.html.

62 *Working towards unity of purpose in public health education: Starting a conversation across three Alberta post-secondary institutions*, Final report from Campus Alberta Health Outcomes.

63 University of Saskatchewan, "About the School," School of Public Health, accessed 11 July 2020, https://sph.usask.ca/about-the-school.php.; Dalla Lana School of Public Health, *Annual Report 2014–2015* (University of Toronto: 2015), http://www.dlsph.utoronto.ca/wp-content/uploads/2015/08/DLSPH-2014-15-Annual-Report_LR.pdf.

64 In addition to the sources noted, this section draws on author LM's own experience as a member of the Department of Community Health Sciences, first as a postdoctoral fellow starting in 2002 and then as a faculty member starting in 2006.

65 The faculty was renamed the Cumming School of Medicine in 2014 following a significant philanthropic donation. University of Calgary, "Our History," Cumming School of Medicine, accessed 11 July 2020, https://cumming.ucalgary.ca/about/cumming-school-medicine/history.

66 The Bachelor of Health Sciences program at the University of Calgary is "an inquiry-based, multidisciplinary, and research-intensive undergraduate health sciences honours degree program." University of Calgary, "Bachelor of Health Sciences," Cumming School of Medicine, accessed 11 July 2020, https://cumming.ucalgary.ca/bhsc.

67 The Health and Society major is one of three within the University of Calgary's Bachelor of Health Sciences program; the others are Biomedical Sciences and Bioinformatics (University of Calgary, "Bachelor of Health Sciences); *Working towards unity of purpose in public health education: Starting a conversation across three Alberta post-secondary institutions*, Final report from Campus Alberta Health Outcomes.

68 Toby Taylor (Administrative Manager, Bachelor of Health Sciences Program), personal communication, 14 May 2020.

69 Ted Schrecker, "What Is Critical about Critical Public Health? Focus on Health Inequalities," *Critical Public Health* 32, Issue 2 (2022); Mike D. Fliss et al., "Public Health, Private Names: Ethical Considerations of Branding Schools of Public Health in the United States," *Critical Public Health* 31, Issue 4 (2021).

70 Social science concentration options for Health and Society students within the University of Calgary's Bachelor of Health Sciences program include: anthropology, community rehabilitation and disability studies, economics, geography, political science, psychology, and sociology. "Health & Society," University of Calgary, "Bachelor of Health Sciences," Cumming Schools of Medicine, accessed 11 July 2020, https://cumming.ucalgary.ca/bhsc/future-students/majors/hsoc.; see also *Working towards unity of purpose in public health education: Starting a conversation across three Alberta post-secondary institutions*, Final report from Campus Alberta Health Outcomes.

71 Ardene Robinson Vollman, interview.

72 Hawe and Shiell expanded population and public health research capacity in the Department of Community Health Sciences, including by recruiting Jim Dunn, an urban geographer who also held a CIHR-PHAC Applied Public Health Chair, and Melanie Rock, a critical qualitative social scientist whose research focuses on societal and cultural dimensions of health with an emphasis on the importance of nonhuman animals for well-being.

73 From a longstanding previous structure of three specializations (i.e., epidemiology, biostatistics, and "health research" which — frustratingly — included everything that did not fall into epidemiology or biostatistics), the graduate program (MSc and PhD) in the Department of Community Health Sciences expanded in the early 2000s and at the time of writing had seven specializations: Biostatistics, Community Rehabilitation and Disability Studies, Epidemiology (including Clinical and Healthcare Epidemiology), Health Economics, Health Services Research, Medical Education, and Population and Public Health. University of Calgary, "Programs and Courses," Department of Community Health Sciences, accessed 11 July 2020, https://cumming.ucalgary.ca/departments/community-health-sciences/education/our-programs/graduate-degrees-community-health-sciences.

74 Ardene Robinson Vollman, interview.

75 Ardene Robinson Vollman, interview.

76 Ardene Robinson Vollman, interview; Chris Hosgood, interview; University of Toronto, "Former UTHealth President Dr. David Low Passes Away.

77 The Association of Schools of Public Health (ASPH) was the U.S. national organization representing deans, faculty and students of accredited schools of public health. The Council on Education for Public

Health, which is responsible for accreditation, was established in 1974 by the ASPH and the American Public Health Association. In 2013, the ASPH became the Association of Schools and Programs of Public Health (ASPPH). Council on Education for Public Health, "About," accessed 11 July 2020, https://ceph.org/about/org-info/.

78 Ardene Robinson Vollman, interview; Chris Hosgood, interview.

79 Alberta. Legislative Assembly of Alberta, 10 May 2006, https://docs.assembly.ab.ca/LADDAR_files/docs/hansards/han/legislature_26/session_2/20060510_1330_01_han.pdf, 1455–1456; 11 May 2006, https://docs.assembly.ab.ca/LADDAR_files/docs/hansards/han/legislature_26/session_2/20060511_1330_01_han.pdf, 1517.

80 According to the records of Ardene Robinson Vollman, in early March of 2006 the provosts at the University of Calgary and the University of Lethbridge had approved the draft memorandum of understanding, but at that time it was still being "reviewed at the highest levels" at the University of Alberta. Therefore, from the point of view of the Universities of Calgary and Lethbridge, the agreement was felt to be in place when the University of Alberta announced its School of Public Health. Ardene Robinson Vollman, personal communication, 21 May 2020.

81 Ardene Robinson Vollman, interview.

82 Ardene Robinson Vollman, interview.

83 At the time of writing, the seven research institutes within the University of Calgary Cumming School of Medicine are,: the Alberta Children's Hospital Research Institute; the Arnie Charbonneau Cancer Institute; the Calvin, Phoebe and Joan Snyder Institute for Chronic Diseases; the Hotchkiss Brain Institute; the O'Brien Institute for Public Health; the Libin Cardiovascular Institute; and the McCaig Institute for Bone and Joint Health. University of Calgary, "Research Institutes," Cumming School of Medicine, accessed 11 July 2020, https://cumming.ucalgary.ca/research/institutes.

84 University of Calgary, "Our History," O'Brien Institute for Public Health, accessed 11 July 2020, https://obrieniph.ucalgary.ca/about/history

85 Hosgood had previously served as Associate Dean of Arts and Sciences, from 2002 to 2005. Chris Hosgood, interview.

86 Chris Hosgood, interview.

87 Chris Hosgood, interview.

88 Chris Hosgood, interview.

89 See *Snapshot: University of Lethbridge School of Health Sciences* 2, Issue 1 (Spring 2009). Originally, the undergraduate program in public health was envisioned as a joint program between the faculties of Health Sciences and Arts and Science. The joint program model did not ultimately materialize but the program retained close ties with Arts and Sciences to ensure that students gained a broad, critical, and multidisciplinary understanding of health.

90 *Snapshot: University of Lethbridge School of Health Sciences* 2, Issue 1 (Spring 2009).

91 The specializations were: applied public health practice; health policy and promotion; and public health administration. *Snapshot: University of Lethbridge School of Health Sciences* 2, Issue 1 (Spring 2009); *Snapshot: University of Lethbridge Faculty of Health Sciences* 4, Issue 1 (Spring 2011). The practicum is not mandatory but is a popular opportunity for which faculty and staff work closely with students. Chris Hosgood, interview.

92 *Snapshot: University of Lethbridge Faculty of Health Sciences* 4, Issue 1 (Spring 2011); *Snapshot: University of Lethbridge Faculty of Health Sciences* 5, Issue 1 (Spring 2012); Chris Hosgood, interview.

93 *Snapshot: University of Lethbridge Faculty of Health Sciences* 4, Issue 1 (Spring 2011).

94 Chris Hosgood, interview; "Bachelor of Health Sciences – Public Health, Academic Quality Assurance Review," Memorandum 2015, accessed 11 July 2020, https://www.ulethbridge.ca/sites/default/files/2017/09/BHSc%20Public%20Health%20review_Closing%20Memo_2015.pdf.

95 Chris Hosgood, interview; University of Lethbridge, "Programs & Degrees," Faculty of Health Sciences, accessed 11 July 2020, https://www.uleth.ca/healthsciences/content/programs-degrees.

96 Peter Catterall, "What (if anything) is Distinctive about Contemporary History?" *Journal of Contemporary History* 32, no. 4 (1997).

97 Ardene Robinson Vollman, interview.

98 Chris Hosgood, interview. According to members of the University of Alberta community, the Council on Education for Public Health's accreditation of a multi-institution arrangement requires that one institution must take the lead, and there was uneasy agreement that the University of Alberta would focus on the master of public health education component. Doug Wilson, personal communication, 20 May 2020.

99 Following the May 2006 memorandum of understanding, the universities continued to work towards a pan-Alberta strategy, including the creation in 2007 of an "Alberta Strategy for Academic Public Health" (unpublished document) which in addition to the Universities of Lethbridge, Calgary, and Alberta, included Athabasca University. The strategy document references the May 2006 memorandum of understanding and includes independent proposals for expansion from each university. The economic recession of 2008 precluded many of the expansion items outlined in the strategy document.

100 Campus Alberta Health Outcomes and Public Health framework, see https://obrieniph.ucalgary.ca/institute/campus-alberta-health-outcomes-and-public-health

101 *Working towards unity of purpose in public health education: Starting a conversation across three Alberta post-secondary institutions,* Final report from Campus Alberta Health Outcomes.

102 Harvey V. Fineberg, "Public Health and Medicine: Where the Twain Shall Meet," *American Journal of Preventive Medicine* 41, no. 4 suppl 3 (2011); Ingrid V. Tyler, et al., "Canadian Medical Students' Perceptions of Public Health Education in the Undergraduate Medical Curriculum," *Academic Medicine* 84 (2009).

103 Jennie Popay, Margaret Whitehead, and David J. Hunter, "Injustice is Killing People on a Large Scale – But What Is To Be Done About It? *Journal of Public Health* 32, Issue 2 (2010); Fran Baum and Matthew Fisher, "Why Behavioural Health Promotion Endures Despite its Failure to Reduce Health Inequities," *Sociology of Health & Illness* 36, no. 2 (2014); Frances Elaine Baum and David M Sanders, "Ottawa 25 Years On: A More Radical Agenda for Health Equity Is Still Required," *Health Promotion International* 26 (suppl 2) (2011); Gemma Carey et al., "Can the Sociology of Social Problems Help us to Understand and Manage 'Lifestyle Drift'?," *Health Promotion International* 32, no. 4 (2016).

104 Daniel Skinner, "Challenges in Public Health Pedagogy," *Critical Public Health* 29, no. 1 (2016).

105 Michael Harvey and Margaret McGladrey, "Explaining the Origins and Distribution of Health and Disease: An Analysis of Epidemiologic Theory in Core Master of Public Health Coursework in the United States," *Critical Public Health* 29, no. 1 (2016).

106 Harvey and McGladrey, "Origins and Distribution of Health and Disease," 14.

107 Harvey and McGladrey, "Origins and Distribution of Health and Disease," 6.

108 Chris Hosgood, interview; Ruth Wolfe, personal communication; *Working towards unity of purpose in public health education: Starting a conversation across three Alberta post-secondary institutions,* Final report from Campus Alberta Health Outcomes.

109 Annalee Yassi et al., "Is Public Health Training in Canada Meeting Current Needs? Defrosting the Paradigm Freeze to Respond to the Post-Truth Era," *Critical Public Health* 31, Issue 4 (2021).

110 For example, the core graduate courses in the Department of Community Health Sciences at the University of Calgary have historically included biostatistics and clinical epidemiology, with qualitative research methods being optional. It has proved to be very difficult to change this longstanding model.

111 Yassi, Lockhart, Gray, and Hancock, "Is Public Health Training in Canada Meeting Current Needs?"

112 Yassi et al., "Is Public Health Training in Canada Meeting Current Needs?" 40.

113 David Opinko, "Province Announces 'Outcomes-based' Funding Model for Post-secondary Education," *LethbridgeNewsNow,* 20 January 2020, https://lethbridgenewsnow.com/2020/01/20/province-announces-outcomes-based-funding-model-for-post-secondary-education/.

114 Lindsay McLaren et al., "Unpacking Vulnerability: Towards Language that Advances Understanding and Resolution of Social Inequities in Public Health," *Canadian Journal of Public Health* 111 (2002).

115 Fliss et al., "Public Health, Private Names".

116 See for example, Anne-Emanuelle Birn, "Philanthrocapitalism, Past and Present: The Rockefeller Foundation, the Gates Foundation, and the Setting(s) of the International/Global Health Agenda," *Hypothesis* 12, no. 1 (2014).

117 Laurie Adkin et al., *Higher Education – Corporate or Public? How the UCP is Restructuring Post-Secondary Education in Alberta* (Edmonton: Parkland Institute, May 2022), https://www.parklandinstitute.ca/higher_education_corporate_or_public

118 The penultimate draft of the memorandum of understanding is in the University of Calgary General Counsel fonds, Accession 2010.047 Box 8 File 8.

NOTES TO TABLE 6.1

1   For the BHSc / BMgt Combined Degree program at the University of Lethbridge, the Health Sciences Major is Public Health, and the Management Majors are General Management *or* Human Resource Management and Labour Relations. "Working Towards Unity of Purpose in Public Health Education: Starting a Conversation across Three Alberta Post-secondary Institutions," Final report from Campus Alberta Health Outcomes and Public Health-funded meeting, 11 February 2019, Calgary.

2   The concentrations within the PhD – Population Studies in Health program are: Diversity, disparities, inequalities, and social determinants of health; Global population health; Life course, aging, and health; Policies, policy analysis, and population health; Population health and demographic change; Sustainability and population health ("Population Studies in Health (PhD)" University of Lethbridge, accessed 11 July 2020, https://www.uleth.ca/future-student/graduate-studies/doctor-philosophy/population-studies-health)

3   The MSc and PhD program specializations in the University of Calgary's Department of Community Health Sciences are: Biostatistics, Community Rehabilitation & Disability Studies, Epidemiology, Health Economics, Health Services Research, Medical Education, and Population & Public Health ("Welcome to the Department of Community Health Sciences," University of Calgary, accessed 11 July 2020, https://cumming.ucalgary.ca/departments/community-health-sciences/about-us/message-department-head)

4   The MSc program specializations at the University of Alberta's School of Public Health are: Clinical Epidemiology, Environmental Health Sciences, Epidemiology, General Public Health, Global Health, Health Policy Research, and Health Promotion and Socio-behavioural Sciences ("MSc Programs," School of Public Health, University of Alberta, accessed 11 July 2020, https://www.ualberta.ca/public-health/programs/msc-programs/index.html)

5   The PhD program specializations at the University of Alberta's School of Public Health are: Epidemiology, Health Promotion and Socio-behavioural Sciences, Health Services and Policy Research, and Public Health ("PhD Programs," School of Public Health University of Alberta, accessed 11 July 2020, https://www.ualberta.ca/public-health/programs/phd-programs/index.html)

6   The MPH program specializations at the University of Alberta's School of Public Health are: Applied Biostatistics, Environmental and Occupational Health, Epidemiology, Food Safety, Global Health, Health Policy and Management, and Health Promotion ("MPH Programs," School of Public Health, University of Alberta, accessed 11 July 2020, https://www.ualberta.ca/public-health/programs/mph-programs/index.html). The MPH in Health Promotion is offered both on campus and by distance ("MPH Health Promotion," School of Public Health, University of Alberta, accessed 11 July 2020, https://www.ualberta.ca/public-health/programs/mph-programs/mph-health-promotion.html)

Stories from First Nation Communities in Alberta: Reconciliation Involves All of Us

Lindsay McLaren and Rogelio Velez Mendoza

> *"In order for [reconciliation] to happen, there has to be awareness of the past, acknowledgement of the harm that has been inflicted, atonement for the causes, and action to change behaviour. We are not there yet."*
>
> — Truth and Reconciliation Commission of Canada[1]

Introduction

The Truth and Reconciliation Commission, which documented the truth of survivors, their families, communities, and anyone personally affected by the residential school experience, released its final report and recommendations in 2015. The report includes ninety-four Calls to Action across social and governmental sectors that are essential to realizing a coherent vision of reconciliation that is fundamentally about "establishing and maintaining a mutually respectful relationship between Aboriginal and non-Aboriginal people in this country."[2]

Seven Calls to Action are explicitly about health (see Table 7.1), and indeed, the implications of the residential school legacy for health and well-being are immense. As described by Indigenous physician and researcher Janet Smylie in a *Canadian Journal of Public Health* editorial, the residential school legacy "violated almost every basic principle of public health, sanitation, and healthy child development."[3] Furthermore, the significant and persistent health inequities experienced by Indigenous Peoples in Alberta and Canada stem directly from government policies that legitimated residential schools, appropriated Indigenous lands, enacted forced community re-locations, replaced Indigenous governments, and outlawed spiritual and cultural practices.[4] The ongoing negative effects of colonial government policies is important for us to acknowledge because colonial governments play a central role in public health, which we consider in some depth throughout this book.

TABLE 7.1: Truth and Reconciliation Commission of Canada — Calls to Action related to health. Source: Truth and Reconciliation Commission, *Honouring the Truth, Reconciling for the Future*, 322–323.

"18. We call upon the federal, provincial, territorial, and Aboriginal governments to acknowledge that the current state of Aboriginal health in Canada is a direct result of previous Canadian government policies, including residential schools, and to recognize and implement the health-care rights of Aboriginal people as identified in international law, constitutional law, and under the Treaties.
19. We call upon the federal government, in consultation with Aboriginal peoples, to establish measurable goals to identify and close the gaps in health outcomes between Aboriginal and non-Aboriginal communities, and to publish annual progress reports and assess long-term trends. Such efforts would focus on indicators such as: infant mortality, maternal health, suicide, mental health, addictions, life expectancy, birth rates, infant and child health issues, chronic diseases, illness and injury incidence, and the availability of appropriate health services.
20. In order to address the jurisdictional disputes concerning Aboriginal people who do not reside on reserves, we call upon the federal government to recognize, respect, and address the distinct health needs of the Métis, Inuit, and off-reserve Aboriginal peoples.
21..We call upon the federal government to provide sustainable funding for existing and new Aboriginal healing centres to address the physical, mental, emotional, and spiritual harms caused by residential schools, and to ensure that the funding of healing centres in Nunavut and the Northwest Territories is a priority.
22. We call upon those who can effect change within the Canadian health-care system to recognize the value of Aboriginal healing practices and use them in the treatment of Aboriginal patients in collaboration with Aboriginal healers and Elders where requested by Aboriginal patients.
23. We call upon all levels of government to: i. Increase the number of Aboriginal professionals working in the health-care field. ii. Ensure the retention of Aboriginal health-care providers in Aboriginal communities. iii. Provide cultural competency training for all health-care professionals.
24. We call upon medical and nursing schools in Canada to require all students to take a course dealing with Aboriginal health issues, including the history and legacy of residential schools, the United Nations Declaration on the Rights of Indigenous Peoples, Treaties and Aboriginal rights, and Indigenous teachings and practices. This will require skills-based training in intercultural competency, conflict resolution, human rights, and anti-racism."

The definition of public health that we embrace in this volume is broad: the science and art of preventing disease and promoting health through organized efforts of society.[5] We chose that definition deliberately because it represents key features that drew some of us to the field in the first place. These include:

- a holistic view of health that incorporates well-being;
- a collective orientation that values social inclusion;
- emphasis on social, economic, political, and ecological determinants of health and well-being;
- concern with ensuring social justice and health equity;
- use of evidence-informed approaches that embrace different ways of knowing; and
- an upstream approach that prioritizes prevention and health promotion.[6]

We humbly suggest that these features of public health have some alignment with the spirit of the Truth and Reconciliation Commission report and recommendations. For example, the commission's assertion that "Reconciliation is not an Aboriginal problem — it is a Canadian problem; it involves all of us"[7] aligns with public health's collective orientation and emphasis on inclusion and social justice.[8] A broad view of public health that embraces social and ecological determinants of health, aligns with the sentiment expressed in the "Treaty 6, 7, and 8 Elders Declaration," and reproduced in the Alberta First Nations Information Governance Centre's 2018 report titled *Indigenous Health Indicators*. The report's authors say, "we understand the 94 Calls to Action [in the Truth and Reconciliation Commission] as a whole, representing not just Calls to Action on Health, but also Calls to Action on Health Determinants."[9]

Grounded in those points of alignment, the purpose of this chapter is to showcase select examples that illustrate this broad view of public health from Alberta First Nation communities. Following a brief background, the chapter is composed of community-based examples, one each from Treaty 6, Treaty 7, and Treaty 8 territories. We were honoured to speak with and learn from individuals from these communities, and to provide a forum to tell these stories.[10]

Background

Putting this volume's hundred-year historical focus into perspective, Indigenous Peoples, including First Nations, Métis, and Inuit, have inhabited the land that we now call Alberta for over ten thousand years, or five hundred generations.[11] Although one could not possibly summarize this rich history concisely,[12] a 2013 Alberta government resource titled *Aboriginal Peoples of Alberta: Yesterday, Today, and Tomorrow* provides a glimpse of that history.

[Indigenous Peoples] in Alberta are culturally diverse — from the Dene in the subarctic north to the Woodland Cree in the boreal forest and the Blackfoot of the southern plains, and the Métis throughout the province. . . . While the Blackfoot gathered in huge camps on the plains, with their lifestyle centred on the great buffalo hunts that provided vast amounts of food,[13] the Dene lived in small groups, gathering edible plants, game animals, and fish in the extensive forests and lakes. . . . For all their diversity, First Peoples have much in common. Foremost was a reverence for the natural world, the web of relationships linking every human to every other thing — be it plant or animal, rock or river, invisible spirit or thunderstorm. Living in harmony with their environment, they made little change in their surroundings for thousands of years.[14]

In an appalling sequence of events (Table 7.2), European colonization of North America, underpinned by settler entitlement and presumed superiority, instigated a drastic change in way of life for Indigenous Peoples that remains at the root of unacceptable health inequities between Indigenous and non-Indigenous persons that persist today.[15] These historical events, individually and collectively, constitute cultural genocide, described in the Truth and Reconciliation Commission summary report as follows:

Cultural genocide is the destruction of those structures and practices that allow the group to continue as a group. States that engage in cultural genocide set out to destroy the political and social institutions of the targeted group. Land is seized, and populations are forcibly transferred and their movement is restricted. Languages are banned. Spiritual leaders are persecuted, spiritual practices are forbidden, and objects of spiritual value are confiscated and destroyed. And, most significantly to the issue at hand, families are disrupted to prevent the transmission of cultural values and identity from one generation to the next. In its dealing with Aboriginal people, Canada did all these things.[16]

One of many important instruments of genocide is the Indian Act, initially passed in 1876, which gave the federal Department of Indian Affairs sweeping powers to intervene in the lives of First Nations Peoples,[17] including to determine who was an Indigenous person; manage Indigenous lands, resources, and moneys; control movement of Indigenous Peoples; outlaw traditional cultural activities; and dictate ways of life — all in the interest of promoting "civilization."

Lest one think that the Indian Act is a distant historical artifact, an important contemporary illustration of its perniciousness is the fact that the otherwise celebrated 1977 Canadian Human Rights Act specifically exempted, under Section 67, decisions or actions made under the Indian Act, meaning that First Nations persons were effectively denied full access to human rights protection. Section 67 was repealed in 2008.[18]

TABLE 7.2: Some key recent historical events at the interface of Indigenous and colonial societies in Alberta and Canada (partial list).[19]

Year	Event
1493	Pope Alexander VI's papal bull, the *Doctrine of Discovery*, which permitted any Christian coming upon land inhabited by non-Christians to claim that land.
1763	*Royal Proclamation*: the King of England acknowledged Indigenous peoples' title over their land and declared a special relationship between First Nations and the Crown that respected their right to occupy their traditional lands.
1867	*British North America Act / Constitution Act*, which unilaterally established Canada's jurisdiction over First Nations and their land.
1869	Red River Resistance: Métis peoples formed a provisional government to assert their rights, in response to the Canadian government's purchase (from the Hudson's Bay Company) of Métis territory in the Red River Valley (in what is now Manitoba) and their assertion of authority over the Métis peoples. Shortly after, Métis peoples began to move west into Saskatchewan and Alberta.
1876	The federal *Indian Act* was originally passed (has been amended several times since).
	Treaty 6 was signed at Carlton and Fort Pitt in what is now called Saskatchewan.
1877	*Treaty 7* was signed at the Blackfoot Crossing of the Bow River in what is now called Alberta
1879	The federal government commissioned the *Davin Report*, which recommended assimilation via removing First Nations children from their families and sending them to residential schools.
1895	The Métis peoples of Alberta were first recognized by the federal government; however, when the province of Alberta was formed in 1905 the colonial government terminated the colony (St. Paul des Métis) and turned over the land for homesteading.
1899	*Treaty 8* was signed at Lesser Slave Lake and Fort Chipewyan in what is now called Alberta.
1900	By the 1900s, colonial settlers decimated First Nations and Inuit communities in Canada by diseases they brought (e.g., smallpox and tuberculosis).
1904	The federal Department of Indian Affairs appointed a general medical superintendent to develop medical programs and facilities.
1922	Dr. Peter Bryce, former Medical Inspector for the federal Department of the Interior and of Indian Affairs, published his scathing report of the failure of the federal government to address the deplorable conditions of residential schools ("Indian Schools") that he had carefully documented. As a result of his efforts, Dr. Bryce was fired and denied appointment as the first Deputy Minister of Health, and he wrote this paper following his involuntary termination in 1921.
1928	Métis peoples began to organize politically in Alberta, including the formation of *L'Association des Métis d'Alberta et les Territoires du Nord-Ouest* which lobbied for a land base and improvements to social and economic conditions for Métis in Alberta.

TABLE 7.2: *(continued)*

Year	Event
1934	The *Ewing Commission* was formed by the Alberta government to investigate the conditions of Alberta Métis peoples. The *Ewing Report*, tabled in 1936, recommended the establishment of Métis settlements on Crown land.
1938	The *Métis Population Betterment Act* was passed, which set aside settlement land for Métis peoples and made Alberta the first province to enact legislation specific to Métis peoples.
1945	Control and supervision of medical care and hospitalization of Indians and Inuit (i.e., Indian Health Service) was transferred to the newly-established (1945) Department of National Health and Welfare.
1960	First Nations peoples acquired the right to vote in federal elections in Canada without having to give up their treaty rights and Indian status.
1962	The *Medical Services Branch* was established within the Department of National Health and Welfare, which assumed the responsibilities of the former Indian Health and Northern Health Services.
1964	First Nations peoples acquired the right to vote in Alberta provincial elections.
1966	*A Survey of the Contemporary Indians of Canada: Economic, Political, Educational Needs and Policies* was published. This report, which was commissioned by the federal government (Ministry of Citizenship and Immigration) and edited by UBC Anthropologist Harry B. Hawthorn, concluded that Indigenous peoples were the most disadvantaged in Canada, and that the disadvantages came from failed government policies, and recommended that Indigenous peoples be considered 'citizens plus' and be provided with opportunities and resources to permit self-determination. Following this publication, the federal government began consulting with First Nations communities across Canada.
1969	The federal government released its *White Paper*, which advocated for increased assimilation of Indigenous peoples and proposed to eliminate Indian Status. Indigenous communities across Canada were shocked that the paper did not address concerns raised during the consultations, and the Paper was ultimately withdrawn (see below). The colonial position of Indian Agent was eliminated (late 1960s), in response to several factors including First Nation activism and the restructuring of the federal Department of Indian Affairs.
1970	The Indian Association of Alberta released its *Red Paper*, which was a detailed response to the 1969 *White Paper*. The *White Paper* was withdrawn.
1972	The *National Indian Brotherhood* issued a policy statement recommending the restructuring of First Nations education around local responsibility and control. By 1975, ten First Nations across Canada were operating their own schools.
1974	*Federal Government Indian Health Policy / Policy of the Federal Government concerning Indian Health Services* was tabled by the Minister of National and Health and Welfare. The policy reiterated that no treaty obligations to provide health services to "Indians" exist, yet the federal government wanted to "ensure the availability of services by providing it directly where normal provincial services were not available, and giving financial assistance to indigent Indians to pay for necessary services when the assistance was not otherwise provided."[1]

Year	Event
1975	The *Alberta Federation of Métis Settlements Association* was formed, with the purpose of representing the interests of the Métis settlements and providing a way for settlement councils to share information and coordinate efforts.
	Prompted by the White and Red papers, *The Canadian Government/The Canadian Indian Relationships* paper was released, which aimed to "define a policy framework for strengthening Indian control of programs and services. In the health sector, under contribution agreements 75% of the Bands became responsible for such programs as the Native Alcohol and Drug Abuse Program and the Community Health Representative Program."[2]
1979	*Indian Health Policy.* This brief document, which is viewed as a culmination of hundred years of efforts by Indigenous peoples, recognized the circumstances and structures that have led to unacceptably low levels of health and well-being. The goal of the policy was "to achieve an increasing level of health in Indian communities, generated and maintained by the Indian communities themselves", which in turn is based on three pillars: (1) community development (i.e., socioeconomic, cultural, and spiritual development to remove conditions that prevent well-being); (2) traditional trust relationship between Indigenous peoples and the federal government; and (3) the Canadian health system including responsibilities of different levels of government, First Nation communities, and the private sector.[3]
1980	The *Alberta Indian Health Care Commission* (AIHCC) was established, "to advocate on behalf of First Nation people to ensure provision of comprehensive health care and assert Treaty Right to Health."[4]
	Report of the Advisory Committee on Indian and Inuit Health Consultation (*Berger Report*) was released; the report recommended methods of consultation that would ensure substantive participation by First Nations and Inuit peoples in the design, management, and control of health care services in their communities.
1982	The federal *Constitution Act* was passed, which recognized *Indian*, *Inuit*, and *Métis* as three distinct groups with unique histories, languages, and cultures; and recognized treaty rights (section 35). Prior to this, reference to "Indians" in the Constitution referred to status First Nation members, and (starting in 1939) Inuit peoples, and did not include Métis peoples nor non-status First Nation peoples.
1983	Release of the Report of the Special Committee on Indian Self-Government (*Penner Report*), which recommended that the federal government establish a new relationship with First Nation and Inuit peoples, with recognition of self-government as an essential element, and health as a key area where this could be pursued.
1984	*Canada Health Act*, which sets out the conditions that provincial health insurance plans must have in order to qualify for full federal transfer payments (publicly administered, comprehensive, universal, portable, and accessible). Insured health services are to be provided to all "insured persons", which is defined as a person who is a resident of that province. "Insured persons" should theoretically include all Indigenous peoples residing in the province (urban, rural, in reserve communities) but there is no mention of Indigenous persons within the Act.
1985	Establishment of the *Assembly of First Nations*, an advocacy organization representing First Nations citizens in Canada.
	Passing of *Bill C-31*; an important amendment to the federal Indian Act, intended to align with the provisions of the Canadian Charter of Rights and Freedoms. The amendment was guided by three principles: (1) removal of discrimination; (2) restoring status and membership rights; and (3) increasing community control. The amendment eliminated some previously discriminatory provisions, such as Indigenous women losing their status when they married non-status men.

TABLE 7.2: *(continued)*

Year	Event
1986	The Non-Insured Health Benefits Directorate was established within the Medical Services Branch of the federal government.
1988	Federal Cabinet approved the policy framework for *Health Transfer*, i.e., the process of transferring health system control to Indigenous communities.
1989	The federal Treasury Board approved the financial resources to support pre-*Health Transfer* planning activities.
1990	Following the signing of the *Alberta-Métis Settlements Accord* in 1989, key legislation was passed in 1990 including the *Métis Settlements Act*. The Act established a land-based governance model including local government for each Métis settlement, an overarching Métis Settlements Council to represent the settlements collectively, and a Métis settlement land registry. The *Act* also includes provisions for health and well being; for example: "A settlement council may make bylaws to promote the health, safety and welfare of the residents of the settlement area."[5]
1996	Release of the *Report of the Royal Commission on Aboriginal Peoples*, which was a massive report that examined social, cultural, and economic challenges of First Nations, Métis, and Inuit peoples in Canada that reflect historical relations between government and Indigenous peoples, and outlined a twenty-year agenda for transformative changes, which included elimination of the federal Department of Indigenous and Northern Affairs (see below).
	The *First Nations – MSB Alberta Region Envelope Co-Management Agreement* was signed in Edmonton, by Chiefs from each Treaty area, the federal Minister of Health, and the Assistant Deputy Minister of the Medical Services Branch.
2000	The Alberta Government's *Aboriginal Policy Framework* was released, which outlined a basic structure for provincial policies that address the needs of Aboriginal peoples in Alberta, and emphasized well-being, self-reliance, effective consultation, and clarification of roles and responsibilities.
	The federal Medical Services Branch was re-named *First Nations and Inuit Health Branch* (FNHIB).
2002	*Romanow Report* (Commission on the Future of Health Care in Canada) was released, which emphasized persistent health disparities between Indigenous and non-Indigenous peoples and recommended increasing the number of Indigenous health workers and creating a fund to support health care integration.
2006	The Alberta Government released *Alberta's First Nations consultation guidelines on land management and resource development*, which outlined the manner in which the Alberta government will consult with First Nations and defines roles and responsibilities (these were updated in 2007).
2007	In response to advocacy by First Nation communities and a large number of abuse claims by residential school survivors, an *Indian Residential Schools Settlement Agreement* was approved and implemented. The agreement included, among other things, financial compensation and establishment of the *Truth and Reconciliation Commission*.
	The United Nations adopted a *Declaration on the Rights of Indigenous People*. Canada, under Prime Minister Stephen Harper, did not endorse the Declaration.

Year	Event
2008	Alberta *Protocol Agreement on Government to Government Relations*, which was signed by the Alberta premier, the minister of Aboriginal Relations, and the Grand Chiefs and Vice-Chiefs of Treaties 6, 7, and 8. The agreement provides a framework for collaboration between First Nations and the Government of Alberta.
	Canadian Prime Minister Stephen Harper issued a public apology to Canada's Indigenous peoples, for the forced assimilation of the Indian Residential School system.
2010	*Memorandum of Understanding for First Nations Education in Alberta*, which was signed by the Government of Canada, the Government of Alberta, and the Assembly of Treaty Chiefs in Alberta, and provides a framework for collaboration to strengthen learning and educational success for First Nations learners in Alberta.
	Bill C-3; another important amendment to the federal Indian Act, intended to further remove discrimination on the basis of gender.[6]
2015	The *Truth and Reconciliation Commission of Canada* released its massive final report which included ninety-four recommendations across sectors to work towards reconciliation, understood as "establishing and maintaining a mutually respectful relationship between Aboriginal and non-Aboriginal peoples" in Canada.[7]
2016	Canada, under Prime Minister Justin Trudeau, removed its objector status for the UN *Declaration on the Rights of Indigenous Peoples* and declared full support for the declaration.
	The *National Inquiry into Missing and Murdered Indigenous Women and Girls* was launched; the final report was released and the inquiry concluded in 2019.
2017	The federal government dissolved the Department of Indigenous and Northern Affairs Canada (which was a recommendation from the *Royal Commission on Aboriginal Peoples*, see above) and created two new federal departments: Indigenous Services Canada, and Crown-Indigenous Relations and Northern Affairs Canada. With this change, the First Nations and Inuit Health Branch (FNIHB) was moved out of Health Canada and will move into the new Indigenous Services Canada department.

The Residential School System was implemented under the Indian Act and the schools were usually administered by churches. There were twenty-five residential schools in Alberta, which is the highest number of any province.[20] Importantly, the dire conditions of the residential schools were known, but this knowledge and accompanying recommendations were actively and deliberately quashed. In his position as medical inspector for the federal Departments of the Interior and of Indian Affairs, Dr. Peter Bryce gathered data from First Nation communities across Canada between 1904 and 1914,[21] including "special inspections" in Alberta and other prairie provinces.[22] His findings were unambiguous: his 1907 report revealed that tuberculosis in residential schools was rampant, and 24 percent of students who had attended the schools were known to be dead.[23] He offered several substantive recommendations, including for the government to take responsibility for "the complete maintenance and control of the schools, since it had promised by treaty to insure such."[24] Yet, those recommendations were not published, and despite repeated attempts over several years, Bryce's efforts to advance "even the simplest effective efforts to deal with the health problem of the Indians" were stymied.[25] This reflected active opposition from church officials[26] and federal leaders, perhaps most infamously Mr. Duncan Campbell Scott of the federal Department of Indian Affairs.[27] Upon his involuntary retirement, Dr. Bryce wrote up his experiences in a highly critical 1922 paper provocatively titled "The Story of a National Crime: An Appeal for Justice to the Indians of Canada," in which he lamented that "this story should have been written years ago and then given to the public."[28]

Between 1871 and 1921, the Canadian government entered into treaties with various First Nations across Canada, of which three pertain to Alberta: Treaty 6, which was signed in 1876 and covers territory in the centre of the province; Treaty 7 (1877) in the south, and Treaty 8 (1899) in the north.[29] Under those historic treaties, First Nations who occupied the territories, who were in some cases facing the devastating challenges brought on by colonization, gave up large areas of land in exchange for promised provisions and goods.[30] However, different intentions and interpretations of what the treaties meant have led to exceedingly complex relationships between First Nation communities and federal and provincial governments. As stated in the summary report, "the negotiation of Treaties, while seemingly honourable and legal, was often marked by fraud and coercion, and Canada was, and remains, slow to implement their provisions and intent."[31] A contemporary map of treaty areas and First Nation communities in Alberta is shown in Figure 7.1 on page 225.

According to the Métis Nation of Alberta, a Métis person is someone "who self-identifies as a Métis, is distinct from other aboriginal peoples, is of historic Métis Nation ancestry, and is accepted by the Métis Nation."[32] Stemming from efforts in the early twentieth century to organize politically, Métis peoples in Alberta have a land base. Briefly, Association des Métis d'Alberta et les Territoires du Nord-Ouest, the precursor of the Métis Association of Alberta and, later, the Métis Nation of Alberta, was formed in 1928 to lobby for improved social and economic conditions and a land base. The lobbying led to land being legally set aside for Métis peoples in Alberta starting in 1938 (Table 7.2), and a governance framework to support local autonomy and self-government was added in the early 1990s. A contemporary map of the eight Métis settlement areas and communities in Alberta is shown in Figure 7.2 on page 226.

Treaty Right to Health

To provide some additional context to the stories that follow, we conclude this background section with a short overview of the colonial structure of health care for Indigenous Peoples in Alberta and Canada (Table 7.2). Importantly, in line with this volume's broad conceptualization of public health, health care is only one of many policy subsystems that is relevant to health and well-being; yet it is intimately connected to Indigenous social and cultural histories. As described in Alberta Health Services' *Indigenous Health Transformational Roadmap*:

> Many Indigenous people consider Inherent Rights to Health and Health Care as granted by the Creator. First Nations are born with Inherent Rights and inherit them from generation to generation based on traditions, customs, practices and connections to the land. . . . The oral assurances . . . of medical aid and the provision of medical care during the Treaty negotiations were important to First Nations and form the basis for our understanding of the Treaty Right to Health.[33]

The Treaty Right to Health has come to signify the failure of colonial government to uphold obligations related to health care as understood in the Treaties. As stated in the Declaration of Treaty 6, 7 and 8 First Nations – Treaty Right to Health:

> As Treaty Indians there is nothing more important than our Treaties, our land and the well-being of our future generations.
>
> All rights are recognized in Treaties between the Crown and Nations or Tribes of Indians in Canada ensuring the wholistic and the spiritual concept of Treaties.
>
> That the medicine chest clause binds the federal government to provide medicines and all that is required to maintain proper health.
>
> Treaty 6, 7 & 8 discussions were based on previous treaties and that all were equally inclusive and applicable.
>
> So long as the sun shines, rivers flow and the grass grows, these words must never be broken.[34]

Contributing to the failed promise by colonial governments to uphold obligations related to health care is Canada's complex jurisdictional arrangements, which stem from its federated structure of government. Briefly, nineteenth-century federal legislation assigned authority for all issues pertaining to Indigenous Peoples, including health care, to the federal government.[35] Initially situated within the federal Department of Indian Affairs (est. 1880),[36] authority for "Indian Health Service" was shifted to the Department of National Health and Welfare upon its establishment in 1945, and in 1962 to the newly created Medical Services Branch within that federal department.[37] However, the creation of that new federal department, and the broader post-WWII government expansion of which it was part — while widely celebrated as ushering in Canada's welfare state — in fact signified intensification of racialized exclusion of Indigenous Peoples. As powerfully described by historian Maureen Lux in her work on Indian hospitals, the use of which are significant in Alberta's history, the post-war expansion could be characterized as pursuing a vision of national health that was based on white citizenship.[38] The Medical Services Branch was renamed the First Nations and Inuit Health Branch in 2000,[39] and has historically held responsibility for funding and/or administering various programs and services including some public health and health promotion programs, non-insured health benefits, and primary care services in remote or isolated communities.[40]

Jurisdictional responsibility for health care for non-Indigenous people has a different administrative structure and history. When coupled with ongoing colonial structures, complications are created that are specific to and manifest most acutely for Indigenous Peoples, particularly First Nations and Inuit because the health care benefits in the treaties are directed at them. Briefly, under Canada's Constitution Act and under parameters enshrined in the Canada Health Act,[41] provincial governments are required to cover insured services, such as hospital and physician services that are deemed medically necessary, for all residents of that province.[42] Although this includes all Indigenous residents of the province, regardless of whether they live in a First Nation reserve community or not, many pertinent pieces of legislation do not make explicit reference to First Nations Peoples.[43] These ambiguities in legislation have created confusion around roles and responsibilities, especially in terms of provincial activities in reserve communities, where there is a common view that the federal government is responsible. These jurisdictional complexities have created significant gaps and problems in health care for Indigenous persons that collectively embody the failed treaty promise of health care.[44]

Following nearly a century of efforts, some slow progress in redressing these colonial-jurisdictional frustrations started to occur in the late 1960s and 1970s.[45] A 1966 report commissioned by the federal government and led by University of British Columbia anthropologist H.B. Hawkins, identified the significant social and economic disadvantages faced by Indigenous Peoples in Canada, attributed them to failed government policies and problematic public attitudes, and recommended that Indigenous Peoples be considered "citizens plus" with additional rights including opportunities and resources to make their own decisions about issues that affect their lives.[46] Following that report, the federal government began consulting with First Nation communities across Canada. However, those activities were highly problematic: when the Pierre Elliot Trudeau government released its "Statement of the Government of Canada on Indian Policy, 1969," colloquially known as the White Paper 1969, First Nations communities across Canada were shocked at the paper's failure to address the concerns their leaders had expressed.[47] Lagace and Sinclair said that "the backlash to the 1969 White Paper was monumental" and included a strong and united response from First Nation communities, including a formal rebuttal in the form of *Citizens Plus*, also known as the Red Paper, which was submitted by the Indian Association of Alberta. This strong and united response led to the withdrawal of the White Paper and empowered a wave of Indigenous leadership and activism that continues to this day.[48]

One outcome of those efforts was the 1979 Indian Health Policy. Although only two pages long, the policy was significant in its recognition of the "intolerably low level of health" in many First Nation communities and its identification of three pillars upon which to build efforts to improve health in those communities: i) the importance of socio-economic, cultural, and spiritual development as the underlying determinants of health; ii) recognition of the traditional relationship between Indigenous Peoples and the Canadian government; and iii) the interrelated nature of the Canadian health system, including active participation by First Nation communities.[49]

Although the process continued to be slow and difficult, the 1979 Indian Health Policy provided a foundation for a health transfer program that gives First Nation communities control of their health services; this includes administration and delivery of public health and insured and non-insured health care services, including those otherwise handled by First Nations and Inuit Health Branch.[50] It also provided a foundation in Alberta for Health Co-Management, which is an agreement signed in 1996 between the First Nation Chiefs of Alberta and the federal government "to work together to make decisions on funding and programs to improve the health of First Nations in Alberta." However, an important backdrop of the transfer activities nationally was concern about growing costs of health care to First Nation communities, especially non-insured health benefits. This led to efforts to try to contain costs, including the 1986 establishment of a federal Non-Insured Health Benefits Directorate, which issued directives that were to be administered regionally within a certain amount of funding, called an "envelope," introduced in 1994. The limited envelope for the Alberta region meant that certain services—particularly within the non-insured bene-fits—would have to be cut, which First Nation communities in Alberta argued was a clear violation of the federal government's treaty obligations.[51] Thus, while transfer and co-management strategies carry the potential for substantive progress toward health and well-being of Alberta First Nation communities, their success hinges on genuine partnerships, which are one key marker of truth and reconciliation. As illustrated in the stories below, and as per the quote from the Truth and Reconciliation Commission with which we opened this chapter, we are not there yet.

Stories from First Nation Communities in Alberta

In this section, we present three stories that illustrate diverse ways in which these historical events and circumstances have played out in Alberta First Nation communities.[52] More importantly, they illustrate the communities' responses, which provide a version of public health where social determinants of health are placed at the forefront of decisions about the public's health; perhaps more so than anywhere else in this book. Arranged in chronological order, the first story considers a Canada-wide initiative, the Community Health Representative program, from a Treaty 6 perspective. The program is a long-standing, and not uncontroversial, initiative in preventive health services in Indigenous communities in Alberta and beyond. The second story showcases vision and leadership by members of Mistassini Nehewiyuk, commonly called Bigstone Cree Nation in Treaty 8 territory in working toward health transfer, to the considerable social and economic (and thus health) benefit of the community. The third story focuses on a recent and ongoing public health crisis — the opioid epidemic — and the courage shown by the Kainai Nation, commonly called the Blood Tribe in Treaty 7 in generating a community response to a devastating experience. The stories speak for themselves, and we conclude our chapter commentary here.

The Community Health Representative Program, Treaty 6

"We're all teachers in some way." — Elder Ella Arcand, Kipohtakaw, Treaty 6 community health representative, retired.[53]

The Community Health Representatives program has provided for public health service delivery in Indigenous communities in Alberta and beyond since the early 1960s. The program is significant in that it represents efforts to provide preventive public health services in a way that recognizes the unique needs and contexts of Indigenous communities. At the same time, it illustrates the long-standing tensions between Indigenous and non-Indigenous peoples, which are caused and perpetuated by settler colonialism. The perspectives of those who served in these front-line roles is thus highly informative from the point of view of the objective of this chapter, which is to share important stories in the history of public health in First Nation communities in Alberta, including social, colonial, and community determinants of health and well-being.

For this story, we are honoured to draw on the experiences of Elder Ella Arcand, a retired community health representative from kipohtakaw, more commonly known as the Alexander First Nation, who has over thirty years of experience working in the field of First Nations health programming. Although the Community Health Representatives program was not unique to Treaty 6 territory, we situate it here within that perspective.[54] Treaty 6 was first signed at Fort Carlton in what is now called Saskatchewan on 23 August 1876, and covers a large area that extends from central western Alberta, through central Saskatchewan, and with a 1898 adhesion, into Manitoba.[55] The territory includes fifty First Nations, of which seventeen are in Alberta (Figure 7.1).

Treaty 6 was negotiated and signed in the context of concerns by Plains Indigenous Peoples over the Canadian government's colonial-capitalist westward expansion, which threatened Indigenous land, along with bison and other game upon which their societies depended.[56] As with other treaties, the signing led to land cession by the First Nation communities to the federal government; however, this was not made clear: the Indigenous signatories believed that they were agreeing to share the land and its resources. Ongoing land claims speak to the unresolved nature of these historical tensions rooted in colonization and capitalism.[57]

Of the numbered treaties that pertain to Alberta, Treaty 6 is the only one that explicitly contains a medicine chest clause. The clause says "that a medicine chest shall be kept at the house of each Indian Agent for the use and benefit of the Indians at the direction of such agent." The Treaty also includes clauses that promise relief in times of famine and pestilence, such as the following:

> That in the event hereafter of the Indians comprised within this treaty being overtaken by any pestilence, or by a general famine, the Queen, on being satisfied and certified thereof by Her Indian Agent or Agents, will grant to the Indians assistance of such character and to such extent as Her Chief Superintendent of Indian Affairs shall

deem necessary and sufficient to relieve the Indians from the ca-
lamity that shall have befallen them.[58]

For many Indigenous Peoples, the medicine chest clause signifies First Nations'
"constitutionally protected, Inherent, and Treaty Rights to Health," which, as
discussed earlier in this chapter, have not been upheld.[59] The Confederacy of
Treaty Six First Nations maintains that "the spirit and intent of the treaties must
be respected and honoured as made sacred by traditional Indian laws and cere-
monies and the involvement of the Crown."[60] The medicine chest clause provides
important context for the Community Health Representative program.

Kipohtakaw (Alexander First Nation) is located northwest of Edmonton in
Treaty 6 Territory.[61] The Alexander Nation speaks nêhiyawêwin (Cree) and the
2020 population was approximately 2,300, including those living on and off reserve, according to an estimate by Indigenous and Northern Affairs Canada.[62]
In a 2010 Health Canada report of First Nation community profiles in Alberta,[63]
the Alexander Nation stands out for its high levels of educational attainment (57
percent high school completion rate), labour force participation (70 percent of
members 15 to 64 years of age), and income (median after-tax family income
of $34,176). Although these statistics compare favourably to other First Nation
communities in Alberta and elsewhere, they are well below those for non-Indigenous populations, which, from the same report, were approximately 72 percent, 74 percent, and $65,000. As discussed throughout this chapter, these per-
sistent inequities reflect a constellation of factors including colonization and the
residential school legacy, which continue to exert negative effects on Indigenous
Peoples' health and well-being.[64] Alexander First Nation is a member of the
Yellowhead Tribal Council, which was established in 1977 to work collectively to
facilitate programs and services for its four member Nations: Alexander, Alexis
Nakota Sioux, O'Chiese, and Sunchild.[65] One of Arcand's many former roles was
as health manager for the Yellowhead Tribal Council.[66]

The origins of the Community Health Representative program in Canada
date back to the late 1950s,[67] when the federal government was "seeking fresh
approaches" to what they saw as "the problems of Indian communities."[68] It was
known that levels of health and well-being in Indigenous communities were
persistently and significantly lower than in non-Indigenous communities,[69] and
there was some growing awareness — albeit painfully slow growth — that unacceptable disparities in social and economic circumstances, themselves rooted
in colonialism, were the cause.[70] Within the international context of the so-called
Development Decade of the 1960s, there was growing faith in the idea and potential of community development, broadly defined as a process intended to

improve social and economic circumstances of a community with their active participation.[71] As applied in Canada, one example was efforts by the federal government to find ways for Indigenous communities to be more involved in their own health care.

In that context, the government decided that they, and in particular the Medical Services Directorate within Canada's Department of National Health and Welfare, would run a pilot project to train community health workers to work in Indigenous communities.[72] While the ultimate goal was to "assist native people to reach and maintain a standard of living comparable to that of the remainder of Canada's population," the program also articulated short-term goals; namely: i) to encourage the participation of local people in the health activities of their communities; ii) to give professional health workers an opportunity to become more effective by providing a link with the local community; and iii) to increase the number of active health workers in the field.[73] However, in her comprehensive study of the program, author Nancy Gerein notes that "although Indians had long talked about employing their own people in community work, no mention was made [in the government planning documents] of consultation with Indian leaders or communities. . . . It remained for Medical Services to explain the program to Indians and to solicit their co-operation."[74] As seen below, this partial or perhaps pseudo version of community engagement is an important theme of the Community Health Representative initiative.

The focus of the Community Health Representative program was public health — that is, prevention, promotion, and protection.[75] In that way, it embodied a broader shift in the federal government's priorities concerning health services for Indigenous communities. As described by Sheila Rymer of the Medical Service Branch, while the department focus in the mid-1940s through the mid-1950s was building and staffing health care facilities on reserves, the late 1950s saw a shift upstream to public health activities, of which the Community Health Representatives program was an example.[76] The trainees enrolled in the pilot project, which was held at Norway House, Manitoba, in 1961, were expected to be "teachers, organizers, promoters, and liaisons *rather than treatment people*" (italics added).[77] Following the pilot project, the program continued and other training sessions were held across western Canada.[78] Arcand's mother was part of that initial wave of training in the mid-1960s.[79]

After attending Olds College and finding limited job prospects, Arcand saw a job advertisement for a community health representative position in Alberta, working for Health Canada.[80] Not surprisingly, Arcand's mother — having been through the training herself — encouraged her to apply. Arcand got the job, and she worked in that capacity for several years, recalling growing interest in the Community Health Representative program at the time from Alberta First Nation communities, including isolated ones.[81] Indeed, the number of community health representatives in Alberta increased from "a few" in 1962, to eighteen in 1974, with an additional twenty-four beginning their training in 1975.[82] In response to the growing interest, Arcand and other community health representative pioneers were involved in efforts to establish a credentialed training program by teaming up with the Alberta Vocational Centre (now called Portage College) at Lac La Biche.[83] The Community Health Representatives program in Lac La Biche started in 1973 as part of the centre's efforts to expand its community-based training programs, and it was the only Community Health Representatives training program in Alberta.[84]

> "Less focused on Treaty right to health; more focused on prevention and promotion." — Ella Arcand

The purview of the community health representatives was broad but consistently focused on prevention and health promotion (Table 7.3).[85] Arcand recalls that health education activities figured prominently, which aligns with one of the original visions of CHRs as "teachers/motivators" who would provide advice and assistance on health issues.[86] With a significant focus on children and mothers, health education activities focused on topics like pre- and postnatal care, nutrition, and personal and home hygiene.[87] It also included family planning, although that could be a "touchy area." Arcand describes her community health representative peers as "really dynamic" people who came up with creative ideas, such as using crafts as teaching tools.[88]

Beyond health education, community health representatives provided or assisted with preventive clinic-based activities like immunization and health assessments.[89] Their activities also extended to health protection activities such as collecting and sending water samples for analysis and advising community members based on the results, home inspections, and dealing with "a lot!" of flies.[90] Providing support to families often involved helping to arrange child care or transportation. Community health representatives like Arcand would often walk between homes within a community and travel between multiple communities, some of which were quite isolated. Overall, these daily activities, which Arcand aptly describes as "24/7," contributed importantly to health and well-being in many Alberta Indigenous communities.

TABLE 7.3: Summary of common / major activities of community health representatives in Alberta, approx. 1970s–early 1990s.[91]

Common Activities of Community Health Representatives
1. Provide health education to families, especially mothers (e.g., nutrition, hygiene, personal care, family planning), including via home visits
2. Provide health education in schools (e.g., dental hygiene, nutrition)
3. Hold or assist with clinics (e.g., pre- and post-natal clinics, well-baby clinics)
4. Provide other forms of health education, e.g., provide information or advice informally, including about available services and supports
5. Assist with immunization
6. Perform health assessments and monitoring (e.g., take temperature, measure height and weight, administer developmental tests)
7. Support families by arranging babysitting, transportation, delivering medicines, etc.
8. Perform water sampling and record results
9. Provide first aid and basic home nursing, and assist with emergencies
10. Contribute to administrative activities such as planning and report-writing
11. Perform house inspections
12. Liaise with Band Council and other community agencies

Another important community health representative role was that of liaison, or cultural bridge between the community and the typically non-Indigenous nurses and other health care personnel and, by extension, the federal government, that served them. In Treaty 6 territory, for example, the Cree language was spoken in all the communities served by community health representatives, which permitted representatives like Arcand to improve upon efforts of the nurses who could not necessarily speak the language of the people they were serving.[92] This bridging role went beyond language: according to Gerein's analysis, CHRs in Alberta advised health care personnel on local culture, values, traditions, and politics. Significantly, they would also help the non-Indigenous health care personnel to become aware of their own personal beliefs, feelings, and biases about Indigenous Peoples. Considering the existence of entrenched and widespread colonial attitudes toward Indigenous Peoples, coupled with the fact that the government-employed nurses during the 1970s "receive[d] practically no formal orientation to Indian culture" in their training, these community health representative activities were extremely important.[93]

As noted above, the context in which the Community Health Representative program was created in the 1960s was one in which problematic ideas of community development were prominent. Accordingly, the community health representative role was envisioned to go beyond delivering health promotion activities and serving as cultural liaison to include advocacy and community mobilization. This role could take various forms.[94] In general it involved active participation in Band Council or other meetings to advocate for resources, facilities, or programs that, based on the Community Health Representatives program's understanding of needs, would benefit the community. Gerein's analysis showed that although some Alberta community health representatives were politically active, such activities were a relatively uncommon part of the community health representative role because the expectation of effective advocacy and community mobilization was fraught, due to the colonial foundations of the program.[95] This is clearly illustrated by a quote from Rymer who identified that, from the perspective of the federal government, CHRs could be "both a help and a hazard." That is, "they were a help when they supervised some of the winter works projects such as building privies or digging wells, but they were a hazard when they called public attention to sanitary conditions in reserve schools or insisted that safe water be supplied."[96] In other words, so long as it was limited to a certain set of largely depoliticized activities, the Community Health Representative program was viewed positively by the federal government, but if CHRs went beyond those activities and engaged with the social determinants of health, it was threatening and unacceptable. This is despite stated program objectives around improving Indigenous health and well-being, and it clarifies exactly how narrow the federal vision of community development was.

The previous paragraphs are not intended to take away from the significant and valued contributions of community health representatives. Those contributions are corroborated by a 1993 survey of graduates from the Community Health Representative program at Portage College in Lac La Biche, which showed some positive findings: of the 92 percent of graduates who were employed, the overwhelming majority were very or fairly satisfied with their job (86 percent) and reported that their training had been very or fairly related to their job (92 percent).[97] However, there have since been some important changes. After nearly forty years, the Community Health Representative training program at Portage College was discontinued around 2010.[98] There have also been changes to public health more generally, upon which Arcand, now retired, is well positioned to reflect, noting, for example, an erosion of public health.

"Public health has sort of disappeared." — Ella Arcand

Drawing on the three pillars from the 1979 Indian Health Policy — community development; the special relationship between First Nation Peoples and the federal government; and the interrelated nature of the Canadian health care system

— Arcand identified changes that signal a disconnect with traditional Indigenous way of life, and a shift toward Western approaches to health and illness.[99] She gave an example of Elders living in care facilities. An Elder who is feeling cold may wear multiple layers of clothing. A care worker who questions the reason for that behaviour, or asks the individual to remove layers, may fail to recognize that the person is mobilizing collective knowledge and practices accrued through a lifetime of experiences, such as living and working on a trap line. Likewise, giving a pharmaceutical sleep aid to an Elder may be experienced as dismissive of Indigenous knowledge and wisdom for understanding the reasons for poor sleep and traditional methods of healing and wellness to help alleviate it. These issues are further complicated by what Arcand describes as "newer" diseases that accompany an aging population, such as dementia or Parkinson's disease, which Arcand did not recall ever encountering during her years working in Treaty 6 communities.[100]

"Everything is not pills." — Ella Arcand

Arcand saw her community health representative work was a stepping-stone to an impressive range of other roles and activities. As a few examples, Arcand was founder and president of the First Nations Health Managers Association, health manager for the Yellowhead Tribal Council, and health director for Enoch Cree Nation. She has also served as a member of the board of directors for the Siksika Medicine Lodge Youth Wellness Centre, as a board member for Stoney Health Services, and as a member of the First Nations, Métis, and Inuit Leadership Committee for the Greater St. Albert Catholic School Division.[101] One of Arcand's particularly treasured experiences was her involvement in The Spirit of Healing initiative, which was a partnership of First Nations representatives from Treaty 6, 7, and 8; the First Nations and Inuit Health Branch; the University of Calgary; the College of Physicians and Surgeons of Alberta; and the Alberta College of Pharmacists, that raised awareness about and addressed the issue of prescription drug misuse and abuse within First Nation communities in Alberta.[102]

Through these significant roles and activities, Arcand has served as a strong champion for public health in Alberta and beyond. The contributions of Arcand and her communities provide a strong illustration of public health as we have defined it for this book — that is, as emphasizing collective approaches to supporting social determinants of health and well-being — and we are honoured to share those contributions here.

The Mistassini Nehewiyuk (Bigstone) Experience: For Our Community, in Our Community, by Our Community, Treaty 8

"There is so much to be done and there's so much opportunity to really make a difference. . . . If they [government] really want to make a difference, if they really want to help reduce costs, if they really want to improve services . . . why can't we be a real partner? We are Albertans and Canadians too." — G. Barry Phillips, former CEO, Bigstone Health Commission[103]

In 1992, then-Chief of Bigstone Cree Nation Gordon T. Auger attended a Treaty 8 meeting of Chiefs in Slave Lake, where he learned that his community of Bigstone was the least healthy First Nation in Alberta. By 2010, the community of Bigstone-Desmarais ranked at the top of the First Nations Community Well-Being Index among communities in Alberta, and it scored above the province's non-First Nations average.[104] The story of how this happened is important and illuminating for public health.

Mistassini Nehewiyuk,[105] commonly known as Bigstone Cree Nation, is a collection of communities in northern Alberta that have been long inhabited by Woodland Cree, an Algonquian people with a history and culture characterized by deep connections to the northern boreal forests and lakes. The region historically spanned a triangular geographic area, with Wapuskaw (more commonly known as Wabasca, which is located approximately 300 km north of Edmonton) and Sandy Lake situated between Calling Lake to the south, Peerless Lake and Trout Lake to the northwest, and Chipewyan Lake to the north.[106] The Bigstone peoples were signatories to Treaty 8 on 21 June 1899 and, as with other First Nation communities, those colonial events and their aftermath caused dramatic disruption in their ways of life. Under the federal Indian Act, for example, there were two residential schools in the Wabasca area,[107] and testimony from those who attended the schools confirm devastating practices such as segregation that divided families and communities by preventing them from talking or interacting.[108]

With the signing of Treaty 8, the Crown established five reserves for the Bigstone people: Reserve 166 at Sandy Lake, 166A along the north side of South Wabasca Lake, 166B on the south side of South Wabasca Lake, 166C on the north end of North Wabasca Lake, and 166D on the south side of North Wabasca Lake; they later established Reserve 183 at Calling Lake.[109] Much later, however, in what would become the largest treaty land entitlement claim in Alberta, Bigstone used early population surveys to successfully argue that they were entitled to more land. That claim, initiated in 1981 and finalized in 2010, led to the creation of new reserves, one for Peerless Lake and Trout Lake communities, and one for the Chipewyan Lake community, as well as additional land for the existing reserve at Calling Lake.[110] Bigstone Cree Nation, with a current population of approximately 7,200, is geographically remote: "there's two highways to Wabasca and they both end there,"[111] and this is a constant theme in the community's efforts to improve health and well-being.

Through exposure to family friends at a young age, Barry Phillips learned about hospital administration and wanted to become a hospital administrator. By pursuing his interests and being open to opportunities, Phillips worked his way to being named administrator of Ste. Catherine's Hospital in Lac La Biche in May 1968, making him the first lay administrator of a Catholic hospital in Alberta. However, his passion lay in functional and strategic design of services that met the needs of communities, and following a winter spent on a trapline with his brother-in-law, Phillips sought out opportunities that better aligned with those values. He became involved in emerging economic development opportunities for Métis peoples in Alberta, and he went on to do consulting contract work for Métis Child and Family Services. When the director of Métis Child and Family Services moved to Bigstone, Phillips's unique set of skills, experiences, and knowledge led to an invitation to follow. In an interview, Phillips told the authors of this book that "perhaps if you are lucky, once in your career you will have a real opportunity to change the way the industry that you work in functions, addresses issues, confronts problems, and meets challenges. Such was my opportunity when I went to work with the Bigstone Cree Nation in northern Alberta."[112]

Phillips's initial job at Bigstone was connected to the federal government's efforts related to the health transfer program. When he arrived in Bigstone in 1992, it took Phillips very little time to recommend not pursuing full health transfer. Although it would have provided much-needed flexibility in terms of how the community could allocate funds and services, the limited resources available would have presented major obstacles.[113]

Fortunately, however, there was another opportunity. The federal government's Medical Services Branch, in conjunction with the Assembly of First Nations, was initiating a pilot project for transfer of non-insured health benefits. In the context of concerns about rising costs of non-insured health benefits noted above, the objective of the pilot was to see if First Nation communities could find innovative ways to effectively deliver those programs. In that first round of projects in the mid-1990s, communities could select one or more programs to test, and Bigstone selected medical transportation for its community members.

That opportunity was significant in that it allowed the community to identify the needs of its members; for example, what services prompted members to leave the community, and where did they go to access those services? With respect to medical transportation, the foundational work undertaken for the first round of pilot projects set the stage for later successes; for example, Bigstone later won a contract to provide medical transportation services in the Edmonton area, approximately 320 km south, which created twelve jobs for Bigstone community members living in Edmonton. Later, when Greyhound bus lines cut back on regional service, Bigstone was able to expand their transportation activities and provide fee-for-service transportation within the community as well as to and from Edmonton.[114]

The knowledge, experience, and confidence gained through that medical transfer project positioned the Bigstone community to then pursue transfer of all non-insured health benefits programs, which was the objective of a second round of projects five years later. Phillips explained that, although making improvements to medical transportation was important, Bigstone's remote location continued to present formidable challenges.

> If I live in Edmonton and I have a vision appointment, say it's going to take me 20 minutes to get there, one hour for the appointment, and 20 minutes to get home. So I only have to make arrangements for two hours. But when, for that vision appointment, [I have to travel from the reserve] I have to get on a medical transportation bus at 7:30 in the morning to get to Slave Lake by 9 a.m. and my appointment isn't until 11a.m., and the bus doesn't leave to come back until 4 p.m., I have breakfast, lunch, and supper for my family I have to worry about; I have all those other normal things in life that have to be taken into consideration, so a lot of people just say "it's not worth it for me so I'll just walk around like this." Access to services is not just "is it even possible to access;" it's, "is it reasonable for me to put in my list of priorities."[115]

There was a need to find ways to strengthen service delivery locally.

The community's efforts were grounded in the social determinants of health. Phillips's thinking was influenced by the 1974 Lalonde Report,[116] along with two other resources — *Why are Some People Healthy and Others Not*, and *Building Communities from the Inside Out*[117] — which Phillips encouraged all members of Bigstone health leadership to read. Informed by these important perspectives and their own experiences, the Bigstone Health Advisory Council developed a vision for the community's health transfer that considered issues of access, income, jobs, education, and living environment: "we see a healthy community where our members receive needed services locally, by our own businesses, staffed by our trained membership."[118] Although the need for adequate funding was recognized, it was also clear that simply expanding the non-insured health benefits budget was not going to solve the problems. For example, even if funds were available to hire health professionals to serve the community, how enticing would such an opportunity be if there was no housing, or housing without running water or a sewer connection? Phillips says that challenges were reconceptualized as opportunities:

- We looked at the fact that we had nothing, and therefore, nothing to lose.
- We looked at the fact of our semi-isolation as a positive geographic factor: we had a captive market.
- We looked at the fact that we had a high unemployment rate and members [who were] eager to find meaningful employment and willing to train.[119]

Mobilizing the resources of the community — including facilities, people, and funds — Phillips and his team developed a capital plan, a human resources plan, and a business plan. Figuring importantly into these plans were the frustrations experienced with current arrangements, in which centralized government decision-making — for example, about what was and was not covered under non-insured health benefits — created rules that felt arbitrary and unfair because they were based on federal resource appropriation rather than on what would meaningfully address needs in the community.

Bigstone's general approach was to create opportunities for community members to train for careers in health service delivery and to provide ways for those educated community members to return home, earn a fair income, and contribute to their community. According to Phillips, "active, educated, and well-paid community members encourage healthier lifestyles and demand services that improve one's living environment. The actual provision of jobs reduces stress among a community where unemployment is high and opportunities are few."[120]

Dental services provide an illustration. The closest available services were 125 kilometres away, presenting the geography-priority trade-off described earlier. The community began by purchasing, for $1, a mobile dental trailer from the provincial government — "this was done even though we were a First Nations organization whose health service was the responsibility of the federal government"[121] — and equipping it with surplus equipment from the University of Alberta's dental program.[122] When the dental services expanded and were moved into the newly built professional centre in Wabasca, the mobile trailer was moved to Trout Lake to provide weekly dental services to the Trout and Peerless Lake communities.

Dental services are one of many under the Bigstone Health Commission,[123] which is the entity responsible for health services for the Bigstone communities and has administered the non-insured health benefits programs for members of the Nation since 2004.[124] From essentially no services in the early 1990s, the community now employs nearly 200 people in health and social service sectors.

> "We provide everything to our members." — former Chief Gordon
> T. Auger[125]

A foundation of Bigstone's efforts to provide public services is data and statistics. Recognizing that high-quality information is often a key catalyst for change, the community embraced a partnership with the First Nations Information Governance Centre and their survey work.[126] Thanks to the efforts of Andy Alook, project coordinator with the Bigstone Health Commission, the community achieved a 92 percent completion rate for First Nations Information Governance Centre's Regional Health Survey, which is one of the highest for any First Nation in Canada. The community has used data from several surveys to support ongoing planning in health and education, such as a proposal to expand their band-operated school, Oski Pasikoniwew Kamik.[127] Further, following a 2010 review of the Health Commission, the community also initiated a local report card that embraces a population health approach and is based on a strong commitment to the importance of continually monitoring and working to improve health in the community.[128]

> "We measure our status against Alberta not just First Nations" —
> G. Barry Phillips[129]

Many factors stand out as contributing importantly to Bigstone's success, including leadership and vision from within the community as well as colleagues from outside the community, including some from the Alberta Region of First Nations and Inuit Health Branch described by Phillips as having "bent over backwards to help us be successful."[130] However, some important challenges remain. One example, continuing with the dental services illustration, concerns a clause within Alberta's Health Professions Act that prohibits dentists from sharing or splitting professional service fees with anyone who is not a dentist registered with the

College of Dental Surgeons of Alberta.[131] Because of the significant expense and financial uncertainty associated with setting up a dental practice in a small, remote community like Bigstone, one way to entice a dentist such as a new graduate to set up a practice is for the community to invest financially. For example, the community could invest funds to build and equip a dental facility, and then set up a volume or fee-based long-term lease agreement with the dentist to recoup that investment over time.[132] This would provide the dentist some financial support and protection to make the venture less risky, and the community would receive a much-needed local service. However, such an arrangement is prohibited under provincial legislation, which leaves the community with no viable choice but to rely on less sustainable arrangements with volunteer dentists.[133]

As per Call to Action number 23 of the Truth and Reconciliation Commission, which pertains to "increase[ing] the number of Aboriginal professionals working in the health care field; [and] ensur[ing] the retention of Aboriginal health care providers in Aboriginal communities," it would be ideal to train and recruit dentists from the community.[134] But until then, as illustrated by the dental example and by health services more generally, the question remains: Why can't we be real partners?[135]

Mobilizing the Community in a Time of Crisis: Kottakinoona Awaahkapiiyaawa, "Bringing the Spirits Home," Treaty 7

> "The Creator has provided us with the gifts, and it is our responsibility to take care of not only our people, but the land and the animals and the environment." — Chief Charles Weaselhead[136]

In a time of crisis, characterized by a terrifying increase in opioid overdoses among their people, the Kainai Nation (commonly called the Blood Tribe) of southern Alberta mobilized to build a community response. It is important not to understate what is meant by a community response — the response was fundamentally grounded in Kainayssini, or guiding principles, that were adopted and prepared by Elders from the past. As powerfully described by Chief Charles Weaselhead,[137] the guiding principles "talk about who we are and what we teach our children, in areas of governance, culture and spirituality, as well as connections and responsibilities to the land, the community, and the spirit of the Creator."

Grounded in these principles, and by extension the rich stories, collective knowledge, and deep wisdom of the community, *Kottakinoona Awaahkapiiyaawa,*

"Bringing the Spirits Home": The Blood Tribe Addiction Framework says that "by knowing the past, in the context of seeing today, we can change the path going forward. We can then take stock, tell our story, and pass it along to future generations as a winter count."[138] We respectfully use these four components of the community's approach to structure their story.

Knowing the Past

> "The Elders recognize that the Blood Indians have always had control over its lands and over its religious, political, economic and cultural destinies." — "Kainayssini," Declaration of the Elders of the Blood Indian Nation[139]

The peoples of the Kainai Nation ("Many Chiefs"), historically known as the Blood Tribe, have a long and rich history in Treaty 7 territory in southern Alberta. Along with the Siksika and two communities of the Piikani (Piegan) people, Aapátohsipikáni in the north and Amskapi Piikani in the south — the Kainai Nation is part of the Siksikaitsitapi (Blackfoot Confederacy), for whom the bison, along with other animals and plants, historically figured prominently for food, housing, clothing, and ceremonial life. The traditional territory of the Niitsitapi (Blackfoot Nation) extends from the North Saskatchewan River in the north to the Yellowstone River in the south, and from the Rocky Mountains in the west to the Eagle Hills in the east. The Kainai Nation, for whom the Siksika language and culture remain strong, inhabits an area of over 1,400 square kilometres located between the Belly and St. Mary's rivers in the southern part of the province and has a population of approximately 14,000 members who live within and outside of the community.[140]

As described by Chief Weaselhead, the Kainai peoples have a very strong connection to Ápistotooki, the Creator, which is the source of traditional spirituality. Community structures, including societies such as the Horn Society and the role of Elders, help to ensure that traditions and beliefs are passed on through generations.[141]

Despite these strong foundations, the Kainai Nation has experienced significant loss. As stated in *Kottakinoona Awaahkapiiyaawa*, "The Blackfoot and Blood Tribe people have been impacted by loss: loss of language, food sources, culture, traditions, land, territory, identity, purpose, and control . . . like ripples in the water [these changes] have far-reaching and continuous effects on every aspect of life, sometimes spanning generations."[142] Colonialism brought an impossible barrage of assaults that are aptly described as cultural genocide.[143] Although the introduction of horses, guns, and tools in the eighteenth century seemed to bring some immediate benefits, the arrival of alcohol and diseases eroded communities to such an extent that when the Northwest Mounted Police arrived in Blackfoot territory in the 1870s, it was seen as a relief. It was in those circumstances of desperation that five Nations — Kainai (Blood), Siksika (Blackfoot), Piikani (Piegan), Nakoda (Stoney), and Tsuu T'ina (Sarcee) signed Treaty 7 in 1877 and agreed to share their land in exchange for various provisions. As with many other communities, the ensuing legacy of institutionalized assimilation was, and continues to be, devastating.[144] Today, the Nation faces persistent and unacceptable challenges including poverty, unemployment, and lack of suitable housing, along with mental and physical health issues including addiction,[145] of which colonial acts and their traumatic and enduring negative impacts are the cause.

Seeing Today

The opioid crisis is a comparatively recent phenomenon that has had destructive effects in communities across Alberta and Canada. This complex public health crisis involves both illegal street drugs that have been laced with fentanyl and prescription opioids. Across Canada, between January 2016 and September 2019, there were over 19,400 opioid-related poisoning hospitalizations and over 14,700 apparent opioid-related deaths.[146] Alberta, like much of the rest of Canada, has seen a steady recent increase in opioid-related deaths,[147] and a 2019 surveillance report estimated that on average, just under two individuals died every day in Alberta as a result of an apparent opioid poisoning. Of all confirmed drug and alcohol poisoning deaths in the province in recent years, opioids were involved in approximately 75 percent.[148]

Statistics for opioid-related harms among First Nations communities in Alberta are available through a collaboration between the Alberta First Nations Information Governance Centre[149] and the Alberta Ministry of Health, in which Bonnie Healy, Kainai Nation member and former executive director of Alberta First Nations Information Governance Centre, played a significant leadership role.[150] Recent statistics stemming from that collaboration indicate that First Nations Peoples have been disproportionately affected by the crisis; for example, despite representing approximately 6 percent of the Alberta population, they represented 13 percent of all opioid-related poisoning deaths from 2016 to 2018. Across the province, opioid-related harms for First Nations Peoples are highest in the Alberta Health Services South Zone, which includes the City of Lethbridge and the Blood Reserve.[151] The contributing factors are a complex mix of the colonial legacy including institutionalized racism and other social determinants of health; one manifestation is that the opioid dispensation rate in Alberta is twice as high for First Nations compared to non-First Nations people.[152]

The Kainai Nation community started to see a considerable number of deaths from opioid overdose around 2014–2015,[153] which led Chief Charles Weaselhead to take the significant step of declaring a local state of emergency. The worst of the situation, however, was yet to come. According to statistics maintained by the Blood Tribe Department of Health, there were thirty overdose calls from the reserve in 2014, and thirty-five in 2015; a concerning number for any community, let alone a small community. However, these numbers foreshadowed a terrifying increase, to 108 in 2016, 180 in 2017, and 335 in 2018. Kevin Cowan, Chief Executive Officer for the Blood Tribe Department of Health, described the changes in numbers as "pretty much a tenfold increase in a fairly short period of time." He continued, "by the fall of 2018, we were simply frustrated by the number that we were seeing."[154] A heartbreaking accompaniment to these statistics is the percentage of babies born exposed to substances: 22 percent in 2014/15, 32 percent in 2015/16, 39 percent in 2016/17, and 51 percent in 2017/18.

An important part of formulating a response to the crisis was recognizing that the existing approach to handling overdoses was not working. If an overdose occurred in the community, first responders would drive the patient thirty kilometres to the nearest medical centre at Cardston or Fort McLeod, or sixty kilometres to the Lethbridge hospital, where they would frequently be released within a few hours. Jacen Abrey, Director-Fire Chief, Blood Tribe Emergency Services, says, "we have seen that in the hospitals: 'oh, they're just high again; oh, they're just drunk again.'"[155] This arrangement was a recipe for disaster. Being alone and away from home, facing racism and discrimination, it is not surprising that some patients relapsed the same day they were admitted.[156] Being in larger towns also provided an opportunity to buy more drugs and bring them back to the reserve.

Since time immemorial, the Blackfoot people have had their healing methods to address mental, spiritual, physical, and emotional ailments.[157] It was time to mobilize those foundations.

Change the Path

In 2018, the work to address the crisis began in earnest. The Blood Tribe Department of Health worked closely with leaders from the Alberta Health Services South Zone, who had been tasked with developing a community-wide, comprehensive, full-continuum of care addiction framework that was based on the Blackfoot culture and context.[158] Lene Jorgensen of Alberta Health Services and Rebecca Many Grey Horses of the Kainai Nation were instrumental in this work. Recognizing the significant strength, wisdom, and resiliency in the community, preparatory work to mobilize those foundations was undertaken between May and November of that year. As stated in *Kottakinoona Awaahkapiiyaawa*, the process of developing the framework involved the following parameters.

- Looking beyond the problem, to consider the role of culture and spirituality.
- Looking beyond evidence and literature, to explore oral history and Indigenous ways of knowing.
- Looking beyond the data, to adhere to ethical considerations about how the data is collected, used and shared.
- Looking beyond environmental scans, to understand jurisdictions, treaties and peace alliances.
- Looking beyond stakeholder input, to develop the art of truly listening to the stories and wisdom.[159]

Kottakinoona Awaahkapiiyaawa was developed through consultations with a wide range of people within and outside the community,[160] and the name signifies two foundations of the framework: i) an invitation to the spirits of those living with addiction, back to the community, and ii) a commitment to bringing back the spirits of those currently living with addiction and those who have lost their lives. The four pillars of the framework — prevention and harm reduction, detoxification, treatment, and aftercare — are grounded in community, healing, wellness, and Blackfoot culture.[161] Yet, while the framework clarified what needed to be in place; the question was how to build it? Approaches used elsewhere, such as larger cities of Calgary or Edmonton, were not necessarily going to work in the Kainai Nation's unique environment.

In late 2018, a meeting was called that brought different departments in the community together. Jacen Abrey, Director-Fire Chief, Blood Tribe Emergency Services, attended that meeting, and had the idea to create a paramedic-run, medically assisted detoxification centre. Paramedic-run was significant: paramedics (and other first responders) have the great advantage of being in the community and closely connected with the people they were helping; there was an important opportunity to strengthen and optimize paramedics' roles.[162] The novel arrangement, which integrated traditional, non-traditional, clinical, and non-clinical knowledge and disciplines, involved protocols whereby patients could enter a detoxification, treatment, and aftercare process without waiting for a referral. Local physicians, including Dr. Esther Tailfeathers and Dr. Susan Christenson, were supportive, and community leaders, notably Elders, were integrally involved in the centre, providing spiritual and cultural guidance, including connection to the Blackfoot language and adherence to the Kainayssini.[163] The efforts to put this idea into practice began.[164]

> "I had done 35 years of front-line paramedic [work]; I'd been in an ambulance, I'd worked for the province in the fire commissioner's office. I knew the layers of bureaucracy in the provincial government, and I'm thinking, there's no way [that this idea will materialize]." — Jacen Abrey[165]

Despite seemingly insurmountable challenges that came with the urgency of the situation, the work unfolded rapidly. Within one week of the community meeting, they had started renovations on an existing Blood Tribe Department of Health facility to expand and transition its functions toward the paramedic-run, medically assisted approach. Within ten days, they had secured provincial funding. After six weeks, the Bringing the Spirit Home detoxification centre opened its doors.

> "[Unlike other programs], we like to think that our community is the centre, and they can open any door and we will bring them in" — Jacen Abrey[166]

A key feature of the program is that it adapts to the individual. For example, in recognition of significant differences in how individuals experience addiction, the duration of the program varies. Another significant example is that babies are welcome and mothers can bring their babies with them. By adapting to circumstances of individuals, including mothers, and working collaboratively with Children's Services, the program plays a critical role in allowing families to stay together as described by Lene Jorgensen: "when I hear about the babies at the site and how some expectant mothers are entering treatment before the baby is born, returning to the site with the baby after and sometimes supported by the grandmother, I know that the spirits are coming home to the community."[167]

Recognizing the need for a range of integrated services and supports, the program includes opportunities for people to access dental care, optometry, and immunizations while in treatment. A routine blood draw permits early detection of sexually transmitted infections, including Hepatitis C and HIV. In addition to services on the reserve, a mobile medical unit operates in Lethbridge where staff will see anyone who needs the services. As part of the aftercare pillar, there are supports for self-care, education, and life- and job skills development.[168] These are a few examples within a holistic initiative that is grounded in community and culture — that is, the Niitsitapi Ways.[169]

A Winter Count

> "In my view, I think we have turned a corner" — Chief Charles Weaselhead

For the Blackfoot people, Winter Counts are a mixture of oral history and pictographs, passed on from one person to the next, which are used to record events and track time.[170] We have respectfully borrowed the concept to situate reflections on the story of the opioid crisis in the Kainai Nation from the point of view of a broad version of public health in which the social determinants of health figure prominently.

There are indications that the Kainai Nation's bold approach is working. The sharp increase in overdose calls has started to level off: following what will hopefully end up being the peak of 335 in 2018, the number of calls went down to 275 in 2019.[171] The percentage of babies born exposed to substances decreased from 51 percent in 2017/18 to 39 percent in 2018/19.[172] Although not specifically measured, there is a sense that the number of incidents of petty crime has gone down, which may reflect the program's success in conveying to clients that the community is there to support them.[173]

> "The [solutions] have to come from within" — Kevin Cowan[174]

More broadly, there are important signs of an empowered community that can serve and support its members. For example, reliance on external agencies is diminishing: according to Jacen Abrey, who has served the reserve in some capacity for over twenty years, 2019 was the first year in memory that the Kainai Nation did not need to call in any outside community for assistance.[175]

This strengthened capacity goes beyond the immediacy of the opioid crisis. For example, under the prevention and harm reduction pillar, activities within *Kottakinoona Awaahkapiiyaawa* extend into the community's schools, where paramedics educate students from pre-kindergarten through grade 12 on a range of topics, including opioids and other substances, fire safety, first aid, and driving safety.[176] Moreover, the Kanai Nation is forging partnerships between the local Red Crow College and other post-secondary institutions such as Lethbridge College and Medicine Hat College to create opportunities to train members as nurses and paramedics to serve their community,[177] thus aligning with Truth and Reconciliation Commission Call to Action #23, for "all levels of government to increase the number of Aboriginal professionals working in the health care field."[178]

"As a health [department], we could try to take care of the opioid crisis. . . . But if we don't take care of those other factors — education, employment, racism, poverty, lack of housing, lack of basic drinking water, all of those, we're spinning our wheels most of the time" — Chief Charles Weaselhead

The Kainai Nation's community response to the opioid crisis is a remarkable story of vision, collaboration, and leadership, grounded in culture and tradition. Yet, as per Chief Weaselhead's words about "spinning our wheels," much greater attention to the social determinants of health — that is, the root causes of addiction and other health problems on a community-wide basis — is needed. Far-reaching challenges, which cannot be addressed by the health department alone, remain. Unacceptable norms of racism and discrimination and circumstances of poverty persist, for the Kainai Nation and for Indigenous Peoples across Alberta. The loss of culture and identity continues to manifest in levels of incarceration and rates of sickness and premature death that are unacceptably high and far higher than in non-Indigenous populations.[179] These circumstances epitomize the concept of health inequities — that is, differences between population groups that are unfair and avoidable that reflect an unequal distribution of health-damaging experiences, and which are "not in any sense a 'natural' phenomenon but [are] the result of a toxic combination of poor social policies and programs, unfair economic arrangements, and bad politics."[180] Although important work is being done, it is not enough. Respectfully, we give the final words of this chapter to Chief Charles Weaselhead.

In my view, the biggest success factor will be in closing that gap [between Indigenous and non-Indigenous peoples]. . . . Our standard of living is third world conditions. And the government and most of our mainstream Canadians are beginning to realize that the Aboriginal people are right: all they have to do is come into the reserve and look.

In a theme that recurs throughout this chapter, we are not there yet.[181]

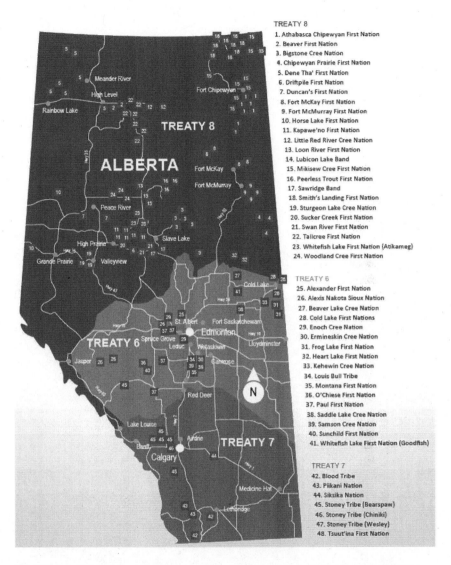

TREATY 8
1. Athabasca Chipewyan First Nation
2. Beaver First Nation
3. Bigstone Cree Nation
4. Chipewyan Prairie First Nation
5. Dene Tha' First Nation
6. Driftpile First Nation
7. Duncan's First Nation
8. Fort McKay First Nation
9. Fort McMurray First Nation
10. Horse Lake First Nation
11. Kapawe'no First Nation
12. Little Red River Cree Nation
13. Loon River First Nation
14. Lubicon Lake Band
15. Mikisew Cree First Nation
16. Peerless Trout First Nation
17. Sawridge Band
18. Smith's Landing First Nation
19. Sturgeon Lake Cree Nation
20. Sucker Creek First Nation
21. Swan River First Nation
22. Tallcree First Nation
23. Whitefish Lake First Nation (Atikameg)
24. Woodland Cree First Nation

TREATY 6
25. Alexander First Nation
26. Alexis Nakota Sioux Nation
27. Beaver Lake Cree Nation
28. Cold Lake First Nations
29. Enoch Cree Nation
30. Ermineskin Cree Nation
31. Frog Lake First Nation
32. Heart Lake First Nation
33. Kehewin Cree Nation
34. Louis Bull Tribe
35. Montana First Nation
36. O'Chiese First Nation
37. Paul First Nation
38. Saddle Lake Cree Nation
39. Samson Cree Nation
40. Sunchild First Nation
41. Whitefish Lake First Nation (Goodfish)

TREATY 7
42. Blood Tribe
43. Piikani Nation
44. Siksika Nation
45. Stoney Tribe (Bearspaw)
46. Stoney Tribe (Chiniki)
47. Stoney Tribe (Wesley)
48. Tsuut'ina First Nation

Fig. 7.1: Map of First Nations in Alberta, which include 48 Nations in three Treaty areas (2018) (reproduced with permission).[182]

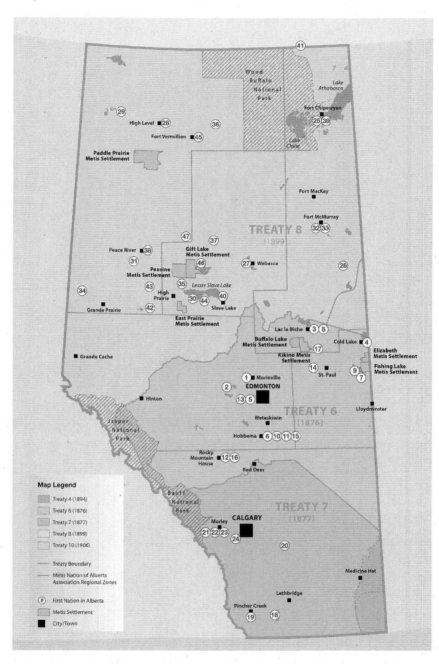

Fig. 7.2: Map of Métis settlements and communities in Alberta.[183]

NOTES

1   Truth and Reconciliation Commission of Canada (TRC), *Honouring the Truth, Reconciling for the Future. Summary of the Final Report of the Truth and Reconciliation Commission of Canada* (Winnipeg: National Centre for Truth and Reconciliation, 2015), 6–7.

2   TRC, *Honouring the Truth*, 6.

3   Janet Smylie, "Approaching Reconciliation: Tips from the Field" (Editorial), Canadian Journal of Public Health 106, no. 5 (2015), e261.

4   TRC, *Honouring the Truth*; Smylie, "Approaching Reconciliation."

5   John Last, ed., *Dictionary of Epidemiology* (4th edition) (Oxford: Oxford University Press, 2001), 145.

6   Canadian Public Health Association (CPHA), *Public Health: A Conceptual Framework*, Canadian Public Health Association Working Paper, Second Edition (Ottawa: CPHA, 2017), https://www.cpha.ca/sites/default/files/uploads/policy/ph-framework/phcf_e.pdf; World Health Organization, Ottawa Charter for Health Promotion (Ottawa: WHO, 1986), https://www.who.int/healthpromotion/conferences/previous/ottawa/en/index1.html.

7   This was expressed by Justice Murray Sinclair, Chair of the TRC. See Chloe Fedio, "Truth and Reconciliation Report Brings Calls for Action, not Words," *CBC News*, posted 2 June 2015, https://www.cbc.ca/news/politics/truth-and-reconciliation-report-brings-calls-for-action-not-words-1.3096863.

8   Lindsay McLaren, "In Defense of a Population-level Approach to Prevention: Why Public Health Matters Today," Canadian Journal of Public Health 110, no. 3 (2019).

9   Paulette Fox, Amelia Crowshoe (editor), and The Alberta First Nations Information Governance Centre, *Indigenous Health Indicators: A Participatory Approach to Co-designing Indicators to Monitor and Measure First Nations Health* (April 2018), http://afnigc.ca/main/includes/media/pdf/digital%20reports/Indigenous%20Health%20Indicators.pdf.

10 Some of the individuals featured in this chapter, while allies to Indigenous communities, are of non-Indigenous ancestry and lived experience.

11 Alberta Government, Ministry of Indigenous Relations, *Aboriginal Peoples of Alberta: Yesterday, Today, and Tomorrow* (November 2013), https://open.alberta.ca/dataset/9a704cab-7510-4796-9301-f373cbc27e30/resource/e7e90b67-7308-4f98-a67b-140bf65c7666/download/6429770-2013-aboriginal-peoples-alberta-2013-11-18.pdf. In an interview, Reggie Crowshoe, Piikani cultural teacher in southern Alberta, referred to his father, Joe Crowshoe, who "often said that when the dominant society understands us like we understand the dominant society, then we'll have a good life." This Alberta government resource was intended to provide "a starting point for moving toward the kind of understanding Joe Crowshoe talked about." Alberta Government, *Aboriginal Peoples of Alberta*, 3.

12 For a much more fulsome treatment of this topic on a national scale, the reader is directed to TRC, *Honouring the Truth* — one of many reliable sources.

13 To the extent that the large gatherings, including the buffalo hunt, occurred with little indication of disease outbreaks, these events perhaps offer early lessons for public health including communicable disease prevention. We are grateful to Dr. Janet Smylie for this insight.

14 Alberta Government, *Aboriginal Peoples of Alberta*, 2.

15 Katherine L. Frohlich, Nancy Ross, and Chantelle Richmond, "Health Disparities in Canada Today: Some Evidence and a Theoretical Framework," *Health Policy* 79 no. 2/3 (2006):; FNIGC, "First Nations Health Trends-Alberta 'One-Pagers,'" accessed 7 August 2020, http://www.afnigc.ca/main/index.php?id=resources&content=FNHTA.

16 TRC, *Honouring the Truth*.

17 The Indian Act does not pertain to Métis peoples.

18 Indigenous and Northern Affairs Canada, "Canadian Human Rights Act — Repeal of Section 67,", date modified 15 September 2010, https://www.rcaanc-cirnac.gc.ca/eng/1100100032550/1622036080282.

19 Compiled from various sources including Alberta Government, *Aboriginal Peoples of Alberta*; Breaker and Smith, "History Prior to Health Co-management"; Government of Canada, *Ten Years of Health Transfer First Nation and Inuit Control* (Health Canada, First Nations and Inuit Health Branch), https://web.archive.org/web/20190925184528/https://www.canada.ca/en/indigenous-services-canada/services/first-nations-inuit-health/reports-publications/funding/years-health-transfer-first-nation-inuit-control-health-canada-1999.html; the Métis Nation of Alberta website (http://albertametis.com/about/history/); Government of Canada, "Indigenous health care in Canada", https://www.sac-isc.gc.ca/eng/1626810177053/1626810219482, date modified 2 May, 2023; Kristin Burnett, "Health of Indigenous Peoples in Canada", *Canadian Encyclopedia*, 7 February 2006, https://www.

thecanadianencyclopedia.ca/en/article/aboriginal-people-health; personal communications from
Bonnie Healey and Eunice Louis.

20 Supreme Court of British Columbia, "List of Residential Schools," Residential School Settlement,
Official Court Notice (27 July 2015), http://www.residentialschoolsettlement.ca/schools.html#Alberta.

21 Dr. Peter Bryce figures prominently in the history of public health in Canada and particularly Ontario.
In addition to his roles and efforts noted here, he was also the first secretary of the Provincial Board of
Health in Ontario in 1882, in which capacity he led the revision of Ontario's Public Health Act; he was
the chief medical officer of health in Ontario from 1887 until he moved into the federal government in
1904; and he chaired the organizing committee that was appointed at the first meeting of the CPHA
in 1919. Christopher Rutty and Sue C. Sullivan, This is Public Health: A Canadian History (Ottawa:
CPHA, 2010); Megan Sproule-Jones, "Crusading for the Forgotten: Dr. Peter Bryce, Public Health, and
the Prairie Native Residential Schools," Canadian Bulletin of Medical History 13 (1996).

22 As per the minister's instruction, this included a "special inspection" of the sanitary conditions and
health status of children from thirty-five "Indian schools" in the three prairie provinces in 1907, and an
examination of 243 children in eight schools in Alberta in 1909. According to Sproule-Jones, this focus
on the prairie provinces was not surprising considering: Bryce's dual responsibility for Indigenous and
immigrant populations; the time frame (namely, the rapid settlement of the prairie region in the early
twentieth century); and the fact that much less attention had been devoted to Indigenous Peoples in
the prairies than to those in older communities in central and eastern Canada. Megan Sproule-Jones,
"Crusading for the Forgotten." Although the requests from the federal minister to undertake these
investigations was prompted in part by health statistics and a need for greater action as expressed by
local medical officers, they were also influenced by money: a letter from the minister to Dr. Bryce in
1909 stated, "as it is necessary that these residential schools should be filled with a healthy class of
pupils in order that the expenditure on Indian education may not be rendered entirely nugatory, it
seems desirable that you should [undertake examinations]." Peter Henderson Bryce, The Story of a
National Crime: An Appeal for Justice to the Indians of Canada (Ottawa: James Hope & Sons, Limited,
1922), 5.

23 The 24% death rate was published in Bryce's 1907 Report on the Indian Schools of Manitoba and the
North West Territories. In one school, located on the File Hills reserve in Saskatchewan, over 65%
of students who had attended in the sixteen years since the school opened were dead, based on "a
complete return" of information from that school. Bryce, The Story of a National Crime; Sproule-
Jonesn "Crusading for the Forgotten."

24 Bryce, The Story of a National Crime, 4; Sproule-Jones, "Crusading for the Forgotten."

25 According to Sproule-Jones, Bryce's 1907 report prompted a 1911 federal memorandum titled
"Correspondence and Agreement Relating to the Maintenance and Management of Indian Boarding
Schools," which outlined regulations for the construction and maintenance of residential schools; the
memorandum did not lead to substantive improvements in the school. Sproule-Jones, "Crusading for
the Forgotten." See also, Bryce, The Story of a National Crime, 4.

26 Church officials who were responsible for managing residential schools in the prairies deflected blame,
asserting that the poor health of students reflected the poor conditions of reserve communities from
which they came and the inadequate government funding for the schools. In one of many examples of
a pervasive theme, the appalling conditions of residential schools were claimed to reflect jurisdictional
confusion within the partnership between church and state, which opened the door for inaction and
deflection of blame by both parties. Further complicating the situation was the existence of different
beliefs about the causes, and thus preventability, of tuberculosis. Despite bacteriological discoveries
such as the identification of the tuberculosis bacterium in 1882, some, including residential school
principals, continued to believe that tuberculosis represented God's punishment for the sins of society
or that it was genetically determined, and that the high rate of tuberculosis among residential school
students reflected the weaker constitution of Indigenous Peoples. Sproule-Jones, "Crusading for the
Forgotten."

27 Mr. Campbell Scott held leadership positions in the federal Department of Indian Affairs including
deputy minister from 1913 to 1932. He has become infamous for his comments about wanting to
"get rid of the Indian problem" and "to continue until there is not a single Indian in Canada that has
not been absorbed into the body politic." Robert L. McDougall, Canadian Encyclopedia, "Duncan
Campbell Scott," last edited 18 January 2018, https://www.thecanadianencyclopedia.ca/en/article/
duncan-campbell-scott.

28 Mr. Campbell Scott, upon his promotion in 1913 to Deputy Superintendent-General of Indian Affairs,
informed Bryce that his statistical reports of conditions of residential schools would no longer be
required, and Bryce was passed over for the appointment as Canada's first deputy minister of health —

a position for which, arguably, he was exquisitely well qualified. Bryce, *The Story of a National Crime*, 15; Sproule-Jones, "Crusading for the Forgotten."

29   Although these were the original signing dates of Treaties 7 and 8, in some cases there were later signings and/or adhesions where additional Nations joined the agreement. Alberta Regional Professional Development Consortium (ARPDC), *Alberta Treaties 6, 7, 8*, accessed 10 August 2020, http://empoweringthespirit.ca/wp-content/uploads/2017/05/Alberta-Treaties-678-1.pdf.

30   For example, prior to signing Treaty 7, First Nations in those territories were confronted with smallpox epidemics and the decline of the buffalo, both instigated by non-Indigenous groups. ARPDC, *Alberta Treaties 6, 7, 8*. On the day Treaty 7 was signed, Blackfoot Chief Crowfoot is widely quoted as saying "Bad men and whiskey were killing us so fast that very few, indeed, of us would have been left to-day" had the police / NWMP not come. Alexander Morris, *The Treaties of Canada with the Indians* (1880; reprint, Saskatoon: Fifth House, 1991), 295.

31   TRC, *Honouring the Truth*.

32   The Métis Nation of Alberta (http://albertametis.com/about/) is the Métis Government for Métis Albertans. Their definition of Métis aligns with that of the Métis National Council.

33   Alberta Health Services, *Population, Public and Indigenous Health SCN, Indigenous Health Transformational Roadmap, 2018–2020* (2 October 2018), https://www.nccih.ca/634/Indigenous_health_transformational_roadmap,_2018-2020.nccih?id=803&col=3

34   Treaty 6, 7 and 8 First Nations. Declaration of Treaty 6, 7 and 8 First Nations — Treaty Right to Health, 16–17 March 2005. Passed by resolution on 17 March 2005, in Edmonton at an Assembly of Treaty 6, 7, and 8 Chiefs. Provided by Eunice Louis, personal communication, 21 May 2020.

35   Colonial federal authority for issues pertaining to Indigenous Peoples is codified in the Constitution Act (1867) and the Indian Act (1876). Chantelle A.M. Richmond and Catherine Cook, "Creating Conditions for Canadian Aboriginal Health Equity: The Promise of Healthy Public Policy," *Public Health Reviews* 37, no. 2 (2016).

36   According to Bryce, medical inspector for the federal Departments of the Interior and Indian Affairs, the first reading in Parliament of the Bill to establish a federal Department of Health, which passed in 1919, contained a provision for including "Indian Medical Service" amongst its services. However, by the second reading that provision was absent. Bryce, *The Story of a National Crime*.

37   Emblematic of the different perspectives on treaty negotiations, federal authorities claimed that they were providing health care to Indigenous Peoples out of a moral or humanitarian sense of responsibility, rather than out of any promise. Maureen Lux, *Canadian Encyclopedia*, "Indian Hospitals in Canada," last edited 31 January 2018, https://www.thecanadianencyclopedia.ca/en/article/indian-hospitals-in-canada.

38   Briefly, there were at least seven racially segregated hospitals established for the treatment of First Nation Peoples in Alberta, including Peigan, Sarcee, Kainai (Blood), Morley/Stoney, Hobbema (now renamed Maskwacis), and Siksika (Blackfoot). Lauren Pelley, "$1.1B Class-action Lawsuit Filed on Behalf of Former 'Indian Hospital' Patients," *CBC News*, 30 January 2018, https://www.cbc.ca/news/canada/toronto/indian-hospital-class-action-1.4508659. Some of these, such as the Kainai (Blood) and Siksika (Blackfoot) hospitals, had their origins as mission hospitals in the late nineteenth century, were rebuilt in the 1920s, and evolved to practice some medical pluralism, such as combining colonial medicine with local healing practices. However, in a colonial context, those early Indian hospitals faced considerable challenges: they were underfunded, understaffed, and underequipped and could scarcely be expected to offset the dismal conditions that created poor health in the first place. During the post-WWII period, the federal government expanded its program of government-owned Indian hospitals, and the first in the expansion was the five hundred-bed Charles Camsell Indian Hospital in Edmonton where unacceptable practices occurred, including medical experimentation and sexual sterilization without consent. Around this period, the government took efforts to close other hospitals including the Kainai (Blood) and Siksika (Blackfoot) hospitals in Alberta. As noted, those hospitals had managed to exert some local autonomy, which made them a threat to the emerging vision of "national health." For a much more fulsome consideration of the complex story of the Indian hospitals, the reader is directed to the work of Maureen Lux, including "Care for the 'Racially Careless:' Indian Hospitals in the Canadian West, 1920–1950s," *The Canadian Historical Review* 91, no. 3 (2010); "We Demand 'Unconditional Surrender': Making and Unmaking the Blackfoot Hospital, 1890s to 1950s," *Social History of Medicine* 25, no. 3 (2012); *Separate Beds: A History of Indian Hospitals in Canada, 1920s–1980s* (Toronto: University of Toronto Press, 2016).

39   In 2017, Prime Minister Justice Trudeau announced organizational changes to the federal government that resulted in the First Nations and Inuit Health Branch being moved out of Health Canada and into the newly-created Indigenous Services Canada department.

40 Government of Canada, "Primary Health Care Authority," Indigenous and Northern Affairs Canada, modified 27 March 2020, https://www.aadnc-aandc.gc.ca/eng/1524852370986/1524852436793.

41 Canada's original Constitution Act (the British North America Act) identified "The establishment, maintenance, and management of hospitals, asylums, charities, and eleemosynary institutions in and for the province, other than marine hospitals" as one of the "exclusive powers of provincial legislatures." The Canada Health Act of 1984 sets out the requirements for provincial health insurance plans to qualify for full federal transfer payments. Specifically, those "insured services" must be administered publicly, and they must be comprehensive, universal, portable, and accessible. Government of Canada, "Canada Health Act," Health Canada, modified 24 February 2020, https://www.canada.ca/en/health-canada/services/health-care-system/canada-health-care-system-medicare/canada-health-act.html.

42 Government of Canada, "Canada Health Act — Frequently Asked Questions," Health Canada, modified 20 October 2020, https://www.canada.ca/en/health-canada/services/health-care-system/canada-health-care-system-medicare/canada-health-act-frequently-asked-questions.html#a3; Alberta Health Care Insurance Act, R.S.A. 2000, c. A-20, current as of 5 December 2019.

43 For example, the Canada Health Act (1984) does not contain any mention of First Nations Peoples (https://laws-lois.justice.gc.ca/eng/acts/C-6/). There is likewise no mention of First Nations Peoples in the Alberta Health Care Insurance Act, the Emergency Health Services Act (which includes ambulance service), or the Regional Health Authorities Act. On the other hand, Alberta's Hospitals Act does stipulate that the provincial health minister may enter into an agreement with the Government of Canada "in respect of the costs incurred . . . in providing insured services to Indians residing in Indian reserves in Alberta." The Regional Health Authorities Act (and the Public Health Act) explicitly reference Métis peoples by including "Métis settlements" within the definition of "municipality."

44 The failed treaty promise (i.e., the failure by colonial governments to uphold their obligations related to health care) takes the form of both insufficient and inadequate care. For example, a First Nation community may use its federal funding to hire medical staff. However, if the funding is only sufficient to hire a small number of staff, and those staff have to align with federal human resource policies, it may be impossible to have 24-hour medical service available in the community. With respect to non-insured benefits, if decisions about what is and is not covered are made centrally and seemingly arbitrarily, they are unlikely to fit the needs of each community. AHS, *Population, Public, and Indigenous Health*.

45 Bonnie Healy, personal communication, 28 November 2019.

46 H. B. Hawthorn (Ed.), *A Survey of the Contemporary Indians of Canada. Part 1: Economic, Political, Educational Needs and Policies* (Ottawa: Indian Affairs Branch, October 1966), https://publications.gc.ca/site/eng/9.700111/publication.html; Robert Breaker and Gregg Smith, "History Prior to Health Co-management" (PowerPoint presentation), 18 February 2014. Provided by William Wadsworth, personal communication, 20 October 2019.

47 Breaker and Smith, "History Prior to Health Co-management."

48 Alberta Government, *Aboriginal Peoples of Alberta*. See also Naithan Lagace and Niigaanwewidam James Sinclair, *Canadian Encyclopedia*, "The White Paper, 1969," last edited 10 June 2020, https://www.thecanadianencyclopedia.ca/en/article/the-white-paper-1969.

49 Government of Canada, "Statement on Indian Health Policy," Health and Welfare Canada (19 September 1979), accessed 14 August 2020, http://publications.gc.ca/collections/collection_2018/sc-hc/H14-296-1979.pdf; T. Kue Young, "Indian Health Services in Canada: A Sociohistorical Perspective," *Social Science & Medicine* 18, no. 3 (1984).

50 A policy framework for Health Transfer was approved by federal cabinet in 1988, and the next year the Treasury Board approved the financial resources to support pre-Transfer planning. Government of Canada, *Ten Years of Health Transfer*. During the 1990s, additional options were advanced to permit communities to take on different levels of transfer activities. For example, in 1994, the federal Treasury Board approved the Integrated Community-Based Health Services Approach, whereby communities could take on a limited or partial version of transfer activities, and in 1995, the federal government announced the Inherent Right to Self-Government Policy, which recognized that First Nation communities have the constitutional right to shape their own forms of government.

51 Breaker and Smith. "History prior to Health Co-Management;" "About Us," Health Co-Management, accessed 10 August 2020, https://torch7.com/hcom/about-us/.

52 While we felt that it was important and valuable to have one story from each Treaty area, we in no way wish to imply that these stories are representative of the diverse communities within Treaty areas or across Alberta.

53 Ella Arcand (Elder, Alexander First Nation), interview by Lindsay McLaren and Rogelio Velez Mendoza, 18 February 2020. All quotations from Ella Arcand are from the interview.

54   The program extended across Canada and the United States. Claudette Lavallée, Catherine A. James, and Elizabeth J. Robinson, "Evaluation of a Community Health Representative program among the Cree of Northern Quebec," *Canadian Journal of Public Health* 82, no. 3 (May/June 1991); U.S. Department of Health and Human Services, "Community Health Representative," Indian Health Service, accessed 10 August 2020, https://www.ihs.gov/chr/.

55   Confederacy of Treaty Six First Nations, "About Us," accessed 10 August 2020, https://www.treatysix.org/.

56   Michelle Filice, *Canadian Encyclopedia*, "Treaty 6," last edited 11 October 2016, https://www.thecanadianencyclopedia.ca/en/article/treaty-6.

57   One Treaty 6 example of an ongoing land claim is the one at Beaver Lake Cree First Nation, which focuses on industrial development related to oil and gas and the impact it has on the Nation's traditional lands and ways of life. Raven Trust, "Defend the treaties", accessed 10 August 2020, https://raventrust.com/campaigns/defend-the-treaties/.

58   Copy of Treaty No. 6 between Her Majesty The Queen and the Plain and Wood Cree Indians and Other Tribes of Indians at Fort Carlton, Fort Pitt and Battle River with Adhesions (Ottawa: Roger Duhamel, Queen's Printer and Controller of Stationery, 1964), http://www.trcm.ca/wp-content/uploads/PDFsTreaties/Treaty%206%20Text%20and%20Adhesions.pdf.

59   Federation of Sovereign Indigenous Nations, "Treaty Right to Health / Medicine Chest Task Force," Health and Social Development Commission, accessed 10 August 2020, https://fsin.ca/hasd/.

60   Confederacy of Treaty Six First Nations, "Fundamental Treaty Principles," accessed 10 August 2020, https://www.treatysix.org/treaty-principles.

61   Alexander First Nation, "Alexander First Nation — Kipohtakaw," accessed 10 August 2020, https://alexanderfn.com.

62   Government of Canada, "Registered Population — Alexander," Indigenous and Northern Affairs Canada, accessed 10 August 2020, https://fnp-ppn.aadnc-aandc.gc.ca/fnp/Main/Search/FNRegPopulation.aspx?BAND_NUMBER=438&lang=eng.

63   N. Lachance et al., *Health Determinants for First Nations in Alberta — 2010* (Health Canada; 2010), http://publications.gc.ca/collections/collection_2011/sc-hc/H34-217-2010-eng.pdf.

64   Naomi Adelson, "The Embodiment of Inequity: Health Disparities in Aboriginal Canada," *Canadian Journal of Public Health* 96, (Suppl. 2) (2005); Kristen M. Jacklin et al., "Health Care Experiences of Indigenous People Living with Type 2 Diabetes in Canada," *Canadian Medical Association Journal* 189, no.3 (2017).

65   Yellowhead Tribal Council, "About," accessed 10 August 2020, https://yellowheadtribalcouncil.ca/about/.

66   Ella Arcand, interview.

67   The program initially referred to both Community Health Workers, to denote working in the community rather than in institutions, and auxiliary health workers, which included community health representatives, who took a community public health approach, and other workers such as Family Health Aides, who took a family approach and may have engaged in some treatment activities depending on location and circumstances. Sheila Rymer, "Community Health Representative Program," *Health Education* 7 (Nov/Dec 1976). For ease, we refer to "community health representative" throughout the section.

68   Initial meetings were held in 1957 and 1958 between the Indian Affairs Branch of the federal Department of Citizenship and Immigration and the Medical Services Directorate of the Department of National Health and Welfare. Nancy Marian Gerein, "The Community Health Representative in Alberta — A Program Evaluation" (M.Sc. thesis, University of British Columbia, 1977), 13. The Medical Services Branch within the Department of National Health and Welfare, upon its establishment in 1962, assumed responsibility for the Indian Health Service.

69   As noted by Gerein, writing in the mid-1970s, "Numerous studies document the poor health of native people in Canada. A quick examination of gross statistics collected by Medical Services of the Federal Government comparing Indian with national health indicators makes obvious the disparities." Gerein, "The Community Health Representative in Alberta," 2.

70   Hawthorn's report, noted earlier in this chapter, laid bare the significant disadvantages faced by Indigenous Peoples in Canada and concluded that those disadvantages were caused by failed government policies. Hawthorn, *Survey of the Contemporary Indians of Canada*.

71   In 1961, the UN declared the 1960s the First Development Decade. Recognizing that economic and social development in "less developed" countries is critical to the well-being of those countries as well as to international peace, security, and prosperity, the designation called on Member States to "intensity their efforts to mobilize and sustain support," primarily to strengthen the economies of those countries. United Nations, "United Nations Development Decade. A Programme for

International Economic Co-operation (I)," accessed 10 August 2020, https://undocs.org/en/A/RES/1710%20(XVI). We acknowledge Nancy Gerein's 1977 work for providing this international contextualization. Gerein, "The Community Health Representative in Alberta," 2.

72   The federal Department of National Health and Welfare had, upon its creation in the mid-1940s, assumed responsibility for Indian Health Services.

73   Gerein, "The Community Health Representative in Alberta," 14.

74   Gerein, "The Community Health Representative in Alberta," 15.

75   As described by Lavallée, James, and Robinson, although community health representatives were involved in primary care in some jurisdictions in Canada, the intention was that those 'curative activities' would be the responsibility of physicians and nurses while the community health representatives would be responsible for prevention and health education. Claudette Lavallée, Catherine A. James, and Elizabeth J. Robinson, "Evaluation of a Community Health Representative Program among the Cree of Northern Quebec," *Canadian Journal of Public Health* 82, no. 3 (May/June 1991).

76   Rymer, "Community Health Representative Program."

77   The pilot project at Norway House included four women and seven men from ten reserves in Manitoba that had medical care available, either at a Medical Services Nursing Station or from nearby private physicians. The trainees had been selected by a joint Medical Services – Indian Affairs Branch committee based on the recommendation of the band councils. Rymer, "Community Health Representative Program,"; Gerein, "The Community Health Representative in Alberta."

78   Writing in 1976, Rymer stated that between 140 and 150 CHRs had been trained in British Columbia since 1963. Rymer, "Community Health Representative Program," 19.

79   Ella Arcand, interview.

80   While community health representatives were initially hired by Health Canada (Medical Services Branch of the Department of National Health and Welfare), over time a growing number were employed by their Band or district council. Rymer, "Community Health Representative Program," 18; Gerein, "The Community Health Representative in Alberta."

81   Ella Arcand, interview.

82   Gerein, "The Community Health Representative in Alberta."

83   Portage College (as it is now called) has an interesting history. According to its website, the college first opened in 1968 as "Alberta NewStart," which was part of federal government efforts to invest in adult education, but it closed without notice in December of 1970 ("they actually used chains to lock the doors, so no one could get in," Corianne Morin, Granddaughter of founder Veronica Morin. Portage College, A People's Success [video], available in "History," Portage College, accessed 10 August 2020, http://www.portagecollege.ca/About/History). Students affected by the closure organized a successful demonstration (a twenty-six-day sit-in), and the federal government provided an additional two-year grant. The community re-named the school "Pe-Ta-Pun" ("New Dawn"). When the federal funding ran out, the provincial government took over the funding and re-opened the school in 1973 as a campus of the Alberta Vocational Centre (AVC) (one of five campuses in the province). During the remainder of the 1970s the institution expanded its programs to include community-based programs; this is the period when the CHR training program began. A new facility was announced (by the provincial government) in 1980 and opened in 1985. In 1999 the institution was re-named Portage College, and the Lac La Biche campus is one of seven across Alberta. "History," Portage College.

84   As described by Akin Bob Adebayo, the CHR training program at the Alberta Vocational Centre was a thirty-week certificate program, including sixteen weeks of instruction and fourteen weeks of practicum work. The courses focused on communication and well-being, environmental health and communicable diseases, health promotion, networking, practical skills, and anatomy and physiology. There were approximately twenty students per year, of whom over 90% were Indigenous. Akin Bob Adebayo, "Characteristics, Employment Status, and Scope of Duties of Community Health Representatives: A Survey of Graduates," *Canadian Journal of Public Health* 86, no. 1 (Jan–Feb 1995).

85   Ella Arcand, interview; Gerein, "The Community Health Representative in Alberta;" Adebayo, "Characteristics, Employment Status, and Scope of Duties."

86   Gerein, "The Community Health Representative in Alberta," 16.

87   CHRs rarely interacted with men in the communities. Gerein, "The Community Health Representative in Alberta," 113.

88   Ella Arcand, interview

89   Ella Arcand, interview; Gerein, "The Community Health Representative in Alberta;" Adebayo, "Characteristics, Employment Status, and Scope of Duties."

90   Ella Arcand, interview.

91 Compiled from several sources. Ella Arcand, personal communication; Gerein, "The Community Health Representative in Alberta – A Program Evaluation," 18; Adebayo, "Characteristics, Employment Status, and Scope of Duties of Community Health Representatives," 16–19. Of course, the breadth and proportionate time spent on different activities depended on various factors, such as the geographic location of the community (CHRs in more isolated communities may have performed a greater breadth of activities) as well as the needs or desires of the (typically non-Indigenous) nurse.

92 Ella Arcand, interview.

93 Gerein, "The Community Health Representative in Alberta."

94 The CHR role also depended on unique local circumstances, such as whether there was an active Band Council. Gerein, "The Community Health Representative in Alberta."

95 Gerein, "The Community Health Representative in Alberta."

96 Rymer, "Community Health Representative Program," 18. This quotation was in reference to the initial set of trainees in the Norway House pilot project in the early 1960s.

97 A questionnaire was distributed via mail to all graduates of the program from 1980 to 1992, and 67% were returned. This high response rate was thought to reflect that "many of the respondents were very enthusiastic about the study and felt that this type of study was long overdue." Adebayo, "Characteristics, Employment Status, and Scope of Duties," 17.

98 Dr. Trent Keough, President and CEO, and Nancy Broadbent, Executive Vice President Academic, Portage College, "Community Information Night" (Power Point presentation), 2 November 2017.

99 Palmer, Tepper and Nolan, "Indigenous Health Services Often Hampered."

100 Ella Arcand, interview.

101 Ella Arcand, interview; For example, see Siksika Medicine Lodge, Youth Wellness Centre, "Our Board of Directors", http://www.siksikamedicinelodge.com/board.html.

102 "Spirit of Healing, Alberta First Nations Conquering Prescription Drug Misuse," accessed 10 August 2020, http://www.abfnspiritofhealing.com.

103 G. Barry Phillips, interview by Lindsay McLaren and Rogelio Velez Mendoza, 22 January 2020.

104 AFNIGC, "The Power of Data," http://www.afnigc.ca/main/includes/media/pdf/news/FNIGC_PoD_Series-Bigstone_FINAL_SCREEN.pdf; Lachance et al., Health determinants.

105 Thanks to Chief Silas Yellowknee for confirming the correct name in Cree.

106 G. Barry Phillips, interview.

107 These were the St. John's Anglican / Church of England Indian Residential School (Wabasca Residential School), which ran from 1895 to 1966, and the St. Martin's Wabasca Roman Catholic Boarding School, which ran from 1901 to 1973. Supreme Court of British Columbia, "List of Residential Schools."

108 TRC, Honouring the Truth, 41.

109 G. Barry Phillips, "The Bigstone Experience: 20 Years to a Healthier Community" (Unpublished manuscript), 4.

110 G. Barry Phillips, interview; Phillips, "The Bigstone Experience"; G. Barry Phillips, personal communication, 18 April 2020; Alberta Government, Aboriginal Peoples of Alberta.

111 G. Barry Phillips, interview.

112 G. Barry Phillips, interview.

113 G. Barry Phillips, interview. Phillips, "The Bigstone Experience."

114 Phillips, "The Bigstone Experience"; Bigstone Health Commission, "Medical Transportation / Referral," accessed 10 August 2020, https://www.bigstonehealth.ca/medical-transportation-referral/.

115 G. Barry Phillips, interview.

116 Marc Lalonde, A New Perspective on the Health of Canadians: A Working Document (Ottawa: Department of National Health and Welfare, 1974), https://www.phac-aspc.gc.ca/ph-sp/pdf/perspect-eng.pdf. Among other things, this report introduced the health field concept, whereby health is influenced by multiple factors including human biology and health care and lifestyle and environment.

117 Robert G. Evans, Morris L. Barer, and Theodore R. Marmor, Why are Some People Healthy and Others Not? The Determinants of Health of Populations (New York: Aldine de Gruyter, 1994); John P. Kretzmann and John L. McKnight, Building Communities from the Inside Out: A Path Toward Finding and Mobilizing a Community's Assets, (Evanston, IL: Institute for Policy Research, 1993). Barry was also influenced by the 1974 Lalonde Report.

118 Phillips, "The Bigstone Experience," 21.

119 Phillips, "The Bigstone Experience," 21-22.

120 Phillips, "The Bigstone Experience," 27.

121   Phillips, "The Bigstone Experience," 38.

122   For these initial steps, which were the first toward providing dental services right in Wabasca, the community is grateful to Dr. Keith Ellis, a retired dentist from Westlock in central Alberta who also helped recruit dental professionals to work in the community. One example was Dr. Joanne Wendell, whose "local presence and personality" in the early years of the dental service inspired members of the Bigstone community to take Dental Assistant training, some of whom became registered to practice in both dental and orthodontic settings. Such double-registration — unusual amongst dental assistants — provided "a reason to hold their head high, a reason to say, 'I can contribute to my community.' " G. Barry Phillips, interview.

123   G. Barry Phillips, interview; Bigstone Health Commission, "About Us," accessed 10 August 2020, https://www.bigstonehealth.ca.

124   Cora Voyageur, Angeline Letendre, and Bonnie Healey, *Alberta Baseline Assessment Report* (AFNIGC, 2015), 23; Bigstone Health Commission, "About Us."

125   Former Chief Gordon T. Auger, as quoted in AFNIGC, "The Power of Data."

126   The First Nations Information Governance Centre has been collecting data about First Nation reserves and northern communities since 1997 through surveys, including the First Nations Regional Health Survey and the First Nations Regional Early Childhood, Education and Employment Survey. The FNIGC, including regional partners, of which AFNIGC is one, is a non-profit organization that "envisions that every First Nation will achieve data sovereignty in alignment with its distinct world view." First Nations Information Governance Centre, "Vision," accessed 10 August 2020, https://fnigc. ca/about-fnigc/vision.html.

127   FNIGC, "The Power of Data."

128   Lorraine Muskwa and Janice Willier, "Bigstone Health Commission Report Card," presentation at FNHMA National Conference, 25 September 2014, https://www.fnhma.ca/archive/conference/2014/ Files/Workshop%20N.pdf.

129   Phillips, "The Bigstone Experience," 33.

130   G. Barry Phillips, interview.

131   Health Professions Act, R.S.A. 2000, c. H-7, current as of 5 December 2019. Health Professions Act, R.S.A. 2000, 79–80.

132   The parameters of the lease could be modeled on those used in other circumstances but adapted for the unique First Nation and non-insured health benefits context. For example, a new dental graduate who sets up a practice within an established practice (working for another dentist) in an urban setting may enter into a 60%–40% (approximate) arrangement where 60% of the amount billed goes to the established dentist to help pay for the space, equipment, etc., and 40% goes to the new dentist as earnings. Adapting this for a First Nation context would take into account the fact that NIHB fees for dental services are lower than Alberta Blue Cross fees. G. Barry Phillips, interview.

133   G. Barry Phillips, interview.

134   TRC, *Honouring the Truth.*

135   G. Barry Phillips, interview.

136   Chief Charles Weaselhead, interview by Lindsay McLaren and Rogelio Velez Mendoza, Standoff, AB, 28 January 2020. All quotations from Chief Charles Weaselhead are from the interview.

137   Charles Weaselhead Jr. served as Chief of the Blood Tribe from 2004 to 2016. During that time he was appointed as the Treaty 7 Grand Chief, and also held the health and education portfolio for the Treaty 7 Chiefs. Amongst numerous other leadership roles, Chief Weaselhead served as the Director of the Blood Indian Hospital in the early 1990s, and as Chief Executive Officer for the Blood Tribe Department of Health until his 2004 election to Chief of the Blood Tribe. "Chancellor Charles Weaselhead," University Secretariat (Governance), University of Calgary, accessed 10 August 2020, https://www.uleth.ca/governance/chancellor-charles-weaselhead.

138   Blood Tribe Department of Health, *Kottakinoona Awaahkapiiyaawa, "Bringing the Spirits Home": The Blood Tribe Addiction Framework,* November 2019, https://btdh.ca/wp-content/uploads/2019/11/ Blood-Tribe-Bringing-the-Spirits-Home-Addiction-Framework_November-2019.pdf. Kottakinoona Awaahkapiiyaawa can be translated as "Bringing the Spirits Home," "Telling Our Spirits to Come Home" or "Calling the Spirits Home." Blood Tribe Department of Health, *Kottakinoona Awaahkapiiyaawa*

139   Kainaysinni, or Guiding Principles, as described in the Declaration of the Elders of the Blood Indian Nation, available at https://crystalgoodrider.weebly.com/blackfoot-values--elders-declarations.html.

140   Blood Tribe Department of Health, *Kottakinoona Awaahkapiiyaawa*; Kevin Cowan (CEO, Blood Tribe Department of Health), personal communication, 28 January 2020.

141 The Horn Society, for example, is a group of spiritual leaders in the community who "come together annually to pray for the protection, for the safety, for the nourishment . . . for our people." Chief Charles Weaselhead, interview; Blood Tribe Department of Health, *Kottakinoona Awaahkapiiyaawa*.

142 Blood Tribe Department of Health, *Kottakinoona Awaahkapiiyaawa*.

143 TRC, *Honouring the Truth*.

144 These include (but are not limited to) the residential schools, of which there were two in the Cardston area, and as the Blood Indian Hospital, which despite evolving to serve the community, was badly affected by a later wave of federal government assimilationist policy, during their post-WWII welfare state expansion. The two residential schools in the area were St. Paul's Anglican school, which opened in 1891 and closed in 1975, and St. Mary's Immaculate Conception Roman Catholic school, which opened in 1898 and closed in 1988. There were several other schools throughout Treaty 7, including St. Joseph's, Ste. Trinité in Cluny (Siksika); Morley (Stony) school in Morley; Old Sun School in Gleichen; Sacred Heart school and St. Cyprian's (Queen Victoria's Jubilee Home), both in Brocket; St. Joseph's school in High River; and St. Barnabas school at T'suu Tina. Supreme Court of British Columbia, "List of Residential Schools." Interestingly, the TRC identified that it was not unusual for parents of an entire community to refuse to take their children to school, and one instance of this resistance was noted in the Blood Reserve: "In October 1927, seventy-five school-aged children from the Blood Reserve in Alberta either had not returned to school or had not been enrolled in school." Although it is not entirely clear, one could speculate that this was an example of strength and resilience in those dire circumstances. TRC, *Honouring the Truth*, 116. For scholarship on the Indian hospitals in general and the Blood Indian Hospital in particular, the reader is directed to the work of Maureen Lux, "Care for the 'Racially Careless,' 407–434; *Separate Beds*.

145 Kevin Cowan, personal communication, 28 January 2020.

146 For current statistics see: Federal, provincial, and territorial Special Advisory Committee on the Epidemic of Opioid Overdoses. Opioid- and Stimulant-related Harms in Canada. Ottawa: Public Health Agency of Canada; https://health-infobase.canada.ca/substance-related-harms/opioids-stimulants/

147 For example, the number of apparent accidental drug poisoning deaths related to fentanyl, a type of opioid, in Alberta was six in 2011, twenty-nine in 2012, sixty-six in 2013, 116 in 2014, 256 in 2015, 347 in 2016, 566 in 2017, and 673 in 2018. "Opioid Surveillance Quarterly Reports," Opioid Reports, Government of Alberta, accessed 11 August 2020, https://www.alberta.ca/opioid-reports.aspx.

148 Government of Alberta, Analytics and Performance Reporting, Alberta Health, *Alberta Opioid Response Surveillance Report, Q3 2019* (December 2019), https://open.alberta.ca/dataset/f4b74c38-88cb-41ed-aa6f-32db93c7c391/resource/c9e430f9-0951-436a-9b36-f372ee476498/download/health-alberta-opioid-response-surveillance-report-2019-q3.pdf.

149 It is essential that data and statistics for First Nation communities reflect First Nations' knowledge and leadership, and this is enshrined in the First Nations' OCAP' (Ownership, Control, Access and Possession) principles. OCAP' is a registered trademark of the First Nations Information Governance Centre (FNIGC), https://fnigc.ca/ocap-training/; Alberta First Nations Information Governance Centre (AFNIGC), accessed 11 August 2020, http://www.afnigc.ca/main/index.php?id=home.

150 In response to a request by Chief Weaselhead, Blood Tribe member Aapooyakii (Bonnie Healy) a, trauma-trained registered nurse with three decades of nursing experience, and executive director of AFNIGC at the time, honoured her ancestral obligation to her people by leading efforts to achieve the AFNIGC mandate from the Alberta Chiefs. The mandate was to create First Nations identifiable data and a First Nations Health Information Governance Agreement with the Alberta Ministry of Health's surveillance unit, which were respectful of OCAP' principles. The Alberta First Nations Opioid Report is significant: it is the first in the world to recode the data in a way that provides more detail including, importantly, separating the prescribed opioids from the illicit drugs (fentanyl). AFNIGC and Government of Alberta, *Alberta Opioid Response Surveillance Report – First Nations People in Alberta*, (December 2019), https://www.alberta.ca/assets/documents/health-first-nations-opioid-surveillance. pdf; Bonnie Healy, personal communication, 25 May 2020.

151 AFNIGC and Government of Alberta, *Alberta Opioid Response First Nations*

152 The discrepancy was three-fold for those aged twenty-five to forty-nine years. AFNIGC and Alberta Government, "Opioid Dispensations to First Nations people in Alberta," 30 August 2016, http://www. afnigc.ca/main/includes/media/pdf/fnhta/HTAFN-2016-08-30-Opioid.pdf.

153 Although our focus here is the opioid crisis, the Blood Tribe people and community have battled other types of addiction as well. Blood Tribe Department of Health, *Kottakinoona Awaahkapiiyaawa*.

154 Kevin Cowan, personal communication, 28 January 28, 2020; Kevin Cowan, interview by Lindsay McLaren and Rogelio Velez Mendoza, Standoff, AB, 28 January 2020.

155 Jacen Abrey, interview by Lindsay McLaren and Rogelio Velez Mendoza, Standoff, AB, 28 January 2020.

156 The racism and discrimination Cardston is deeply rooted. When the federal government stepped up their assimilationist policies in the post-WWII period, including efforts to force the closure of the Blood Indian Hospital in Cardston, they recommended that the local First Nation people instead attend the municipal hospital in Cardston. Members of the Blood Tribe resisted, citing the discrimination against the Indigenous Peoples by the people of Cardston. Maureen K. Lux, *Separate Beds.*

157 Blood Tribe Department of Health, *Kottakinoona Awaahkapiiyaawa.*

158 The task was initially to develop an opioid response plan, which included detoxification, treatment, and aftercare. However, because opioids are merely the major drug of choice, it was determined that it would be more appropriate to create a broader addiction framework that included dimensions of prevention and harm reduction. Lene Jorgensen, personal communication.

159 Blood Tribe Department of Health, *Kottakinoona Awaahkapiiyaawa,* 7.

160 Including those on the front line of the crisis, within and outside the community; those providing other programs and services to members; Elders and Knowledge Keepers; those living with addiction; those in recovery; those who have recovered; and family members. Blood Tribe Department of Health, *Kottakinoona Awaahkapiiyaawa.*

161 Blood Tribe Department of Health, *Kottakinoona Awaahkapiiyaawa.*

162 Lene Jorgensen, personal communication.

163 Lene Jorgensen, personal communication.

164 Dr. Tailfeathers had advocated for a safe withdrawal site in the community as early as 2015, which provided an important foundation for the 2018 efforts. Personal communication, Lene Jorgensen, March 29 2020.

165 Jacen Abrey, interview.

166 Jacen Abrey, interview.

167 Lene Jorgensen, personal communication, 2 April 2020.

168 Jacen Abrey, interview.

169 Blood Tribe Department of Health, *Kottakinoona Awaahkapiiyaawa*

170 Details of the evaluation, of the activities that we have partially described here, have not been fully worked out; however, they will involve quantitative service data as well as Blackfoot ways of knowing, including the Winter Count. In the Winter Count, symbols illustrate the most significant events, and are painted – often on buffalo hides – starting in the centre and spiraling outward. The importance of the information captured in the Winter Count is more about the story contained within, than about the chronological order. Blood Tribe Department of Health, *Kottakinoona Awaahkapiiyaawa.*

171 Kevin Cowan, personal communication, 28 January 2020.

172 Lene Jorgensen, personal communication.

173 Jacen Abrey, interview.

174 Kevin Cowan, interview.

175 Kevin Cowan, interview.

176 Jacen Abrey, interview.

177 Jacen Abrey, interview.

178 TRC, *Honouring the Truth.*

179 Charlotte Reading and Fred Wien, *Health Inequalities and Social Determinants of Aboriginal Peoples' Health* (Prince George, BC, National Collaborating Centre for Aboriginal Health, 2009), https://www.ccnsa-nccah.ca/docs/determinants/RPT-HealthInequalities-Reading-Wien-EN.pdf; AFNIGC and Government of Alberta, "Mortality Rates in First Nations in Alberta" (23 February 2016), https://www.afnigc.ca/main/includes/media/pdf/fnhta/HTAFN-2016-02-23-AllCauseMortality.pdf

180 National Collaborating Centre for Determinants of Health, "Let's Talk: Health Equity" (Antigonish, NS: NCCDH, St. Francis Xavier University, 2013), http://nccdh.ca/images/uploads/Lets_Talk_Health_Equity_English.pdf; Commission on Social Determinants of Health (CSDH), *Closing the Gap in a Generation: Health Equity through Action on the Social Determinants of Health. Final report of the Commission on Social Determinants of Health* (Geneva: World Health Organization, 2008), https://www.who.int/social_determinants/thecommission/finalreport/en/.

181 TRC, *Honouring the Truth.*

182 Alberta Health Services, Population, Public and Indigenous Health Strategic Clinical Network, Esther Tailfeathers, *Indigenous Health in Alberta: A Primer 101* (May 31, 2018), 4.

183 Alberta, Legislative Assembly, MLA Committee on the First Nations, Metis and Inuit Workforce Planning Initiative, *Connecting the Dots: Aboriginal Workforce and Economic Development in Alberta* (Edmonton: Government of Alberta, 2010), 12-13, https://open.alberta.ca/publications/9780778559726. Contains information licensed under the Open Government Licence – Alberta.

NOTES TO TABLE 7.2

1   "History of Providing Health Services to First Nations people and Inuit," First Nations and Inuit Branch, Government of Canada, accessed 14 August 2020, https://web.archive.org/web/20191012164923/https://www.canada.ca/en/indigenous-services-canada/corporate/first-nations-inuit-health-branch/history-providing-health-services-first-nations-people-inuit.html.

2   Health Canada, First Nations and Inuit Health Branch, Ten Years of Health Transfer First Nation and Inuit Control (1999), https://web.archive.org/web/20190925184528/https://www.canada.ca/en/indigenous-services-canada/services/first-nations-inuit-health/reports-publications/funding/years-health-transfer-first-nation-inuit-control-health-canada-1999.html.

3   Government of Canada, Indian Health Policy (1979), accessed 14 August 2020, http://publications.gc.ca/collections/collection_2018/sc-hc/H14-296-1979.pdf

4   Breaker and Smith, "History Prior to Health Co-management."

5   *Metis Settlement Act*, R.S.A. 2000, c. M-14, 132, current as of 1 September 2019.

6   Bill C-3 (2010) amended the federal Indian Act to entitle individuals in the following circumstances to register: those whose mother lost Indian status upon marrying a non-Indian man; those whose father is a non-Indian; those who were born after the mother lost Indian status (with date restrictions); those who had a child with a non-Indian (with date restrictions. Alberta Government, Ministry of Indigenous Relations, *Aboriginal Peoples of Alberta: Yesterday, Today, and Tomorrow.* The amendment was in response to a British Columbia Court of Appeal decision that section 6 of the Indian Act contained gender discrimination.

7   Truth and Reconciliation Commission of Canada, *Honouring the Truth, Reconciling for the Future.*

Health Protection — Climate Change, Health, and Health Equity in Alberta

Lindsay McLaren, Cristina Santamaria-Plaza, and Dennis Slater

Introduction

> [There is] an unprecedented surge in awareness of and engagement with the climate emergency. . . . Yet, the link made by individuals between health issues and climate change is weak.[1]

Health protection, one of the core functions of public health practice, refers to "important activities of public health, in food hygiene, water purification, environmental sanitation, drug safety and other activities, that eliminate as far as possible the risk of adverse consequences to health attributable to environmental hazards."[2] Sometimes used interchangeably with *environmental health*, health protection is a long-standing aspect of public health practice.

Widely considered to have emerged out of the sanitary movement in mid-nineteenth-century England in response to health problems caused by industrialization and urbanization, health protection activities have evolved to include a breadth of issues including occupational hazards and working conditions; built environments including housing, land-use patterns and roads; and agricultural methods.[3] These issues are significantly intertwined with structural drivers of inequity. For example, environmental hazards in the workplace often result from employment characteristics typical of neoliberal capitalism, such as precarious employment and inadequate pay and benefits (see Chapter 9).[4]

Partly because of their relatively long history, health protection activities concerning quality and safety of air, water, and food occupy a dominant place in public health practice: to a large extent they underpin public health's broad and institutionalized approach, including the professional practice of health inspection. Indeed, the historical prominence of health protection activities in public health has led to a common — but inaccurate — perception that the two are synonymous, or in other words that public health is reducible to health protection activities.[5]

While the current chapter considers one of these long-standing concerns — namely, air pollution — it does so with the intent of providing a historical backdrop for a newer and complex topic in public health: climate change, the persistent, long-term changes to the state of the climate, driven by both natural and human and industrial factors that release CO_2 and other greenhouse gases into the atmosphere.[6] Along with biodiversity loss and ecosystem destruction more generally, the health implications of climate change are significant. An example of a direct implication is the sickness and death caused by extreme weather. Indirect impacts include health consequences stemming from changes to food growing conditions and to water quality and quantity, zoonotic disease emergence, and mental health impacts following climate-related disasters or forced climate migration.[7] Moreover, within and between countries, the health impacts of climate change are highly inequitable. Therefore, a *climate justice* orientation — that is, a just, or fair, response that considers the complex social and political dimensions — is essential.[8] A climate justice perspective is theoretically consistent with public health's "values of social justice and fairness for all, and its focus on the collective actions of interdependent and empowered peoples and their communities."[9] However, as Buse and others have written, certain assumptions and beliefs embedded within public health practice can present a challenge to the field's ability to substantively engage with these socio-political aspects.[10]

Following a brief overview of national and international milestones, the chapter proceeds in two main sections. The first considers the first two-thirds of the twentieth century, when provincial environmental policy in Alberta was focused on pollution. The second section presents our analysis of provincial government deliberations on climate change policy since 2000; in particular, we explore whether and how concepts of health and equity have been mobilized in those deliberations. Overall, our analysis contributes to a rapidly growing literature on public health and climate change, and on contemporary health protection more generally, by adding a historical perspective aimed at articulating and strengthening a broad, coherent vision of public health in the Alberta context.[11]

National and International Milestones in Environmentalism

To help situate the chapter content, a partial list of key events in international and national climate change history is shown in Table 8.1.

TABLE 8.1: Summary of some key international and national milestones in climate change.[12]

Decade	Event or Initiative
1820s	• First recorded inquiry into the greenhouse gas effect by French mathematician, Joseph Fourier (1824)
1860s	• British physicist John Tyndall established that there were several types of gases (including water vapour) that contributed to the greenhouse gas effect (1861)
	• Early federal conservation-oriented legislation, the *Act for the Regulation of Fishing and Protection of Fisheries*, was passed by the Canadian Government to regulate "sea-coast and inland fisheries, to prevent or remedy the obstruction and pollution of streams" (1868)
1880s	• Banff National Park (Canada's first National Park in Alberta) was created by the federal government (1885)
1890s	• Swedish chemist Svante Arrhenius observed a correlation between CO_2 and temperature change, thus demonstrating that coal burning during the industrial revolution contributed to the greenhouse gas effect (1895)
1930s	• The *National Parks Act* was passed by the Canadian government in 1930, which provided for parks to be maintained and used in such a way that left them "unimpaired for the enjoyment of future generations"
	• British engineer Guy Callendar showed that temperatures in the United States had increased significantly since the industrial revolution. This was most likely due to rising CO_2 emissions, which had increased during the same period (1938)
1950s	• Canadian physicist Gilbert Plass examined the infrared absorption of different gases, and concluded that doubling of greenhouse gases (i.e., CO2) would raise temperatures by 3 to 4 degrees (1955)
	• American scientist Charles Keeling developed a way to record CO_2 levels at a research station in Hawaii, and demonstrated that annual atmospheric CO_2 emissions had steadily risen between 1958 and 1964. The research station continued to collect data which confirmed Keeling's findings (1958)

TABLE 8.1: (*continued*)

Decade	Event or Initiative
1970s	• The first United Nations Conference on the Environment was held (Stockholm, 1972).
	• *Canada's Water Act* was enacted in 1970; it provided for "the management of water resources of Canada, including research and the planning and implementation of programs relating to the conservation, development and utilization of water resources" (1970)
	• The *Arctic Waters Pollution Prevention Act* was enacted, which aimed to "prevent pollution of areas of the arctic waters adjacent to the mainland and islands of the Canadian arctic" (1970)
	• Canada's *Clean Air Act* was passed, which aimed to "promote and achieve uniform approach to air pollution control across the country" (1971)
	• Canada's first Environment Ministry was created in 1971; it was responsible for, among other things, "preserving and enhancing the quality of the natural environment", and "coordinating policies and programs" to do so.
1980s	• In 1983 the United Nations convened the World Commission on Environment and Development (*Brundtland Commission*) to examine issues relating to economic development, labour practices and environmental protection. The Commission's report, Our Common Future, established three pillars: economic growth, environmental protection, and social equality.
	• The United Nations created the *Montreal Protocol on Substances that Deplete the Ozone Layer* (1987), in which 197 UN Member States including Canada, aimed to "phase out [the different] groups of [ozone depleting substances (ODS)], control of ODS trade, annual reporting of data, national licensing systems to control ODS imports and exports"
	• The Intergovernmental Panel on Climate Change (IPCC) was created by the World Meteorological Organization (WMO) and the United Nations Environment Programme (UNEP) (1988), with a main goal to comprehensively review and make recommendations concerning "the science of climate change; the social and economic impact of climate change, and potential response strategies and elements for inclusion in a possible future international convention on climate"
	• The *Canadian Environmental Protection Act* was passed in 1988, with the aim to prevent pollution and protect the environment and human health
1990s	• The United Nations Framework Convention on Climate Change (UNFCCC), signed by Canada in 1992, aimed to keep the global average temperature from rising to levels that would damage the environment
	• The *Canadian Environmental Assessment Act* was passed, which required all ministries to conduct environmental assessments for projects to protect the environment (1992)
	• The Kyoto Protocol was created in 1997 and aimed to engage member countries in committing to the UNFCCC's mandate. In signing, Canada agreed to GHG emission target reductions over the period 2008–2012.

TABLE 8.1: *(continued)*

Decade	Event or Initiative
2010s	• Under Prime Minister Stephen Harper, Canada withdrew from the Kyoto Protocol (2011) and the original *Canadian Environment Assessment Act* was repealed (2012)
	• Justin Trudeau was elected prime minister in 2015, after running on a campaign focused on climate change action including a carbon tax. The J. Trudeau administration signed the Paris agreement, to keep global temperature increases to 1.5°C above pre-industrial levels, in 2016. Also under the federal Liberals, the Pan Canadian Framework on Clean Growth and Climate Change was released (2016) and the Impact Assessment Agency of Canada was established (2019).
	• The *North American Climate Clean Energy and Environment Partnership Act* was created between Canada, the United States and Mexico to continue building their efforts to address climate change. (2016)
	• Greta Thunberg, Swedish climate activist, started a worldwide climate-related political movement by protesting in front of the Swedish Parliament with a sign titled "School Strike for Climate". Greta Thunberg received the Nobel Peace Prize in 2019 (2018–2019)

The Industrial Revolution and its capitalist underpinnings is considered to mark the point where human activity became the most important contributor to climate change, beginning with shifts toward coal-burning technologies that enabled mass textile production and transportation, such as railways, canals, and iron ships, in the late eighteenth and early nineteenth centuries. Waves of industrialization between the 1860s and 1940s, which were more pertinent to the North American context, were characterized by a colonial, extractive transition toward economies of scale through growth of the automotive industry, rail transportation, and consumer goods. Concurrent with these developments were rising deforestation and resource extraction of oil, gas, and coal.[13]

Public and political concern about environmental preservation and conservation has evolved over time. In terms of settler-dominated activities, popular sources describe Canada's environmental movement as occurring in four waves.[14] During the late 1800s and early 1900s, European colonization and rapid exploitation of Canada's natural resources, which were incorrectly perceived as inexhaustible, prompted some limited awareness, particularly within the forestry industry, of the need for protections to allow long-term harvesting to continue.[15] Otherwise, organized conservation was not very prominent in Canada at that time, and some activities that resembled environmental protection were in fact driven by economic goals (Banff National Park, for example, was created to generate tourism revenue).[16]

A second wave started in the 1960s and represented somewhat of an inflection point in environmental preservation and activism. Important organizations were formed, including the National and Provincial Parks Association of Canada (now the Canadian Parks and Wilderness Society) in 1963, the World Wildlife Fund Canada in 1967, and Greenpeace (including a Canadian contingent) in 1971.[17] Growing pressure from these and other groups contributed to important legislative and administrative changes, including in Alberta. The federal government context for air pollution included the 1969 creation of a new division of the Department of National Health and Welfare devoted to health aspects of air pollution; the 1970 federal Motor Vehicle Safety Act, which allowed vehicle emissions to be regulated; the 1970 introduction of incentives to reduce air pollution under federal Income Tax Regulations; and the 1971 introduction of a national Clean Air Act and establishment of a federal Department of Environment.[18]

Following a third era of the 1980s and 1990s, which significantly included the 1983 creation of the Green Party of Canada,[19] the fourth era — aligning with this chapter's focus — is characterized by the climate change preoccupation of the 2000s that started with the 1997 Kyoto Protocol. The nations that signed the accord, including Canada, committed to reducing their greenhouse gas emissions by 6 percent between 2008 and 2012. However, in one of many important illustrations of the need to situate these issues in socio-political context, progress stalled in Canada under the federal Conservative government of Stephen Harper (2006–2015), which withdrew Canada from the accord in 2011; cut funding to environmental research and organizations; repealed and replaced key environmental legislation, such as the Canadian Environmental Assessment Act; and effectively silenced environmental non-profit organizations, such as by placing severe limits on "political activity" that impede the organizations' normal activities. Upon their majority election in 2015, the federal Liberal government under Justin Trudeau signed the 2016 Paris agreement, which signified a commitment to work toward limiting global temperature rise during the current century to 1.5° Celsius above pre-industrial levels. Also in 2016, the federal government released the *Pan-Canadian Framework on Clean Growth and Climate Change*, which outlined a plan to "to meet emissions reduction targets, grow the economy, and build resilience to a changing climate." In 2019 they created the Impact Assessment Agency of Canada, which — consistent with a broad, intersectoral version of public health — examines positive and negative environmental, economic, social, and health impacts of major resources projects.[20] However, despite these initiatives, whether or the extent to which the federal Liberal government is serious about taking substantive action on climate change is questionable and remains to be seen.[21]

Pollution Control and Public Health in Alberta During the Twentieth Century

We first consider environmental policy around air pollution in Alberta during the twentieth century. See Table 8.2 for a summary of provincial milestones.[22] Notably, from 1907 until 1970, public health and pollution control were administratively connected: the Provincial Board of Health was responsible for processes and legislation concerning safe and healthy environments including clean air.

TABLE 8.2: Timeline of some major milestones in Alberta environmental policy as it intersects with public health, 1905–1970s.

Year	Event
1907	• Alberta's first provincial *Public Health Act* authorized the provincial Board of Health to create regulations to prevent water pollution, for the purpose of preventing communicable diseases.
1919	• The provincial Department of Public Health was created, which assumed responsibility for the provisions of the *Public Health Act* (including prevention of water pollution).
1944	• In the context of population and industrial growth in Alberta cities, an amendment to the provincial *Public Health Act* acknowledged water used "for agricultural, domestic or industrial purposes"; water pollution control measures in Alberta subsequently intensified.
1947	• Imperial Oil struck oil near Leduc, Alberta, marking the beginning of Alberta's petroleum industry (a significant impact on Alberta's economy was not apparent, however, until the 1960s).
1955	• An amendment to the provincial *Public Health Act* added "pollution of atmosphere" to the list of items that could be regulated by the provincial Board of Health, thus signaling a shift of attention to air pollution.
1961	• Alberta implemented a program of air pollution control measures, including emissions standards and regulations focused on industrial plants and operations.
1960s	• The provincial *Public Health Act* acknowledged "pipelines" as a source of pollution
1971	• A new provincial Department of Environment was created, which took over responsibility for pollution-related activities from the provincial Department of (Public) Health.
1970s	• Reference to "pollution" disappeared from the provincial *Public Health Act*. • Substantive early efforts to protect the environment (e.g., the 1970 creation of an "independent watchdog" for the environment – the Environment Conservation Authority) gave way to an emphasis on economic and industrial growth. Significant negative environmental impacts of oil sands development were apparent by the mid-1970s.

Until around the 1940s, government pollution legislation focused primarily on water pollution, which was a concern from Alberta's first Public Health Act of 1907.[23] This arrangement remained largely the same from the 1920s to the 1940s. In 1944, in an early indication of the ongoing intersection between environmental concerns and extractive industry, an amendment to the act acknowledged uses of source water "for agricultural, domestic or industrial purposes," in addition to water for drinking.[24] In the context of population growth and industrial expansion in Alberta cities, water pollution control measures in the province intensified in the 1950s and 1960s.[25]

The 1950s signalled a shift in attention to air pollution. A 1955 amendment to the Public Health Act added "pollution of atmosphere" to the list of items that could be regulated by the Provincial Board of Health. Specifically, the board's authority was extended to include "prevention of the pollution, defilement or fouling of the atmosphere and the regulation of plants or industries discharging chemical or other waste matter into the atmosphere."[26] During the 1960s, that wording was amended to say "regulation of plants, industries *and pipe lines*" (emphasis added); as discussed below, the expansion of the oil and gas industry figured prominently, and problematically, in the evolution of Alberta's environmental policy starting in the 1960s.[27]

Government recognition of the connection between air pollution and health during the 1950s is clear from the description of "pollution of atmosphere" in the 1955 Public Health Act, which addressed

> [circumstances where] dust, vapour, fumes or smoke is being discharged into the atmosphere either within or outside the confines of any building, and that as a result of such discharge the quality of the air is being impaired or corrupted *and the comfort or health of the public or a portion of the public is being injuriously affected.*[28] (emphasis added)

Following the regulatory authority established by the 1955 act, in 1961 Alberta implemented what was described as a broad program of air pollution control. This included emissions standards and regulations focused on industrial plants and operations where, under Alberta Regulation 262/61 (O.C. 1327-61) plans for the construction of pipelines and plants "likely to contribute to air pollution" had to be submitted to the Provincial Board of Health for approval.[29] An explicit concern with health, which persisted in this new program, expanded to include plant and animal life.[30]

1971: Creation of a Provincial Department of Environment

From the point of view of the intersection of provincial public health and environmental policy, circumstances changed with the 1971 creation of a new provincial Department of Environment. The new department, which was one of the first of its kind in Canada,[31] took over air- and water pollution control activities from the Department of (Public) Health.[32] Likewise, references to "pollution" in the Public Health Act, which had been present since the very first act in 1907, disappeared during the 1970s, and did not return. When the new Department of Environment inherited the Division of Environmental Health from the Department of Public Health, it was renamed the Division of Pollution Control; "health" was removed from the name.[33]

The creation of the new Department of Environment must be situated in the development of the Alberta oil and gas industry. In what has become provincial lore, Imperial Oil struck oil near Leduc, Alberta, in February 1947, which, ominously, "marked the beginning of a petroleum boom that rapidly transformed Alberta's impoverished agricultural economy and drew thousands of people to the province."[34] Although the 1947 date is significant, the transformation of Alberta's economy took some time. Within an extractive colonial context, a growing human-centric demand for oil led to the production of synthetic oil from the massive Athabasca bitumen deposit in northeastern Alberta.[35] However, because of technical challenges associated with mining and upgrading the bitumen into synthetic crude oil, commercial production of bitumen did not occur until the 1960s. This perhaps explains why reference to "pipelines," in the context of pollution, did not appear in Alberta's Public Health Act until that decade.[36]

In the context of significant environmental concerns from scientists and citizens that accompanied the development of the oil industry and growing community pressure to address them, legislation to establish a provincial Department of Environment was passed in early 1971 by the Social Credit government of Harry Strom (1968–1971) and implemented under the PC government of Peter Lougheed (1971–1985) upon their election later that year.[37] As discussed by historians, Alvin Finkel, and Hereward Longley, while the SC party originated in the post-Depression context as a social reform party that focused on the rights of workers and farmers and was opposed to big business including oil, their position shifted over the course of their long tenure toward an increasingly laissez-faire orientation toward the oil industry; at the same time they were seen as increasingly representing right-wing religious fundamentalism.[38] In the light of that ideological shift, Finkel argues that the Social Credit's flurry of environmental initiatives in 1970 was a last-ditch and somewhat disingenuous effort to gain public support and, unsuccessfully, avoid losing the 1971 election.[39]

Overall, explicit concern with human health and well-being was not prominent in government discourse on environmental policy around the time of the creation of the provincial Department of Environment. Perhaps the closest thing would be a somewhat general reference to "quality of life" in the 1971 Strom administration throne speech: "The quality of life depends substantially on the availability of a wide variety of natural resources . . . the land itself for agricultural and recreational purposes, the water, the air we breathe."[40]

The dominant focus on the capitalist economy — and the pride of place of extractive industries within the economy — continued under the Lougheed administration. After winning the 1971 provincial election, the PCs brought in a "sweeping array of environmental research programs, standards and approvals procedures, and a pollution control judiciary."[41] This included the potentially noteworthy Environment Conservation Authority, an "independent watchdog for the environment" that reportedly, upon its establishment in the early 1970s, was the first of its kind within or outside of Alberta.[42] However, and perhaps predictably in hindsight, the administration's early caution about the environment shifted to an orientation focused on quickly developing the oil industry, which led to environmental matters being marginalized.[43]

Significant harmful environmental impacts of oil sands development were apparent by the mid-1970s and had worsened by the 1980s.[44] In addition, the global energy crises of the 1970s caused by political unrest in the Middle East, and the subsequent introduction of Canada's National Energy Program under Pierre Trudeau's Liberals in the 1980s, which was marketed as aiming to stabilize and promote self-sufficiency of oil supplies but was experienced as highly unfair to Alberta because of its impact on provincial oil surpluses, strongly and negatively influenced federal-provincial relations.[45] This federal-provincial animosity, which continues today, is the context in which attention shifted to climate change.

1990s–2019: Climate Change and Health Equity in Alberta

This section is based on references to "climate change" in the *Alberta Hansard*, and especially — in line with the broad definition of public health embraced by this volume — comments and statements that also mobilized concepts of health, conceptualized broadly to include well-being and equity.[46] Pertinent comments were summarized thematically, situated within the main elements of the debate, and presented using illustrative quotations. The bills, along with the individual politicians who engaged in the debates and are referenced below, are summarized in Table 8.3a and Table 8.3b.

TABLE 8.3A: List of bills referenced in our analysis of climate change, health, and equity in Alberta legislative debates, 1990s–2019 (chronological). Note: PC = Progressive Conservative; NDP = New Democratic Party; UCP = United Conservative Party.

Year (Governing party)	Bill
1991 (PC)	Bill 209: *Air Quality Act* (did not pass)
2002 (PC)	Bill 32: *Climate Change and Emissions Management Act* (did not pass)
2003 (PC)	Bill 37: *Climate Change and Emissions Management Act* (passed)
2007 (PC)	Bill 3: *Climate Change and Emissions Management Amendment Act* (passed)
2008 (PC)	Bill 8: *Climate Change and Emissions Management Amendment Act* (passed)
2016 (NDP)	Bill 20: *Climate Leadership Implementation Act* (passed)
2019 (UCP)	Bill 1: *Act to Repeal the Carbon Tax* (passed)

TABLE 8.3B: List of individuals referenced in our analysis of climate change, health, and equity in Alberta legislative debates, 1990s–2019 (alphabetical by last name).

Name	Party Affiliation and Constituency (during time period referenced)
Wayne Anderson	Wildrose, MLA for Highwood
Laurie Blakeman	Liberal, MLA for Edmonton-Centre
William Bonko	Liberal, MLA for Edmonton-Decore
David Broda	PC, MLA for Redwater
Debby Carlson	Liberal, MLA for Edmonton-Ellerslie
Greg Clark	Alberta Party, MLA for Calgary-Elbow
Scott Cyr	Wildrose, MLA for Bonnyville-Cold Lake
Richard Gotfried	PC, MLA for Calgary-Fish Creek
Ernest Isley	PC, MLA for Bonnyville
Brian Jean	Wildrose, MLA for Fort McMurray-Conklin
Arthur Johnson	PC, MLA for Calgary-Hays
Ralph Klein	PC, Premier and MLA for Calgary-Elbow
Gary Mar	PC, Health Minister and MLA for Calgary Nose Creek
Brian Mason	NDP, MLA for Edmonton-Highlands
Don MacIntyre	Wildrose, MLA for Innisfail-Sylvan Lake
Grant Mitchell	Liberal, MLA for Edmonton-Meadowlark
Jason Nixon	Wildrose, MLA for Rimbey-Rocky Mountain House-Sundre
Rachel Notley	NDP, Premier and MLA for Edmonton-Strathcona

Name	Party Affiliation and Constituency (during time period referenced)
Ronald Orr	Wildrose, MLA for Lacombe-Ponoka
Raj Pannu	NDP, MLA for Edmonton-Strathcona
Shannon Phillips	NDP, Environment Minister and MLA for Lethbridge-West
Angela Pitt	Wildrose, MLA for Airdrie
Robert Renner	PC, MLA for Medicine Hat
Dave Rodney	PC, MLA for Calgary-Lougheed
Ed Stelmach	PC, Premier and MLA for Vegreville-Viking
David Swann	Public health physician and Medical Officer of Health in Southern Alberta; later MLA for Calgary-Mountain View and Leader of the Alberta Liberal Party
Kevin Taft	Liberal, MLA for Edmonton-Riverview
Bob Turner	NDP, MLA for Edmonton-Whitemud
Glenn van Dijken	Wildrose, MLA for Barrhead-Morinville-Westlock

Following infrequent reference to "climate change" in the *Hansard* during the 1970s and 1980s (indeed, there were fewer than ten references to "climate change" in the *Alberta Hansard* between 1970 and 1989), references started to increase in the 1990s coinciding with national and international milestones noted above. There was indication that some members of government were not taking climate change seriously. For example, during question period in a 1990 sitting, the PC Minister of Agriculture, Ernest Isley, described driving in from his constituency of Bonnyville in cold weather when the temperature was "minus 45, and my constituents were saying, 'Hey, we'd like to see some evidence of this global warming.'"[47]

In general, references to health in relation to climate change in the 1990s were inconsequential and infrequent.[48] Perhaps the most prominent example was private member Bill 209, the Air Quality Act, introduced by Grant Mitchell (Liberal, MLA for Edmonton-Meadowlark) in 1991.[49] One of the two objectives of the bill was "to ensure that the air in Alberta is of excellent quality and presents no hazard to human health;" indeed, in making a case for the bill Mr. Mitchell itemized health consequences of gases being emitted into the atmosphere: "Alberta has the highest rate of death due to asthma in Canada today . . . because there is a direct relationship between the nature of the air we breathe, what's in it — the pollutants, the irritants, the toxic gases that are in it — and the propensity for people to get asthma and to die from asthma attacks."[50] Accordingly, Bill 209 called for a much more significant leadership role by the health minister in establishing strong air quality standards to protect human health.[51]

Bill 209 timed out prior to second reading, with one point of PC opposition being that the bill was redundant with initiatives already in place, and was therefore unnecessary.[52] Regarding the alleged "initiatives already in place," environmental historian Longley describes the 1990s as a period when the governing PCs created a perception that they were appropriately managing environmental issues while in fact they were expediting industrial development. This problematic "symbolic policy discourse," as Longley calls it,[53] persisted in climate change debates in the new millennium, of which we consider two prominent examples: the Climate Change and Emissions Management Act of the first decade of the twenty-first century and the Climate Leadership Implementation Act of 2016.

2000s: Climate Change and Emissions Management Act

The Climate Change and Emissions Management Act deliberations unfolded under the PC governments of Ralph Klein (1992–2006), a period that was immensely problematic for the public's health as described in Chapter 4, and then Ed Stelmach (2006–2011). Premier Klein's intention to introduce a bill dealing with environmental concerns was conveyed in his government's throne speech of 26 February 2002, with reference to health and well-being: "The health of Alberta's unmatched natural environment is also critical to the province's overall health and to individual health and well-being. In 2002 the government will further encourage practices that prevent pollution and other environmental problems."[54] Before getting into the deliberations on Bill 32, the Climate Change and Emissions Management Act (2002), that followed, two significant events of late 2002 must be pointed out. First, the federal Liberal government, which had signed the international Kyoto accord in 1997, was in the process of ratifying it; the Klein government vehemently opposed the accord. Second, and pertinent to our focus on the intersection of environmental policy and public health, in October 2002 Dr. David Swann, public health physician and medical officer of health in southern Alberta, was fired for speaking out in favour of the accord (see also Chapter 13).[55]

BILL 32: CLIMATE CHANGE AND EMISSIONS MANAGEMENT ACT, 2002

Key elements of Bill 32 included gas emission intensity targets, an emission trading system, mandatory reporting, and the establishment of a Climate Change and Emissions Management Fund.[56] Consistent with his vitriol toward the Kyoto deliberations, Klein, when introducing the bill at second reading, spent several minutes criticizing the federal government before getting into the bill's substance. This was not lost on opposition members such as Debby Carlson (Liberal), who characterized Bill 32 as "a bill that's targeted at setting up a constitutional battle with the federal government [while] minimizing any kind of contribution Alberta would have."[57] In this context, it is perhaps not surprising that the concept of fairness or equity primarily arose in comments describing initiatives such as Kyoto as economically unfair to Alberta, as argued by David Broda (PC): "The protocol is not a fair or equally binding agreement. Even though Canada puts out only 2 percent of the world's greenhouse gas emissions, the economic risk to Canada would be four times that of the European Union and 10 times that of Japan."[58]

Consistent with Longley's notion of symbolic policy discourse noted above, opposition members saw Bill 32 as disingenuous and ineffective. They took particular issue with the emission targets, which focused on reducing emission *intensity* as opposed to absolute reductions. Raj Pannu (NDP) argued that "the most flawed aspect of Bill 32 is . . . that emissions will be reduced relative to GDP. . . . In other words, the faster our economy grows, the more emissions will be allowed to go up." Referencing an analysis by the Pembina Institute, a national think-tank focused on clean energy, Pannu argued that under the emission intensity approach, greenhouse gas emissions could be expected to increase by over 80 percent compared to 1990.[59]

In terms of reference to health and well-being during the Bill 32 deliberations, one interesting example comes from an exchange between Kevin Taft (Liberal) and PC Minister of Health and Wellness, Gary Mar, during question period on 20 November 2002. Referencing deaths from West Nile Virus in Ontario due to mosquitoes spreading north into Canada as a result of climate change, Taft queried whether the government had attempted to measure the health impact of climate change on Albertans. Mar responded: "I think that the Minister of Environment is well on this particular file, Mr. Speaker. We do co-ordinate with work that is being done out of his department. Our focus has really been on things that are much more closely associated with issues related to health care . . . ensuring, for example, that people get the highest level of cardiac care in this province."[60] This response conveys a problematic separation between health problems caused by climate change on the one hand, and the purview of the Ministry of Health, that is, health care, on the other.

Another illustration of such a disconnect came from Premier Klein himself. In describing his government's intention to introduce Bill 32, he described it as legislation that

> not only serves to reduce greenhouse gases and address the issue of climate change but will ensure that the economy is sustained. . . .

You know, jobs mean a lot to people, Mr. Speaker, a *healthy lifestyle* where people can grow up in a family secure in the knowledge that the breadwinner of that family will have secure employment is just as important as the issue of climate change.[61] (emphasis added)

Here, Klein frames action on climate change as a competing policy priority to other actions that promote health — which he framed narrowly as achieving a healthy lifestyle — such as actions to sustain the neoliberal capitalist economy. This framing, which obscures the interconnected social, economic, and political determinants of health, occurred repeatedly in climate change deliberations and we return to it later in the chapter. Bill 32 passed second reading but did not progress at that time.[62] Meanwhile, the federal Liberal government, under Jean Chretien, ratified the Kyoto accord on 17 December 2002.[63]

BILL 37: CLIMATE CHANGE AND EMISSIONS MANAGEMENT ACT, 2003

In April 2003, the governing PCs once again introduced the Climate Change and Emissions Management Act; this time as Bill 37. Bill 37 was largely similar to Bill 32, which raised the ire of some opposition members who felt that it ignored important interim events such as the federal ratification of the Kyoto protocol and served only as "fed-bashing."[64]

One reference to health and well-being was made by Laurie Blakeman (Liberal; see also Chapter 12) while commenting on the bill's lack of attention to motor vehicle driving as a cause of emissions. She remarked, "Let's look at helping the individual to drive their car less and use public transportation more or, heck, walk. We've had a $3 million ad campaign come out of the Department of Health and Wellness about how people should be healthier and should walk more. Do we make it more attractive for people to walk around, especially in the urban areas? No."[65] Mobilizing a broader version of health and well-being than seen to date in the climate change deliberations, Blakeman noted the policy incoherence between different areas of government, where the activities of the Department of Health and Wellness, which promoted walking, were undermined by the failure of Bill 37 to consider and try to reduce emissions from driving, despite the potential for synergy between public health and emissions reduction efforts; for example, more walking and wider public transit use could contribute to fewer emissions and improved health. Despite considerable opposition, Bill 37 passed quickly in November 2002.[66]

BILLS 3 AND 8: CLIMATE CHANGE AND EMISSIONS MANAGEMENT AMENDMENT ACTS, 2007 AND 2008

During the window between Bill 37 and Bill 3, an amendment to the Climate Change and Emissions Management Act that was introduced in 2007, public health physician David Swann entered politics. Fuelled by his experience with the Kyoto accord, he was elected to the Alberta legislature in November 2004 as a Liberal and served as Critic for the Environment for the opposition from 2004 to 2009, during which time he also won the Liberal leadership.

When introducing Bill 3 in March 2007, PC Environment Minister Robert Renner described it as "ground-breaking legislation" that would establish "Canada's first legislated greenhouse gas emission targets for large industrial emitters."[67] Once again, however, and in another illustration of Longley's notion of symbolic policy discourse, opposition members criticized the disingenuous nature of the bill and its anticipated lack of effectiveness, characterizing it as "lip service."[68] There were a few references to health and well-being during the Bill 3 deliberations,[69] including, not surprisingly, from Swann (Liberal), who argued that " we are paying millions every day now as a result of inaction on climate change.... We are also paying the health costs which industry is imposing on all of us as a result of the decline in air quality and the impacts on human health."[70] In addition, Arthur Johnson (PC) commented: "Albertans value their economic prosperity; however, it should not impede their quality of life."[71] Johnson's comment is worth noting because it conveys recognition — unusual among PC members — that quality of life, although a broad concept, is not synonymous with economic prosperity. Ultimately, despite several attempted amendments and impassioned pleas from opposition members,[72] Bill 3 passed, thus placing Alberta first in Canada for "legislated greenhouse gas emission reduction targets;" although as noted above this title is highly misleading.[73]

Bill 8, the final element of the Climate Change and Emissions Management Amendment Act, passed in October 2008, creating the infrastructure to administer the Climate Change and Emissions Management Fund established as part of Bill 37. Opposition members expressed resigned support, again lamenting the bill's inadequacy in terms of having any impact on emission reductions.[74]

Climate Leadership Implementation Act

Following the historically significant election of the NDP government of Rachel Notley in 2015, Bill 20, the Climate Leadership Implementation Act was introduced, deliberated, and passed after a marathon session during May and June of 2016.[75]

Bill 20 included three key components: the Climate Leadership Act, which implemented a carbon levy; the creation of a new agency called Energy Efficiency Alberta; and amendments to existing legislation to align with the government's overall Climate Leadership Plan.[76] The amendments permitted carbon revenue funds to be used for a broader array of activities than previously, including to support initiatives to reduce greenhouse gas emissions and to provide rebates to consumers, businesses, and communities. Introducing the flagship legislation, Premier Notley signalled the significant change from previous governments when she said, "we are proud that we are taking steps to finally establish Alberta not only as a participant but as a world leader on environmentally responsible energy development."[77]

The Bill 20 deliberations were aggressive and focused most prominently on the carbon levy. Opposition members were patronizing and dismissive in their comments. Two examples of such remarks are:

> It's the shrill finger pointing and the chicken clucking and all the rest that discredit your entire message.[78]

> The Member [Notley] . . . has once again demonstrated a profound lack of understanding of the business world.[79]

Opposition members attacked the governing NDP as ideological and anti-Albertan.[80] Comments invoked a caricatured version of "Albertans" as hard-working — in a "pioneer" sense — heterosexual, car-driving families, as illustrated by this comment from Ronald Orr (Wildrose), referencing the added fuel costs from the carbon levy:

> honestly, how many Albertan families do you know that have only one car? Most people have two cars. The wife has a car. The husband has a car. In many cases kids have their own cars. The average family house in Alberta has a two-car garage. I wonder why. . . . Well, it's because the typical family in Alberta actually has two cars.[81]

Within this context of Bill 20, our two concepts of interest — health and equity — were present in ways that are informative for advancing a broad vision of public health focused on upstream determinants of population well-being and health equity.

HEALTH AND WELL-BEING

To some extent, health was embedded in Bill 20. The bill itself did not mention health, nor did it provide new levers for the public health sector to engage with climate change.[82] However, during the deliberations, health implications were noted. For example, during first reading, Shannon Phillips (NDP), Minister of Environment and Parks, identified that the Climate Leadership Plan would "diversify our economy, create new jobs, improve the health of Albertans, and erase any doubt about our environmental record."[83] Other members likewise acknowledged anticipated health benefits with respect to reducing particulate damage from coal plants and new infectious diseases caused by a warming climate.[84]

In contrast, and similar to the Taft/Mar exchange of 2002 noted earlier, several opposition members framed investment in climate change and investment in health— which was interpreted in a downstream manner and conflated with health care — as competing policy priorities. One pernicious line of argument was that investment in action on climate change would harm health care by imposing additional costs on that sector or by diverting money away from it. For example, Scott Cyr (Wildrose) argued that "the NDP love to talk about how . . . they would never hurt health care. . . . Well, that's really interesting because the last time I checked, ambulances use diesel, and this [carbon levy] raises the costs on all fuels."[85] Likewise, Don MacIntyre (Wildrose) argued that "the good people of Innisfail-Sylvan Lake are a little bit concerned that this government can put $3.4 billion earmarked toward a box named Other, but they can't seem to find a nickel for an urgently needed urgent care facility in Sylvan Lake."[86] Cyr was taking issue with the "economy-wide" nature of the carbon levy, which meant that no sector, including health care, was exempt, while MacIntyre opposed the amendment that would permit broader use of carbon levy revenue, which he connected with the NDP's failure to invest in health care facilities in his constituency.

Other opposition members took a different tack, misleadingly drawing attention to potential negative consequences for health that could ensue from implementation of the carbon levy. Ronald Orr (Wildrose), for example, opposed the levy on the basis that it would impact families' abilities to heat their homes, which in turn would negatively impact their health:

> the World Health Organization has done a number of significant studies . . . on the health impacts of low indoor temperatures. . . . It relates to acute respiratory diseases, that are among the leading causes of death in Europe. . . . We're taxing [families'] natural gas, which is the essential service by which they're to heat their home, and now we're going to be pushing them to turn their thermostats down to the point where we may be actually causing health impacts.[87]

Likewise, Dave Rodney (PC) spoke about possible consequences of the carbon levy for social and emotional dimensions of health: "I don't know if it's because of my previous portfolio in wellness or as chair of the Alcohol and Drug Abuse Commission, but people [knowing about the impending carbon levy] are telling me: 'You know what? I've turned to a little self-medication. I'm in a lot of trouble,' and/or 'My spouse and I are disagreeing to the point where there's domestic abuse.'"[88] Comments from Orr and, especially, Rodney illustrate a pernicious invocation of the social determinants of health, where the levy was framed as creating health-damaging financial precarity for families. This sets the stage for our second concept of interest — equity.

EQUITY AND VULNERABILITY

A prominent point of opposition to the carbon levy was the assertion that it would unfairly burden Alberta families and that this was intensified in the context of an economic recession.[89] These comments frequently and misleadingly drew attention to "vulnerable" Albertans, as noted for example by Scott Cyr (Wildrose) during second reading of Bill 20 when he said, " how can you not see . . . how it's going to affect our most vulnerable? Are we going to see seniors on the streets? Are we going to see children and single mothers put on the streets because . . . the unintended consequences of this carbon tax could really impede Albertans' way of life?"[90]

Such comments were coupled with those focusing on the burden on charities. One example came from Glenn van Dijken's (Wildrose) comments focusing on the fact that charities were not exempt from the levy:

> Charitable organizations play a critical role in our society. . . . They support the basic needs of our most vulnerable and are currently swamped trying to attend to the needs of the thousands of Albertans that have lost their jobs in the last year and need some extra help. . . . How can this government justify increasing the costs to charities when our province needs them now more than ever before?[91]

Notable, with respect to the purposes of this chapter, is van Dijken's assertion of the "critical" role of charities — versus robust public sector initiatives by government — vis-à-vis Albertans' well-being. Comments of this nature intensified during deliberations over a proposed amendment to Bill 20 to designate the charitable sector as eligible for a carbon rebate. Indicative of the depth of commitment to charity as a viable solution to social and economic problems, Angela Pitt (Wildrose) introduced the amendment as something that would have broad support when she argued that "all sides of the House can support [this amendment] . . . to show our commitment to the most vulnerable people in Alberta. . . . This is an opportunity for this House to show these hard-working individuals that we support them, that we've got their backs."[92]

These comments from conservatives who did not support climate change legislation invoke social and economic factors affecting Albertans' well-being. However, and problematically, they do so in a way that frames economic disadvantage and its solutions as private matters. In contrast to a social justice orientation, where inclusive public institutions are key factors in supporting and empowering citizens, conservative comments align with a market justice orientation, which views charity as a viable way to address economic well-being among those who cannot achieve it through the market (see also Chapter 12).[93] For these reasons, these comments are significant from the point of view of an overall objective of this volume: to illustrate and strengthen a broad vision of public health.

BILL 20: THIRD READING

The deliberations continued through a marathon session on 6 June 2016, during which over twenty amendments to Bill 20 were put forth by various members of non-governing parties and lost. In addition to points of opposition noted above, a significant one that transcended the opposition parties concerned a lack of detail and accountability that would result in the bill being ineffective. For example, Alberta Party member Greg Clark argued that "there are no details in this bill . . . there are some very significant gaps. . . . We're essentially in many ways being asked to sign a blank cheque here, and I'm very uncomfortable with that."[94] David Swann (Liberal) had raised this concern throughout the debate.[95] Ultimately, and significantly, Swann, a public health leader who had entered politics because of his commitment to the issue of climate change, did not support the bill on this basis. Although this must be interpreted within the dynamics of politics, we close with excerpts from his eloquent commentary:

> I really, really want to support this bill. This is, to me, a sea change that has been so important in my political life.
>
> There is no single item in this bill that's particularly egregious . . . but the amalgamation of a number of weak points in the bill leaves the bill open to becoming as ineffective as the previous PC attempts at a carbon intensity tax [which] had the predictable outcome of no change.
>
> [T]his is a new government. They're trying to do the right thing. I don't know about the next government, though.
>
> It's with a heavy heart that I must say that I cannot support the bill at this time.[96]

With the majority NDP government, Bill 20 passed third reading on 7 June 2016, with a vote of 42 to 29. Three years later, the act was predictably repealed by the United Conservative Party government of Jason Kenney in their flagship legislation, Bill 1 of 2019.[97]

Conclusions

Anchored in the long-standing public health function of *health protection*, this chapter explores the historical and contemporary connection between policy domains of environment and (public) health in Alberta. We acknowledge limitations to our focus and analysis. Because of our particular interest in how concepts are mobilized by provincial governments, a key decision-making level, we did not examine municipal government initiatives or community-led activities in the non-profit sector.[98] We also did not examine how recent environmental activities, including climate change, were understood or navigated from the perspective of local, regional, and provincial health services authorities in Alberta, including how changes such as regionalization impacted these issues.[99] In the context of intensifying concerns around the integrity of our ecosystems, all of these would be excellent topics for future research in the Alberta context.

With regards to our analysis here, we conclude with two main points. First, from the contemporary point of view of a broad, intersectoral version of public health and the challenges presented by isolated government departments,[100] it is interesting and potentially informative to consider that up until 1971, there was a built-in administrative connection between policy domains of environment, such as pollution, and health in Alberta when the provincial Department of Public Health was responsible for preventing and controlling air pollution. Not surprisingly, health was an explicit concern in those policies. The Department of Environment, created in 1971, marked a separation of the two policy domains, which weakened or at least changed the relationship between environment and health on an administrative level. The creation of the Department of Environment was one part of a general historical trend of a growing number of increasingly specialized government entities. However, that does not mean that it is insignificant; as historian Frits Pannekoek notes, "some may well think that the changing organization of various units into ministries really is not relevant, but these nuanced structures have had a profound impact on Alberta."[101] Indeed, as also discussed in Chapter 12, from the perspective of a broad vision of public health, these nuanced structures would appear to represent an informative focus for further historical analysis with a critical, socio-political orientation.

The 1971 creation of the provincial Department of Environment signalled increased attention to environmental concerns, which is a positive development in terms of public sector leadership for important problems. However, in the context of ideologically driven intensification of colonial extractive industries and capitalist economic growth, it is perhaps not surprising that environmental policy in Alberta quickly became weak, and worse, disingenuous. Against that backdrop, our analysis of climate change deliberations in the early 2000s showed our second concluding point, which is that some members framed climate change and health as competing policy priorities; for example, arguing that investment in climate change meant less money for health care. Embedded in this argument was a conflation of health and health care, as well as a dissociation of health from its upstream or root causes including social equity and healthy environments. These dynamics continue to hinder a broad vision of public health today. In terms of equity, the conviction and persistence with which many members mobilized a downstream and depoliticized version of equity as being about a static population of inherently "vulnerable" Albertans who depend on charities for well-being is significant in terms of its striking contrast with how equity is conceptualized from a social determinants of health point of view. Illustrative of the latter, a 2008 report from the World Health Organization's Commission on Social Determinants of Health argued that health inequity is "not in any sense a 'natural' phenomenon but [is] the result of a toxic combination of poor social policies and programmes, unfair economic arrangements, and bad politics."[102] We recognize of course that comments in government deliberations constitute "playing politics." However, the points of view advanced in those comments would not be mobilized if they did not powerfully resonate with at least some Albertans.

These observations illuminate challenges for public health. They illustrate and shed light on the weak link made by individuals, and governments, between health issues and climate change noted in the *Lancet* quotation that opened this chapter. Strengthening the link will require, among other things, efforts to revisit entrenched forms of public health practice that perpetuate a downstream orientation and conflate public health with health care.[103] Research in climate change and public health practice indicates that activities are dominated by *adaptation*, or adjusting to or moderating harms from climate change, such as climate change and health vulnerability assessments.[104] While it is certainly important to plan for adaptation responses, these efforts must be accompanied by *mitigation*, that is, political engagement to demand reduction of emissions, including by ceasing extractive activities altogether. The upstream orientation of mitigation is, in theory at least, strongly aligned with public health's stated focus on efforts to address upstream determinants of health and well-being in populations.[105] Guidance may be found in the Canadian Public Health Association's work on the ecological determinants of health, led by Dr. Trevor Hancock, who was the first leader of the Green Party of Canada, which explicitly rejects the view that humans are inherently more important than other life forms and outlines an agenda for action that demands "explicit re-engagement with the values of public health" including to challenge prevailing economic norms that promote economic growth as the solution to social problems.[106]

To return to the core public health function of health protection with which we began this chapter, climate change illustrates that there is an important opportunity for public health communities to push the boundaries of health protection to embrace new and emergent priorities and ways of thinking, while continuing to respect and strengthen the long-standing focus on water, air, and food safety. Substantive engagement around ecosystem integrity, social equity, and the political economic systems that obstruct them would enable the field of public health to remain relevant and to meet its core mandate around the public's health. For a field that is lamented as weakening, that is an important opportunity for public health indeed.[107]

NOTES

1   "Health and Climate Change: Making the Link Matter [Editorial]," *The Lancet* 394, no. 10211 (2019): 1780.

2   Public Health Agency of Canada, *Core Competencies for Public Health in Canada: Release 1.0* (Public Health Agency of Canada, 2008), https://www.phac-aspc.gc.ca/php-psp/ccph-cesp/pdfs/cc-manual-eng090407.pdf.

3   Annette Prüss-Üstün et al., *Preventing Disease through Healthy Environments: A Global Assessment of the Burden of Disease from Environmental Risks* (Geneva: World Health Organization, 2016); Chris G. Buse et al., "Public Health Guide to Field Developments Linking Ecosystems, Environments and Health in the Anthropocene," *Journal of Epidemiology and Community Health* 72 (2018).

4   National Collaborating Centre for Determinants of Health, *Determining Health: Decent Work Issue Brief* (Antigonish, NS: NCCDH, St. Francis Xavier University, 2022).

5   Trevor Hancock et al., "There is Much More to Public Health than COVID-19," *Healthy Debate*, 15 June 2020, https://healthydebate.ca/opinions/more-to-public-health-than-covid; Jean-Louis Denis et al., "On Redesigning Québec Public Health: Lessons Learned from the Pandemic," *Canadian Journal of Public Health* 111, Issue 6 (2020).

6   Chris G. Buse and Rebecca Patrick, "Climate Change Glossary for Public Health Practice: From Vulnerability to Climate Justice," *Journal of Epidemiology and Community Health* 74, no. 10 (2020): 867–871; Intergovernmental Panel on Climate Change, "Glossary of terms," in *Managing the Risks of Extreme Events and Disasters to Advance Climate Change Adaptation. A Special Report of Working Groups I and II of the Intergovernmental Panel on Climate Change (IPCC)*, eds. C.B. Field, et al. (Cambridge, UK, and New York: Cambridge University Press, 2012).

7   Buse and Patrick, "Climate Change Glossary;" Intergovernmental Panel on Climate Change, "Summary for Policymakers," in *Global Warming of 1.5°C. An IPCC Special Report on the Impacts of Global Warming of 1.5°C Above Pre-industrial Levels and Related Global Greenhouse Gas Emission Pathways, in the Context of Strengthening the Global Response to the Threat of Climate Change, Sustainable Development, and Efforts to Eradicate Poverty*, eds. V. Masson-Delmotte et al. (Cambridge, UK and New York: Cambridge University Press NY, 2018).

8   Buse and Patrick, "Climate Change Glossary;" Chris G. Buse, "Health Equity, Population Health, and Climate Change Adaptation in Ontario, Canada," *Health Tomorrow* 3 (2015).

9   Richard Horton, et al., "From Public to Planetary Health: A Manifesto," *The Lancet* 383, no. 9920 (2014): 847.

10   Chris G. Buse et al., "Public Health Guide to Field Developments Linking Ecosystems, Environments and Health in the Anthropocene," *Journal of Epidemiology and Community Health* 72 (2018).

11   Buse and Patrick, "Climate Change Glossary."

12   Compiled from various sources; for example: BBC (https://www.bbc.com/news/science-environment-15874560); History.com (https://www.history.com/topics/natural-disasters-and-environment/history-of-climate-change); The Canadian Encyclopedia (https://www.thecanadianencyclopedia.ca/en/article/environmental-and-conservation-movements). See also *Act for the Regulation of Fishing and Protection of Fisheries*, Statutes of Canada, 1868, c. LX; Kevin Mcnamee and Maxwell W. Finkelstein, "National Parks of Canada," in *The Canadian Encyclopedia. Historica Canada*, article published 12 January 2012, https://www.thecanadianencyclopedia.ca/en/article/national-parks-of-canada; *An Act respecting National Parks*, S.C. 1930, c. 33; Trevor Hancock, Donald W. Spady, and Colin L. Soskolne, *Global Change and Public Health: Addressing The Ecological Determinants Of Health*, Canadian Public Health Association Discussion Paper (Ottawa: Canadian Public Health Association, 2015), https://www.cpha.ca/sites/default/files/assets/policy/edh-discussion_e.pdf; Larry Booth and Frank Quinn, "Twenty-five Years of the Canada Water Act," *Canadian Water Resources Journal* 20, no. 2 (1995); 65–90; *Canada Water Act*, S.C. 1969–1970, c. 52; *Arctic Waters Pollution Prevention Act*, S.C. 1969–1970, c. 47; R. J. Powell and L. M. Wharton, "Development of the Canadian Clean Air Act," *Journal of the Air Pollution Control Association* 32, no. 1 (1982): 62–65; "Acts," Acts & Regulations, Environment and Climate Change Canada, accessed 27 October 2020, https://ec.gc.ca/default.asp?lang=En&n=E826924C-1&wbdisable=true; "Conventional Oil," Alberta Culture and Tourism, accessed 27 October 2020, http://history.alberta.ca/energyheritage/oil/default.aspx; "History of the IPCC," The Intergovernmental Panel on Climate Change, accessed 27 October 2020, https://www.ipcc.ch/about/history/; "Overview of Canadian Environmental Protection Act," Government of Canada, modified 2 August 2017, https://www.canada.ca/en/environment-climate-change/services/canadian-environmental-protection-act-registry/general-information/overview.html; "About Montreal Protocol," United Nations Environment Programme, accessed 27 October 2020, https://www.unenvironment.org/ozonaction/who-we-are/about-montreal-protocol; "United Nations Framework Convention on Climate Change," Government of Canada, modified 27 April 2020, https://www.canada.ca/en/environment-climate-change/corporate/international-affairs/partnerships-organizations/united-nations-framework-climate-change.html; *Canadian Environmental Assessment Act*, S.C. 1992, c. 37; "What is the Kyoto Protocol?," United Nations Framework Convention on Climate Change, accessed 27 October 2020, https://unfccc.int/kyoto_protocol; "Leaders' Statement on a North American Climate, Clean Energy, and Environment Partnership," Justin Trudeau, Prime Minister of Canada, published 26 June 2016, https://pm.gc.ca/en/news/statements/2016/06/29/leaders-statement-north-american-climate-clean-energy-and-environment

13   Canadian Public Health Association, *Position Statement: Climate Change and Human Health* (October 2019), https://www.cpha.ca/climate-change-and-human-health; "Causes of Climate Change," Environment and Natural Resources, Government of Canada, modified 28 March 2019, https://www.canada.ca/en/environment-climate-change/services/climate-change/causes.html; Dimitry Anastakis, "Industrialization in Canada," in *The Canadian Encyclopedia*, last edited 14 March 2017, https://thecanadianencyclopedia.ca/en/article/industrialization.

14   Monte Hummel, "Environmental Movement in Canada," in *The Canadian Encyclopedia*, last edited 16 October 2020, https://www.thecanadianencyclopedia.ca/en/article/environmental-and-conservation-movements.

15   Hummel, "Environmental Movement in Canada."

16   Hummel, "Environmental Movement in Canada."

17   "Our history," Canadian Parks and Wilderness Society (CPAWS), accessed 28 October 2020, https://cpaws.org/about/about-cpaws/history/; "Our Story," Greenpeace Canada, accessed 28 October 2020, https://www.greenpeace.org/canada/en/about-us/history-successes/; "About Us," World Wildlife Fund Canada, accessed 28 October 2020, https://wwf.ca/about-us/.

18   R.J. Powell and L.M. Wharton. "Development of the Canadian Clean Air Act," *Journal of the Air Pollution Control Association* 32, no. 1 (1982). These federal initiatives formed part of the complex, inter-jurisdictional governance arrangements under which environmental policy in the provinces and territories operates today. Jeff Surtees, "Who's The Boss? — Jurisdiction Over the Environment in Canada," *LawNow*, 2 March 2017, https://www.lawnow.org/whos-the-boss-jurisdiction-over-the-environment-in-canada/; Penny Becklumb, *Federal and Provincial Jurisdiction to Regulate Environmental Issues*, Background Paper (Publication No. 2013-86-E) (Ottawa: Library of Parliament, 24 September 2013, revised 29 October 2019), https://lop.parl.ca/staticfiles/PublicWebsite/Home/ResearchPublications/BackgroundPapers/PDF/2013-86-e.pdf.

19 "History," Green Party of Canada, accessed 28 October 2020, https://www.greenparty.ca/en/party/ history. The first leader of the Green Party of Canada was public health physician Trevor Hancock. See Trevor Hancock, *Ecological Economics and Public Health: An Interview with Dr. Trevor Hancock* (Montréal, QC: National Collaborating Centre for Healthy Public Policy, 2019), http://www.ncchpp. ca/867/Publications.ccnpps?id_article=2052.

20 Vanessa Hrvatin, "A Brief History of Canada's Climate Change Agreements," *Canadian Geographic*, 30 May 2016, https://www.canadiangeographic.ca/article/brief-history-canadas-climate-change-agreements; Government of Canada, *Pan-Canadian Framework on Clean Growth and Climate Change: Canada's Plan to Address Climate Change and Grow the Economy* (2016), http://publications.gc.ca/ collections/collection_2017/eccc/En4-294-2016-eng.pdf; "Mandate," Impact Assessment Agency of Canada, accessed 28 October 2020, https://www.canada.ca/en/impact-assessment-agency/corporate/ mandate.html. The Impact Assessment Act of 2019, which created the agency, replaced the weak 2012 version of the Canadian Environmental Assessment Act passed under the Harper government.

21 Shannon Daub et al., "Episodes in the New Climate Denialism," in *Regime of Obstruction: How Corporate Power Blocks Energy Democracy*, ed. William K. Carroll (Edmonton, AU Press, 2021).

22 In light of our contemporary focus on climate change, we focus on air pollution as the logical historical precursor because climate change reflects human activities that release CO2 and other greenhouse gases into the atmosphere; it is therefore related to, but is not the same as, air pollution. We consider the historical overlap between this version of environment and health and well-being.

23 For example, Alberta's inaugural (1907) Public Health Act included the following clause among the items for which the provincial board of health could create regulations for the purpose of preventing the spread of communicable diseases: "The prevention of the pollution, defilement, discolouration or fouling of all lakes, streams, pools, springs and waters, and to ensure their sanitary condition and to regulate the cutting and storage of ice." *Act respecting Public Health*, S.P.A., 1907, c. 12. A 1919 amendment further added "prevention of the pollution of soil" to the list (*Act to Amend the Public Health Act*, S.P.A. 1919, c. 46).

24 *Act to Amend the Public Health Act*, S.P.A. 1944, c. 53.

25 For examples of water pollution measures, see R.H. Ferguson, "Water Pollution Control in Alberta," in H.L. Hogge et al., "Air and Water Pollution Control Programs in Alberta: A Panel Presentation," *Canadian Journal of Public Health* 57, no. 2 (February 1966); PAA (PAA), *An Administrative History of the Government of Alberta, 1905–2005* (Edmonton: PAA, 2006).

26 *Act to Amend the Public Health Act*, S.P.A. 1955, c. 30. See also "Alberta will spend more on highways," *Edmonton Journal*, 18 February 1955, Alberta Legislature Library, Scrapbook Hansard, https:// librarysearch.assembly.ab.ca/client/en_CA/search/asset/161992/0; "New legislation would curb disputes over mineral rights", *Edmonton Journal*, 24 February 1955, Alberta Legislature Library, Scrapbook Hansard, https://librarysearch.assembly.ab.ca/client/en_CA/search/asset/162014/0

27 *Public Health Act*, R.S.A. 1970, c. 294.

28 *An Act respecting Public Health*, R.S.A. 1955, c. 255.

29 Alberta Department of Public Health, *Annual Report 1961* (Edmonton: Printed by L.S. Wall, Printer to the Queen's Most Excellent Majesty, 1963), 2; Powell and Wharton, "Development of the Canadian Clean Air Act;" Hogge et al., "Air and Water Pollution Control Programs in Alberta."

30 S.L. Dobko, "Air Pollution in Alberta," in H.L. Hogge et al., "Air and Water Pollution Control Programs in Alberta."

31 PAA, *An Administrative History*.

32 Specifically, the Department of Environment took over responsibility for: i) assessment of the pollution control facilities at all new or expanding industries or other activities; ii) measurement of the air quality in those areas of the province in industrial and urban centres where air contaminants are being released in significant amounts; iii) measurement of the rates of release of contaminants (stack surveys) at larger industries; iv) review of air quality and contaminant release rate information submitted by industries, as required in the Air Pollution Control Approvals; and v) Evaluation and follow-up on reports and complaints related to air quality. Alberta Department of Health and Social Development, *A Summary Report 1971* (Edmonton, 1972), 19.

33 PAA, *An Administrative History*.

34 Hereward Longley, "Conflicting Interests: Development Politics and the Environmental Regulation of the Alberta Oil Sands Industry, 1970-1980," *Environment and History* 27, no. 1 (1February 2021), https://doi.org/10.3197/096734019X15463432086919.

35 Longley, "Conflicting Interests."

36 *Public Health Act*, R.S.A. 1970.

37   An an example of citizen concern, Longley notes that three Edmonton-based environmental groups were formed in 1969 or 1970 and pressured government for environmental policy and legislation. Longley, "Conflicting interests;" STOP — Save Tomorrow Oppose Pollution fonds, PR1502. PAA, Edmonton, Alberta.

38   Alvin Finkel, *The Social Credit Phenomenon in Alberta* (Toronto: University of Toronto Press, 1989); Longley, "Conflicting Interests."

39   Finkel, *The Social Credit Phenomenon.*

40   Throne Speech, 11 February 1971 (Harry Strom, Social Credit administration). Jack Lucas and Jean-Philippe Gauvin, "Alberta Throne Speeches 1906–2017 (Comparative Agendas Project)," 2019, https://doi.org/10.5683/SP2/0WH5FH, Borealis, V1.

41   Longley, "Conflicting Interests."

42   Retrospective description of the Environment Conservation Authority: Alberta. Legislative Assembly of Alberta, 26 November 1990 (Bob Hawkesworth, NDP). All Alberta Hansard transcripts are available at https://www.assembly.ab.ca/assembly-business/transcripts/transcripts-by-type. The Environment Conservation Authority, which was created through *An Act respecting Environment Conservation,* S.A. 1970, c. 36, was responsible for reviewing and reporting on government policies and programs on matters pertaining to environmental conservation. Environment Council of Alberta records, GR0053.0001F. PAA, Edmonton, Alberta.

43   As an example of environmental matters being marginalized, in 1977 the Environment Conservation Authority was replaced by the Environment Council of Alberta, which was later described as "largely impotent" in its ability to advocate for the environment. Alberta. Legislative Assembly of Alberta, 26 November 1990 (Bob Hawkesworth, NDP).

44   As an example of increasingly harmful oil sands activity, Longley states that by 1976 the GCOS company's tailings pond leached over 1.5 million litres per day of toxic effluent into the Athabasca River. Longley, "Conflicting Interests."

45   "Conventional Oil," Alberta Culture and Tourism, accessed 29 October 2020, http://history.alberta.ca/energyheritage/oil/default.aspx.

46   In focusing our analysis in this way, and in the interest of coherence, we omit other concepts and dimensions that figured prominently in the climate change debate, many of which would constitute an interesting, informative analysis.

47   Alberta. Legislative Assembly of Alberta, 8 June 1990 (Ernest Isley, PC), to which Grant Mitchell (Lib) replied, "It's just appalling that a minister of this government would joke about something as critical as this." 1749.

48   Substantive reference, in the Hansard, to equity or fairness vis-à-vis climate change was absent during the 1990s.

49   Alberta. Legislative Assembly of Alberta, 18 March 1991, first reading; 23 May 1991, second reading (did not pass second reading).

50   Alberta. Legislative Assembly of Alberta, 23 May 1991 (Grant Mitchell, Lib).

51   Alberta. Legislative Assembly of Alberta, 23 May 1991 (Grant Mitchell, Lib).

52   Alberta. Legislative Assembly of Alberta, 23 May 1991 (Donald Tannas, PC).

53   Longley, "Conflicting Interests."

54   Throne Speech, 26 February 2002 (Ralph Klein, PC administration). Lucas and Gauvin, "Alberta Throne Speeches."

55   Brad Mackay, "Firing Public Health MD Over Pro-Kyoto Comments a No-no, Alberta Learns," *Canadian Medical Association Journal* 167, no. 10 (2002): 1156. See also multiple stories in the *Edmonton Journal,* 5 October 2002.

56   Bill 32: Climate Change and Emissions Management Act, 2002; Alberta. Legislative Assembly of Alberta, 19 November 2002, first reading; 26 November 2002, second reading.

57   Alberta. Legislative Assembly of Alberta, 26 November 2002 (Debby Carlson, Lib).

58   Alberta. Legislative Assembly of Alberta, 18 November 2003 (David Broda, PC).

59   Alberta. Legislative Assembly of Alberta, 26 November 2002 (Raj Pannu, NDP).

60   Alberta. Legislative Assembly of Alberta, 20 November 2002 (Kevin Taft, Lib, Gary Mar, PC).

61   Alberta. Legislative Assembly of Alberta, 19 November 2002 (Ralph Klein, PC).

62   Alberta. Legislative Assembly of Alberta, 26 November 2002.

63   Bill Doskoch, "Canada and the Kyoto Protocol – a Timeline," *CTVNews,* 5 December 2011, https://www.ctvnews.ca/canada-and-the-kyoto-protocol-a-timeline-1.732766.

64   Alberta. Legislative Assembly of Alberta, 18 November 2003 (Brian Mason, NDP).

65   Alberta. Legislative Assembly of Alberta, 18 November 2003 (Laurie Blakeman, Lib).

66   Alberta. Legislative Assembly of Alberta, 18 November 2003, second reading, committee of the whole; Alberta. Legislative Assembly of Alberta, 20 November 2003, third reading.

67   Alberta. Legislative Assembly of Alberta, 8 March 2007 (Robert Renner, PC).

68   Alberta. Legislative Assembly of Alberta, 20 March 2007, second reading, Bill 3 (William Bonko, Lib).

69   For example: Alberta. Legislative Assembly of Alberta, 10 April 2007 (Harry Chase, Lib; David Eggen, NDP).

70   Alberta. Legislative Assembly of Alberta, 20 March 2007, second reading, Bill 3 (David Swann, Lib).

71   Alberta. Legislative Assembly of Alberta, 8 March 2007 (Arthur Johnston, PC).

72   Proposed changes included several amendments designed to make the bill stronger, including those put forth by David Eggen, NDP (Alberta. Legislative Assembly of Alberta, 5 April 2007, amendment A1; 10 April 2007, amendments A2, A3, and A4) and by Swann (Alberta. Legislative Assembly of Alberta, 11 April 2007; 12 April 2007). See also "Environmental Sustainability", Alberta. Legislative Assembly of Alberta, 12 April 2007.

73   Bill 3: Alberta. Legislative Assembly of Alberta, 3 April 2007, second reading; 11 April 2007, Committee of the Whole; 17 April 2007, third reading.

74   Alberta. Legislative Assembly of Alberta, 16 October 2008 (Laurie Blakeman, Lib); 20 October 2008 (David Swann, Lib).

75   Alberta. Legislative Assembly of Alberta, 24 May 2016, first reading; 1 June 2016, second reading; 7 June 2016, third reading.

76   Alberta. Legislative Assembly of Alberta, 25 May 2016, Bill 20 – second reading (Phillips, NDP).

77   Alberta. Legislative Assembly of Alberta, 24 May 2016 (Rachel Notley, NDP).

78   Alberta. Legislative Assembly of Alberta, 2 June 2016 (Ronald Orr, Wildrose).

79   Alberta. Legislative Assembly of Alberta, 6 June 2016 (Don Macintyre, Wildrose).

80   Alberta. Legislative Assembly of Alberta, 25 May 2016 (Richard Gotfried, PC).

81   Alberta. Legislative Assembly of Alberta, 31 May 2016, (Ronald Orr, Wildrose).

82   Bill 20: Climate Leadership Implementation Act. The Legislative Assembly of Alberta, Second Session, 29th Legislature, https://docs.assembly.ab.ca/LADDAR_files/docs/bills/bill/legislature_29/session_2/20160308_bill-020.pdf.

83   Alberta. Legislative Assembly of Alberta, 24 May 2016 (Shannon Phillips, NDP).

84   Examples include comments from Bob Turner, NDP and David Swann, Lib: Alberta. Legislative Assembly of Alberta, 25 May 2016 and 31 May 2016.

85   Alberta. Legislative Assembly of Alberta, 25 May 2016 (Scott Cyr, Wildrose).

86   Alberta. Legislative Assembly of Alberta, 1 June 2016 (Don Macintyre, Wildrose).

87   Alberta. Legislative Assembly of Alberta, 31 May 2016 (Ronald Orr, Wildrose).

88   Alberta. Legislative Assembly of Alberta, 7 June 2016 (Dave Rodney, PC).

89   Alberta. Legislative Assembly of Alberta, 24 May 2016 (Brian Jean, Wild Rose).

90   Alberta. Legislative Assembly of Alberta, 25 May 2016 (Scott Cyr, Wildrose).

91   Alberta. Legislative Assembly of Alberta, 25 May 2016 (Glenn van Dijken, Wildrose).

92   Alberta. Legislative Assembly of Alberta, 6 June 2016 (Angela Pitt, Wildrose).

93   Ahmed M. Bayoumi and Adrian Guta, "Values and Social Epidemiologic Research," in Rethinking Social Epidemiology: Towards a Science of Change, eds. Patricia O'Campo and James R. Dunn (Dordrecht: Springer, 2012).

94   Alberta. Legislative Assembly of Alberta, 31 May 2016 (Greg Clark, Alberta Party).

95   Alberta. Legislative Assembly of Alberta, 31 May 2016 (David Swann, Lib).

96   Alberta. Legislative Assembly of Alberta, 7 June 2016 (David Swann, Lib).

97   Bill 1: An Act to Repeal the Carbon Tax (Kenney). Alberta. Legislative Assembly of Alberta.

98   Examples of climate change related in municipal government and non-profit sectors include: "Calgary's Climate Change Program," The City of Calgary, accessed 28 October 2020, https://www.calgary.ca/uep/esm/energy-savings/climate-change.html; "Climate Action," Town of Canmore, accessed 28 October 2020, https://canmore.ca/residents/stewardship-of-the-environment/climate-change-adaptation-plan; "Home," Alberta Environmental Network, accessed 28 October 2020, https://www.aenweb.ca.

99   For example, "Environmental Public Health," Alberta Health Services, accessed 28 October 2020, https://www.albertahealthservices.ca/eph/eph.aspx. For an example of an analysis of public health adaptation to climate change from the perspective of practitioners, see Chris G. Buse et al., "'We're All

Brave Pioneers on this Road:' A Bourdieusian Analysis of Field Creation for Public Health Adaptation to Climate Change in Ontario, Canada," *Critical Public Health*, 31, Issue 1 (2021).

100 For example, see Evelyne de Leeuw and Dorothee Peters, "Nine Questions to Guide Development and Implementation of Health in All Policies," *Health Promotion International* 30, no. 4 (2014).

101 PAA, *An Administrative History of the Government of Alberta*.

102 Commission on Social Determinants of Health, *Closing the Gap in a Generation: Health Equity through Action on the Social Determinants of Health*, Final Report of the Commission on Social Determinants of Health (Geneva: World Health Organization, 2008), https://www.who.int/social_determinants/ thecommission/finalreport/en/.

103 Buse, "Health Equity, Population Health;" Buse et al., "'We're All Brave Pioneers on this Road.'"

104 Stephanie E. Austin et al., "Public Health Adaptation to Climate Change in OECD Countries." *International Journal of Environmental Research and Public Health* 13, no. 9 (2016); Malcolm Araos et al. "Public Health Adaptation to Climate Change in Large Cities: A Global Baseline," *International Journal of Health Services* 46, no. 1 (2016). We were surprised to read in these publications that "in the public health context, adaptation is synonymous with prevention and may constitute policies (etc.) to avert the negative health impacts of climate change." This sounds like tertiary prevention at best. Chris G. Buse, "Why Should Public Health Agencies Across Canada Conduct Climate Change and Health Vulnerability Assessments?" [commentary], *Canadian Journal of Public Health* 109, no. 5-6 (2018).

105 Adaptation strategies can in some cases directly conflict with mitigation. One example is the adaptation strategy of air conditioning to reduce heat-related illnesses when air conditioning also contributes to greenhouse gas emissions and climate change. Younger et al., "The Built Environment, Climate Change, and Health: Opportunities for Co-benefits;" Canadian Public Health Association (CPHA), *Public Health: A Conceptual Framework*, CPHA Working Paper, Second Edition (Ottawa: CPHA, 2017), https://www.cpha.ca/public-health-conceptual-framework; "Glossary," National Collaborating Centre for Determinants of Health, accessed 30 October 2020, https://nccdh.ca/index. php?/glossary/entry/upstream-downstream.

106 Trevor Hancock, Donald W. Spady, and Colin L. Soskolne, *Global Change and Public Health: Addressing the Ecological Determinants Of Health*, CPHA Discussion Paper (Ottawa: Canadian Public Health Association, 2015), https://www.cpha.ca/sites/default/files/assets/policy/edh-discussion_e.pdf. See also Margot W. Parkes et al., "Preparing for the Future of Public Health: Ecological Determinants of Health and the Call for an Eco-social Approach to Public Health Education," *Canadian Journal of Public Health* 111 (2020).

107 Louise Potvin, "Canadian Public Health under Siege" [editorial], *Canadian Journal of Public Health* 105, no. 6 (December 2014), doi:10.17269/cjph.105.4960; Ak'ingabe Guyon et al., "The Weakening of Public Health: A Threat to Population Health and Health Care System Sustainability," *Canadian Journal of Public Health* 108, no. 1 (2017).

9

Mobilizing Preventive Policy

Lindsay McLaren, Rogelio Velez Mendoza, and Donald W. M. Juzwishin

Introduction

Prevention, broadly defined as actions aimed at eliminating or reducing the occurrence and impact of illness, is a fundamental concept in public health.[1] Public health, with its emphasis on populations, equity, and addressing underlying determinants of health, is especially aligned with *primary prevention*, that is, actions to prevent the occurrence of illness or injury in the first place, by reducing or eliminating exposure to hazards or risks at the population level. Primary prevention includes what some call *primordial prevention*, which are efforts that are often in the domain of public policy and redress health-damaging environmental, economic, social, and cultural conditions.[2] However, as we illustrated in Chapter 2, there is indication of a downstream shift over time in the use of the term *prevention* in the Alberta context. The shift is increasingly toward attention to secondary prevention efforts to reduce risk among those with elevated risk, who may be identified via screening, and tertiary prevention efforts to slow disease progression, such as disease management occurring within health care settings.[3] This apparent shift, we argue, presents an important barrier to a broad vision of public health as embraced by this volume.

Case Examples

In this chapter, we build on the general analysis of *prevention* from Chapter 2 by considering three examples in more depth: tobacco control, community water fluoridation, and workers' health. Together, these examples illustrate the important tensions that can accompany efforts to prevent health problems at the population level.

Tobacco Control[4]

Tobacco control is widely described as a public health success story.[5] Whereas approximately half of Canadian adults smoked in 1965, the 2017 estimate was 15 percent (18.9 percent in Alberta).[6] These population-level reductions reflect several factors, including anti-smoking campaigns that mobilize scientific evidence on harms of tobacco use; regulatory actions, such as clean indoor air bylaws, restrictions on tobacco product advertising, and restrictions on tobacco sales; increased taxes on smoking products; and broader societal trends, which have collectively contributed to a context in which not smoking has become a dominant social norm.[7]

The social norm element speaks to an important counter-narrative on tobacco control from critical public health scholarship, which has identified that the "de-normalizing" nature of tobacco reduction interventions — for example leveraging social pressure to make smoking less desirable, acceptable, and accessible — has created a new set of ethical concerns.[8] Intersecting with a complex layering of the social determinants of health, de-normalization has contributed to an epidemiologic profile of tobacco use where overall prevalence is low, but distribution is highly and increasingly inequitable. For example, nationally in 2017, smoking prevalence was approximately 12 percent among households in the highest income quintile, versus 21.7 percent in the lowest quintile.[9] A broad vision of public health embraces critical perspectives as an important reminder of tensions that can accompany the dual public health goals of maximizing population-level impacts and redressing social inequities in health.[10]

Our focus here is tobacco-related legislation, including that which restricts smoking in public places, because it is recognized as a cornerstone of comprehensive tobacco control efforts.[11] In Alberta and elsewhere, the adoption of tobacco-related legislation reflects important contributions by local and provincial advocacy groups, thus illustrating the important role and contribution of activism in mobilizing a broad vision of public health. We are grateful to Les Hagen, executive director of Action on Smoking & Health, for his input to this section (see also Chapter 13).

MUNICIPAL LEGISLATION: EARLY SUCCESS IN EDMONTON

Smoking-related legislation[12] across Canada owes its origins to grassroots efforts by non-smokers in the early 1970s who spoke up for the right to breathe clean air.[13] Instrumental in the early Edmonton legislation was the Group Against Smokers' Pollution. Initially formed in 1971 in the United States,[14] chapters of the organization emerged across North America during the 1970s, including in Edmonton, Calgary, Medicine Hat, and Lethbridge.[15]

The Edmonton chapter of the Group Against Smokers' Pollution was formed in approximately 1975 and initially set its sights on provincial legislation.[16] In March 1977, Progressive Conservative MLA Eric Musgreave introduced private member's bill, Bill 221, An Act Respecting Smoking in Public Places, which the organization supported via a petition that Musgreave presented in the legislature on 21 April 1977.[17] Second reading of Bill 221 took place one week later, and the lengthy discussion included indications of both support for and opposition to restricting smoking in public places.[18] Points of opposition included concern about whether it was reasonable to "destroy a custom of smoking that has been built up over the centuries" just because it is "offensive to the senses."[19] The bill did not pass, and the Edmonton chapter of the Group Against Smokers' Pollution turned its attention to municipal government.

Based on frequent and prominent mentions in the print media, the Edmonton chapter of the Group Against Smokers' Pollution was active throughout the late 1970s and had a strong presence in local debate.[20] In their public messaging, the group maintained that their aim was not to eliminate smoking, but rather to protect the rights of non-smokers from second-hand smoke. This also served as a useful response to the frequent point of opposition that a municipal smoking bylaw would infringe on smokers' rights.[21] There were, however, indications that the group at times went too far for the likings of some. For example, in 1977, the Group Against Smokers' Pollution sold small, battery-powered fans that were intended to be used in instances where smokers insisted on smoking despite polite requests to stop, to blow smoke back in smokers' faces.[22] By 1980 the organization had stopped selling the fans as part of efforts to adopt a "less militant image."[23]

In May 1980, organization spokesperson Wally Gloeckler presented to Edmonton City Council's public affairs committee in support of a draft bylaw on smoking restrictions in public places.[24] In September of that year, after hearing presentations from the Group Against Smokers' Pollution and three other groups — the Alberta Restaurant and Food Services Association, Edmonton Northlands racetrack, and the Alcohol-Drug Education Association of Alberta — the committee recommended approval of the bylaw.[25] In January of 1981, although five aldermen voted against the legislation, Edmonton City Council passed a no-smoking bylaw (Bylaw 6177, as amended) that made it illegal to smoke in some public places.[26] Edmonton thus became one of the first cities in western Canada to pass a municipal smoking bylaw.[27]

Following the 1981 municipal legislation, the Edmonton chapter of the organization continued to meet throughout the early 1980s[28] and to speak up for tobacco control efforts.[29] In the context of growing public support for the existing restrictions, the group envisioned stronger regulations. A proposed amendment to the bylaw, which was supported by Edmonton's Medical Officer of Health, Dr. James Howell, passed at city council by a seven to four margin and went into effect on 9 April 1985.[30] The new bylaw required restaurants to set aside 35 percent of their seating for non-smokers (up from 15 percent); it also contained smoking restrictions in new settings, including city buses, the light rail transit system, and taxis, unless both driver and passengers agreed otherwise. Although the Edmonton chapter's president at the time, Dr. Roger Hodkinson, was pleased with the improvements, he expressed disappointment that the revised bylaw did not mandate a "stated preference rule" for restaurants where they must ask patrons whether they wish to sit in smoking or non-smoking areas, and that it did not require restaurants to place no-smoking signs directly on tables.[31] Nonetheless, not to be defeated by these perceived omissions, the Edmonton chapter of the Group Against Smokers' Pollution worked within the parameters of the revised bylaw, including filing complaints about restaurants that were not obeying the new bylaw, and serving as a resource for members of the public who wished to do the same.[32] These efforts contributed to Edmonton's smoking restrictions being further strengthened in the early 1990s.[33]

Like Edmonton, a Calgary chapter of the organization was also formed around 1975 and held several meetings throughout through 1977.[34] According to a February 1977 item in the *Calgary Herald*, the Calgary chapter persuaded the city's parks and recreation board to discourage smoking in public arenas, including stands, dressing rooms, and concourses, via announcements asking spectators not to smoke, and by arena staff asking violators to extinguish their cigarettes.[35] Beyond that modest change, however, the Calgary chapter's impact seemed limited, and they appear to have disbanded in early 1980.[36] Calgary eventually passed a municipal smoking bylaw in 1985, although it was felt by some to be overly lenient.[37] Nonetheless, a few years later — with significant support from Calgary pediatrician Dr. John Read — the city hosted the world's first smoke-free Olympics in 1988.[38] These milestones were achieved under Mayor Ralph Klein, who was himself a smoker.

SHIFT TO A PROVINCIAL FOCUS FOR TOBACCO REDUCTION

With municipal anti-smoking legislation established in Edmonton, advocacy groups shifted their focus back to the provincial context.[39] In the late 1980s, the Edmonton chapter of the Group Against Smokers' Pollution evolved into Action on Smoking & Health,[40] a non-profit organization that is still active today and embraces a broader tobacco control agenda including public awareness, advocacy, tobacco control programs and research, public policy development, community mobilization, and tobacco counter-marketing.

Action on Smoking & Health's shift to a provincial focus in the mid to late 1980s was prompted by circumstances occurring nationally. The federal Liberal government under Prime Minister Pierre Trudeau (1968–1979 and 1980–1984) had not been particularly supportive of tobacco reduction legislation; indeed, in an illustration of the politics of health, one journalist referred to the federal Liberal Party at that time as the Tobacco Party.[41] In contrast, the health minister of Brian Mulroney's Progressive Conservative government (1984–1993), Jake Epp, was reportedly a strong champion of tobacco reduction.[42] In June 1988, federal tobacco-related legislation was passed including the Non-Smokers Health Act, which regulated smoking in federal workplaces and on "common carriers," such as aircraft, ships, and trains, and the Tobacco Products Control Act, which prohibited advertising and promotion of tobacco products.[43] As Les Hagen notes, there was "tremendous national progress on tobacco control in the late 1980s."[44]

Coupled with this federal legislation was Action on Smoking & Health's recognition that, in the light of changes to funding arrangements for health care during the late 1970s and early 1980s,[45] provincial governments increasingly had a stake in tobacco reduction, because they were responsible for financing the costly medical consequences of tobacco-related morbidity. Against this backdrop, the Alberta Interagency Council on Smoking and Health was formed in approximately 1984, which included representatives from the Canadian Cancer Society, the Alberta Cancer Board, the Alberta Lung Association, the Alberta Medical Association, the Alberta Alcohol and Drug Abuse Commission, the Group Against Smokers' Pollution, and three boards of health.[46] Perhaps not surprisingly, there was friction within the council between the advocacy groups, such as the Group Against Smokers' Pollution, on the one hand and the health charities on the other, over which tobacco reduction efforts would be pursued. For example, in September 1985 the organization's president Dr. Roger Hodkinson criticized the Alberta Lung Association's Lungs Are for Life campaign because it emphasized an educational, rather than a political, strategy.[47]

A few days later, Dr. Hodkinson took aim at the council more broadly, asserting that the council was "sidestepping its mandate to combat tobacco use by shying away from aggressive action," which he attributed to organizations' fear of alienating potential donors.[48] In what Hagen describes as a "huge turning point" for the Group Against Smokers' Pollution, the group staged a demonstration outside the Jubilee Auditorium in Edmonton to protest the tobacco company du Maurier's sponsorship of arts and cultural events including local performances by the Alberta Ballet Company.[49] The "du Maurier Dance of Death," which was one of the first instances of tobacco industry sponsorships being publicly challenged, drew national media attention to the concerns of advocacy groups about the disproportionate attention and resources being devoted to public awareness and medical research (e.g., lung cancer research versus substantive efforts to prevent smoking).[50] In this, the Group Against Smokers' Pollution was supported by the broader public health community: at the 1985 Alberta Public Health Association annual meeting, noted scientist and environmental activist David Suzuki commented, "I do not damn well want to spend one cent" on lung cancer research until action is taken on smoking.[51]

Throughout the 1990s, Action on Smoking & Health established itself as a key player in tobacco reduction policy in Alberta and western Canada.[52] In the early 1990s, despite strong support from provincial Health Minister Nancy Betkowski (PC), the Tobacco Control Act, Bill 207, which would prohibit sales of tobacco products to youth, did not pass,[53] and the change in provincial leadership to Ralph Klein (PC) in 1992 meant going back to square one. During Klein's government, there was substantive discussion in the legislature around Bill 215, the Non-Smokers Health Act, which included restrictions on smoking in workplaces and public buildings, and Bill 208, the Prevention of Youth Tobacco Use Act; in both cases, time ran out before a vote could occur.[54] In 1995, Action on Smoking & Health and other organizations established the Alberta Tobacco Reduction Centre, which Hagen describes as "a formative step in the development of a more meaningful provincial strategy," and in 1998 the provincial government made a significant investment in the Alberta Tobacco Reduction Alliance, which was tasked with creating a provincial tobacco reduction strategy.[55]

These events set the stage for considerable progress on tobacco legislation in Alberta in the first decade of the twenty-first century, which occurred against the backdrop of the 2003 World Health Organization Framework Convention on Tobacco Control.[56] Significant for tobacco control in Alberta was Klein's 2000 appointment of Gary Mar as minister of health and wellness, who was supportive of tobacco control.[57] In 2002, the Klein government implemented a tax increase of $2.25 per pack of twenty-five cigarettes — the largest single tobacco tax increase in Canadian history[58] — and there was a reduction in the volume of cigarettes sold in Alberta the following year.[59] In the days following the tax increase, and reflecting many years of hard work by Action on Smoking & Health and other organizations, Mar announced the Alberta Tobacco Reduction Strategy, which was launched in 2002 with a $12 million annual budget.[60] Five years later, in 2007, the provincial government under Ed Stelmach approved Bill 45, the Smoke-free Places (Tobacco Reduction) Amendment Act. The act was described by Hagen as one of the strongest tobacco control laws in Canada and perhaps the world that represented a milestone in what Hagen calls "transforming Canada's Marlboro

Country." A newer emphasis, at the time of writing, was expansion of existing legislation to flavoured tobacco products.[61]

From the non-smokers rights movement of the 1970s to the broader contemporary tobacco control movement, efforts to prevent and reduce smoking in Alberta shed light on dynamics of primary and primordial prevention, including how they intersect with the socio-historical context of the province. In reflecting on this history, Hagen identifies health ministers who are — for whatever reason — strong champions of tobacco reduction, coupled with a strong coalition of health organizations, as key elements. He cautions, however, that with the continued affordability of tobacco products, limited funding for tobacco control efforts, the absence of a robust and continuous mass media campaign, and unimplemented legislation, significant challenges to population-level reductions in smoking remain.[62]

Community Water Fluoridation

A prominent feature of dental services in Alberta and across Canada is that they overwhelmingly fall into the private sector in terms of financing and delivery, with contemporary estimates of less than 5 percent of services financed publicly.[63] Reflecting a highly politicized history,[64] dental services are downstream in orientation (largely individualized and treatment-oriented) and there are significant and inequitable barriers to access.[65] In this context, it is important to consider primary prevention approaches for dental health. Here we consider community water fluoridation, which is the controlled adjustment of the fluoride content of a public drinking water supply for the purpose of preventing tooth decay in populations.[66] We provide provincial historical context as well as a more detailed narrative of events in the city of Calgary.

FLUORIDATION: THE PROVINCIAL AND NATIONAL CONTEXT

Archival sources suggest that Alberta's fluoride story started as early as the 1930s, within a broader context of international research that linked a mottled tooth appearance (i.e., dental fluorosis) to resistance to tooth decay, both of which in turn could be traced to naturally-occurring fluorine in drinking water.[67] Local reports of mottled enamel in southern Alberta prompted members of the University of Alberta, the provincial Department of Public Health, and the provincial laboratory, to conduct a large survey to study the issue.[68] The survey involved collecting data via questionnaires sent to dentists and doctors, dental exams of all new students entering the University of Alberta in the fall of 1936, and water samples. Results, published in 1937, confirmed an association between high fluorine in the water and the prevalence of mottled enamel; they also identified two areas where mild mottled enamel was endemic: one around Lethbridge and the other around Red Deer.[69]

The early observations signalled by mottled teeth led to the idea of community water fluoridation (fluoridation) as a deliberate population-level intervention to prevent tooth decay. Fluoridation was first implemented in Canada in 1945 in the context of a research trial in Ontario.[70] The "Brantford experiment," which has been well-described elsewhere, had Alberta connections.[71] In 1942, a committee on dental research was struck within Canada's National Research Council, and Dr. H.R. MacLean (dentist) represented Alberta on that committee.[72] According to Alberta dentists G. Clarke and C.R. Castaldi, MacLean introduced the subject of fluoridation at the inaugural meeting, which prompted discussion about the need for controlled studies, including in Alberta, to determine whether fluoride added to water would have the same benefits for teeth as naturally-occurring fluoride.[73] Unfortunately, national funding for an Alberta study was not forthcoming, and leadership of the initial trials in Ontario fell to the Department of National Health and Welfare and the University of Toronto's Faculty of Dentistry. Still, an Alberta connection existed. The Brantford experiment was led by Dr. Harry Knowlton Brown in his capacity as Chief of the Dental Division at the Department of National Health and Welfare. Dr. Brown was a graduate (1930) of the School of Dentistry at the University of Alberta who, prior to enlisting to serve in WWII, practised dentistry in the municipality of Barrhead, Alberta, and represented Barrhead in the provincial legislature for the governing Social Credit party.[74]

Early results from the Brantford experiment and other early trials in North America released in the mid-1950s, showed reductions in rates of children's tooth decay following initiation of fluoridation.[75] However, reaction to the new idea of fluoridation was decidedly mixed. On the one hand, many Alberta communities wanted to implement the practice and took action to do so. On the other hand, some individuals and groups expressed opposition, including concerns about safety, possible influence on health professionals of large corporations, and opposition to fluoridation's violation of individual liberties.[76] Calgary's medical officer of health from 1933 to 1960, Dr. William H. Hill, who also served as the inaugural (1943–1944) president of the Alberta Public Health Association, was a vocal opponent of fluoridation, which was and is somewhat of an unusual stance in the public health professional community.[77]

For Alberta communities that wished to implement fluoridation in the 1950s, a practical challenge was quickly encountered: there was no legislation in place to permit or regulate the measure (see Table 9.1 for a summary of key provincial fluoridation legislation in Alberta).[78] In 1952, the provincial Public Health Act was amended to permit fluoridation. Specifically, a new clause allowed for "the purification and treatment of public water supplies and the addition of a chemical thereto" as part of the Provincial Board of Health's regulatory authority to take action to prevent and mitigate disease.[79] As explained by Deputy Minister of Health Dr. W.W. Cross, prior to the amendment, the provincial board's authority concerning the addition of chemicals to water was limited to purification purposes; the amendment extended the authority to include prevention of disease, such as tooth decay. Around the same time, the provincial lieutenant governor commissioned the Research Council of Alberta to prepare a report on "all aspects of fluoridation," which upon its release was described as "unconditionally endors[ing] fluoridation as a means of preventing tooth decay in children."[80] Nonetheless, there was hesitation in advancing supportive legislation, which reflected the controversial nature of the issue,[81] including the fact that the governing Social Credit party was not supportive of the measure.[82]

TABLE 9.1: Timeline of changes to Alberta provincial legislation concerning fluoridation

Year	Change to provincial legislation concerning fluoridation
1952	The *Public Health Act* was amended to permit chemicals to be added to water systems for reasons other than purification and treatment of water, thus permitting the addition of fluoride to prevent tooth decay.
1956	The *Public Health Act* was amended to include a new section outlining the parameters and processes for Alberta municipalities to implement fluoridation. Municipalities could pass or rescind a fluoridation bylaw, but they were first required to hold a plebiscite and secure the approval of 2/3 of voters. If such approval was not achieved, municipalities had to wait at least one year before holding another plebiscite.
1958	The *Public Health Act* was amended to extend the waiting period following a failed plebiscite from one year to two. This made it consistent with the two-year waiting period required between passing a fluoridation bylaw and rescinding it.
1964	The *Public Health Act* was amended to clarify the fluoridation parameters and processes in circumstances where a communal water supply provided water to only a portion of a municipality (in that case, which mainly pertained to rural areas, the municipality still had authority to pass a bylaw in the manner described above).
1966	The *Public Health Act* was amended to 1) accept a simple majority (instead of a two-thirds majority) in a municipal plebiscite to pass or rescind a fluoridation bylaw, and 2) grant authority to the Minister of Health to provide fluoride in tablet or other form, for distribution without charge to residents, to any health unit or city health department.
1984	A new *Public Health Act* was passed, which was described as a "total rewrite." Provision for fluoridation bylaws was transferred from the *Public Health Act* to the *Municipal Government Act*. The requirement for a plebiscite remained.
1994	A new *Municipal Government Act* was introduced, which removed the requirement for municipalities to hold a plebiscite to pass or rescind community water fluoridation (and other municipal decisions).
	The *Regional Health Authorities Act* was passed, which gave Regional Health Authority Boards the responsibility "to promote and protect the health of the population in the health region, and work towards the prevention of disease and injury". In Calgary, in the absence of a plebiscite requirement, this new legislation was used to argue that the Health Authority, and not municipal council, should have a primary role in fluoridation decisions.

In March 1956, another amendment to the provincial Public Health Act was passed; the amendment assigned fluoridation decision-making to municipalities and outlined the processes for municipalities to implement fluoridation. Specifically, the new section of the act stated that, to pass or rescind a fluoridation bylaw, municipalities must hold a plebiscite and secure the approval of two-thirds of voters.[83] On the issue of delegation to municipalities, Cross expressed that he did not believe that the provincial government had the right to prevent fluoridation if a municipality wanted to implement it.[84] Under this new legislation, several Alberta municipalities held fluoridation plebiscites in the late 1950s; some, such as Fairview, Grande Prairie, Innisfail, and Red Deer, secured the necessary two-thirds majority to introduce fluoride into the water.[85] However, there were several municipalities for which the two-thirds majority was a barrier. Edmonton, for example, held four fluoridation plebiscites between 1957 and 1964, all of which fell short of the required 66.6 percent (support was approximately 65 percent in 1957, 56 percent in 1959, 62 percent in 1961, and 65 percent in 1964).[86] A survey of medical officers of health in 1960 revealed that of fourteen plebiscites held in Alberta, only six had achieved the required two-thirds majority approval.[87]

Perhaps unsurprisingly, some viewed the two-thirds majority requirement as unnecessarily restrictive and lobbied to reduce it to a simple majority.[88] Legislation permitting a simple majority ultimately passed eight years later in 1966, but in a different form than anticipated by some. Specifically, in what was described in the *Hansard* as a "surprise move," when the simple majority amendment was put forth, Health Minister J. Donovan Ross added an amendment for a provincially-funded initiative to provide oral fluoride in the form of tablets or drops to health units or departments, which could be distributed to individuals for free with a prescription from a family doctor or dentist.[89] Calgary was one municipality that embraced that option, introducing the Calgary Health Services Fluoride Supplement Program in 1966; the program remained in place until 1989. Meanwhile, in Edmonton, a fifth fluoridation plebiscite was held and easily passed under the new simply majority legislation. Edmonton implemented fluoridation in 1967.

Provincial fluoridation legislation in Alberta remained largely the same through the 1970s and early 1980s under the Progressive Conservative government of Peter Lougheed. However, with the "complete rewrite" of the provincial Public Health Act in 1984 (see Chapter 4), fluoridation legislation was moved from the Public Health Act to the Municipal Government Act.[90] From the point of view of articulating the contours of public health, the transfer of fluoridation and other legislation out of the Public Health Act is important to note. In the case of fluoridation, the change meant that, although a municipal bylaw to pass or rescind fluoridation still required a plebiscite, there were now two avenues to a plebiscite: city council could initiate one (as had been the case under the Public Health Act); or a plebiscite could be prompted by a petition from at least 10 percent of electors.[91] The implications of this change, as well as subsequent legislation changes in the mid-1990s, are illustrated by a consideration of fluoridation in Calgary.

THE EBB AND FLOW OF COMMUNITY WATER FLUORIDATION IN CALGARY

Calgary held fluoridation plebiscites in 1957, 1961, 1966, and 1971; however, unlike some other municipalities such as Edmonton, support hovered much closer to, or below, 50 percent each time.[92]

After a lengthy hiatus, efforts led by Calgary Health Services, the contemporary version of the city's health services authority, ramped up significantly in preparation for a 1989 plebiscite. Some members of public health communities felt optimistic that changes to Calgary's population, which had become larger and more diverse since the previous vote in 1971, would lead to a different outcome.[93] As described by historian Catherine Carstairs, one impetus for the 1989 plebiscite was a grade 11 science class at Diefenbaker High School, which, after completing a unit on dental health, wrote to then-Mayor Ralph Klein to encourage a reconsideration of fluoridation.[94] By way of encouraging city council, Calgary Health Services pointed out the very limited reach of the fluoride supplement program that was currently in place; for example, in 1988 the fluoride supplement program was estimated to reach only 16 percent of Calgary children.[95] After making it clear that they were not endorsing fluoridation but rather giving residents of Calgary an opportunity to vote on the issue, Calgary City Council supported a plebiscite, at which Calgarians voted in favour of fluoridation (53 percent). Bylaw 37M89 was passed in November 1989, and the fluoride supplement program was stopped. However, due in part to a failed attempt by individuals and groups who were opposed to fluoridation to prompt a discontinuation plebiscite with a petition, which was newly permissible in 1984 when fluoridation legislation was moved to the Municipal Government Act, implementation was delayed until 1991.[96]

Efforts by fluoridation opposition groups in Calgary continued unabated following fluoridation's 1991 implementation, and those efforts came to some degree of fruition in the late 1990s in the form of another plebiscite, this time on the question of whether to continue fluoridation. As described by authors Catherine Pryce and Jackie Smorang, in 1997, the City of Calgary sponsored a review of fluoridation, prompted by a group of citizens who had expressed concern about fluoridation's safety based on new scientific evidence that included research concerning osteosarcoma, a type of bone cancer, in rats exposed to sodium fluoride in drinking water.[97] An expert panel was assembled; the members reviewed and assessed scientific information published since the 1989 plebiscite.[98] Four of the five panel members agreed that there was not sufficient new evidence to suggest a change in fluoridation policy, and the Calgary Regional Health Authority, the health services authority that had been created in the interim in 1994, reaffirmed its support for fluoridation, although at a reduced concentration of 0.7 parts per million (down from 1.0 ppm), as recommended by the panel. Although the City had indicated that they would follow the recommendation of the health authority, the presence of a dissenting perspective on the panel introduced some doubt and the City opted to hold a plebiscite anyway (which, under contemporary legislation they were no longer obligated to do, see below) in conjunction with the 1998 municipal election. Despite a considerably shortened lead up time, the Calgary Regional Health Authority once again mobilized a large campaign in support of fluoridation, with Medical Officer of Health, Dr. Brent Friesen, serving as an effective spokesperson (see Figure 9.1). Although anti-fluoridation efforts were present, Calgarians voted 55 percent in favour of continuing fluoridation.[99]

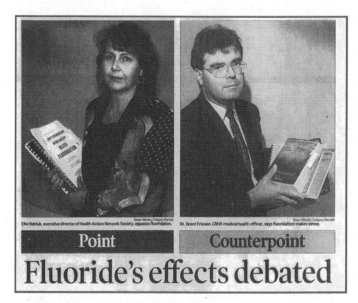

Fig. 9.1: Medical Officer of Health, Brent Friesen, served as a key spokesperson on fluoridation for the Calgary Regional Health Authority during the 1990s. He appeared frequently in print news media around this time, facing significant attacks from those (including journalists) who opposed fluoridation. He was sometimes pitted against a vocal opponent of fluoridation, Elke Babiuk. Source: "Fluoride's Effects Debated," *Calgary Herald*, 4 October 1998, 40.

Between Calgary's 1989 and 1998 fluoridation plebiscites, a new Municipal Government Act was introduced in 1994, which reflected the contemporary trend of devolution of authority and was much less prescriptive than previous iterations of the act in terms of what municipal governments could and could not do.[100] Significantly, from the point of view of fluoridation, the new act removed the requirement for municipalities to hold a plebiscite when passing or rescinding a fluoridation bylaw. In 1997–1998, as discussed above, the Calgary Regional Health Authority, working within this new legislation, tried to support city council in making a decision to retain fluoridation without holding a plebiscite. In doing so, they drew on another new piece of legislation, the Regional Health Authorities Act of 1994, to argue that the health authority's recommendations should hold considerable weight in council's decision, specifically referencing the mandate of health authorities "to promote and protect the health of the population in the health region, and to work toward the prevention of disease and injury."[101] Nonetheless, council opted to hold a plebiscite.

In 2011, however, and speaking to the importance of context, these legislative circumstances permitted Calgary's City Council to explicitly reject a plebiscite and vote on their own to discontinue fluoridation in the city. Several sources analyze this more recent situation more thoroughly than we can do here.[102] With Calgary's 2011 decision to cease fluoridation, the percentage of Albertans receiving fluoridated water went from 74.6 percent, one of the highest in the country, to approximately 43 percent,[103] to the detriment of dental health.

Workers' Health

Our final example of prevention in Alberta's history concerns workers' health. This topic is informative because it permits bringing together traditional public health concerns in the domain of occupational health and safety, such as hazardous exposures and ergonomic considerations on the one hand, with broader social, economic, and political factors on the other. These broader factors include the dominant industries and sectors of work; how workers are treated, including wages, working conditions, and job security; the intersecting structures that shape work, including capitalism, colonialism, and racism; and forms of worker resistance, such as organized labour activism.[104]

These intersecting political economic factors have immense importance for the public's health including health equity.[105] Yet, they are largely absent from mainstream public health discourse.[106] For instance, in the Public Health Agency of Canada's 2008 core competencies document, references to "work" focus on decontextualized "workplace hazards" and "harmony" in the workplace; practical examples of meeting the competencies include evaluating a smoke-free workplace program and forwarding workplace health information from a health promotion listserv to members of a workplace health committee.[107] Consideration of the broader political economic context is absent.

Accordingly, this section considers workers' health in Alberta's history through the lens of political economy. Briefly, this is a framework for understanding health and other phenomena in terms of the way our economy is organized, the politics surrounding it, and the resulting distribution of power that is highly unequal. Within capitalism, especially the neoliberal variety, the political economy of health foregrounds the imperative of private profit accumulation, the practices mobilized in support of this goal, including government deregulation of extractive and polluting industries and privatization and austerity around public services, and the significant and highly inequitable consequences of those practices for health and well-being.[108] Work figures prominently in this framework, in that the profit imperative construes workers as expendable and incents exploitation of workers through cost-saving measures such as poor wages, unsafe working conditions, and precarious work, all of which strongly and negatively affect health. Moreover, low-paid, poor-quality jobs are not distributed randomly but reflect the intersection of capitalism with racism, colonialism, ableism, sexism, gender binarism, and other categories and are disproportionately held by members of communities that dominant society has already marginalized. Under capitalism, most of us are workers, and employment and working conditions are well-established social determinants of health and health equity,[109] making an analysis of workers' health from a political economy perspective highly relevant to a broad version of public health.

In writing this section we have benefited greatly from emeritus professor of history, Alvin Finkel, and colleagues' 2012 volume, *Working People in Alberta: A History*, to which the reader is directed for a richer and more in-depth analysis.[110] We bring our lens of population well-being and health equity and its structural causes — that is, a broad version of public health — to that important work.

CAPITALISM, THREATS TO WORKER WELL-BEING, AND WORKER RESISTANCE – HISTORICAL EXAMPLES IN ALBERTA

The intersecting goals of early capitalism and colonialism — to settle the land and extract its natural resources — led to a massive influx of immigrants to western Canada between the late 1800s and early 1900s. Researcher and historian Jim Selby describes four job environments in that context that shed light on the political economy of workers' health: railway construction projects, where tens of thousands of mostly un/semi-skilled workers were situated in temporary camps; single-industry coal towns, where workers tended to put down roots; workers in sectors and industries demanded by growing urban centres, such as construction; and waged farmworkers.[111] Within a capitalist context, these jobs shared in common elements that are highly detrimental to health such as poor pay, job precarity and unpredictability, and demanding and/or dangerous working conditions. Coal miners, for instance, faced extremely dangerous conditions, which were made worse by cost-saving measures by mine operators. For example, miners had to buy their own explosives, and low wages put safer but more expensive explosives out of reach for the average miner. Indeed, weekly accidents were "a fact of life" in early Alberta mines.[112] The intersection of capitalism and racism resulted in some workers, such as Chinese railroad labourers, being seen as especially expendable and thus holding the most dangerous and deadly jobs.

Health inequities are rooted in power inequities; thus, workers' efforts to rebalance power via collective mobilization is highly pertinent to a broad version of public health. Collective resistance by workers during this early period sheds light on tactics they used and challenges they encountered — both practical and political. Railway workers, for example, faced challenges to organizing due to the isolation of work camps and the work's migratory nature, which made it difficult to bring large numbers of workers together. Organizing by urban construction workers, who were very poorly paid, often took the form of endorsing political candidates who were union members, to varying degrees of success. Labour organizing was prominent among coal miners, but many acts of resistance serve to illustrate the power of private companies in shaping the state, to the detriment of workers. For example, an important 1906 strike by workers at the Galt mine in Lethbridge, then owned by Toronto financiers, faced invasive and intensive opposition by the North-West Mounted Police, and led to federal tabling of the Industrial Disputes Investigation Act. The act undermined unions and empowered employers by, for example, mandating compulsory arbitration and permitting — by not prohibiting — employer tactics such as arbitrary wage changes and firing or intimidating union supporters.[113]

Depressed economic conditions at the onset of WWI prompted many young men to sign up for paid military service. For those who stayed behind, the 1915 lifting of the recession that had begun four years earlier meant that jobs and wages generally increased, although they did not keep up with wartime inflation; income, and the forces shaping it, is a well-established social determinant of health.[114] Moreover, poor working conditions persisted and were amplified due to so-called enemy aliens (a term used to describe citizens of states legally at war with the British Empire and who resided in Canada during the war), whom employers viewed as a vulnerable, non-complaining, and thus exploitable, workforce. Amid these challenges, relatively lower unemployment during the war empowered important labour activism, with some successes. For example, pushed by job action, in 1917 the provincial Liberal government passed the Factory Act which established a minimum wage of $1.50/day. Although a victory in important respects, the act largely excluded women, both because women were less likely to work in factories, but also through a loophole where women were hired as apprentices — who did not qualify for minimum wage — and then fired once the apprentice period had ended.[115] This is one of many examples of employment conditions, and the political economic factors that shape them, intersecting with social identities (in this case, gender) to worsen inequities in health and well-being.

When the war ended and many veterans returned home, a new set of political economic challenges materialized. Labour shortages became labour surpluses, and the government's failure to support workers in the context of post-war unemployment was evident. A social determinants of health perspective reminds us that a robust public sector, with universal and generous forms of public services and supports, is a foundation for population well-being and health equity.[116] Many workers were furthermore angry that the war, which had been framed as democratic, in fact served to benefit the economic elite. This anger and disillusionment underpinned short-lived efforts to build worker solidarity across sectors and industries including — perhaps most famously — the Winnipeg General Strike of 1919, which was accompanied by sympathy strikes throughout Alberta. Although the Winnipeg strike faced violent suppression by the Royal North-West Mounted Police and ended with no demands met, the Alberta sympathy strikes are, importantly, thought to have helped to bridge some divisions within the labour movement.[117]

Worker resistance continued even during the Great Depression when up to 15 percent of workers in Calgary, Edmonton, and Lethbridge were receiving municipal relief. Under a residualist welfare model, which views government assistance as a last resort, only the most destitute qualified for relief and thus the number of workers suffering was almost certainly much higher. A Hunger March on 20 December 1932, where farmers, farm labourers, and town workers converged on Edmonton, where they faced a formidable Royal Canadian Mounted Police (RCMP) presence, signified both the persistence of workers in dire circumstances and the aggressive pushback by authorities. These tensions set the stage for the 1933 founding of the Co-Operative Commonwealth Federation, the forerunner of the New Democratic Party, and of the Social Credit party which won a majority government in the 1935 provincial election. Although the Social Credit government under Premier William Aberhart initially passed some pro-labour legislation, such as the 1937 bill that granted legal status to collective bargaining, they soon backtracked and by the 1940s had embraced a firm stance favouring capitalists over workers, to the detriment of workers including their health and well-being.[118]

The post-WWII context of expanded social programs and relative union security — both important contributors to the public's health — interacted in Alberta with the growing prominence of the oil industry, which began to overtake other extractive industries including farming and coal mining. Although oil brought considerable economic prosperity to the province, that prosperity was poorly distributed and workers' ability to benefit from it was limited by the Social Credit government's alliance with the fossil-capitalist nexus and its anti-union sentiment. These dynamics once again speak to inequities in power and resources, which are the root causes of health inequities. Under Premier Ernest Manning, in 1947 the Social Credits amended the Alberta Labour Act and made it more difficult for workers to form unions by stipulating that union certification required the support of a majority of workers, versus a majority of voters. Further changes in 1948 stipulated that organizing could only take place at work during work hours, with employer consent; penalties for violations were described by legal history scholar James Muir as "draconian." (see Chapter 2 for other examples of how Ernest Manning was detrimental to a broad vision of public health in Alberta).[119]

Although the 1960s and 1970s brought a groundswell of activism around issues of social and environmental justice, capitalist imperatives meant that government anti-union sentiment and poor working conditions persisted. In 1962, for example, the Manning government-backed Board of Industrial Relations exempted "inexperienced employees" from the minimum wage, which in practice excluded large numbers of workers in certain industries, such as the garment industry which was dominated by racialized women. In male-dominated jobs, such as construction, companies continued to organize work in such a way that so-called accidents were inevitable. The word "accident" implies that an event was unavoidable, but in fact these are largely preventable had better working conditions been in place; the failure to do so is a political decision. While women were less likely than men to die at work, they likewise faced poor wages and working conditions: one example came from a worker at a private daycare in Calgary in the 1970s who was solely responsible for ten infants with no ability to take breaks. Although increasing unionization of women workers accompanied their increasing labour force participation, this was not without tension in the context of the traditionally male-dominated macho union culture where an influx of any workers, including women, was seen as a threat to union goals of good work for good pay.[120]

The Social Credit government was defeated in 1971. In the context of a period of strong labour influence, the Progressive Conservative government under Peter Lougheed (1971–1975) passed, in 1973, a potentially promising Occupational Health and Safety Act, following the lead of other provinces. The act contained some important items with respect to health and well-being, such as granting workers the right to know about occupational health hazards and to refuse unsafe work. However, it was far from perfect, and it mainly benefited unionized workers who had mechanisms to demand that the items were implemented and enforced. Overall, and despite some initially promising and health-promoting labour-related initiatives, the Lougheed government was not very different from its predecessors in terms of anti-worker sentiment. For example, in response to indications of growing militancy among provincial workers, in 1977 the Lougheed government passed the Public Service Employee Relations Act, which aimed to curtail union power by banning strikes in favour of arbitration; removing issues such as work organization, promotion, training, and termination from the scope of arbitration; and extending the restrictive legislation to include teaching staff of universities and colleges, thus curtailing their union power as well. The Lougheed government remained committed to the Labour Act even though it violated the United Nations' International Labour Organization's Freedom of Association and Protection of the Right to Organize Convention, which Canada had signed.[121] All of these activities served to disempower workers, with negative implications for their health, safety, and well-being.

INTENSIFICATION OF THREATS TO WORKER WELL-BEING – THE NEOLIBERAL PERIOD IN ALBERTA

While anti-labour sentiment and action were clearly present in Alberta prior to 1980, the neoliberal turn made things considerably worse for workers, including for their health and well-being. As noted earlier in this section and throughout this volume, there are well-established connections between neoliberal policies and health inequity including via austerity and privatization which erode public services upon which most people depend; deregulation of health-damaging industries (e.g., food industry; fossil fuel industry); and economic policy that treats workers as commodities to be exploited for profit.[122]

As described by labour history researcher Winston Gereluk, the global recession of the early 1980s affected Alberta particularly badly because of the province's excessive dependence on oil and gas. Oil companies laid off thousands of employees. In Alberta's capital city of Edmonton, which was further affected by cuts to government jobs, the unemployment rate in 1987 was over 11 percent, and almost 24,000 residents required social assistance and food banks. Rationalized by the misguided view that addressing government deficit (versus supporting peoples' well-being) should guide policy, the Progressive Conservative governments of Lougheed and then Don Getty (1985–1992) responded with aggressive neoliberal economic and social policy reforms of cutbacks, privatization, and labour-unfriendly legislation that collectively threatened working conditions and worker quality of life. Workers in construction were very badly affected when contractors took advantage of large numbers of unemployed workers to destroy unions. When collective agreements expired, employers locked out workers, declared the agreement no longer in effect, then offered workers their jobs back at significantly reduced pay. In cases where agreements had not yet expired, some employers set up spin-off companies, which allowed them to transfer work and workers to non-unionized environments. These changes were devastating for workers and led in some cases to very negative outcomes for health and well-being such as marital breakdowns, lost homes, and suicides.[123]

Circumstances for workers worsened further in the 1990s. In a global context of shifting power to transnational corporations and a provincial economic context focused almost exclusively on oil, Ralph Klein's success in winning the Progressive Conservative party leadership and shortly thereafter becoming premier (1992–2006) signalled the beginning of what labour studies scholar Jason Foster describes as some of the most tumultuous years in Alberta's history. As discussed in Chapter 4 of this volume, the Klein government's intensified agenda of austerity, privatization, and deregulation led to significant job elimination in core government jobs, nursing, education, and advanced education. He gutted occupational health and safety during the 1990s through a 42 percent budget reduction. In 1993, the Klein government asked all public sector workers to voluntarily accept a 5 percent wage reduction, which was followed by a two-year wage freeze. Meanwhile, minimum wage under Klein was the lowest in Canada for most of the 1990s. Beyond the direct effects of these decisions, Foster highlights the insidious effects of Klein's agenda in terms of an enduring weakening of the public sector and reframing of the dominant narrative so that the destructive neoliberal activities seemed reasonable.[124]

Workers, with the help of supporters, continued to fight back, to some success.[125] In 1994, for example, sixty laundry workers from the Canadian Union of Public Employees at Calgary General Hospital, after having accepted a 28 percent pay cut and then being informed that their jobs were being privatized, staged an illegal wildcat strike for which they were joined in solidarity by other hospital workers. After ten days, the government delayed privatization by eighteen months. In 2000, ten thousand Alberta Union of Provincial Employees health care workers staged an illegal walkout, which led to wage increases and a guarantee of no further contracting. In 2002, teachers, who were still reeling from dramatic 1994 provincial government cuts to education funding, abandoned their formerly moderate stance and built a province-wide coordinated and overtly political bargaining strategy. A thirteen-day strike, which affected two-thirds of all students in Alberta, eventually led to a sizable wage increase but did not improve classroom conditions, which the Alberta Teachers' Association maintained was the biggest issue. And in 2004, deplorable working conditions at the Lakeside Packing Plant in Brooks, Alberta, prompted a wildcat protest by the mostly Sudanese workers, which ultimately led to unionization by a narrow majority. Despite these successes, however, workers' energy waned under the immense weight of the Klein government's broad-based attacks on workers, and most unions ultimately negotiated settlements that entrenched poor conditions, job losses, and wage reductions, which in turn weakened unions further by reducing their membership.[126]

Although Klein's provincial leadership ended in 2006, circumstances for workers, and thus the implications of those circumstances for health and well-being, did not improve. In 2008, when Alberta reached the peak of one of its many economic booms based on oil, 166 workers died in industrial accidents.[127] When the global financial crisis of 2008 hit, Alberta was once again especially badly impacted due to its single-industry economy when 80,000 jobs were lost in ten months.[128] These enduring economic, political, and social challenges, and their significant implications for well-being and health equity, formed the context for the historic 2015 provincial election of the NDP under Rachel Notley. Compared to previous governments, the provincial NDP achieved some important gains for workers such as increasing the minimum wage from one of the lowest in Canada at $10.20/hour to one of the highest at the time at $15/hour and in updating safety rules for farms. On other issues, such as environmental policy, evaluation of the NDP's legacy is decidedly less positive (see also Chapter 8) and this is a crucially important issue as we transition to a more sustainable economy that is supportive of workers in Alberta and beyond.[129]

Overall, despite significant implications of work for well-being and health equity,[130] engagement of mainstream public health with the broader political economic factors that shape the landscape and quality of work and the power and dignity of workers is limited. It is with the goal of strengthening this intersection, which is integral to a broad version of public health, that we have include a section on worker health from a political economy perspective in this volume. The dynamics outlined here have only persisted in the context of the COVID-19 pandemic where those jobs with the highest risk of exposure to the virus also tended to be poorly paid and precarious and were disproportionately held by women, racialized populations, and immigrants. An important recent analysis showed that these workers were more likely to contract the virus *despite* being equally or more likely to be vaccinated than comparison groups, thus pointing to the need to focus on improving working conditions and pay for essential workers rather than a narrow and reductive focus on individual's decisions around whether or not to be vaccinated.[131] Shifting upstream in this way, to centre root causes of poor health in their social, economic, and political systems and structures, rather than place dominant reliance on technical biomedical solutions such as vaccines and their uptake by individuals, is a long-standing challenge for public health.[132]

This history also contains important examples of resistance by workers; that is, efforts to rebalance power inequities which are the root causes of health inequities. Examples of worker resistance likewise continue to accrue, such as the pandemic-inspired collective efforts that prompted legislated paid sick days in British Columbia and federally (but not in Alberta).[133] While the challenges of capitalism may seem overwhelming, historical political economy analysis makes clear the imperative of collective mobilization even if it is not always successful. Indeed, if our concern is population well-being and health equity and its structural causes, there is no alternative.

Conclusions

With the aim of showcasing *prevention* as a fundamental public health orientation and activity, we summarized some aspects of the history of prevention in Alberta using three examples: tobacco control, community water fluoridation, and workers' health. Our range of examples collectively illustrate the intersectoral nature of prevention, which includes roles for different levels of government, academic researchers, and civil society; the imperative of collective action, by citizens and organizations; and the continuing need for prevention — especially in its upstream primary and primordial forms — as a key part of a broad vision of public health. [134]

We titled this chapter "Mobilizing Preventive Policy." Preventive policy is a broad concept that can range from specific legislation around discrete issues — such as tobacco and fluoridation — to an overarching re-orientation of government, economy, and society to be much more attuned to upstream drivers of poor health and health inequity, as illustrated by our example of workers' health.[135] The latter is especially well-aligned with a broad vision of public health that anchors this volume, and to which we hope our analysis here can contribute.

NOTES

1   Canadian Public Health Association (CPHA), *Public Health: A Conceptual Framework,* CPHA Working Paper (Ottawa: CPHA, 2017), https://www.cpha.ca/public-health-conceptual-framework; Public Health Agency of Canada, *Core Competencies for Public Health in Canada: Release 1.0* (Public Health Agency of Canada, 2008), https://www.phac-aspc.gc.ca/php-psp/ccph-cesp/pdfs/cc-manual-eng090407.pdf. John Last, ed., "Prevention," *A Dictionary of Epidemiology,* fourth ed. (New York: Oxford University Press, 2001).

2   Last, *A Dictionary of Epidemiology,* "Primordial prevention"; CPHA, *Public Health: A Conceptual Framework.*

3   Centers for Disease Control and Prevention (CDC), "Prevention," https://www.cdc.gov/pictureofamerica/pdfs/picture_of_america_prevention.pdf.

4   At Les Hagen's request, this section of the chapter is dedicated to the memory of the Honourable Stanley Schumacher, Q.C., Honorary Patron of Action on Smoking & Health (ASH) 1993 to 2008.

5   "History of the Surgeon General's Reports on Smoking and Health," Smoking & Tobacco Use, CDC, accessed 34 September 2020, https://www.cdc.gov/tobacco/data_statistics/sgr/history/index.htm.

6   Jessica Reid et al., *Tobacco Use in Canada: Patterns and Trends,* 2019 ed. (Waterloo, ON: Propel Centre for Population, Health Impact, University of Waterloo, 2019), https://uwaterloo.ca/tobacco-use-canada/sites/ca.tobacco-use-canada/files/uploads/files/tobacco_use_in_canada_2019.pdf. Notwithstanding the steady decline in smoking prevalence since the 1960s, the 2017 national prevalence estimate (15%) was significantly higher than in 2015 (13%).

7   Christopher Rutty and Sue C. Sullivan, *This Is Public Health: A Canadian History* (Ottawa: CPHA, 2010); Alan Davidson, *Social Determinants of Health: A Comparative Approach* (Don Mills, ON: Oxford University Press, 2015); Margot Shields, "Smoking Bans: Influence on Smoking Prevalence," *Health Reports* 18, no. 3 (2007).

8   Kirsten Bell, Amy Salmon, and Darlene McNaughton, "Alcohol, Tobacco, Obesity and the New Public Health," *Critical Public Health* 21, no. 1, (2011); Kirsten Bell et al., "'Every Space is Claimed': Smokers' Experiences of Tobacco Denormalisation," *Sociology of Health & Illness* 32, no. 6 (2010); Katherine L. Frohlich et al., "Creating the Socially Marginalized Youth Smoker: The Role of Tobacco Control," *Sociology of Health & Illness* 34, no. 7 (2012).

9   "Health Fact Sheets, Smoking, 2017," Statistics Canada, accessed 4 September 2020, https://www150.statcan.gc.ca/n1/pub/82-625-x/2018001/article/54974-eng.htm. Estimates refer to the national average excluding the territories, as drawn from the 2017 Canadian Community Health Survey, in which coverage in the territories was partial.

10   Lindsay McLaren, "In Defense of a Population-Level Approach to Prevention: Why Public Health Matters Today," *Canadian Journal of Public Health* 110, no. 3 (June 1, 2019), https://doi.org/10.17269/s41997-019-00198-0.

11   The World Health Organization Framework Convention on Tobacco Control provides a foundation for countries to implement and manage tobacco control, which includes six components: monitor tobacco use and prevention policies; protect people from tobacco smoke; offer help to quit tobacco use; warn about the dangers of tobacco; enforce bans on tobacco advertising, promotion and sponsorship; raise taxes on tobacco. "MPOWER," Tobacco Free Initiative (TFI), World Health Organization, accessed 4 September 2020, https://www.who.int/tobacco/mpower/en/.

12   This section largely begins in the 1970s; however, interest in tobacco control in Alberta may have begun quite a bit earlier than this. According to *Towards a Healthier City: A History of the Edmonton Board of Health,* in the 1940s, the Women's Christian Temperance Union put forth a proposal for restrictions on smoking in public places to Edmonton City Council. Although a civic regulation was apparently already in place for smoking in 'public conveyances,' Council declined the proposal on the basis that the Board of Health did not consider smoking to be a public health problem. Maureen Riddell and Richard Sherbaniuk, *Towards a Healthier City: A History of the Edmonton Board of Health, 1871–1995* (Edmonton: 1995), 51.

13   Les Hagen, interview by Rogelio Velez Mendoza, 30 November 2018; Rutty and Sullivan, *This Is Public Health.* Another key non-profit group was the Non-Smokers' Rights Association, which began in Toronto in 1974 and has been active in campaigning for tobacco legislation and regulation at the municipal, provincial, and federal levels ever since. "What We Do What is the NSRA?," Non-Smokers' Rights Association, accessed 7 September 2020, https://nsra-adnf.ca/what-we-do/what-is-the-nsra/.

14   Sarah Milov, "Grass Roots Activists Won the War on Smoking. Can They Win the War on Climate Change?" *Washington Post,* 29 June 2017, https://www.washingtonpost.com/news/made-by-history/wp/2017/06/29/grass-roots-activists-won-the-war-on-smoking-can-they-win-the-war-on-climate-change/?noredirect=on&utm_term=.827c9b7d331e.

15 "Not Fast Enough for GASP. Statistics Show Smokers are Becoming a Dying Breed," *Calgary Herald*, 21 May 1979;.

16 "Getting a G(R)ASP on the Problem," *Edmonton Journal*, 2 October 1975, 23. The *Edmonton Journal* reported that GASP-Edmonton presented to the deputy minister of health, Dr. Jean Nelson in February 1977. They proposed that smoking be completely banned areas such as elevators, libraries, and supermarkets and at least partially banned places like arenas, restaurants, and, planes. They presented a petition containing 13,136 names collected by GASP groups in Edmonton and Calgary. "The GASP Message: Smokers Beware of Fines in the Air," *Edmonton Journal*, 8 February 1977, 25.

17 Alberta. Legislative Assembly of Alberta, 21 April 1977 (Eric Musgreave, PC); "Getting a G(R)ASP on the Problem," *Edmonton Journal*.

18 Alberta, Legislative Assembly of Alberta, 28 April 1977. All Hansard Transcripts are available at https://www.assembly.ab.ca/assembly-business/transcripts/transcripts-by-type.

19 John Gogo, PC MLA for Lethbridge-West, and John Ashton, PC MLA for Edmonton-Ottewell. Alberta, Legislative Assembly of Alberta, 28 April 1977. The enforcement comment echoes points of opposition made during the seatbelt debate (see Chapter 3).

20 The meeting announcements described the group as an "Environmental action group supporting the rights of the non-smoker" (e.g., "Public Notices," *Edmonton Journal*, 24 January 1977, 32). To illustrate its strong presence, in 1980 alone, GASP was mentioned explicitly at least seven times in the *Edmonton Journal* in the context of the municipal bylaw deliberations, where they were often portrayed as the main or only anti-smoking group.

21 "The GASP Message: Smokers Beware of Fines in the Air," *Edmonton Journal*, 8 February 1977, 25; "Council in Brief," *Edmonton Journal*, 22 May 1980, 30.

22 "You and Your Heart. Smoke can Cause Irritation," *Edmonton Journal*, 6 April 1977, 27.

23 "GASP Group Wants Bylaw to Segregate the Smokers," *Edmonton Journal*, 12 June 1980, 25.

24 "Council in Brief," *Edmonton Journal*, 22 May 1980, 30.

25 "Cloud of Smoking Controls Hovers over Council Session," *Edmonton Journal*, 16 September 1980, 13.

26 Barb Livingstone, "Curb your Puffing or Pay the Penalty," *Edmonton Journal*, 14 January 1981, 1.

27 Ottawa was the first city to pass a municipal bylaw in 1976, and Toronto passed theirs in 1979. "Key Issues: Municipal Bylaws," Non-Smokers' Rights Association, accessed 7 September 2020, https://nsra-adnf.ca/key-issues/second-hand-smoke/municipal-bylaws/. Vancouver city council passed a bylaw in late 1986 banning smoking in many public places. The city ban was extended to restaurants and cafes in 1996. Maryse Zeidler, "30 Years Ago Smoking in Public Places was Banned in Vancouver – and Smokers were Outraged," *CBC News*, 4 December 2016, https://www.cbc.ca/news/canada/british-columbia/smoking-bylaw-vancouver-history-1.3875548.

28 Public notices of regular GASP meetings continued to appear in the *Edmonton Journal* throughout 1981, 1982, and 1983.

29 In December 1981, for example, GASP spoke in support of efforts to remove the University of Alberta's exemption from the city's smoking bylaw. "Smoking May be Out for U's Faculty Council," *Edmonton Journal*, 9 December 1981, 25.

30 "Butt-out Backers Rewarded for Huffing about Puffing," *Edmonton Journal*, 25 April 1984, 18.

31 David Howell, "Bylaw gets Tougher on Public Smokers," *Edmonton Journal*, 10 April 1985, 15.

32 "Bylaw Charges GASP-inspired," *Edmonton Journal*, 10 July 1985, 22; Judy Schultz, "Be Sure to Complain about Rude Smokers (Feedback)," *Edmonton Journal*, 17 July 1985, 48.

33 Mike Sadava, "Council Toughens Smoking Bylaw: Anti-smoking Group Applauds Council's Efforts," *Edmonton Journal*, 25 March 1991, 15.

34 "Nonsmokers Set to Unite," *Calgary Herald*, 23 April 1975, 28; "Anti-smoke Group Aims Pollution Blow," *Calgary Herald*, 1 May 1975, 25.

35 "Arenas Plan Crackdown on Smoking," *Calgary Herald*, 26 February 1977, 27.

36 Don Martin, "Ryan Runs Out of Puff on Bylaw," *Calgary Herald*, 23 January 1980, 1; "Passing Anti-smoking Torch (letter)," *Calgary Herald*, 31 January 1980, 8.

37 Portia Priegert, "No-smoking Regulations Lack Teeth, Says Pears," *Calgary Herald*, 19 March 1985, 17. In terms of "lacking teeth", Calgary's initial bylaw appears to have been more lenient than Edmonton's: while it required restaurants and lounges to establish non-smoking areas, it left the amount of designated non-smoking space or number of seats to the discretion of the operators of the businesses.

38 Starting with Calgary in 1988, all Olympic Games have been declared tobacco-free. "Tobacco Free Olympics," Tobacco Free Initiative (TFI), World Health Organization, accessed 7 September 2020, https://www.who.int/tobacco/free_sports/olympics/en/; Les Hagen, interview; Carmen Chai, "50 Years after Historic Report, Canadian Officials Reflect on Anti-smoking Efforts," *Global News*, 10 January

2014, https://globalnews.ca/news/1074275/50-years-after-history-making-report-canadian-officials-reflect-on-anti-smoking-efforts/.

39   Provincial legislation concerning smoking existed in Alberta prior to the 1970s. This included: An Act respecting the Use of Tobacco by Minors (1922, 1942), which prohibited sales of tobacco to minors except under written request from a parent, guardian or employer; An Act respecting the Welfare of Children (1925), which outlined the powers of officers and others to confiscate cigarettes from a child, and to detain and search a child suspected to have cigarettes; An Act to License and Regulate Public Vehicles on Highways (1927), according to which drivers of public vehicles carrying passengers are not permitted to smoke while driving; and An Act to Provide for the Imposition of a Tax on Purchasers and Users of Tobacco (1969) that outlines amounts and parameters of provincial tax on tobacco products.

40   The overlap and continuity between GASP-Edmonton and ASH is illustrated by common members, such as Dr. Roger Hodkinson who served as president of GASP-Edmonton and spokesperson for ASH in the mid-1980s. See for example Paul Cashman, "GASP Wants Puffers to Pay for Anti-smoking Agency," Edmonton Journal, 9 April 1985, 15. The name change from GASP to ASH occurred in 1987. Les Hagen, interview.

41   Daniel Stoffman, "The Ability of the Tobacco Industry to Stay Healthy While its Customers Get Sick is One of the Most Amazing Marketing Feats of All Time," Globe and Mail, Report on Business Magazine, September 1987; Garfield Mahood, "Warnings that Tell the Truth: Breaking New Ground in Canada," Tobacco Control 8, no. 4 (1999). For example, federal legislation for a total ban on cigarette advertising was proposed in 1971, but the decision was made under federal Liberal leadership to go with voluntary guidelines for industry at that time. That said, the Canadian Charter of Rights and Freedoms, which became law under the federal Trudeau government in 1982, helped set the stage for legal protection of non-smokers from tobacco smoke in public areas. Rutty and Sullivan, This Is Public Health: A Canadian History.

42   Les Hagen, interview. Within the Canadian public health community, Epp is perhaps most known for the 1986 report, Achieving Health for All: A Framework for Health Promotion, also known as the Epp Report, which makes reference to tobacco reduction as an example of the strategy of healthy public policy. Jake Epp, Achieving Health for All: A Framework for Health Promotion (Ottawa: Health and Welfare Canada, 1986), https://www.canada.ca/en/health-canada/services/health-care-system/reports-publications/health-care-system/achieving-health-framework-health-promotion.html.

43   Non-smokers' Health Act, Statutes of Canada 1988, c. 21 (vol. 1); Tobacco Products Control Act, S.C. 1988, c. 20 (vol. 1).

44   Les Hagen, interview.

45   Briefly, the federal Established Programs Financing (EPF) plan, introduced in 1977, provided funding to provinces and territories for health care and post-secondary education. Upon the enactment of the Canada Health Act of 1984, EPF funding was made conditional on provinces' alignment with the criteria of the act. In 1995, the EPF and the Canada Assistance Plan (established in 1966 to fund social assistance programs) were combined into the Canada Health and Social Transfer (CHST), and then in 2004 the CHST was restructured into the Canada Health Transfer and the Canada Social Transfer. "History of Health and Social Transfers," Department of Finance Canada, modified 15 December 2014, https://www.canada.ca/en/department-finance/programs/federal-transfers/history-health-social-transfers.html.

46   Dene Creswell, "Non-smokers Forge Restaurant Campaign," Edmonton Journal, 6 February 1984, 11; Katherine Dedyna, "Smoking Council Draws GASP Fire," Edmonton Journal, 3 October 1985, 22.

47   Katherine Dedyna, "Smokers May be Threat to their Fellow Workers," Edmonton Journal, 30 September 1985, 45.

48   Dedyna, "Smokers May be Threat," Edmonton Journal; Dedyna, "Smoking Council Draws GASP Fire," Edmonton Journal.

49   Richard Helm, "'Death and Disease' Funds Ballet — Anti-smoking Group," Edmonton Journal, 13 November 1985, 17; "Dancers Protest Cigarette Sponsors," Edmonton Journal, 18 February 1986, 2.

50   See for example, "'Dance of Death' Protests du Maurier Aid for Ballet," The Citizen, Ottawa, 18 February 1986, B8; Les Hagen, interview.

51   Katherine Dedyna, "Group Wants Anti-smoking Agency," Edmonton Journal, 28 April 1985, 2. Suzuki's comment was in the context of discussions around lobbying the provincial government to create a new provincial agency to focus on reducing smoking, whose efforts, it was argued, could be funded by a modest tax increase on cigarette products.

52   Action on Smoking & Health was present in the legislature and/or explicitly mentioned in the Alberta Hansard, during debates on Bill 42, The Tobacco Tax Amendment Act (Alberta. Legislative Assembly of Alberta, 17 and 18 June 1991); Bill 207, the Tobacco Control Act (14 May 1992); Bill 258, the Tobacco

Control Act, 27 October 1993); Bill 215, the Non-Smokers' Health Act (25 October 1994); and Bill 208, the Prevention of Youth Tobacco Use Act (7 December 1999).

53   Alberta. Legislative Assembly of Alberta, 14 May 1992.

54   Alberta. Legislative Assembly of Alberta, 25 October 1994; 7 December 1999.

55   The Alberta Tobacco Reduction Centre started in 1995 and ran for about three years, and the Alberta Tobacco Reduction Alliance began in 1998/99 and ran for about four years. Les Hagen, interview; Alberta Ministry of Health, *Annual Report 1998–99* (Edmonton, 1999), 40.

56   The World Health Organization Framework Convention on Tobacco Control was developed in response to the globalization of the tobacco epidemic, and emphasizes the importance of price and tax measures, measures to protect people from exposure to tobacco smoke, regulation of the contents of tobacco products, and regulation of tobacco product disclosures. The framework convention is significant in that it was the first treaty negotiated under the auspices of the World Health Organization, and it "represents a paradigm shift in developing a regulatory strategy to address addictive substances". World Health Organization, *WHO Framework Convention on Tobacco Control* (Geneva: World Health Organization, 2003, updated reprint 2004, 2005), https://www.who.int/fctc/text_download/en/.

57   This is a good illustration of the complexity of public health and its intersections with politics. Although the Klein government was supportive of substantive tobacco control measures, which contribute importantly to population morbidity and mortality, his government was in most other ways devastating to a broad vision of public health due to its ideologically driven restructuring and cuts to public services.

58   Alberta. Legislative Assembly of Alberta, 19 March 2002. Taxes on cigarettes had increased steadily between the mid-1980s and the early 1990s, with provincial tax in Alberta increasing from $3.07 per carton in 1985–1986 to $11.01 per carton in in 1991–1992, after which it levelled off. W. Kerry Mummery and Les C. Hagen, "Tobacco Pricing, Taxation, Consumption and Revenue: Alberta 1985–1995," *Canadian Journal of Public Health* 87, no. 5 (September / October 1996).

59   Alberta Cancer Board, *Snapshot of Tobacco Facts: A Resource to Guide Tobacco Control Planning in Alberta*, First Edition (September 2007), 10–11, https://www.biodiversitylibrary.org/item/246940#page/21/mode/1up.

60   Les Hagen, interview. According to Campaign for a Smoke-Free Alberta, the Alberta Tobacco Reduction Strategy was renewed in 2012 "with a revised 10-year plan and new performance targets but no specified budget." "Alberta Tobacco Reduction Strategy," Campaign for a Smoke-Free Alberta, accessed 7 September 2020, https://protectalbertakids.ca/issues/alberta-tobacco-reduction-strategy/; Alberta Health, *Creating Tobacco-free Futures: Alberta's Strategy to Prevent and Reduce Tobacco Use 2012–2022* (Edmonton: Government of Alberta, 2012), https://open.alberta.ca/dataset/5e2a807f-1045-45d6-82eb-946ed25fcdd7/resource/d39bb973-48c1-4288-9656-8b2152e595b0/download/6906901Creating-tobacco-free-futures-2012-2022-Strategy.pdf.

61   Les Hagen, "Transforming Canada's Marlboro Country," PowerPoint presentation, 16 November 2016.

62   Les Hagen, interview.

63   Jodi L. Shaw and Julie W. Farmer, *An Environmental Scan of Publicly Financed Dental Care in Canada: 2015 Update* (Prepared under the direction of the Chief Dental Officer, PHAC), https://caphd.ca/wp-content/uploads/2022/06/FINAL-2015-Environmental-Scan-ENGLISH-16-Feb-16.pdf; Alberta Health Services (AHS), Provincial Oral Health Office, *Oral Health Action Plan (OHAP)* (AHS, 2016), https://www.albertahealthservices.ca/assets/info/oh/if-oh-action-plan.pdf.

64   Carlos Quiñonez, *The Politics of Dental Care in Canada* (Toronto: Canadian Scholars, 2021).

65   Canadian Academy of Health Sciences (CAHS), *Improving Access to Oral Health Care for Vulnerable People Living in Canada* (Ottawa: CAHS, 2014), https://cahs-acss.ca/improving-access-to-oral-health-care-for-vulnerable-people-living-in-canada/; Canadian Institute for Health Information (CIHI), *Treatment of Preventable Dental Cavities in Preschoolers: A Focus on Day Surgery under General Anesthesia* (Ottawa: CIHI, 2013), https://secure.cihi.ca/free_products/Dental_Caries_Report_en_web.pdf; Cynthia Weijs et al., "Advancing Public Health Communication in the Era of Empowered Health Consumerism: Insights from Dental Hygienist-Client Interactions Around Community Water Fluoridation," *Critical Public Health* (online) (2020), doi.org/10.1080/09581596.2020.1791315.

66   "Position Statement on Community Water Fluoridation," PHAC, Government of Canada, modified 8 February 2018, https://www.canada.ca/en/services/health/publications/healthy-living/fluoride-position-statement.html.

67   M. Bellemare, P. Simard, L Trahan, "Summary on Fluoridation of Drinking Water," *Le Journal Dentaire du Québec* 16 (1979); William L. Hutton, Bradley W. Linscott, and Donald B. Williams, "Final Report of Local Studies on Water Fluoridation in Brantford," *Canadian Journal of Public Health*

9 | Mobilizing Preventive Policy   *291*

47, no. 3 (1956); Pammie R Crawford, "Fifty Years of Fluoridation," *Journal of the Canadian Dental Association* 61 (1995); CDC "Achievements in Public Health, 1900-1999: Fluoridation of Drinking Water to Prevent Dental Caries," *MMWR (Morbidity and Mortality Weekly Report)* 48 (1999); R. Allan Freeze and Jay H. Lehr, *The Fluoride Wars: How a Modest Public Health Measure Became America's Longest-Running Political Melodrama* (Hoboken, N.J.: J. Wiley & Sons, 2008).

68   Reports of mottled enamel in Grassy Lake and in Granum, in southern Alberta, came in around 1935 from the provincial travelling clinic and from a local school principal. G. Clarke and C.R. Castaldi, "Fluorine, Fluorides and Fluoridation in Alberta," *Canadian Journal of Public Health* 52 (1961); Osman James Walker and Elvins Yuill Spencer, "The Occurrence of 'Mottled Enamel' of Teeth in Alberta and its Relation to the Fluorine Content of the Water Supply," *Canadian Journal of Research* 15, Sec. B (1937).

69   Walker and Spencer, "The Occurrence of 'Mottled Enamel.'"

70   The three Ontario communities were: Brantford, where fluoride was added to the drinking water system at a concentration of 1.0 ppm, Sarnia, where no was fluoride added and there were negligiblelevels of naturally-occurring fluoride in the water, and Stratford, where no fluoride was added and there were high levels (1.2–1.6 ppm) of naturally-occurring fluoride in the water.

71   H. K. Brown et al., "The Brantford-Sarnia-Stratford Fluoridation Caries Study 1955 Report," *Canadian Journal of Public Health* 47, no. 4 (1956); Lindsay McLaren and Lynn McIntyre, *Drinking Water Fluoridation in Canada: Review and Synthesis of Published Literature*, report prepared for PHAC, April 2011, https://www.albertahealthservices.ca/poph/hi-poph-surv-phids-drinking-water-fluoridation.pdf.

72   H.R. MacLean, dentist, president of the Alberta Dental Association (1943, 1952, and 1953), and later dean of the Faculty of Dentistry at the University of Alberta (1958–1970), Provincial Archives of Alberta, "H.R. MacLean fonds," No. PR3398, https://hermis.alberta.ca/paa/Details.aspx?st=edmonton&cp=2053&ReturnUrl=%2Fpaa%2FSearch.aspx%3Fst%3Dedmonton%26cp%3D2053&dv=True&DeptID=1&ObjectID=PR3398.

73   G. Clarke and C.R. Castaldi, "Fluorine, Fluorides and Fluoridation in Alberta;" Riddell and Sherbaniuk, *Towards a Healthier City.*

74   MacLean, *History of Dentistry in Alberta*; Harry Knowlton Brown, "Mass Control of Dental Caries by Fluoridation of a Public Water Supply," *Journal of the Canadian Dental Association* 17, no. 11 (November 1951).

75   For example, Brown et al. presented data for the three communities from 1948 to 1955. Overall, findings indicated that prevalence of dental caries among children fluctuated at a high level over time in Sarnia (not fluoridated), fluctuated at a low level in Stratford (naturally fluoridated), and improved significantly in Brantford (fluoride added). Brown, McLaren, Josie, and Stewart, "The Brantford-Sarnia-Stratford Fluoridation Caries Study 1955 Report;" David B. Ast, Sidney B. Finn, and Isabel McCaffrey, "The Newburgh-Kingston Caries Fluorine Study; Dental Findings after Three Years of Water Fluoridation," *American Journal of Public Health* 40 (1950).

76   Catherine Carstairs, "Cities without Cavities: Democracy, Risk, and Public Health," *Journal of Canadian Studies* 44, no. 2 (2010); Catherine Carstairs and Rachel Elder, "Expertise, Health, and Popular Opinion: Debating Water Fluoridation, 1945–80," *Canadian Historical Review* 89 (2008); Lisa Watson, "The Edmonton Fluoridation Controversy," *Alberta History* 38 (1990). These points of opposition have been remarkably consistent over time and place. See for example McLaren and McIntyre, *Drinking Water Fluoridation in Canada.*

77   Carstairs, "Cities without Cavities;" "Obituary: Dr. William H. Hill," *Canadian Medical Association Journal* 89, (September 7, 1963), 526; "Past Presidents," Alberta Public Health Association; W.H. Hill, "Fluoridation of Water" [Letter to the Editor], *Canadian Journal of Public Health* 43, no. 7 (July 1952), 320-321.

78   Specifically, around 1951 or 1952, the city of Edmonton wished to implement fluoridation. Deputy Minister of Health W.W. Cross had checked the legislation and found that there was nothing to prevent the city from taking such action. "Plebiscite by Municipalities May Settle Fluoridation Issue," *Calgary Herald*, 18 February 1956, 1.

79   *An Act to Amend the Public Health Act*, S.P.A. 1952 c. 68.

80   Clarke and Castaldi, "Fluorine, Fluorides and Fluoridation in Alberta." The report was authored by O.J. Walker, professor of chemistry at the University of Alberta and H.R. MacLean.

81   Watson, "The Edmonton Fluoridation Controversy;" "Water Fluoridation Attack Launched By Woman MLA," *Edmonton Journal*, 4 March 1954; "Mrs. Wood Scores Water Fluoridation," *Calgary Herald*, 5 March 1954; "Member Opposes Water Fluoridation," *Edmonton Journal*, 29 March 1955.

82   MacLean, *History of Dentistry in Alberta*; Clarke and Castaldi, "Fluorine, Fluorides and Fluoridation in Alberta;" Watson, "The Edmonton Fluoridation Controversy."

83   *An Act to Amend the Public Health Act*, S.P.A 1956, c. 42. The amendment also stipulated that if approval for fluoridation was not secured, the municipality must wait at least one year before holding another plebiscite. In 1958, a further amendment extended this waiting period to two years to make it consistent with the two-year mandatory waiting period before rescinding a fluoridation bylaw. *An Act to Amend the Public Health Act*, S.P.A 1958, c. 63; "Fluorine Bill Would Limit Bylaw Voting," *Edmonton Journal*, 27 February 1958, 19.

84   "Plebiscite by Municipalities May Settle Fluoridation Issue," *Calgary Herald*; "34-Day Session of House Ends," *Edmonton Journal*, 31 March 1956, 1.

85   Clarke and Castaldi, "Fluorine, Fluorides and Fluoridation in Alberta;" Alberta Department of Public Health, *Annual Report 1957* (Edmonton: Printed by L.S. Wall, Queen's Printer, 1959), 8.

86   D. G. Fish, E.S. Hirabayashi and G.K. Hirabayashi, "Voting Turn-out at A Fluoridation Plebiscite," *Journal of the Canadian Dental Association* 31, no. 2 (February 1965): 88–96; Watson, "The Edmonton Fluoridation Controversy."

87   Clarke and Castaldi, "Fluorine, Fluorides and Fluoridation in Alberta."

88   For example, in 1960 the Union of Alberta Municipalities passed a motion that was initiated by the town of Hinton to urge the provincial government to amend the legislation to require a simple majority. Clarke and Castaldi, "Fluorine, Fluorides and Fluoridation in Alberta." According to Riddell and Sherbaniuk, *Towards a Healthier City*, the Edmonton Board of Health also lobbied the Alberta government to reduce the required majority.

89   "Fluoride Battle Averted," *Edmonton Journal*, 19 April 1966; *An Act to Amend the Public Health Act*, S.P.A 1966, c. 77.

90   *Public Health Act*, S.A. 1984, c. P-27.1. See item 101 "The Municipal Government Act is amended" on page 251.

91   28 June 1988 Commissioners' Report to Community Service Committee, City of Calgary, AHS – Historical Collections. There is no accession number available for materials from AHS Historical Collections cited in this chapter.

92   Carstairs, "Cities without Cavities;" Clarke and Castaldi, "Fluorine, Fluorides and Fluoridation in Alberta."

93   Preparatory efforts in Calgary initially ramped up in anticipation of a fluoridation plebiscite to be held in conjunction with the 1986 municipal election, but that did not materialize. Calgary fluoridation files, held at AHS — Historical Collections.

94   Carstairs, "Cities without Cavities."

95   Therefore, although the estimated costs for the community water fluoridation and fluoride supplement programs were approximately $3/child age 0–13 for each program, when one takes into account the differential reach (100% vs 16%), the supplement program is much costlier (>$20/child age 0–13). Calgary fluoridation files, held at AHS — Historical Collections.

96   The "rescinding fluoridation petition", which was initiated by the fluoridation opposition group Health Action Network Society, was ultimately deemed legally invalid by city solicitors, but this took bit of time to sort out. The delay also reflected engineering delays. Calgary fluoridation files, held at AHS — Historical Collections.

97   Catherine Pryce and Jackie Smorang, "Continuing Water Fluoridation in the City of Calgary, Alberta, 1997–1998," *Journal of the Canadian Dental Association* 65, no. 2 (1999).

98   The panel included members with expertise in bone health, pediatrics and community health, toxicology, environmental design, and biostatistics. The members, all from the University of Calgary, were David Hanley (Medicine), Hossein Joe Moghadam (Medicine), Miloslav Nosal (Science), Sheldon Roth (Medicine), and Dixon Thompson (Environmental Design).

99   Pryce and Smorang, "Continuing Water Fluoridation in the City of Calgary, Alberta."

100   "A Brief History of Planning Legislation in Alberta," Alberta Urban Municipalities Association, accessed 7 September 2020, https://auma.ca/advocacy-services/programs-initiatives/municipal-planning-hub/historical-context/brief-history-planning-legislation-alberta.

101   Brian Brennan, "Fluoride: Is it Right to Put it in our Drinking Water?" *Calgary Herald*, 4 October 1998, 16.

102   Weijs et al., "Advancing Public Health Communication;" Brenda O'Neill, Taruneek Kapoor, and Lindsay McLaren, "Politics, Science, and Termination: A Case Study of Water Fluoridation Policy in Calgary in 2011," *Review of Policy Research* 36, no. 1 (2018), https://doi.org/10.1111/ropr.12318; Salima Thawer et al., "Exploring Reported Dental Hygiene Practice Adaptations in Response to Water Fluoridation status," *Canadian Journal of Dental Hygiene* 52, no. 2 (2018); Lindsay McLaren and Rachel

Petit, "Universal and Targeted Policy to Achieve Health Equity: A Critical Analysis of the Example of Community Water Fluoridation Cessation in Calgary, Canada in 2011," *Critical Public Health* 28, no. 2 (2018), https://doi.org/10.1080/09581596.2017.1361015; Lindsay McLaren et al., "Fluoridation Cessation and Children's Dental Caries: A 7-year Follow-up Evaluation of Grade 2 Schoolchildren in Calgary and Edmonton, Canada," *Community Dentistry and Oral Epidemiology* (2021), https://doi.org/10.1111/cdoe.12685; Lindsay McLaren et al., "Fluoridation Cessation and Oral Health Equity: A 7-year Post-cessation Study of Grade 2 Schoolchildren in Alberta, Canada," *Canadian Journal of Public Health* (2022), https://doi.org/10.17269/s41997-022-00654-4.

103   Public Health Agency of Canada, *The State of Community Water Fluoridation across Canada, 2017 Report*, Prepared by the Public Health Capacity and Knowledge Management Unit, Quebec Region for the Office of the Chief Dental Officer of Canada, PHAC, accessed 7 September 2020, https://publications.gc.ca/collections/collection_2018/aspc-phac/HP35-97-2018-eng.pdf.

104   For a contemporary example of traditional occupational health and safety concerns, see the description of AHS' Workplace Health and Safety program in "Workplace Health & Safety," AHS, accessed May 5, 2023, https://www.albertahealthservices.ca/findhealth/service.aspx?Id=4867&facilityId=1025102.

105   Commission on Social Determinants of Health, *Closing the Gap in a Generation: Health Equity through Action on the Social Determinants of Health*, Final Report of the Commission on Social Determinants of Health (Geneva: World Health Organization, 2008).

106   National Collaborating Centre for Determinants of Health, *Core Competencies for Public Health in Canada: An Assessment and Comparison of Determinants of Health Content* (Antigonish, NS: National Collaborating Centre for Determinants of Health, St. Francis Xavier University, 2012), https://nccdh.ca/images/uploads/Core_competencies_EN_121001.pdf.

107   PHAC, *Core Competencies*.

108   Robert Chernomas and Ian Hudson, *To Live and Die in America: Class, Power, Health and Healthcare*, (Halifax and Winnipeg: Fernwood Publishing, 2013); Michael Harvey, "The Political Economy of Health: Revisiting its Marxian Origins to Address 21st-Century Health Inequalities," *American Journal of Public Health* 111, no. 2 (2021).

109   National Collaborating Centre for Determinants of Health, *Determining Health: Decent Work Issue Brief* (Antigonish, NS: NCCDH, St. Francis Xavier University, 2022), https://nccdh.ca/resources/entry/determining-health-decent-work-issue-brief.

110   Alvin Finkel, with contributions from Jason Foster, Winston Gereluk, Jennifer Kelly, Dan Cui, James Muir, Joan Schiebelbein, Jim Selby, and Eric Strikwerda, *Working People in Alberta: A History* (Edmonton: AU Press, 2012).

111   Jim Selby, "One Step Forward: Alberta Workers 1885–1914," in Finkel et al., *Working People in Alberta*.

112   To illustrate the frequency of accidents, these dangerous conditions led to 1,435 serious accidents in Crowsnest mines between 1904 and 1928; when "slight" accidents" were factored in, the overall accident rate increased to an average of two per week between 1906 and 1928 (Selby, "One Step Forward," 58).

113   Selby, "One Step Forward."

114   Dennis Raphael et al., *Social Determinants of Health: The Canadian Facts* (2nd ed.) (Oshawa: Ontario Tech University Faculty of Health Sciences and Toronto: York University School of Health Policy and Management, 2020), http://www.thecanadianfacts.org/

115   Eric Strikwerda and Alvin Finkel, "War, Repression, and Depression, 1914–1939," in Finkel et al., *Working People in Alberta*.

116   Raphael et al., *Social Determinants of Health: Canadian Perspectives*.

117   Strikwerda and Finkel, "War, Repression, and Depression."

118   Strikwerda and Finkel, "War, Repression, and Depression."

119   James Muir, "Alberta Labour and Working-class Life, 1940–1959, in Finkel et al., *Working People in Alberta*.

120   Alvin Finkel, "The Boomers Become the Workers: Alberta, 1960-1980," in Finkel et al., *Working People in Alberta*.

121   Finkel, "The Boomers Become the Workers."

122   Arne Ruckert and Ronald Labonté, "The Global Financial Crisis and Health Equity: Early Experiences from Canada," *Globalizatino and Health* 10 (2014); Ted Schrecker and Clare Bambra, *How Politics Makes us Sick: Neoliberal Epidemics* (New York: Palgrave McMillan, 2015).

123   Winston Gereluk, "Alberta Labour in the 1980s," in Finkel et al., *Working People in Alberta*.

124   Jason Foster, "Revolution, Retrenchment, and the New Normal: The 1990s and Beyond," in Finkel et al., *Working People in Alberta*.

125 Key partners included the Parkland Institute, which was founded in 1996 in response to the need for different voices and perspectives in the context of 25 years of uninterrupted Progressive Conservative party rule in Alberta. (https://www.parklandinstitute.ca/about)

126 Foster, "Revolution, Retrenchment, and the New Normal."

127 Alvin Finkel, "Conclusion: A History to Build Upon," in Finkel et al., *Working People in Alberta.*

128 Foster, "Revolution, Retrenchment, and the New Normal."

129 See Geoff Dembicki, "What Rachel Notley Actually Achieved: The Complex Legacy of Alberta's First NDP Premier," *The Tyee*, 19 February 2019, https://thetyee.ca/News/2019/02/19/Rachel-Notley-Actually-Achieved/. See also Alook et al., *The End of this World.*

130 Commission on Social Determinants of Health, *Closing the Gap in a Generation.*

131 Naomi Lightman and Hamid Akbary, "New Data Provide Insight into Pandemic Inequalities, *Policy Options*, 27 March 2023, https://policyoptions.irpp.org/magazines/march-2023/new-data-provide-insight-into-pandemic-inequalities/.

132 Fran Baum and Matthew Fisher, "Why Behavioural Health Promotion Endures despite Its Failure to Reduce Health Inequities," Sociology of Health & Illness 36, no. 2 (February 2014), https://doi.org/10.1111/1467-9566.12112.

133 National Collaborating Centre for Determinants of Health, *Determining Health.*

134 Canadian Network of Public Health Associations, "A Collective Voice for Advancing Public Health: Why Public Health Associations Matter Today," *Canadian Journal of Public Health* 110, no. 3 (2019), https://doi.org/10.17269/s41997-019-00197-1.

135 Paul Cairney and Emily St Denny, *Why Isn't Government Policy More Preventive?* (Oxford: Oxford University Press, 2020).

10

Health Promotion and the Ottawa Charter in Alberta: A Focus on Maternal and Child Health

Temitayo Famuyide, Benjamin Sasges, and Rogelio Velez Mendoza

> *"It shall be the duty of the department . . . to disseminate information in such manner and form as may be found best adapted to promote health and to prevent and suppress disease."*
>
> — An Act respecting the Department of Public Health, 1919

Introduction

Initiatives such as educating new mothers in rural areas on how to care for their babies, enacting legislation to reduce financial pressures for new parents, and providing health-promoting resources at school theoretically follow the principle of enabling people to have control over their health. Health and well-being are facilitated if supportive knowledge, skills, resources, and settings are in place that permit people to achieve their needs and aspirations throughout their lifespan. The creation of these conditions is the essence of health promotion.

In this chapter, we illustrate how health promotion principles have played out over the course of Alberta's public health history, using the Ottawa Charter for Health Promotion as a framework. Although the strategies and action areas of health promotion as articulated in the charter are contemporary notions, we argue that their essence was apparent much earlier. By using a contemporary framework such as the Ottawa Charter to shed light on history, we can explore how health promotion principles intersect with the socio-historical context.

We begin the chapter with an overview of the Ottawa Charter for Health Promotion — including some key points of critique — and a brief historical overview of health promotion's evolution within the Alberta government. Anchored in that overview, the rest of the chapter is devoted to three case examples that we believe illustrate health promotion principles over the past one hundred years. The examples are united by a focus on the mother/child dyad, which is one of many focal areas that we could have chosen.[1] Our three examples from Alberta's history are: i) preventive health services for mothers and children aimed at reducing infant and maternal mortality, where the health promotion action areas of developing personal skills and reorienting health services were apparent; ii) the introduction of maternity and parental leave legislation and mother's allowances, as examples of building healthy public policy; and iii) school health promotion, focusing on health inspections, vaccination efforts, and shifts in the provincial junior high health curriculum, which we examine through the lens of developing personal skills and building healthy public policy from the perspective of children. In this third example, we also note the significant, albeit historically more recent, trend toward comprehensive school health.[2]

We conclude that, first, although principles of health promotion are apparent in activities to improve maternal/child health prior to the creation of the Ottawa Charter, such efforts incrementally became more encompassing, including efforts to incorporate social determinants of health, after the creation of the charter, suggesting that the charter had some impact, at least symbolically. For example, Alberta lawmakers did not initially make a connection between mothers' allowances and parental leaves on the one hand, and health benefits on the other, but eventually used that connection to justify them. A second key conclusion is that schools in settler-colonial settings have long acted as primary settings for health promotion, and they continue to do so.

Health Promotion and the Ottawa Charter

The Ottawa Charter for Health Promotion has served as a foundation for individual-, community-, sector/system- and societal-level approaches to improving health and well-being for over thirty-five years.[3] Adopted in 1986 by a group of health professionals and representatives of governmental, voluntary, and community organizations from thirty-eight countries, the charter aimed to situate health as a product of daily life, which it described as follows: "to reach a state of complete physical, mental and social well-being, an individual or group must be able to identify and to realize aspirations, to satisfy needs, and to change or cope with the environment. Health is therefore, seen as a resource for everyday life, not the objective of living."[4]

The charter proposed core values and principles and outlined strategies and action areas that went beyond the traditional boundaries of the health care sector and treatment-oriented practices at that time.[5] The strategies for promoting health are i) advocacy, toward making political, economic, social, cultural, environmental, and behavioural conditions favourable for all citizens; ii) mediation, or coordinating between differing interests in society such as government (including health and other sectors), non-governmental and voluntary organizations, and industry; and iii) enabling, or reducing differences in health status and ensuring equal opportunities and resources to enable all people to achieve their fullest health potential.[6] The action areas are:

- Build healthy public policy, which requires policy-makers to be aware of the health consequences of their decisions;
- Create supportive environments by generating safe, stimulating, and enjoyable living and working conditions;
- Strengthen community actions, which involves enhancing social support, and developing systems for strengthening public participation in health matters;
- Develop personal skills, by providing information and education for health, and enhancing life skills; and
- Reorient health services, by moving the health sector beyond curative services and respecting difference in cultural needs.

Although the contemporary notion of *health promotion* is commonly traced to the publication of the Ottawa Charter in 1986, three prior documents inspired the charter.[7] As discussed by researchers Potvin and Jones, the first is the preamble of the 1946 World Health Organization constitution, which contains a positive definition of health where health is not merely the absence of disease, but rather a complete state of physical, mental, and social well-being.[8] Second is *A New Perspective on the Health of Canadians* (better known as the Lalonde Report) of 1974, which was notable for, among other things, the *health field* concept, which recognized determinants of health outside of the health care system, stating that "future improvements in the level of health of Canadians lie mainly in improving the environment, moderating self-imposed risks and adding to our knowledge of human biology."[9] Finally, the Alma Ata Declaration, adopted at the 1978 International Conference on Primary Health Care, called for health as a human right and a responsibility of every nation; the declaration asserted that health is achieved by involving concerned populations and coordination among different sectors.[10]

The first International Conference on Health Promotion, held in Ottawa in November 1986, signified growing expectations for a new public health movement around the world.[11] At the time, some members of the public health community saw the field as overly reliant on a medical model and oriented toward infectious diseases and not going far enough in terms of environmental, social, and economic challenges.[12] Conceived now as an agenda-setting document, the charter took ideas from inside and outside of the health sector and transformed them into a set of possible actions. In essence, it provided a framework for public health communities to seek alliances with other sectors.[13]

Importantly, health promotion and the Ottawa Charter are not without critique. First, it is well recognized that, despite the charter's acknowledgement of equity as a prerequisite for health,[14] health promotion has tended to over-emphasize individual health behaviours and the mechanisms that enable healthy choices.[15] Such behaviourally oriented health promotion strategies concentrate efforts on reducing health risks via behaviour change such as smoking and physical activity to improve health status. However, these efforts, when applied at the population level, are shown to be minimally effective in reducing social inequities as the root causes of poor health and well-being.[16]

A second major critique of the charter concerns its embedded systems of power and privilege, which can be seen through a critical analysis of the context of its development. For example, despite the charter's positioning as globally relevant and committed to "Health for All," the charter's core authors did not reflect global representation.[17] With primary authorship from Europe and Canada and lack of representation from non-western countries, the charter's development and some of its content reflect global inequities of power and privilege.[18] Using Canada as an example, the colonial causes of inequities among Indigenous Peoples (rooted in legacies of racism and white supremacy), along with the immense significance of Indigenous world views around health and ways of knowing, were largely ignored in the Canadian contribution to the charter.[19] Notably, more recent efforts are working to try to redress these earlier failures.[20]

Government Health Promotion in Contemporary Alberta

In Alberta, health promotion efforts have taken different forms, which have varied in the extent of their alignment with Ottawa Charter principles. From a government administration point of view, in 1981, the provincial department responsible for public health created a Health Promotion and Protection Directorate comprising six programs, which gives some insight into what health promotion was (narrowly) understood to entail at that time in government: community health nursing, environmental health, nutrition, dental services, family planning, and health promotion/lifestyle programs.[21] Following the 1986 release of the Ottawa Charter, Alberta's health units, which formed the health services delivery infrastructure in the province until the mid-1990s, shifted their language to adopt health promotion tenets. Importantly, however, as argued by Nancy Kotani and Ann Goldblatt, and consistent with broader critiques of health promotion noted above, in reality the health units remained focused on educational campaigns designed to modify risk behaviours in individuals.[22]

In 1989, the Premier's Commission on the Future of Health Care in Alberta published their final report, The Rainbow Report: Our Vision for Health (The Rainbow Report), which presented a conceptual vision for health in Alberta. The Rainbow Report appeared to embrace the notion of health promotion, but once again it reduced the concept to a rather narrow focus on health education and lifestyle changes, leaving aside the other actions areas outlined in the Ottawa Charter, such as those that focused on strengthening environments and empowering communities.[23] Moreover, and consistent with equity-related critiques of health promotion noted earlier in this chapter, although the rainbow as a symbol of LGBTQ2S+ pride and allyship dates to 1978, the use of rainbow in this 1989 report does not appear to embrace that allyship, but rather speaks to optimism and diversity more generically.[24]

In 1990, the provincial Health Promotion Directorate was renamed the Health Promotion Branch and was included under the Public Health Division of the Department of Health.[25] The branch disappeared in name during the department's restructuring in the mid-1990s, but health promotion activities in the province continued.[26] Notably, one of the main goals for the provincial Department of Health (1988–1999) and then Health and Wellness (1999–2012) was to "improve the health and wellness of Albertans through provincial strategies for protection, *promotion* and prevention" (italics added).[27] Importantly, however, and as discussed in chapters 2 and 4, that language during that time period in particular reflected an ideological orientation that was highly contrary to a broad version of public health because it focused on individual responsibility for health as a way to save money in the health care system. When the department was renamed Alberta Health in 2012, Public Health and Wellness was included as a division within health services, and after the NDP election victory of 2015, the department was reorganized once again to include a Health and Wellness Promotion Division within Public Health and Compliance.[28] At least in the general structure of the department, the public health administration, including health promotion, seems to have moved up one administrative level during the NDP government period, perhaps (pending future critical analysis with the benefit of hindsight) speaking to health promotion's importance from the point of view of that government.

Focal Area: Maternal and Child Health

We next describe three examples of health promotion strategies across Alberta's history in our focal area of maternal/child health. We define maternal health as the health of women during pregnancy, childbirth, and the postpartum period.[29] We define child health as "the extent to which individual children or groups of children are able or enabled to i) develop and realize their potential, ii) satisfy their needs, and iii) develop the capacities that allow them to interact successfully with their biological, physical, and social environments."[30] This definition echoes the principles of the Ottawa Charter, including a view of health as a positive concept and as a resource for everyday life, with the important contemporary recognition that this positive concept of health is not the lived experience of many children, especially children from Black, Indigenous, or racialized communities in health and social care systems.[31]

Pregnancy, childbirth, and childhood have significant implications for the physical, mental, and socio-economic well-being of women and children, families, and societies more generally; indeed, the early childhood period is considered to be a key social determinant of health.[32] While much effort has been placed on the clinical management of maternal and child health and illness, our focus in this chapter is those non-clinical interventions, including school health promotion, preventive health services for mothers and children, and maternal and parental leave allowances, which potentially align with a broad version of public health as conceptualized for this book.

Example 1: Preventive Health Services for Mothers and Children

Early efforts to improve maternal and child health in Alberta were prompted in part by statistics on infant (see Figure 10.1) and maternal mortality, both of which were high in the early decades of the twentieth century. For example, Alberta's maternal mortality rate in 1921 was 6.7 per 1,000 live births, which was higher than all other Canadian provinces (excluding Québec, which did not report maternal mortality that year).[33] In a 1930 publication, Deputy Minister of Public Health, Dr. Malcolm Bow raised alarm about maternal mortality, arguing that "if, during the year 1928, ninety-four mothers in Alberta had been burned to death or more than 1,300 mothers in Canada [the number of pregnancy related deaths in Canada] had been drowned, the shock of such a tragedy would have swept the nation. The lives of our mothers have been held far too cheaply."[34]

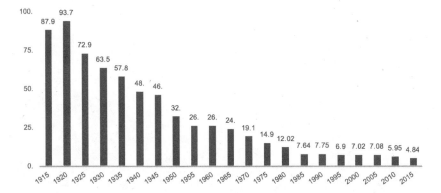

Fig. 10.1: Infant mortality in Alberta, 1915 to 2015. Number of deaths under one year of age, per 1,000 live births, per year. Source: Alberta Provincial Vital Statistics Reports and publications, 1915 to 2015.

The earliest and perhaps clearest example of organized health promotion-like activities on a provincial level is the work of public health nurses. Public health nurses utilized what we might now refer to as health promotion activities to improve maternal and child health across Alberta, including in rural areas. Importantly, although urban/rural disparities in access to preventive health services were a stated concern of government at the time, the absence of a strong social justice orientation is evident in the fact that inequities across other intersecting social identities — such as class, gender, race, and ethnicity — were largely perpetuated by a government and service orientation that assumed a uniform, white Anglo-Saxon, middle-upper class population, with relatively high levels of power and privilege; departures from this norm were viewed as a problem to be solved (see Chapter 1). Additionally, the concentration on educational health promotion activities, with the end goal of behaviour change, is an early signal of an enduring overemphasis on behavioural health promotion strategies noted above.

The early 1920s saw the establishment of child welfare clinics, which were intended to reduce infant mortality by providing education to mothers regarding the care of their children; the clinics illustrate an assumption that lack of knowledge, rather than other factors, was at the root of maternal and child health problems.[35] The first provincial child welfare clinic was established in Edmonton in 1920 and operated twice a week for four hours, at no cost to mothers.[36] Children of pre-school age were "kept well" by the clinic nurses, while cases that required treatment were referred to a family doctor. Child welfare clinics in Medicine Hat and Calgary opened in 1922, and in Vegreville in 1926.[37] By the end of the 1920s it was estimated that approximately 11,000 Albertans (mothers and their children) had been served by these clinics.[38] Speaking to power dynamics built into the service infrastructure, the 1929 annual report of the Department of Public Health expressed pride at the large numbers of "young mothers of foreign birth, especially Ukrainian" — seen as particularly in need of the service due to embedded classism and racism — who had attended the clinics that year.[39]

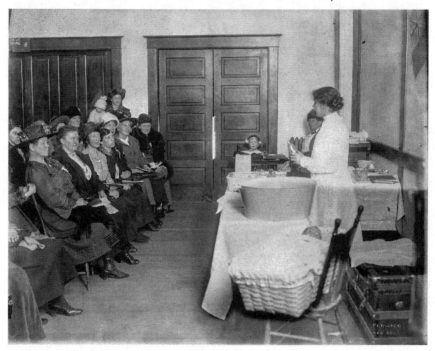

Fig. 10.2: An Alberta public health nurse holding a child welfare clinic (between 1920 and 1927). Source: Provincial Archives of Alberta (Image: A6949).

The largely educational nature of the clinic work, with the stated intent of assisting mothers to raise "better babies and healthier school children, thus giving all a better chance in life,"[40] aligns with the health promotion action area of developing personal skills, that is, supporting personal and social development through providing information, education for health, and enhancing life skills, although in a way that belies the significant inequities embedded in Alberta society and institutions of the time.[41] Contextualized in this way, nurses performed a wide range of activities, including screening and examination for a wide range of concerns including malnutrition, defective teeth, infected tonsils and eye problems. In cases where poor diet or malnutrition was observed in babies, they gave specific advice to mothers about how, when, and what to feed their babies, and breastfeeding was emphasized in most cases. For older children, mothers were given healthy eating tips and educational resources.[42] Other related efforts that align with developing personal skills within this socio-historical context include baby welfare weeks, which included instruction on sterilizing milk bottles, preparing healthy foods, supervision of playtime, breastfeeding as long as possible, and avoiding overuse of medicines; and Travelling Child Welfare Clinics, which provided services in remote rural areas.[43] Public health nurses also made home visits and delivered lectures upon requests from rural school districts.[44]

In addition to recommending improved clinical interventions, such as better obstetrical training and practice, Deputy Health Minister Bow emphasized the importance of adequate and efficient prenatal and postnatal health services in rural areas.[45] This idea aligns to an extent with the health promotion action area of reorienting health services, where the health sector has the responsibility to move beyond clinical and curative services. Indeed, in the context of Alberta's evolving rural public health unit infrastructure, prevention- and promotion-oriented activities for maternal/child health were prominent. Reorienting health services in the Ottawa Charter was intended to "support the needs of individuals and communities for a healthier life, and open channels between the health sector and broader social, political, economic, and physical environmental components." Although embedded assumptions around class and ethnicity meant limited attention to the broader social, political, and economic components now recognized as essential to health promotion, these historical efforts convey an understanding that different groups and sectors, including governments and institutions, had a shared responsibility to "work together toward a health care system which contributes to the pursuit of health."[46] Notably, by the 1960s, there had been a significant decrease in overall maternal mortality. In that year, only seven maternal deaths were registered with a rate of 1.8 deaths per 10,000 live births, the lowest of all the provinces.[47]

In 2018, Alberta Health Services provides well child services in clinics in urban and rural areas around the province. As in the past, the contemporary clinics are staffed by public health nurses and provide both standardized immunization, such as vaccinations for children after two months of age, and non-immunization services. However, service delivery is now considerably more streamlined, specialized, and "patient/family-centered."[48] These trends have occurred within a broader neoliberal context of public sector cuts and individualization of responsibility for health as they have intersected with regionalization of health care services in Alberta. Compared to the past, concerns around diverse aspects of equity are now explicit in at least some areas of public health service delivery.[49] However, considering the harmful legacies of the past, and the neoliberal context of the present, a considerable amount of work remains to be done.

Example 2: Mothers' Allowances and Parental Leaves

Notwithstanding criticisms for overconcentration on behavioural health promotion strategies, the intention of health promotion as expressed in the Ottawa Charter includes healthy public policy, which recognizes that health and well-being are strongly influenced by public policy in various domains, not just health care. Healthy public policy is similar to the contemporary notion of a "health-in-all policies" orientation, where health and health equity implications of policy and legislation in all sectors — not just health — are considered.[50] A healthy public policy aims to overcome the formidable obstacles presented by political, social, or economic power disparities that create inequitable access to health-promoting resources (see also Chapter 12).

One example of public policy to foster equity and promote health for mothers and children is government-mandated support for parents during the first years of their child's life. *Parental leaves* are a contemporary version of support that usually consists of a timeframe away from the workplace with a guarantee of job protection, accompanied in some circumstances by partial wage replacement and benefits.[51] Importantly, despite their supportive intentions, these arrangements can create and perpetuate social inequity: some parents are excluded because their work is part-time, they are self-employed, or they have not worked for a sufficient length of time to qualify; these circumstances, moreover, may intersect with other social axes associated with more limited power and privilege.[52] Mothers' allowances, which refer to financial benefits received from governments when fathers were absent, were a precursor to contemporary parental leaves, which allow mothers to better take care of their children by alleviating financial concerns.

In the paragraphs below, we track the historical evolution of these two policies in Alberta and examine the rhetoric behind them to explore whether or the extent to which they were conceived as a healthy public policy. A main source used is the *Alberta Legislative Hansard*, which provides a marker of the ways in which policy makers in Alberta understood and discussed such issues.

MOTHERS' ALLOWANCES

Physical and psychological damages from the First World War and high mortality rates from the influenza pandemic of 1918–1919 led to the absence or incapacity of many husbands in Albertan families.[53] Within the gendered and heteronormative context of the time, Alberta's Mothers' Allowance Act, ascended in 1919, stated that widows or wives of incapacitated husbands who had children could apply for relief in their municipality.[54] The act specified that any widow or wife of a person committed to a sanatorium or jail, who had children in her custody, and who was "unable to take proper care" of her child or children, may "apply to an inspector of the city or town of which she is a resident for assistance." The inspector would present the case to the Superintendent of Neglected and Dependent Children for approval, who would in turn recommend to the attorney general the amount of payment to be given weekly. More and more mothers joined the program as time passed, and by 1925, 825 women in the province were receiving allowances.[55]

At first, within the racially unequal context, the rhetoric behind the mothers' allowances appealed to the white patriarchal view (there is far less attention to the experiences of non-white people in Alberta at that time) that it was the main job of women to raise children to be productive members of society. Both Liberal and United Farmers of Alberta governments viewed children as assets of the province.[56] In cases where husbands could not fulfill their role as providers, the state had to step in to help mothers in their responsibility for "the creation of a valuable product: healthy, morally upstanding children."[57] Recipients were expected to pursue gendered and Anglo middle-class ideals of mothers and housekeepers, and were subject to supervision accordingly.[58] According to Canadian historian Amy Kaler, mothers' allowances were emblematic of the belief that children made it impossible for women to be self-sufficient because care of children was to take precedence over paid work; women receiving the allowance were expected to be good (paid) workers and engage in paid labour to the extent it did not interfere with childrearing.[59] That said, in some jurisdictions such as Ontario, the allowances were deliberately set at low levels, thus necessitating paid work and illustrating the reality that women's paid work could not usually support a family.[60]

Some acknowledgement of a relationship between mothers' allowances and health of children was present early on; the Alberta program was even housed within the provincial Department of Public Health during the late 1930s and early 1940s.[61] However, this connection was made more evident after World War II; in 1945, for example, one MLA stated that "Mothers' allowances should be used for the purpose they were first intended, for children's health. They should not be considered a donation."[62] Although this statement suggests somewhat of a shift in government perspective — from entrusting mothers with the responsibility of raising good citizens during the previous decades to a concern for raising healthy ones — the underlying gendered rhetoric persisted. Infant mortality was an important concern and putting responsibility on women, in a way that assumed and conveyed class and racial uniformity, was seen as one way to address it.[63]

PARENTAL LEAVES

The evolution of parental leave benefits in Alberta and Canada is complex. Briefly, as increasing numbers of women entered the labour market during the 1960s and 1970s, the model of support for mothers and parents changed; this was part of the broader welfare state development in the second half of the twentieth century.[64] In Canada, the federal government initiated a national program in 1971, where new mothers could claim up to fifteen weeks of maternity leave including benefits, such as extended health benefits. Two decades later, in 1990, ten weeks of parental leave were introduced with the new provision that either parent could use them and that mothers could add them to the existing maternity leave provision.[65] In December 2000, parental leave was increased further to thirty-five weeks, such that mothers could take up to a full year (fifteen weeks maternity leave plus thirty-five parental leave). During the maternal / parental leave periods, employees under the federal legislation were to receive 55 percent of their salary from federal funds through the Employment Insurance program.[66] Finally, in 2017 the federal government extended the benefits to eighteen months, if the employees chose to, but in this case, parents would receive 33 percent of their original salary during the final six months, with the continued guarantee of having their job back.[67] Nonetheless, and significant from an equity point of view, the benefits continue to be restricted to a subset of parents because qualifying for employment insurance parental benefits requires a minimum accumulation of six hundred insured hours of paid employment.[68] It thus excludes or obstructs those who are not in the paid labour force, and those in precarious work circumstances, which tends to co-occur with other marginalized social identities.[69]

As the seventh province in Canada to do so, Alberta was a laggard in enacting parental leave legislation.[70] In 1975, the provincial government introduced an amendment to the Alberta Labour Act (passed in 1976), stating that the Labour Board had the power to order an employer to grant a maternity leave without pay (that guaranteed job protection) for up to twelve weeks before and six weeks after the birth of the child.[71] However, this legislation did not apply to all employers until 1980 when it became "universal and mandatory," albeit with the significant proviso that the mother had been an employee for at least twelve months.[72] In 1998, a *Calgary Herald* newspaper article stated, "while the length of maternity leave in Alberta is in line with other provinces, this is the only province that doesn't also provide for parental leave."[73] It was not until 2001 that the provincial government saw fit to extend the leave to both parents, thereby matching the federal legislative context and showing some indication of a (belated) shift away from the relatively privileged and cis-gendered views that childcare responsibility primarily lies with the mother. At the time of writing, in Alberta, and again significant from an equity point of view, leaves continue to be contingent on employment circumstances, and employees are eligible for maternity and parental leave if they have been employed at least ninety days with the same employer. Employers are not required to pay wages or benefits during leave, in which case the funds come from the federal Employment Insurance program.[74] These parameters are out of step with prominent characteristics of the contemporary labour market, including growing numbers of poorly-paid, insecure, and non-unionized jobs with no benefits, which are disproportionately held by racialized people who are most negatively affected during periods of crisis, such as the COVID-19 pandemic.[75]

PARENTAL LEAVES AS HEALTHY PUBLIC POLICY

Several studies have demonstrated the health benefits, and to a lesser extent, health equity benefits, of parental leaves. For example, using data from sixteen Organisation for Economic Co-operation and Development countries from 1969 to 1994, economist Christopher Ruhm showed that longer parental leave was linked to marked decreases in pediatric mortality, especially for health outcomes "where a causal effect is most plausible," that is, outcomes seen to be preventable via supportive policy, including post neonatal mortality (deaths between twenty-eight days and one year of age) and child fatalities (deaths between the first and fifth birthdays).[76] Effects on perinatal mortality (fetal deaths and deaths in the first week), neonatal mortality (deaths in the first twenty-seven days), and the incidence of low birth weight, were less pronounced, thus speaking to the validity of the effect.[77] Economist Sakiko Tanaka extended Ruhm's data to 2005 and confirmed the noticeable decrease in child mortality rates with longer parental leave periods.

A study published that same year by social work researcher Lawrence Berger found that mothers' early return to work was substantially linked to reduced breastfeeding and immunizations rates, based on data from the United States.[78] On the other hand, economists Qian Liu and Oskar N. Skans found no impact of increasing parental leaves from twelve to fifteen weeks in Sweden on child health.[79] Economist and health researcher Maya Rossin-Slater and others found that longer maternity leave duration had positive effects on child health outcomes, but only as long as mothers had family support or a secondary income during the leave duration.[80] Overall, there is evidence to support the benefits of parental leaves on child health outcomes, but the effects may depend on context, such as the presence of other forms of support, including policy-level and interpersonal, and vary by health outcome, speaking to an ongoing need for robust equity-oriented research in healthy public policy.

Alberta legislators did not make the connection between health and maternity or parental leave explicitly until the early 2000s. Prior to that, they appeared to believe they were unconnected. For example, during the first session of the 1975 legislature, Alberta NDP Leader Grant Notley inquired about the introduction of maternity leaves and what the conservative government was doing about it. Notley mentioned that he first directed his inquiries to the minister of social services and health, which was responsible for public health at the time, but was referred to the minister of labour, suggesting that maternity leaves were not viewed as falling within the domain of health.[81]

In recent years, in contrast, health has been mobilized to justify increasing the length of parental leaves. For example, when debating the province's Employment Standards Amendment Act relating to Parental Leave (Bill 209) in 2000, MLA Wayne Cao (PC) stated that the potential benefits of the bill were clear when he said, "study after study shows that the early relationship between parent and child is one of the most critical factors in determining the future health and happiness and success of a child."[82] LeRoy Johnson (PC) likewise spoke in support of increasing parental leave, on health grounds when he stated that "long leaves of over 20 weeks are associated with better maternal health, as measured by mental health, vitality, and role function, whereas the reverse is true for short to moderate leaves of 12 to 20 weeks." Johnson remarked on the benefits of longer leaves for breastfeeding and, in turn, decreasing disease incidence. He cited statistics from Ruhm's report, arguing that "those numbers cannot be ignored." Consistent with a healthy public policy perspective, Johnson furthermore acknowledged broader benefits of extended parental leave, "not only for children and parents but also for employers and the wider society. These advantages include better maternal and child health and well-being, increased time investment of parents in their children's early years, increased retention of female employees, decreased recruitment costs, and improved labour market status for women."[83]

While Alberta lawmakers did not initially recognize the health and health equity implications of mothers' allowances and parental leaves, years after they were first proposed or debated, health benefits were mobilized to justify both policies. These examples suggest a shift in this policy domain, albeit a slow and partial one, toward a health-in-all-policies orientation, which recognizes that "government objectives are best achieved when all sectors include health and well-being as a key component of policy development" and — along with health equity — the orientation is a central tenet of health promotion under the action area of building healthy public policy.

Example 3: Health Promotion in Schools

Our final example of health promotion deals with efforts to improve the health of young people in schools. For better or for worse (with colonial residential schools being the clearest example of the latter), schools have long been at the forefront of state-directed efforts regarding health. However, the ways in which these efforts were deployed changed throughout the twentieth century, reflecting shifting cultural attitudes and priorities. We first describe some early public health interventions in a settler-colonial context that focused on school-based immunization. Then, to demonstrate the changing nature of how health was addressed in schools, we examine a shift that occurred in Alberta's provincial junior high health curriculum during the 1950s and 1960s, followed by acknowledgement of a much more recent shift toward the adoption of the comprehensive school health approach. Overall, these health interventions are seen through the lens of the Ottawa Charter for Health Promotion's action areas of developing personal skills and building healthy public policy. These events played out in contexts that were largely ignorant to or exclusionary with respect to social inequities along dimensions such as class and race.

MEDICAL INSPECTIONS AND IMMUNIZATION IN SCHOOLS

Some of the earliest settler school-based public health initiatives in Alberta perhaps align more with prevention than with health promotion; nonetheless, they are illustrative of the long-standing importance of the school setting in public health. Edmonton's first city health officer, Dr. Thomas H. Whitelaw, wrote in 1914 that "medical inspection of school children has come to stay, and . . . it is to become an increasingly important factor in obtaining the maximum of mental and physical efficiency for future generations."[84] Whitelaw thus conveyed the viewpoint that schools represented an institution well suited to the aims of those who concerned themselves with public health.

Whitelaw's comments stemmed, in part, from his experience about six years earlier, when he had been at the forefront of one of the earliest major public health interventions in Alberta that affected schools: compulsory smallpox vaccinations.[85] In response to considerable backlash from parents who were opposed to their children being vaccinated, Whitelaw authored a piece in the *Edmonton Bulletin* where he doubled down on the importance of vaccinations for school-aged children.[86] For proponents of vaccination, especially those working within the Department of Public Health, making vaccination mandatory was seen as the most effective way to control smallpox, and the benefit of vaccinating children in particular was emphasized.[87] Indeed, Alberta's inaugural Public Health Act of 1907 included a provision that allowed educational authorities, such as school boards, to pass regulations to deny admittance to schools for unvaccinated pupils.[88]

In response to this call, and speaking to the power held by the early, medically focused version of public health, school boards moved to pass rules to make schools the sites of mandatory vaccinations. An early example was the Bowden Public School District in Central Alberta, which implemented compulsory smallpox vaccination of all pupils attending school sometime before 1906. In the absence of a doctor, the vaccinations were performed by pupils, taught by one of the teachers, with some of the very young students being vaccinated by their parents.[89] In 1908, the Edmonton School Board ruled that students had to have proof of vaccination against smallpox to be allowed to attend school.[90]

These efforts tied early public health and education systems together intimately: schools were not just passive sites of public health intervention, but active partners in the public health apparatus. Now, if parents wanted their children to attend school, they had to buy into a certain version of community-based and expert (largely physician) driven conceptualization of health. This conceptualization was often challenged to varying degrees of success. For example, the 1915 Edmonton School Board policy was quickly challenged and subsequently ruled irreconcilable with the Truancy Act by the Alberta Supreme Court as it prohibited students from attending school despite the act making school attendance mandatory.[91] The policy was repealed and the School Board was ordered to admit students without proof of vaccination.[92] Overall, the story of mandatory vaccination for Alberta school children illustrates ways in which the school could be a battleground — for public health officials, teachers, parents, and politicians — over the direction of public health, and should prompt thoughtful consideration of how to build healthy public policy while respectfully engaging stakeholders with differing views and different levels of power and voice.[93]

Schools remained central to public health during the mid-twentieth century. In a contrasting example, we next examine changes in Alberta's provincial curriculum for health in the 1950s and 1960s.

HEALTH AND THE CURRICULUM

Using curriculum guides for junior high schools that applied to all public schools in the province, we identify a particular turn in approach and content that illustrates the interplay between the nature of public health promotion in schools and popular, and at times hegemonic, conceptualizations of health.

The Junior High School Curriculum Guides for Health and Personal Development are used by all public schools at the junior high level in Alberta. Generally formed through close consultation between the Department of Health and the Department of Education, these documents reflect the high-level vision for health education in schools, as well as granular direction on, for example, the type of videos to show, guest speakers to invite, and books to read. Evidence suggests that throughout the 1950s, the Department of Public Health had considerable impact on the curriculum and revisions suggested by various members of that department were incorporated.[94] Therefore, a close examination of these curricula permits exploration of approaches to public health promotion in schools over time, including embedded dimensions of equity and power.

In the 1950s, the provincial health curricula seemed to place considerable emphasis on the individual as the main site of responsibility for health, somewhat humorously typified by an assignment from 1952 that encouraged students to write an essay on the topic Others are Inconvenienced When I am Ill.[95] This individual orientation was furthermore infused with a moral dimension. In 1951, for example, the Junior High School Curriculum Guide *for Health and Personal Development* (italics added) proclaimed its mandate as, "to encourage the objective analysis of personal problems common to adolescents and to foster the development of wholesome attitudes."[96] Subsequent curriculum guides produced during the 1950s emphasized personal responsibility for health through the development of a moral toolkit. Through the lens of the Ottawa Charter, and consistent with the critique of overemphasis on behaviourally oriented health promotion, these actions can be understood as early, historically situated attempts to build personal skills, teaching students to understand their own agency and responsibility within their community. However, as historian of education Mona Lee Gleason has noted in the context of sexual education, "sex educators . . . continued to conflate sex education with lessons in acceptable moral conduct."[97] Although teachers were encouraged to "avoid moralizing," the expectation was that students would develop a strong set of core values, with "faith in ideals" through the careful guidance of their educators.[98]

In these curricula, although health was tied to the morals of the individual, it was also associated with acceptance in the community. As the 1953 curriculum guide put it, "everyone wants to be popular — to be liked for himself. The relationship of popularity to one's personal habits, to the way he talks, and acts in 'company,' to the impression he gives to those around him can well be discussed in the group . . . [the curriculum] suggests ways in which the individual can 'sell' himself to the world with which he is in contact."[99] This is not to suggest that schools were in the business of legislating personalities, but instead to highlight the extent to which health was viewed as one part of a certain, holistic definition of self. A morally well-developed student would be popular (as a reward for their morally appropriate behaviours) and, in turn, would be a student who made positive choices for their health.

By the next decade, however, things had changed. By 1961, health and personal development had been separated, and the curriculum guide was titled *Junior High School Curriculum Guide for Health* (italics added). The name change reflects the shift in content, as principles of individual morality ceded ground to the pragmatic idea of helping students "come to know health principles which they can apply in daily living."[100] By at least the mid-1960s, students were encouraged to see themselves as part of a greater concept of "national health," and there was a focus on enabling students to navigate their larger communities armed with knowledge of "functional health."[101] This new model emphasized students' role as members of somewhat homogenous communities, an identity that carried rights and responsibilities relevant to both individual and community health.

Illustrative of this shift is the changing ways in which curriculum guides discussed the concept of overweight. In 1952, the curriculum guide admonished teachers to "discuss the causes of overweight. Emphasize that it usually results from overeating."[102] By 1964, teachers were instead encouraged to get students to think about diet using Canada's Food Guide to ensure regular meals, and appreciate that "concern about being overweight or underweight should be discussed with one's doctor."[103] The earlier, somewhat singular approach that centered on individualized preventive behaviours such as not overeating, gave way to a more medically grounded regimen of health promotion that was based around a systematized understanding of nutrition, codified by Canada's Food Guide and in consultation with experts, including health professionals and scientists. While remaining largely exclusionary and/or ignorant of many dimensions of equity, these resources allowed school-based health interventions to transform from a moral and individual appeal to an apparently scientifically rigorous and community-based appeal. Overall, the efforts described in the junior high health curricula illustrate subtle shifts in how efforts to enable school children to take control over their health may manifest, including which perspectives are privileged or excluded.

Since the 1990s, and illustrative of growing alignment with health promotion principles, there has been a significant trend in Alberta toward comprehensive school health, which is an internationally recognized, evidence-based approach for building healthy school communities. At the time of writing, Alberta Health Services supported all school authorities in the province in using the comprehensive school health approach to improve student health and educational outcomes.[104] The approach uses a community development process and has four components: teaching and learning, social and physical environments, partnerships and services, and policy to create healthy school communities. With this broad orientation, use of the comprehensive school health framework may help to address a variety of health issues, such as healthy eating, substance use, mental health, tobacco use reduction, injury, and physical activity. The comprehensive school health approach is heavily anchored in the Ottawa Charter, and its strengths include its attention to multi-level and intersectoral processes.[105] Another example of comprehensive school health is Ever Active Schools, a charity that works directly with Alberta schools to support wellness education and build capacity through projects and competency-based based learning to improve health and social outcomes of children and youth in Alberta. Through collaborative partnerships and knowledge exchange, Ever Active Schools uses a multi-sectoral approach, centres Indigenous populations, and is funded through a collaboration between government ministries, thus providing an example of healthy public policy.[106]

To ensure its ambition of student well-being, critical analysis of comprehensive school health initiatives — which to date is relatively limited — is important to ensure, for example, that the focus on behavioural health promotion, such as physical activity and healthy eating, does not preclude careful attention to population-level equity considerations that may be at play before students come to the school setting. [107] Moreover, such initiatives must always be situated critically within the broader — and currently highly problematic — ideological and political economic context of Alberta education.[108]

Conclusions

In this chapter we provide examples of what are now called health promotion actions that occurred throughout Alberta's public health history and which must be situated critically within socio-historical context including concern — or lack thereof — with dimensions of equity and inclusion. Preventive health services to new mothers and their children, deployed by public health nurses in local settings such as child welfare clinics, illustrate some elements of health promotion strategies of reorienting health services and developing personal skills, although in a context that was largely exclusionary or ignorant to equity along dimensions such as class and race. The mothers' allowance and subsequent parental leave legislation served as examples of building healthy public policy, where a connection with health was not initially recognized but evolved over time. Finally, health promotion in schools resembles the health promotion action areas of developing personal skills — in some cases with explicit moral connotations — and healthy public policy where early experience in Alberta provides a lesson of where policies such as tying vaccinations to school attendance, contributed to or emphasized fault lines of conflict. Although recent trends concerning comprehensive school health may indicate growing alignment with health promotion principles, these must be interpreted in the broader political economic context of public sector cuts and orientations that threaten to erode health and well-being for all Albertans.[109]

NOTES

1   For examples of health-promotion activities in Alberta, see Wilfreda E. Thurston et al., *Health Promotion Effectiveness in Alberta: Providing the Tools for Healthy Albertans: Summary Report on the Review of the Effectiveness of Health Promotion Strategies in Alberta* (Edmonton: Alberta Health and Wellness, 1999).

2   Alberta Health Services, "The Comprehensive School Health Approach," accessed 22 August 2020, https://www.albertahealthservices.ca/info/csh.aspx.

3   "The Ottawa Charter for Health Promotion," WHO Global Health Promotion Conferences, World Health Organization, accessed 22 August 2020, https://www.who.int/healthpromotion/conferences/previous/ottawa/en/.

4   World Health Organization (WHO), "Ottawa Charter for Health Promotion — Charte D'ottawa pour la Promotion de la Santé," *Canadian Journal of Public Health / Revue Canadienne de Santé Publique* 77, no. 6, Special Health Promotion Issue (November/December 1986).

5   Louise Potvin and Catherine M. Jones, "Twenty-five Years after the Ottawa Charter: The Critical Role of Health Promotion for Public Health," *Canadian Journal of Public Health* 102, no. 4 (2011); WHO, "Ottawa Charter."

6   WHO, "Ottawa Charter."

7   Potvin and Jones, "Twenty-five Years," 244.

8   Potvin and Jones, "Twenty-five Years," 244; WHO, *Constitution of the World Health Organization*, adopted by the International Health Conference, New York, 19 June to 22 July 1946.

9   Marc Lalonde, *A New Perspective on the Health of Canadians: A Working Document* (Ottawa: Government of Canada, Queen's Printer, 1974).

10   Potvin and Jones, "Twenty-five Years," 244; Lalonde, *A New Perspective*; WHO, *Constitution*; WHO, *Declaration of Alma-Ata. International Conference on Primary Health Care*, Alma-Ata, USSR, 6–12 September 1978, https://cdn.who.int/media/docs/default-source/documents/almaata-declaration-en.pdf?sfvrsn=7b3c2167_2.

11   WHO, "Ottawa Charter."

12   Trevor Hancock, "The Ottawa Charter at 25," *Canadian Journal of Public Health* 102, no. 6 (2011): 404.

13   Hancock, "Charter at 25," 404; Potvin and Jones, "Twenty-five Years," 245.

14   WHO, "Ottawa Charter."

15   Fran Baum and Matthew Fisher, "Why Behavioural Health Promotion Endures despite Its Failure to Reduce Health Inequities," *Sociology of Health & Illness* 36, no. 2 (2014), https://doi.org/10.1111/1467-9566.12112.

16   Baum and Fisher, "Behavioural Health Promotion."

17   Karen McPhail-Bell, Bronwyn Fredericks, and Mark Brough, "Beyond the Accolades: A Postcolonial Critique of the Foundations of the Ottawa Charter," *Global Health Promotion* 20, no. 2 (June 1, 2013), https://doi.org/10.1177/1757975913490427.

18   McPhail-Bell, Fredericks, and Brough, "Beyond the Accolades."

19   McPhail-Bell, Fredericks, and Brough, "Beyond the Accolades."

20   Brittany Wenniserí:iostha Jock et al., "Dismantling the Status Quo: Promoting Policies for Health, Well-Being and Equity: An IUHPE2022 Prelude," *Global Health Promotion* 29, no. 1 (0 March 2022), https://doi.org/10.1177/17579759211019214.

21   Alberta Department of Social Services and Community Health, *Annual Report 1981–1982* (Edmonton, 1983), 27.

22   Nancy Kotani and Ann Goldblatt, "Alberta: A Haven for Health Promotion," in *Health Promotion in Canada: Provincial, National & International Perspectives*, eds. Ann Pederson, Michel O'Neill, Irving Rootman (Toronto: Saunders, 1994), 169.

23   Kotani and Goldblatt, "Alberta: A Haven for Health Promotion," 172.

24   "Rainbow Flag: Origin Story," Gilbert Baker (blog), accessed 17 September 2022, https://gilbertbaker. com/rainbow-flag-origin-story/; Lesbian & Gay Community Services Center (NY), *The Gay Almanac* (New York: Berkley Books, 1996), 94; Premier's Commission on Future Health Care for Albertans and Marion A. Saffran, *The Rainbow Report: Our Vision for Health* (Edmonton: The Commission, 1989), http://archive.org/details/rainbowreportourprem.

25   Alberta Department of Health, *Annual Report 1990–1991* (Edmonton, 1992); Provincial Archives of Alberta, *An Administrative History of the Government of Alberta, 1905–2005* (Edmonton: Provincial Archives of Alberta, 2006), 288.

26   For a small sampling of examples of health promotion activities, see Sharlene Wolbeck Minke et al., *The Evolution of Integrated Chronic Disease Prevention in Alberta, Canada, Preventing Chronic Disease* 3, no. 3, [serial online] (July 2006), http://www.cdc.gov/pcd/issues/2006/jul/05_0225.htm; Kim Raine et al., "Healthy Alberta Communities: Impact of a Three-Year Community-Based Obesity and Chronic Disease Prevention Intervention," *Preventive Medicine* 57, no. 6 (1 December 2013), https://doi.org/10.1016/j.ypmed.2013.08.024); Candace I. J. Nykiforuk et al., "Community Health and the Built Environment: Examining Place in a Canadian Chronic Disease Prevention Project," *Health Promotion International* 28, no. 2 (June 2013), doi.org/10.1093/heapro/dar093.

27   Alberta Ministry of Health and Wellness, *Annual Report 2003/2004*, 15.

28   Alberta Ministry of Health, *Annual Report 2013–14* (Edmonton, 2014), 6; Alberta Ministry of Health, *Annual Report 2018–2019* (Edmonton, 2019), 11; Alberta Ministry of Health, *Annual Report 2016–17* (Edmonton, 2017), 11.

29   "Maternal Infant Health (0–2 Yrs)," Canadian Best Practices Portal, Public Health Agency of Canada, modified 19 June 2015, http://cbpp-pcpe.phac-aspc.gc.ca/public-health-topics/maternal-infant-health/.

30   National Research Council, *Children's Health, the Nation's Wealth: Assessing and Improving Child Health* (Washington, D.C.: National Academies Press, 2004), https://www.ncbi.nlm.nih.gov/books/NBK92198/.

31   WHO, "Ottawa Charter for Health Promotion," National Collaborating Centre for Aboriginal Health, *Indigenous Children and the Child Welfare System in Canada* (Prince George, BC: National Collaborating Centre for Aboriginal Health, 2017), https://www.nccih.ca/docs/health/FS-ChildWelfareCanada-EN.pdf; National Collaborating Centre for Determinants of Health, *Let's Talk: Racism and Health Equity (Rev. ed.)* (Antigonish, NS: National Collaborating Centre for Determinants of Health, St. Francis Xavier University, 2018).

32   Clyde Hertzman and Tom Boyce, "How Experience gets under the Skin to Create Gradients in Developmental Health," *Annual Review of Public Health* 31 (2010).

33   Canada Dominion Bureau of Statistics, *The Canada Year Book 1922–23* (Ottawa: Minister of Trade and Commerce, F.A. Acland, 1924), 203.

34   Malcolm Bow, "Maternal Mortality As A Public Health Problem," *Canadian Medical Association Journal* 23, no. 2 (1930): 172.

35   Adelaide Schartner, *Health Units of Alberta* (Edmonton: Health Unit Association of Alberta, 1982).

36   Janet C. Ross-Kerr, *Prepared to Care: Nurses and Nursing in Alberta* (Edmonton: University of Alberta Press, 1998), 77.

37   Sharon Richardson, "Alberta's Provincial Travelling Clinic, 1924–42," *Canadian Bulletin of Medical History* 19, no. 1 (2002).

38   Paul Victor Collins, "The Public Health Policies of the United Farmers of Alberta Government, 1921–1935" (Ph.D. diss., University of Western Ontario, 1969).

39   Alberta Department of Public Health, *Annual Report of the Department of Public Health, 1929* (Edmonton: W.D. McLean, King's Printer, 1931).

40   Edna Kells, "Travel Clinic Does Fine Work," *Calgary Herald*, 5 November 1929, 17.

41   WHO, "Ottawa Charter."

42   Edna Kells, "Over Twenty-Five Hundred Children Pass Through Clinics," *Edmonton Journal*, 1 November 1929, 22.

43   Amy Kaler, *Baby Trouble in the Last Best West: Making New People in Alberta, 1905–1939* (Toronto: University of Toronto Press, 2017), 155.

44   Richardson, "Alberta's Provincial Travelling Clinic," 6.

45   Collins, *Public Health Policies*, 119.

46   WHO, "Ottawa Charter."

47   Alberta Department of Public Health, "Annual Report of the Division of Vital Statistics," *Annual Report 1962* (Edmonton: L. S. Wall, Printer of the Queen's Most Excellent Majesty, 1964), 4.

48   Alberta Health Services, *Alberta Health Services Well Child Clinic Standardization and the Postpartum Depression Screening Policy — Information for Physicians* (June 2019), https://www.albertahealthservices.ca/assets/info/hp/hcf/if-hp-hcf-wccs-ppd-info-for-physicians.pdf.

49   Michelle Kilborn et al., "Addressing health inequities in environmental public health in Alberta," *Environmental Health Review* 62, no. 4 (2019).

50   Marcello Tonelli, Kwok-Cho Tang, and Pierre-Gerlier Forest, "Canada needs a "Health in All Policies" action plan now," *Canadian Medical Association Journal* 192, no. 3 (Jan 2020), https://www.cmaj.ca/content/192/3/E61.

51   In Alberta, birth and adoptive parents can take up to sixty-two weeks of unpaid parental leave and receive salary and benefits through Canada's federal Employment Insurance (EI). In Canada, paid leave is usually at 55 percent of the salary. *Employment Standards Amendment Act*, S.A., 2001, c. 6. In Quebec, mothers can receive thirty weeks at 70 percent pay, complemented with twenty-five weeks at 55 percent pay.

52   Jody Heymann and M. S. Kramer, "Public Policy and Breast-Feeding: A Straightforward and Significant Solution," *Canadian Journal of Public Health* 100, no. 5 (2009).

53   Kaler, *Baby Trouble*, 115–116.

54   *Act Granting Assistance to Widowed Mothers Supporting Children*, S.P.A., 1919, c. 6.

55   Kaler, *Baby Trouble*, 113.

56   Kaler, *Baby Trouble*, 121.

57   This "historical" rhetoric is interesting from the perspective of contemporary events in Alberta. The 'women in politics' essay competition was held in 2022 as an initiative of the provincial United Conservative Party, which unearthed quite similar views about women by some of the contestants. Jessika Guse, "Status of Women Minister Apologizes for Racist, Sexist Essay Contest in Alberta," *Global News*, 9 August 2022, https://globalnews.ca/news/9047574/ucp-essay-contest-winner-ndp-reaction-outrage/; Kaler, *Baby Trouble*, 110.

58   James Struthers, *The Limits of Affluence: Welfare in Ontario, 1920--1970* (Toronto: University of Toronto Press, 1994), 34.

59   Kaler, *Baby Trouble*, 108.

60   Struthers, *The Limits of Affluence*.

61   Alberta Department of Public Health, *Annual Report 1938* (Edmonton: A. Shnitka, King's Printer, 1939).

62   "House Discusses Future of Grant Paid to Mothers," *Edmonton Bulletin*, 21 March 1945.

63   Kaler, *Baby Trouble*, 148–149.

64   For comparison to parental leave in European countries, see "Detail of Change in Parental Leave by Country," OECD Family Database, accessed 21 August 2020, https://www.oecd.org/els/family/PF2_5_Trends_in_leave_entitlements_around_childbirth_annex.pdf; Christopher J. Ruhm, "The Economic Consequences of Parental Leave Mandates: Lessons from Europe," *Quarterly Journal of Economics* 113, no. 1 (February 1998).

65   Katherine Marshall, "Benefiting from Extended Parental Leave," *Perspectives on Labour and Income* 4, no. 3 (2003), https://www150.statcan.gc.ca/n1/pub/75-001-x/00303/6490-eng.html#:~:text=Starting%20in%201971%2C%20mothers%20with,between%20them%20(HRDC%201996).

66   Marshall, "Benefiting from Extended Parental Leave."

67   Erica Alini, "Federal Budget 2017: Liberals Extend Parental Leave to 18 Months, Boost Childcare Funding," *Global News*, 22 March 2017, https://globalnews.ca/news/3328107/federal-budget-2017-liberals-extend-parental-leave-to-18-months-boost-childcare-funding/; "More Choice for Parents," Employment Insurance Improvements, Employment and Social Development Canada, accessed 21 August 2020, https://www.canada.ca/en/employment-social-development/campaigns/ei-improvements/parental-choice.html.

68   Marshall, "Benefiting from Extended Parental Leave."

69   "Precarious Work on the Rise," Canadian Union of Public Employees, accessed 17 September 2022, https://cupe.ca/precarious-work-rise; "Precarious Employment," Gender & Work Database, accessed 17 September 2022, http://www.genderwork.ca/gwd/thesaurus-main/thesaurus/?term=PRECARIOUS%20EMPLOYMENT&exact=YES.

70   Only Quebec, Prince Edward Island and Newfoundland lacked such legislation at that point. "Maternity Leave Standards Approved," *Edmonton Journal*, 2 December 1976, 25; Alvin Finkel, *Working People in Alberta: A History* (Athabasca, AB: Athabasca University Press, 2012), 259.

71   "Maternity Leave Standards Approved," *Edmonton Journal*.

72	This new maternity leave legislation was included in the Employment Standards Act assented in 1980. *Employment Standards Act*, S.P.A 1980, c. 62 (Division 7); Finkel, *Working People in Alberta*, 259.

73	"Alberta Only Province with No Provision for Parental Leave," *Calgary Herald* (Index-only), 11 July 1998, J1.

74	"Maternity and Parental Leave," Alberta Employment Standards Rules, Alberta Government, accessed 22 August 2020, https://www.alberta.ca/maternity-parental-leave.aspx.

75	Sheila Block and Grace-Edward, Galabuzi. "Canada's Colour Coded Labour Market: The Gap for Racialized Workers". Canadian Centre for Policy Alternatives, March 21, 2011, https://policyalternatives.ca/publications/reports/canadas-colour-coded-labour-market.

76	Christopher J. Ruhm, "Parental Leave and Child Health," *Journal of Health Economics* 19, no. 6 (2000).

77	Leave entitlements are also unrelated to the death rates of senior citizens, suggesting that the models adequately control for unobserved influences on health that are common across ages.

78	Lawrence M. Berger, Jennifer Hill, and Jane Waldfogel, "Maternity Leave, Early Maternal Employment and Child Health and Development in the US," *The Economic Journal* 115, no. 501 (2005).

79	Qian Liu and Oskar Nordstrom Skans, "The Duration of Paid Parental Leave and Children's Scholastic Performance," *The BE Journal of Economic Analysis & Policy* 10, no. 1 (2010).

80	Maya Rossin-Slater et al., "The Effects of California's Paid Family Leave Program on Mothers' Leave-taking and Subsequent Labor Market Outcomes," *Working Paper Series (National Bureau of Economic Research)*, Working Paper No. 17715 (Cambridge, Mass.: National Bureau of Economic Research, 2011).

81	Alberta. Legislative Assembly of Alberta, 13 June 1975 (Grant Notley, NDP), 688, 696.

82	Alberta. Legislative Assembly of Alberta, 15 November 2000 (Wayne Cao, PC), 1891.

83	Alberta. Legislative Assembly of Alberta, 22 November 2000 (LeRoy Johnson, PC), 2062.

84	T. H. Whitelaw, "Medical Inspection of Schools in Edmonton, Alberta," *The Public Health Journal* 5, no. 12 (December 1914): 714; Heber C. Jamieson, *Early Medicine in Alberta: The First Seventy-Five Years* (Edmonton: Canadian Medical Association, Alberta Division, 1947), 147.

85	Schartner, *Health Units of Alberta*, 33.

86	T.H. Whitelaw, "On the Subject of Vaccination," *The Edmonton Bulletin*, 26 September 1908, 8; Schartner, *Health Units of Alberta*, 33.

87	Alberta Department of Public Health, *Annual Report of the Department of Public Health, Province of Alberta, 1921* (Edmonton: J.W. Jeffery, King's Printer, 1922), 12.

88	*Act respecting Public Health*, S.P.A. 1907, c. 12.

89	Violet Friesen, *Schools of the Parkland* (Red Deer: Red Deer District Local A.T.A. No. 24 Centennial Project, 1967), 27.

90	"Forty-Five Teachers will Resume Work on Monday," *Edmonton Evening Journal*, 29 August 1908, 1.

91	"Edmonton School Board Ordered to Admit Gordon Clowes Without Child Submitting to Vaccination," *Edmonton Journal*, 6 November 1915, 1.

92	"Edmonton School Board Ordered to Admit Gordon Clowes," *Edmonton Journal*.

93	Nuffield Council on Bioethics, *Public Health: Ethical Issues* (London: Nuffield Council on Bioethics, 2007), http://nuffieldbioethics.org/wp-content/uploads/2014/07/Public-health-ethical-issues.pdf.

94	Alberta Department of Public Health, *Annual Report 1956* (Edmonton: A. Shnitka, Queen's Printer, 1958), 27.

95	Alberta Department of Education, *Junior High School Curriculum Guide for Health and Personal Development* (Edmonton, 1952), 195.

96	Alberta Department of Education, *Junior High School Curriculum Guide for Health and Personal Development* (Edmonton, 1951), 5.

97	Mona Lee Gleason, *Normalizing the Idea: Psychology, Schooling, and the Family in Postwar Canada* (Toronto: University of Toronto Press, 1999), 72.

98	Alberta Department of Education, *Junior High School Curriculum Guide for Health and Personal Development* (Edmonton, 1953), 113, 172.

99	Alberta Department of Education, *Junior High School Curriculum Guide for Health and Personal Development* (Edmonton, 1951), 92.

100 Alberta Department of Education, *Junior High Health: Curriculum Guide for Junior High Health* (Edmonton, 1964), 7.

101 Alberta Department of Education, *Junior High Health* (Edmonton, 1964), 7.

102 Alberta Department of Education, *Junior High School Curriculum Guide for Health and Personal Development* (Edmonton, 1952), 195.

103 Alberta Department of Education, *Junior High Health: Curriculum Guide for Junior High Health* (Edmonton, 1964), 53.

104 Alberta Health Services, *Framework for the Comprehensive School Health Approach.*

105 "Comprehensive School Health," Concepts, Pan-Canadian Joint Consortium for School Health, accessed 17 September 2022, http://www.jcsh-cces.ca/en/concepts/comprehensive-school-health/; Charlotte Beaudoin, "Twenty Years of Comprehensive School Health: A Review and Analysis of Canadian Research Published in Refereed Journals (1989–2009)," *Revue PhénEPS / PHEnex Journal* 3, no. 1 (March 18, 2011), https://ojs.acadiau.ca/index.php/phenex/article/view/1409.

106 Ever Active Schools (EAS) is a special project of the Health and Physical Education Council of the Alberta Teachers' Association. EAS received funding from the Government of Alberta, Alberta Health, Alberta Education and Alberta Culture, Multiculturalism and Status of Women. "Ever Active Schools," Health & Physical Education Council, accessed 21 August 2020, https://www.hpec.ab.ca/ever-active-schools18.

107 Beaudoin, "Twenty Years of Comprehensive School Health;" Paul J. Veugelers and Margaret E. Schwartz, "Comprehensive School Health in Canada," *Canadian Journal of Public Health* 101, no. 2 (July 1, 2010), https://doi.org/10.1007/BF03405617.

108 See articles by University of Alberta professor Dr. Carla Peck at "Carla Peck, PhD,' Alberta Curriculum Analysis, accessed 17 September 2022, https://alberta-curriculum-analysis.ca/author/peck99/.

109 Eva Ferguson, "UCP Budget Freezes K-12 Education Funding, Cuts Post Secondaries," *Calgary Herald* (online), 25 October 2019, https://calgaryherald.com/news/local-news/ucp-budget-freezes-k-12-education-funding-cuts-post-secondaries.

Disaster Mitigation, Preparedness, Response and Recovery: Lessons from Trains, Fires, Tornadoes and Floods

Donald W.M. Juzwishin

Introduction

Disasters can come in several forms, including natural disasters and disasters caused by humans, which may be purposeful or accidental. The capacity to protect the public from disaster-related harms is a foundation of a society concerned with the well-being of its citizens and communities. A society's disaster response entails government efforts to control, contain, and learn from previous successes and failures. The context is important: what may be an emergency in an urban setting might be a disaster in a remote setting, depending in part on resources available for response and recovery.

Although it was the influenza epidemic of 1918–1919 that prompted the act that led to the creation of the provincial Department of Public Health (see Chapter 4), several notable disasters preceded the proclamation of that act. These were the Frank Slide of 1903, which claimed seventy to ninety lives, the Rogers Pass avalanche of 1910, which claimed sixty-two lives, and 1914 the Hillcrest mine disaster, where 189 workers were killed.[1] Proactive steps toward improved avalanche safety and the creation of occupational mine safety standards (see also Chapter 9), helped to mitigate future risks associated with these early forms of disaster in the province.[2] In this chapter, we focus on disasters that occurred since the 1980s. Our rationale is that the level of scrutiny that governments undertook in the recent past, to learn how response and recovery could be improved, has been deliberate and well documented, and may thus be particularly informative for drawing lessons for the future.

The inextricable link between human beings and the ecosystem we live in is clear (see also Chapter 8). As stated in a 2015 Canadian Public Health Association discussion document:

> In the late 20th and early 21st centuries, myriad threats to the health of the Earth's environment have become apparent. There is a growing recognition that the Earth is itself a living system and that the ultimate determinant of human health (and that of all other species) is the health of the Earth's life-supporting systems. The ecosystem-based 'goods and services' that we get from nature are the ecological determinants of health. Among the most important of these are oxygen, water, food, fuel, various natural resources, detoxifying processes, the ozone layer and a reasonably stable and habitable climate.[3]

The intrinsic relationship of humans and their ecosystem has reached an unprecedented level of understanding.[4] We can no longer think of natural disasters as being unrelated to the activities of humans on the planet, and this insight forms crucial context for this discussion.

In this chapter, we focus on four types of disasters — train crashes, fires, tornadoes, and floods — that impacted the province of Alberta's disaster and emergency preparedness. Emergency preparedness and disaster response is a core public health function in Canada and is defined by the Canadian Public Health Association as "those activities that provide the capacity to respond to acute harmful events that range from natural disasters to infectious disease outbreaks and chemical spills."[5] The chapter has the following objectives.

- Identify and analyze the impact and consequences of the selected disasters on Albertans.
- Draw lessons from the preparedness for, and response and recovery to, each disaster to identify strengths, weaknesses, opportunities, and threats in the province's disaster preparedness plans.
- Identify and analyze the laws, regulations, policies, measures, and practices that were instituted as a result of the lessons learned from earlier disasters.
- Evaluate how future preparedness can be improved to minimize disruption to Alberta citizens and their communities.

Our four examples are: i) the Hinton train collision of 1986, which resulted in twenty-three deaths; ii) tornadoes in Edmonton in 1987 with twenty-seven deaths and in Pine Lake in 2000 with twelve deaths; iii) the Slave Lake and Wood Buffalo fires of 2011 and 2016 respectively, which had no direct fatalities but immense property loss and dislocation of communities; and iv) the 2013 southern Alberta flood that caused five deaths. Although there have been other disasters (Table 11.1), these four were selected because of the role of government in taking more responsibility for understanding the lessons to be learned from the response and recovery to protect the public's health. We therefore viewed these examples as well-aligned with the volume's overall focus on ways to strengthen public health — the science and art of preventing disease, prolonging life, and promoting health through organized efforts of society[6] — in Alberta by learning from past disasters.

TABLE 11.1: Disastrous events in Alberta, 1910–2019, and consequences.

Event	Year(s)	Deaths/Injuries or displacement	Damages
Frank Slide	1903	70–90 deaths; unknown injuries	Unknown
Rogers Pass Avalanche	1910	62 deaths	Unknown
Hillcrest Mine Disaster	1914	189 deaths	Unknown
Spanish Flu	1918–1919	2,800 deaths	Unknown
Lamont train crash	1960	17 deaths; 25 injured	Unknown
Hinton train derailment	February 1986	23 deaths; 95 injured	$30 million
Mindbender rollercoaster	June 1986	3 deaths; 4 injured	Unknown
Edmonton tornado	July 1987	27 deaths; 300 injured	$ 332 million
Pine Lake Tornado	July 2000	12 deaths; 100+ injured	$ 13 million
Slave Lake Fire	May 2011	7,000 people evacuated	$750 million
Southern Alberta Flood	June 2013	5 deaths; 100,000 displaced	$ 5 billion
Wood Buffalo Fire	May 2016	80,000 evacuated	$ 8.9 billion
Opioid crisis	2011–2018	1,720 deaths	Unknown

Sources: Diana Wilson, *Triumph and Tragedy in the Crowsnest Pass* (Nanoose Bay: Heritage House Publishing, 2000); Jennifer Dunkerson, "The White Death: The Rogers Pass Avalanche of 1910," *British Columbia History* 43, no. 1 (2010): 10–12; Crowsnest Pass Historical Society, *Crowsnest and Its People*, (Coleman, AB: Crowsnest Pass Historical Society, 1979); "Bus-Train Collision Toll Increases to 17," *Edmonton Journal*, 30 November 1960, 1; "Carnage at Hinton: 30–50 Die in Alberta's Worst Rail Accident," *Edmonton Journal*, 9 February 1986, 1; "Coaster Crash Tied to Errors in Design," *Edmonton Journal*, 22 October 1986, B1; Environment Canada; "Tornado Damage Pegged at $13 Million," *CBC News*, 18 July 2000; "The Flood of 2013," The City of Calgary; KPMG, *Lesser Slave Lake Regional Urban Interface Wildfire - Lessons Learned* (6 November 2012); KPMG, *May 2016 Wood Buffalo Wildfire: Post-Incident Assessment Report* (May 2017);" "Opioid Reports," Government of Alberta, accessed 30 August 2020, https://www.alberta.ca/opioid-reports.aspx.

Origins of Emergency Preparedness in Alberta

Although the province had emergency provisions for circumstances of disease outbreak since the Public Health Act of 1907, provincial provisions for disaster and emergency preparedness and response started later.[7] The first such provincial act —the Act to Provide for the Organization and Administration of Civil Defence and Disaster — was assented in 1951 and fell under the responsibility of the Department of Municipal Affairs. The act permitted the minister of that department to enter into agreements with the federal government to develop a comprehensive disaster preparedness plan; it also allowed local authorities to establish their own organizations to respond to disasters.[8]

Thereafter, responsibility for the provisions of the act resided within different departments. In 1957, responsibility for disaster planning was transferred from the Department of Municipal Affairs to the Department of Agriculture. In 1959, Alberta Civil Defence became a branch of that department, and in 1960, the branch was renamed the Emergency Measure Organization, which in 1962 was assigned to Public Welfare.[9] In 1967, the Emergency Measure Organization once again became the responsibility of the minister of agriculture. The Emergency Measure Organization was re-established under Municipal Affairs from 1968 to 1971 and then once again transferred to agriculture.[10] In 1973, the Emergency Measure Organization was renamed the Alberta Disaster Services Division, and three years later, it became independent of agriculture.[11] This movement of the emergency response function from department to department and back again was indicative of the uncertainty in government as to where responsibility should be housed, and perhaps demonstrates the inherently cross-ministerial nature of emergency preparedness and response.

In 2007, the provincial government established the Alberta Emergency Management Agency within Municipal Affairs.[12] The agency leads the "coordination, collaboration and cooperation of all organizations involved in the prevention, preparedness and response to disasters and emergencies."[13] In addition, at the time of writing, Alberta Health Services had an Emergency Coordination Centre, and the Government of Canada had a Health Portfolio Emergency Operations Centre.[14] The existence of these centres and agencies, coupled with other administrative and jurisdictional entities such as municipal governments, Indigenous communities, Emergency Social Services, and industry, underscores the complexity of and challenges associated with disaster response.

Example 1: Hinton Train Collision

Alberta is no stranger to fatalities due to train collisions. For example, on 29 November 1960, seventeen students from Chipman High School near Edmonton were killed and twenty-five were injured when their school bus was struck by a freight train in Lamont, Alberta.[15] The case study for this chapter is the Hinton railway collision of 8 February 1986, when twenty-three people were killed and seventy-one were injured sixteen kilometres east of Hinton, Alberta. Westbound Canadian National Railway freight train collided with an eastbound Via Rail passenger train (the Super Continental).[16] The two crew members on Train 413 and two on Train 4 were killed. Eighteen occupants in the day coach of Train 4 and one occupant of the dome car also perished. The estimated property damage was over $35 million.[17]

On 10 February 1986, the governor general-in-council appointed Honourable Mr. Justice René Paul Foisy of the Court of Queen's Bench of Alberta to lead a commission of inquiry. The commission was charged with examining three aspects of the collision: the specific circumstances and causes of the crash, the conditions relating to railway safety, and recommendations to improve rail safety and reduce risk of such collisions in the future.[18]

Based on the inquiry, the commission determined that "the collision occurred because the westbound freight train (Train 413) failed to obey signals along the track calling for it to stop, and ran a switch governing its entry onto a single-track section where it came into collision with passenger train (Train 4)."[19] The report indicated that the signals governing the movement of the two trains operated satisfactorily and no mechanical deficiencies were found in the train or track. It was, in the conclusions of the commission, the inability of the engineer, conductor, and trainman of Train 413 to observe and obey signals along the track that led to the collision. Brakes were not applied prior to the collision, leading to the conclusion that the engineer, trainman, and conductor were individually incapacitated in their roles and responsibilities.

The commission identified several conditions affecting the crew of Train 413 that contributed to the collision. First, the crew were fatigued, due to performing monotonous work in long and irregular shifts. Additionally, the engineer suffered from medical conditions that the commission concluded may have contributed to his actions. Finally, the engineer's personnel records revealed past behaviour in which disciplinary action would have been warranted.[20]

The commission estimated that there were nineteen seconds during which Trains 413 and 4 would have been visible to one another. Train 4 did not engage the emergency brakes and there was no explanation why: "All that can be said is that the front-end crew were either in a state of frozen shock as they saw the freight train approaching or were not looking forward so that they did not know that the freight train was approaching."[21]

LESSONS LEARNED

The commission concluded that human error contributed to the collision and that "management shares in the responsibility for the conditions that contributed to the human errors involved in this case." Canadian National Railway management failed to take appropriate action on "a variety of performance and rules violations."[22] For example, the commission determined that the railway did not give enough priority to its policy of replacing the dead man's pedals, a basic failsafe, with the more effective reset safety controls, which would automatically stop the train if the engineer were to become incapacitated.[23] Finally, a dismissive culture of employees, the union, and management that demonstrated a disregard for safety, was also a factor in the collision. Recommendations from the Foisy inquiry were extensive, with an overall focus on the weak safety norms in railroad culture. Specifically, recommendations focused on a need for improvements with respect to rest, medical supervision, and the employee assistance program. Other recommendations were to enhance the company's supervision and discipline policies and practices, get government involved in regulating railroad operations, and install modern safety control appliances in all trains.[24]

The Lac-Megantic rail disaster in Québec on 6 July 2013, in which forty-seven people were killed, is a sober reminder that rail safety still has much room for improvement.[25] Opportunities for improvement are highlighted in the 2018 federal Railway Safety Act review final report, which identified three elements necessary for an effective rail safety program: i) compliance with technical regulations and standards; ii) safety management systems; and iii) a safety culture.[26] The challenges to improve rail safety have been taken on by Transport Canada and they, along with the Government of Canada, have called for collaboration between railways, governments, and communities to address the issues.[27]

With the Alberta political economy so focused on petroleum and its products, and as public concern with transportation of petroleum by pipeline continues to grow, government and industry have a serious responsibility to ensure that safety regulations and culture in rail transportation meet the highest standards of practice. Important resources, training and infrastructure for transportation disaster and emergency circumstances have been developed,[28] however, additional supports and leadership around preventive upstream thinking are needed. The public health imperative of humanity living in harmony within its habitat in a safe and secure manner demands urgent and substantive steps to respect and mitigate harms to the health of all species and our environments.

The Hinton train collision was largely due to human error. In contrast, the next three disasters are considered natural disasters, defined as "a natural event such as a flood, earthquake, or hurricane that causes great damage or loss of life."[29] We acknowledge legal terms like "act of god" or "force majeure," which describe events caused by the effect of nature or natural causes and without human interference;[30] however, we also recognize the increasingly fuzzy boundaries between "human" and "natural," such as natural disasters that stems from climate change caused by human activity.

Example 2: Edmonton and Pine Lake Tornadoes

Canadians can expect an average of over sixty recorded tornadoes per year, and Canada ranks second to the U.S. globally for annual occurrence of tornadoes.[31] Table 11.2 identifies the most fatal tornadoes in Alberta's history.

TABLE 11.2: Tornadoes with loss of life in Alberta.

Year	Location	Deaths/Injuries	Damage (Est.)
1915	Medicine Hat	2 deaths; unknown injuries	$500,000
1918	Vermilion	3 deaths; unknown injuries	Unknown
1972	Bawlf	1 death; 2 injured	$112.000
1987	Edmonton	27 deaths; 253 injured	$332.27 million
2000	Pine Lake	12 deaths; 100+ injured	$13 million

Sources: "Tornado in Canada," Colonist lvii, issue 13805, 28 June 1915; "Tornado Barely Misses Calgary," Edmonton Journal, 7 July 1965; "Small Tornado Hits Near Nanton," Calgary Herald, 13 June 1966; "Alberta Farms Hit by Tornado," Calgary Herald, 31 July 1972; "Top Weather Events of the 20th Century," Environment and Climate Change Canada, modified 8 August 2017, https://www.ec.gc.ca/meteo-weather/default.asp?lang=En&n=6A4A3AC5-1; "Tornado Damage Pegged at $13 Million," CBC News, 18 July 2000, https://www.cbc.ca/news/canada/tornado-damage-pegged-at-13-million-1.228502.

Below, we focus on two tornadoes in Alberta: Edmonton in 1987 and Pine Lake in 2000, which together resulted in thirty-nine deaths, over 353 injuries, and $345 million in damages.

Edmonton and Pine Lake Tornadoes

Black Friday, as it became known to Edmontonians, passed through the eastern part of the city and parts of neighbouring counties on 31 July 1987. The tornado was classed as an F4,[32] reaching wind speeds of up to 420 km/h and leaving a path of destruction that measured thirty kilometres in length and 1.3 kilometres at the widest point. Twenty-seven people were killed, over three hundred were injured, and more than three hundred homes were destroyed. Monetary estimates of damage at four major disaster sites ranged from $260,000,000 to $332,000,000.[33]

Weather conditions during the last week of July that year were hot and humid, with frequent thunderstorms throughout the province.[34] Fourteen tornadoes were eventually reported between July 25 and July 30. Weather maps showed a weak low-pressure trough over Central Alberta at the surface and a strong flow of air from the southwest high altitudes; "As the week progressed, surface dew-point temperatures (a measure of the absolute humidity or moisture content of the air) rose to near–record levels at 20 degrees C."[35] On July 31, severe thunderstorms were forecast during the day with a weather watch commencing at noon. At 2:45 p.m. a severe weather warning was issued after a tornado touched Leduc, just south of Edmonton, at 2:55 p.m. The tornado suddenly retracted and touched down northeast of Leduc, near Beaumont, remaining on the ground for an hour over a forty km path. In total, the tornado destroyed homes across its path, including two hundred trailers in Edmonton's Evergreen Mobile Home Park, and killed fifteen people.

Thirteen years later, on 14 July 2000 at 7 p.m., an F3 tornado with winds up to 300 km/h killed twelve people and injured more than one hundred others at the Green Acres Campground and RV Park in Pine Lake, Alberta. The Pine Lake tornado formed out of a severe thunderstorm emerging from the eastern slopes of the Rocky Mountains at approximately 4 p.m., which moved rapidly eastward and collided with a narrow stretch of low-level moisture, causing the thunderstorm to develop into a supercell.[36] Environment Canada issued a severe thunderstorm warning at 6:18 p.m. The Pine Lake tornado touched down five kilometres west of the campground and travelled along the ground for twenty kilometres. It destroyed more than three hundred homes and caused an estimated $13 million in damage at the campground and trailer park.[37]

LESSONS LEARNED AND RESPONSES

In 1987, the meteorological technology for monitoring weather systems and public warning were relatively rudimentary. An identified need for a better severe weather warning system led to the creation in 1992 of the Alberta Emergency Public Warning System,[38] which was "the first warning system of its kind, using existing media outlets to broadcast critical life-saving information directly to the public as a joint operation between government and broadcasters."[39] The system was renamed Alberta Emergency Alert in 2011, when radio and television migrated from analog to digital systems, and the Alberta government promoted the Alberta Emergency Alerts smartphone application as a way of increasing public awareness of disaster warnings.[40] On 6 April 2018, the Canadian Radio-television and Telecommunications Commission ordered that all smartphones would automatically receive emergency alerts.[41]

The role of the non-profit sector in collaborating with government in emergencies is crucial. With the Edmonton tornado, the Red Cross responded quickly to help citizens deal with the devastation by making phone lines available to the public and mobilizing a team of more than 1,300 registered volunteers. According to a Red Cross report: "Red Cross stations quickly became hubs for coordinating emergency social response, processing more than 11,000 inquiries from those affected, distributing food and beverages to displaced families and relief workers, organizing temporary housing for eighty-nine displaced families in the aftermath and set up a Victim Assistance Centre used by roughly 482 families."[42]

The Pine Lake tornado in 2000, among other disasters, contributed to the creation of a more centralized provincial emergency social services framework, which seeks to coordinate the many stakeholders in these efforts.[43] The study, occurrence, and damage of tornadoes has also had an impact on the development and implementation of tornado resiliency measures in the National Building Code of Canada.[44]

Example 3: Slave Lake and Wood Buffalo Wildfires

According to a 2012 report on the Slave Lake wildfire of May 2011, "never have so many people been evacuated, or so much property been lost" in the province.[45] One helicopter pilot died when he crashed battling the fire and the total cost was estimated at $750 million. The RCMP concluded that the reason for the fire was arson.[46] Five years later, in May 2016, the Wood Buffalo fires presented an even greater threat. Although no one was killed, the amount of property damage was immense, and recovery efforts are still taking place at the time of writing.

Slave Lake Fire

The spring of 2011 was dry, and on Saturday, May 14, the Alberta Emergency Management Agency was monitoring several wildfires across the province. Although fires in the Lesser Slave Lake region were noted, their urgency was not realized until later in the day when two more wildfires started in the region. At that point, both the Town of Slave Lake and the Municipal District of Lesser Slave River No. 124 declared states of local emergency and activated their respective emergency operations centres.

By the next day, as the two wildfires burned out of control, a combination of weather and other conditions emerged that would result in a disaster that could not be halted. That morning, Alberta Health Services evacuated the Slave Lake Healthcare Centre.[47] The Municipal District evacuated many of its residents to

Slave Lake and moved its Emergency Operations Centre into the town for safety reasons. Under mandatory evacuation on Sunday afternoon and night, an estimated 7,000 people fled their homes, driving through flames that compromised visibility on the roads. Highways into and out of the town were closed due to flames and smoke. Highway 2 eastbound was re-opened Sunday afternoon. Aircraft that were assisting with the evacuation and fighting the fire were grounded due to the smoke. Water, gas stations, electricity, and telephone infrastructures began to fail. Evacuees began arriving in Westlock, Athabasca, Edmonton, and other Alberta communities early Monday morning. The mandatory evacuation lasted until June 1. The recovery began on June 2 and extended for several years. The provincial government instituted a recovery plan in early August of that year.[48]

LESSONS LEARNED

The Alberta government's ministry of Sustainable Resources Development was responsible for wildfire suppression within forest protection areas of the province. At the time, they were fighting numerous fires across the province, and high winds exacerbated the situation. As the situation near Slave Lake worsened, provincial staff were preparing to assist local communities with no expectation that the fires would threaten the town itself; however, the winds picked up dramatically on Sunday afternoon to gusts of over 100 km/h, surprising everyone with their rapid advance toward the town.[49]

The magnitude of the efforts was significant, involving thirty separate entities and thirty-eight fire departments, with limited coordination.[50] Evacuee support in the form of reception centres was provided from neighbouring municipalities with little notice. The Canadian Red Cross was contracted and provided support to reception centre services.[51] Housing was needed, and the Alberta government mobilized temporary short-term housing until homes could be replaced.[52] Being prepared for sudden unexpected changes of conditions, coordinating information exchange and being able to quickly mobilize voluntary and government efforts to provide for the necessities of life were all important lessons learned.

The Alberta Emergency Management Agency is responsible for providing strategic policy direction and leadership during disasters and for coordinating collaboration between emergency management partners such as local first responders, disaster relief agencies and all levels of government. In order to learn the lessons from the response to the fire the province hired KPMG to conduct a review and assessment of the response. The analysis found that "Alberta's emergency management system reflects a network between different levels and orders of government, industry and other public safety partners that often respond independently to a hazard."[53] The report provided recommendation for improving coordination efforts, focusing on those that would strengthen the horizontal management of services among those that are providing a response at the local level, better integrate the response, and identify single points of accountability.[54]

The Municipal District of Slave Lake, the Town of Slave Lake, and the Sawridge First Nation formed a tri-council with a shared governance structure to begin planning and implementing the recovery phase of the disaster. The Alberta NGO Council and their partners mobilized support for the residents of the region. An important lesson from the experience is that communities affected by disaster need continued support and respect that it is "their community" because, as the KPMG report noted, community leadership in recovery efforts enhance the long-term success of that recovery.[55] The Lesser Slave Lake Regional Wildfire Recovery Plan was developed and released in August 2011.[56]

The economic impact of the fires was unprecedented in Alberta's history. The Alberta government responded with a revenue stabilization plan, providing $50 million early in the response followed by two additional allocations of $50 million and $189 million in the following three months. Provision of emergency funds to residents, responders, and communities included, for example, debit cards to permit discretionary spending without having to wait for prior approvals. On the other hand, the collection, storage, distribution, and destruction of donations became an overwhelming challenge for community responders.[57]

From the Slave Lake fires came many lessons on the safety and health of the public and how the province could prepare for the future. Preparedness, with a scalable emergency and command structure that would facilitate collaboration among the players, is key. Coordination of people and resources is essential, and establishing clear jurisdictional boundaries avoiding unnecessary conflict. Evacuation plans with defined roles and responsibilities need to be developed, and communications between responders from a consistent source need to be established to reduce confusion during emergencies. The fires taught that financial support needs to materialize quickly so that residents can return to a life of normalcy whereas responders require resources to enable critical decisions quickly. A mechanism for coordinating donations can ensure that needs of victims are met.

Wood Buffalo Wildfire

Five years after the Slave Lake fire, in 2016, a dry winter, coupled with a spring with record high temperatures and a dry air mass created another summer of combustible forest in northern Alberta. Over one hundred wildfires were burning in Alberta, a quarter of which were out of control, and the majority were located in the Lesser Slave Lake area. Temperatures hovered around 31 to 32 degrees Celsius in early May and humidity was as low as 12 percent. Winds gusted up to 72 km/h. On May 1, a fire broke out in a remote area seven kilometres southwest of Fort McMurray. The fire spread northeast, and by May 3 it encroached on the city, causing the evacuation of 88,000 residents from their homes. The fire's extremely rapid expansion took everyone by surprise. The fire destroyed 2,400 homes and buildings, and burned 589,552 hectares of forest, causing $8.9 billion in damages, making it the costliest disaster in Canadian history to date.[58] There was only one road leading out of the city forcing people to drive through smoke and flames to escape the fire. No deaths occurred as a direct result of the fire but two people died in a car crash during the evacuation.[59] Having impacted oil production for a period of time, the fire stimulated a conversation about the association between human induced climate change and wildfires.[60] The cause of the fire was deemed most likely to be the result of human activity, but no charges have been laid.

LESSONS LEARNED

No one could have guessed that a community in Alberta would ever have to evacuate its entire population. Fort McMurray did so in one day.

As with the Slave Lake fire, the Alberta government, through the Alberta Emergency Management Agency, commissioned KPMG to assess the performance of the province in responding. The assessment found that there were many positive attributes to the response; however, opportunities for improvement were also identified. These included: i) investing in and reinforcing the province's preparations and readiness for each hazard season; ii) building depth and capacity within local authorities to enable communities to support one another; iii) ensuring that enhanced decision-making capacity is in place at all levels of the response and iv) enhancing the public's understanding of engagement for emergency preparedness.

According to the KPMG report, different approaches to management across organizations in response to the disaster led to some confusion. It was recommended that local authorities be mandated to adopt the incident command system model. The standardized model is used to manage emergencies and disasters by enhancing coordination and cooperation among participants, simplify reporting and decision-making processes, and facilitate the seamless flow of information. The aim is to minimize harm, reduce the potential for confusion or unnecessary duplication in response efforts, and ensure an organized and effective response. The report also recommended that the Provincial Emergency Social Services Framework continue to be strengthened and refined by collaborating on identifying the unmet needs for emergency social supports based on a situational awareness and that a disaster resiliency strategy be developed to help mitigate the effects of disasters and help in the recovery phase. Because coordination among many different levels of responder partners can be a challenge, the report's authors recommended that internal communications between key stakeholders be enhanced with technology.[61] Other lessons related to the value of a psychosocial response framework to support citizens and responders encompassing psychological first aid, skills for psychological recovery, grief and loss, along with recognition of the role that pet rescue and reconnection plays in recovery.

Two catastrophic fires within a five-year span tested the emergency responsiveness of the province; they also taught valuable lessons on how to plan, prepare, train, and develop robust decision-making and command centres with clear roles and responsibilities.

Example 4: Southern Alberta Floods

Floods are not uncommon in Canada; they are considered by Public Safety Canada to be the most common natural hazard in the country. Alberta's most devastating floods have occurred recently. In 2005, heavy rainfall caused rivers to flood in southern Alberta, forcing 7,000 people to evacuate and costing $400 million in damages.[62] Leading up to 19 June 2013, Alberta experienced heavy rainfall, which triggered the most severe flooding in Alberta and Canadian history to date. Thirty-two states of emergency were declared, and twenty-eight emergency operations centres were activated. There were five confirmed deaths and over 100,000 people evacuated. The Alberta government commissioned a review and analysis of the 2013 flood. The review, which was prepared by MNP LLP, a Canadian national professional services firm, stated "the 2013 floods cut off dozens of Alberta's communities and necessitated the largest evacuation in Canada in more than sixty years. An estimated 100,000 Albertans were instructed to evacuate their homes, and approximately 14,500 homes and 1,100 small businesses were impacted. In select areas of the province, entire neighborhoods were under water for weeks."[63] The total damage was estimated at over $5 billion, and in insurable terms it was the costliest disaster in Canadian history to date.[64]

LESSONS LEARNED

The MNP report, commissioned by the Alberta government, serves as a powerful tool for not only documenting the trajectory of the disaster but also assessing the response to it, including whether and how the response could have been better. By most accounts, everything that could have been done, was done. In the words of one person badly impacted by the flood, "we are lucky to live in Alberta and lucky to live in Canada, compared to anywhere else on earth where this could have happened."[65] As described in the MNP report:

In the face of this catastrophic event response was swift and co-ordinated. The Provincial Operations Centre (POC), was activated at its highest level, Level 4, for 24 days and over 2,200 members of the Canadian forces and numerous other agencies were deployed throughout the province to help with the response. The Flood Recovery Task Force, led by Municipal Affairs and with key representation from across the provincial government and a direct link to the provincial Treasury Board, was quickly formed and managed recovery efforts. Showcasing their signature determination and independence, Albertans responded by pulling together to help their neighbors and fellow citizens through offers of food, temporary shelter, clothing and other supplies."[66]

The MNP report assessed and analyzed the disaster using five themes: i) people, attitude, and approach, ii) provincial government legislation, organization structures, processes and plans, iii) emergency management capacity, iv) communications, and v) continuous improvement. The report's authors made sixteen recommendations,[67] of which several are particularly aligned with a theme of this book, namely, to reflect on ways to strengthen public health in Alberta. One is the recognition that Albertans themselves are in an important position to protect the public's health, and that empowering Albertans to do so should be encouraged. However, these efforts require the guidance of an Alberta Emergency Plan that clearly defines roles and responsibilities with a robust provincial emergency social services framework. Additionally, it is paramount not to lose sight of the social determinants of health, which create inequitable disaster vulnerability and impact. Finally, being prepared to monitor and report to the public on the progress being made by governments and other groups is essential to ensure that the public stay informed and governments remain accountable.

Concluding Remarks

Over the last one hundred years, we have witnessed a shift from the most severe disasters in Alberta occurring in mining and occupational circumstances, to human error and weather being the most significant threats. The lesson from the 1986 Hinton train collision is that human error due to a dismissive railroader culture had a significant effect on how people behaved and performed their roles. Railroad safety was not a serious consideration of management or employees, hence the Foisy Commission recommendation to improve those conditions. When the focus of an enterprise in a neoliberal economic context is simply maximizing profit and shareholder value at the cost of public safety, unfortunate

— and foreseeable — consequences may arise. Unfortunately, implementation of improvement at the federal level was slow, with important consequences such as the Lac-Megantic train derailment twenty-six years later.

The Edmonton and Pine Lake tornadoes motivated the government to introduce improvements in technologies, including severe weather monitoring and public warning systems. Keeping Albertans safe by communicating threatening and high-risk weather systems became a priority. In addition, provincial and municipal governments updated building codes to increase the resiliency of buildings in case of severe weather events. These efforts are excellent examples of the intersectoral nature of the public health system core function of emergency preparedness and response.[68]

The Slave Lake and Wood Buffalo wildfires highlighted for Albertans the importance and necessity of social cohesion and solidarity, coupled with political will to respond with the social determinants of health foremost in mind. Two catastrophic fires within a five-year span were a wake-up call for Albertans and tested the resiliency of the province's emergency response and recovery programs. The fires, tornados and floods collectively contributed to a heightened public discourse around the links with climate change that is induced by human activity. This raises serious questions about the respective role and responsibilities of citizens, landowners, the provincial government, municipalities, and insurance companies as to who is to bear the cost of responding to and recovering from the disasters. The fires taught us that an uncoordinated, fragmented and rudderless system is bound to be limited in its effectiveness; and a health-in-all-policies approach holds promise in that regard. Finally, the southern Alberta flood of 2013 reinforced the need for continuing to monitor and report to the government and public on the implementation of recommendations and whether they are achieving the goals identified in the post-incident assessments. A periodic reporting of progress by the provincial government to the public is encouraged.

The approach that Albertans have used to address improvements to disaster response might be considered for application to other public health policy responses to issues such as the opioid crisis, chronic illnesses, and the climate crisis; all of which reflect the interconnectedness between human behaviour, ecosystems, and political economy.

NOTES

1   Diana Wilson, *Triumph and Tragedy in the Crowsnest Pass* (Nanoose Bay, BC: Heritage House Publishing, 2000); Jennifer Dunkerson, "The White Death: The Rogers Pass Avalanche of 1910," *British Columbia History* 43, no. 1 (2010); Thomas MacGrath, "Sacrifice, Fate, and a Working-Class Heaven: Popular Belief in the Crowsnest Pass" (MA thesis, University of Calgary, 2017).

2   See, for example, the "Mining Operations and Mining Certificates" section of the Occupational Health and Safety Regulation R.A, 62/2003 of the *Occupational Health and Safety Act*, R.S.A. 2000, c. O-2, https://search-ohs-laws.alberta.ca/legislation/occupational-health-and-safety-code/part-36-mining/.

3   Canadian Public Health Association, "Global Change and Public Health: Addressing the Ecological Determinants of Health," Discussion Paper (Ottawa: Canadian Public Health Association, 2015).

4   Nick W. Watts et al., "Health and Climate Change: Policy Responses to Protect Public Health," *The Lancet* 386, no. 10006 (2015): 1861–1914.

5   Canadian Public Health Association, *Public Health: A Conceptual Framework*, Canadian Public Health Association Working Paper (Ottawa: CPHA, 2017), 12.

6   Donald Acheson, *Public Health in England. The Report of the Committee of Inquiry into the Future Development of the Public Health Function* (London: HMSO, 1988).

7   *Act respecting Public Health*, S.P.A. 1907, c. 12.

8   *Act to Provide for the Organization and Administration of Civil Defence and Disaster within the Province of Alberta*, S.A. 1951, c. 10.

9   Provincial Archives of Alberta, (PAA) *An Administrative History of the Government of Alberta 1905–2005* (Edmonton: The PAA, 2006), 48.

10 PAA, *An Administrative History*, 48.

11 PAA, *An Administrative History*, 49.

12 *Disaster Services Amendment Act*, S.A. 2007, c. 12, section 5.

13 "Alberta Emergency Management Agency," Government of Alberta, accessed 30 May 2010, https://www.alberta.ca/alberta-emergency-management-agency.aspx.

14 "Alberta Emergency Management Agency," Government of Alberta; "Emergencies and Disasters," Health Canada, Government of Canada, modified 3 January 2019, https://www.canada.ca/en/health-canada/services/health-concerns/emergencies-disasters.html; Pan-Canadian Public Health Network, *Federal/Provincial/Territorial Public Health Response Plan for Biological Events* (Ottawa: Pan-Canadian Public Health Network, 2018), https://www.canada.ca/en/public-health/services/emergency-preparedness/public-health-response-plan-biological-events.html.

15 "Bus-Train Collision Toll Increases to 17," *Edmonton Journal*, 30 November 1960, 1; "Nov. 29, 1960: Seventeen Students Killed when School Bus, Train Collide near Lamont," *Edmonton Journal*, 28 November 2012.

16 "Carnage at Hinton: 30–50 Die in Alberta's Worst Rail Accident," *Edmonton Journal*, 9 February 1986, 1.

17 René P. Foisy, *Commission of Inquiry, Hinton Train Collision: report of the Commissioner, the Honourable Mr. Justice René P. Foisy*, (Edmonton: The Commission, Minister of Supply and Services Canada, 1986), 32, http://publications.gc.ca/collections/collection_2016/bcp-pco/T22-72-1986-1-eng.pdf.

18 Foisy, *Commission of Inquiry*, 3.

19 Foisy, *Commission of Inquiry*, 3.

20 Foisy, *Commission of Inquiry*, 155.

21 Foisy, *Commission of Inquiry*, 79.

22 Foisy, *Commission of Inquiry*, 5.

23 Foisy, *Commission of Inquiry*, 7.

24 Foisy, *Commission of Inquiry*.

25 "Lac-Mégantic Runaway Train and Derailment Investigation Summary," Investigations and Reports, Transportation Safety Board of Canada, accessed 28 August 2020, https://www.bst-tsb.gc.ca/eng/rapports-reports/rail/2013/r13d0054/r13d0054-r-es.html.

26 Government of Canada, *Enhancing Rail Safety in Canada: Working Together for Safer Communities* (Ottawa: Her Majesty the Queen in Right of Canada, represented by the Minister of Transport, 2018), 1, https://publications.gc.ca/site/eng/9.854166/publication.html.

27 Railway Safety Act Review (RSAR) Panel, Minister of Transport, *Enhancing Rail Safety in Canada: Working Together for Safer Communities* (Ottawa: Her Majesty the Queen in Right of Canada, represented by the Minister of Transport, 2018).

28   Emergency Management Training, Government of Alberta, accessed 3 April 2024, https://www.
      alberta.ca/emergency-management-training.

29   "Natural Disaster," English Oxford Living. n.d. Oxford Living Dictionaries, accessed 20 May 2019,
      https://en.oxforddictionaries.com/definition/natural_disaster.

30   Stephen Gerard Coughlan, John A. Yogis, and Catherine Cotter, *Canadian Law Dictionary*, 7th ed.
      (Hauppauge, New York: Barrons Educational Series, 2013).

31   Shelby Blackley, "Are Tornadoes in Canada on the Rise? A Look at the Dangerous Storms," *The Globe
      and Mail*, 27 September 2018, https://www.theglobeandmail.com/canada/article-are-tornadoes-in-
      canada-on-the-rise-a-look-at-the-dangerous-storms/; Ian Livingston, "10 Years Later, Canada's Only
      F5 Tornado Remains in a Class of its Own," *Washington Post*, 22 June 2017; "Tornadoes," Emergency
      Management, Public Safety Canada, accessed 30 August 2020, https://www.publicsafety.gc.ca/
      cnt/mrgnc-mngmnt/ntrl-hzrds/trnd-en.aspx; Vincent Y.S. Cheng et al., "Probability of Tornado
      Occurrence across Canada," *Journal of Climate* 26, no. 23 (2013), doi.org/10.1175/JCLI-D-13-00093.1.

32   A Fujita Scale system classifies tornadoes based on wind damage. The scale is from F-0 for weak
      tornadoes (light damage caused by winds up to 32 m/s) to F-5 for the strongest tornadoes (heavy
      damage from winds 116 m/s) with wind speeds topping 500 km/h. "The Fujita Scale of Tornado
      Intensity," *A Dictionary of Environment and Conservation* (Oxford: Oxford University Press), accessed
      on 15 May 2019, https://www.oxfordreference.com.

33   "Canadian National Tornado Database: Verified Events (1980–2009)," Environment and Climate
      Change Canada, Open Government, accessed 30 May 2019, https://open.canada.ca/data/en/dataset/
      fd3355a7-ae34-4df7-b477-07306182db69.

34   Alberta Public Safety Services, *Tornado: A Report, Edmonton and Strathcona County, July 31st 1987*
      (Edmonton: Alberta Public Safety Services, 1991), 13.

35   Alberta Public Safety Services, *Tornado: A Report*, 13.

36   A supercell is a thunderstorm that lasts longer than one hour, which feeds off a rising current of air that
      is tilted and rotating. This rotating updraft could be as large as 10 miles in diameter and up to 50,000
      feet tall and can be present as much as 20 to 60 minutes before a tornado forms. "Severe Weather 101 —
      Thunderstorms," The National Severe Storms Laboratory, accessed 28 August 2020, https://www.nssl.
      noaa.gov/education/svrwx101/thunderstorms/types/.

37   Sunil Sookram et al., "Tornado at Pine Lake, Alberta — July 14, 2000: Assessment of the Emergency
      Medicine Response to a Disaster," *CJEM: Journal of the Canadian Association of Emergency
      Physicians* 3, no. 1 (2001), https://caep.ca/periodicals/Volume_3_Issue_1/Vol_3_Issue_1_Page_34_-
      _37_Sookram.pdf; "Tornado Damage Pegged at $13 Million," *CBC News*.

38   Jonny Wakefield, "Can You 'Over Warn' About a Tornado? Improvements since 1987 Created a World
      with (Potentially) Too Much Weather Info," *Edmonton Journal*, 31 July 2017, https://edmontonjournal.
      com/news/local-news/can-you-over-warn-about-a-tornado-improvements-since-1987-created-a-
      world-with-potentially-too-much-weather-info.

39   "Tornado — A Report," Canadian Red Cross, accessed 30 May 2019, http://www.redcross.ca/history/
      artifacts/tornado-a-report.

40   Janet French, "Technology Would Change Edmonton's Tornado Response Today, Officials Say,"
      Edmonton Journal, updated 31 July 2017, https://edmontonjournal.com/news/local-news/technology-
      would-change-edmontons-tornado-response-today-officials-say.

41   Canadian Radio-television and Telecommunications Commission, "Implementation of the National
      Public Alerting System by Wireless Service Providers to Protect Canadians," Telecom Regulatory
      Policy CRTC 2017-19, Ottawa, 6 April 2017, https://crtc.gc.ca/eng/archive/2017/2017-91.pdf.

42   "Tornado — A Report," Canadian Red Cross.

43   Alberta Government, *Provincial Emergency Social Services Framework* (2016), http://www.aema.
      alberta.ca/documents/PESS-Framework-Final-Document-01182016.pdf; City of Calgary, "ESS
      Integration in Municipal Emergency Planning with Non-Profit Organizations" (Power Point
      presentation, 2019), accessed 28 August 2020, http://aema.alberta.ca/documents/D4.pdf.

44   David Sills et al., "Using Tornado, Lightning, and Population Data to Identify Tornado Prone Areas in
      Canada," 26th Conference on Severe Local Storms, Manuscript, https://ams.confex.com/ams/26SLS/
      webprogram/Paper211359.html.

45   KPMG, *Lesser Slave Lake Regional Urban Interface Wildfire — Lessons Learned, Final Report*, 6
      November 2012, https://open.alberta.ca/publications/lesser-slave-lake-regional-urban-interface-
      wildfire-lessons-learned; Lessons-Learned-Final-Report.pdf; Alberta Municipal Affairs, *Annual
      Report 2011–2012* Edmonton, June 2012, 6, http://www.municipalaffairs.alberta.ca/documents/2011-
      2012-MA-Annual-Report.pdf.

46   "RCMP Seek Six People in Slave Lake Fire Investigation," *CTV News*, 8 February 2012, https://www. ctvnews.ca/rcmp-seek-six-people-in-slave-lake-fire-investigation-1.765506.

47   KPMG, *Lesser Slave Lake Regional Urban Interface Wildfire*, 73.

48   KPMG, *Lesser Slave Lake Regional Urban Interface Wildfire*, 7.

49   "RCMP Seek Six People in Slave Lake Fire Investigation," *CTV News*.

50   KPMG, *Lesser Slave Lake Regional Urban Interface Wildfire*, 8.

51   KPMG, *Lesser Slave Lake Regional Urban Interface Wildfire*, 14.

52   KPMG, *Lesser Slave Lake Regional Urban Interface Wildfire*, 11.

53   "RCMP Seek Six People in Slave Lake Fire Investigation," *CTV News*.

54   Shih-Hsuan Hong, "Slave Lake Recovery: Whole-Of-Government Disaster Response," Institute of Public Administration of Canada (IPAC) Case Study Program, 1, accessed 3 April 2040. https://ipac. ca/Revamp/iCore/Store/StoreLayouts/Item_Detail.aspx?iProductCode=726&Category=DIGITAL.

55   KPMG, *Lesser Slave Lake Regional Urban Interface Wildfire*, 13, 116.

56   KPMG, *Lesser Slave Lake Regional Urban Interface Wildfire*, 7.

57   KPMG, *Lesser Slave Lake Regional Urban Interface Wildfire*, 125.

58   KPMG, Prepared for Alberta Emergency Management Agency, Final Report, May 2017, accessed 30 May 2019, https://open.alberta.ca/dataset/accfd27e-5e08-4f6c-8cd9-188be0e1e1b2/resource/541f276f-2fb4-4789-a41f-ef5ce7c0eec5/download/2016-wildfire-kpmg-report.pdf.

59   "2 Die in Fiery Crash on Highway 881 South of Fort McMurray," *CBC News*, 4 May 2016, https:// www.cbc.ca/news/canada/edmonton/2-die-in-fiery-crash-on-highway-881-south-of-fort-mcmurray-1.3567142.

60   John Paul Tasker, "'Of Course' Fort McMurray Fire Linked to Climate Change, Elizabeth May Says," *CBC News*, updated 4 May 2016, https://www.cbc.ca/news/politics/elizabeth-may-fort-mcmurray-climate-change-1.3566126.

61   KPMG, *May 2016 Wood Buffalo Wildfire*, 112–124.

62   Ian Burton, "Floods in Canada," in *The Canadian Encyclopedia. Historica Canada*, article published 7 February 2006, edited 4 March 2015, https://www.thecanadianencyclopedia.ca/en/article/floods-and-flood-control.

63   MNP, "Review and Analysis of the Government of Alberta's Response to and Recovery from 2013 Floods," July 2015, accessed 30 May 2019, http://www.aema.alberta.ca/documents/2013-flood-response-report.pdf.

64   Gary Lamphier, "Alberta Flood Tab Could Run as High as $5B: Too Early for Insurer of 278 Municipalities to Estimate Costs," *Edmonton Journal*, 19 October 2013.

65   MNP, "Review and Analysis," 33.

66   MNP, "Review and Analysis," 20.

67   MNP, "Review and Analysis," 82–89.

68   Canadian Public Health Association, *Public Health: A Conceptual Framework*, 2nd edition, March 2017, accessed 3 April 2024, https://www.cpha.ca/sites/default/files/uploads/policy/ph-framework/phcf_e.pdf.

Social Determinants of Health in the Alberta Government: Promising and Pernicious Historical Legacies

Lindsay McLaren

Introduction

Health and well-being are fundamentally shaped by the quality of the circumstances in which we are born, grow, live, work, and age; these are the social determinants of health. Inequitable distribution of the determinants, which reflects inequities in power and resources that are inherent to our political, economic, and colonial systems and structures, creates and perpetuates health inequities, which are unfair and avoidable differences in health between social groups.[1] Health equity occurs when people are not disadvantaged by social, economic, political, and environmental conditions, including how those conditions intersect with social identities based on factors such as ability, age, gender, race, sexuality, and social status.[2]

The social determinants of health and health equity are integral to a broad definition of public health; that is, the art and science of promoting health and preventing illness through organized efforts of society.[3] Yet, the extent to which this knowledge and perspective is embraced in Alberta (and indeed across Canada, and beyond) is limited. The 2008 final report of the World Health Organization Commission on Social Determinants of Health boldly asserted that addressing the social determinants of health required action to improve peoples' daily living conditions; to tackle the inequitable distribution of power, money, and resources;

and to measure and understand the problem and assess the impact of action. Yet, analyses of the report's impact ten years later show a persistent tendency — by researchers, practitioners, and governments — to embrace downstream, de-politicized versions of the social determinants of health that emphasize individual-level, bio-behavioural explanations for, and responses to, health inequities.[4]

One foundation of the social determinants of health concept is that the primary determinants of well-being and health equity reflect public policy decisions in government ministries other than health. A health-in-all-policies approach — and its historical precursor of healthy public policy — that systematically considers the implications for health, well-being, and health equity of policies across government ministries, theoretically provides a way to operationalize this foundation. Anchored in contemporary calls for a health-in-all-policies approach,[5] the objective of this chapter is to consider examples of how the social determinants concept has manifested across Alberta's history in the provincial government, such as how the provincial Department of (Public) Health was organized, and how legislative assembly deliberations that transcended health and other sectors played out. Key sources included annual reports of the provincial department or ministry responsible for public health and the *Alberta Hansard*. We were particularly interested in whether, or the extent to which, an upstream approach that was social justice-oriented and focused on root causes of poor and inequitable health, was evident.

Following some brief historical framing around societal approaches to addressing poverty and need, we first provide some examples of how the administrative lines separating health and social policy domains were (appropriately) blurred during the first half of the twentieth century in Alberta. Next, we consider a period during the 1970s and 1980s when health and social policy were merged into one provincial government ministry and which, on the surface, could embrace consideration of the health implications of social policy decisions and vice versa, in line with a health-in-all-policies approach. Finally, to shed light on more recent discourse, tensions, and opportunities for a broad vision of public health, we examined instances where "social determinants of health" was mentioned in the provincial legislature, including by whom and in what circumstances. Alberta provides an interesting context for this study. The province's recent history, particularly since the 1970s, is largely characterized by a precarious boom-bust economy dominated by fixation on extractive resource revenue and politically conservative leadership which — notwithstanding the range of beliefs within conservatism — tends to be at odds with a social determinants of health approach. Indeed, Alberta's record on public policy, which has almost universally worsened social and economic inequality, poverty, and the quality and availability of public services and supports, has been highly problematic from the point of view of well-being and health equity.[6]

Conceptual Framing: Societal Responses to Poverty and Need

In his review of milestones in Alberta's public welfare history, social worker and historian Baldwin Reichwein provided examples from ancient history of societies feeling a duty to "help the poor." For most of human history, this sentiment took the form of charity, or voluntary acts of giving, to those deemed "in need" by those with social and economic advantage.[7]

This sentiment, and its underpinnings in classical political conservativism, evolved into different approaches to social policy within organized state administration which, as per the social determinants of health approach, have significant implications for well-being and health equity. The post-WWII development of Canada's welfare state is a relatively recent example; although, as discussed elsewhere in this volume, the welfare state has not prevented a broad array of services and supports from falling to the private and non-profit sectors (Chapter 5), nor has it embodied the inclusivity that it is widely believed to symbolize (Chapters 1 and 7).

A much earlier historical example is England's "poor laws." The poor laws of the sixteenth and seventeenth centuries took the form of a parish-level tax administered locally, which provided relief for the aged, sick, and infant poor, with leftover funds to be used to create jobs for "able-bodied" people, often in workhouses.[8] The poor laws and subsequent versions of them are relevant to this chapter and to public health more generally because some of the tensions embedded in the contemporary social determinants of health discourse have roots in those early activities. For example, having state infrastructure to collect and redistribute public taxes raises pragmatic but value-laden questions about who is and is not eligible for assistance, how much they should receive, and the criteria for evaluating need. Notions of eligibility have long been infused with tensions around deservingness and what constitutes appropriate generosity. For example, a fourteenth-century English statute made a distinction between the "worthy poor" — which included older people, people with disabilities, widows, and dependent children — and the "unworthy poor" — those who were able-bodied but unemployed.[9] A problematic belief that the "able-bodied poor" could and should work for pay has long underpinned a view that the generosity of aid should not exceed a certain limit, to ensure that there is no incentive to remain on public assistance.[10]

In Canada, these tensions have materialized in what Danish welfare state scholar Gøsta Esping-Andersen has called a liberal welfare orientation.

Underlying Esping-Andersen's liberal regime is a key belief, whether implicit or explicit, that the state should only intervene in the economic lives of individuals if the capitalist market fails. Welfare benefits in liberal regimes, according to Esping-Andersen, accordingly tend to be modest, that is low enough that they do not present a disincentive to working for private wages, and/or means-tested where one must prove their eligibility.[11] Alberta's recent historical alignment with this liberal orientation is succinctly conveyed by the subtitle of Reichwein's public welfare review noted above: "history rooted in benevolence, harshness, punitiveness, and stinginess."[12] These styles and modes of governance and approaches to public policy have demonstrable implications for health, well-being, and health equity;[13] they are thus integral rather than peripheral to public health as a field of scholarship and applied practice.

Social Determinants of Health in the Provincial Government: Insights from Alberta's History, 1919–2019

"As part of its commitment to community health during the early 1900s, the [Edmonton] Board of Health helped administer the limited social service programs offered by the city [including] the distribution of relief funds necessary to tide destitute citizens over the difficult winter months. Efforts were made, starting in 1908, to develop an effective system of assessing relief cases and supplying provisions to citizens who qualified for assistance." — Toward a Healthier City: A History of the Edmonton Board of Health, 1871–1995[14]

The quotation about the Edmonton Board of Health shows that local public health authorities were involved in efforts related to social determinants of health — in this case, poverty relief — during Alberta's earliest years as a province. Although one should not over-interpret this involvement — in the early phases of the province, all government departments had a wide range of responsibilities (see Chapter 4) — it does not seem unreasonable to speculate that officials were attuned to the (likely obvious) health effects of economic destitution, especially during winter in a northern climate.

An administrative connection between health and social policy continued and, perhaps not surprisingly, expanded during the depression years of the late 1920s through the 1930s. Starting in 1926, under the United Farmers of Alberta government, the provincial minister of public health was given responsibility for the provision of poverty relief in Improvement Districts of the province (relief in urban areas was the responsibility of the individual municipalities). The Social Credit government, elected in 1935, continued to build social welfare infrastructure. They consolidated provincial relief efforts into a Bureau of Public Welfare which, along with the Child Welfare and Mothers' Allowance Branch, was under the authority of the Department of Public Health starting around 1937. This arrangement, with the provincial public health department having responsibility for social welfare, continued until 1944 when the bureau and the branch moved to a newly created provincial Department of Public Welfare.[15]

There are indications that public health authorities of the time were aware that social and economic factors were important for health. One example is Alberta Deputy Minister of Health Dr. Malcolm Bow's 1937 address to the Canadian Public Health Association, of which he was president at the time, where he said, "if our ideal is a full measure of physical and mental health for all, then the housing problem ought to be one of the first to receive attention."[16] Bow identified housing —in particular, unsanitary housing — as the first of "eight major health problems facing us to-day," thus providing an illustration of early attention to what we now call the social determinants of health.

The 1970s and 1980s: The Health and Social Merger Period

> "You will, therefore, be asked to consider legislation to create a new Department of Health and Social Development, laying the foundation for an integrated approach to preventive, as well as active and rehabilitative health and social services at the community level." — 1971 Alberta government throne speech, Harry Strom (SC).[17]

In 1971, as announced in the quotation from the Strom government's throne speech, provincial health and social policy domains were brought together into the Department of Health and Social Development. The arrangement theoretically signified attention to health implications of social policy and vice versa and is thus potentially informative from a contemporary health-in-all-policies perspective. The department was renamed Social Services and Community Health in 1975.[18] To accompany this section, a timeline of key events is provided in Table 12.1.

TABLE 12.1: Summary of some milestones concerning intersectoral (health and social policy domains) activities and arrangements in the province of Alberta, 1905–2010s.

Year	Event
Early 1900s	The Edmonton Board of Health helped to administer the limited social service programs offered by the city at the time
1926	The Minister of Public Health was made responsible for provision of relief (social assistance) in Improvement Districts of the province
1937	The Bureau of Public Welfare and the Child Welfare and Mothers' Allowance Branch fell under the authority of the Department of Public Health (until 1944)
1966	The provincial *Preventive Social Service* program was introduced as part of a broader Social Credit reform of welfare services. The program aimed to empower local governments to deliver preventive social programs.
1967	The *Preventive Health Services* report, commissioned in 1965, was released. Its mandate was to make recommendations on preventive health services in Alberta including ways to coordinate and integrate preventive health services with other services including social services. With the passing of the *Department of Health Act*, the provincial *Department of Public Health* (est. 1919) was replaced by the *Department of Health*, which was divided into two sections each with its own deputy minister: Health Services, and Hospital Services.
1969	Within a broader context of deinstitutionalization, the *Blair Report* on mental health, commissioned in 1967, was released. One of the report's key recommendations was to integrate social services and health services at the local level.
1971	The provincial *Department of Health and Social Development* was created under the Social Credit government of Harry Strom and unfolded under the Progressive Conservative government of Peter Lougheed, elected in 1971.
1975	The department was re-named *Social Services and Community Health*, and functions related to hospitals and health care insurance were transferred to a separate, newly established provincial *Department of Hospitals and Medical Care*.
1986	*Social Services and Community Health* was dissolved with the creation of the provincial *Department of Community and Occupational Health*, which absorbed the public health programs (but not the social service programs) from the former department.
1989	With the passing of the *Department of Health Act*, the Department of Community and Occupational Health and the Department of Hospitals and Medical Care were dissolved. All of "health" (i.e., public health, medical care, and hospitals) was back together under one ministerial roof, separate from social services (and other social determinants of health).
2012	The provincial *Ministry of Human Services* was created, which consolidated several people-centered departments and programs
2013	Alberta's *Social Policy Framework* was released, one of the main goals of which was to coordinate activities within and between government and ensure that there is policy alignment and consistency. "Social policy" was defined as extending beyond social services, to consider how we work, live, and spend our time, thus showing some alignment with a social determinants of health approach
2014	The *Social Policy Framework* disappeared with the election of Jim Prentice

THE ALBERTA DEPARTMENT OF HEALTH AND SOCIAL DEVELOPMENT: CONTRIBUTING FACTORS

Although the new department existed almost entirely during Peter Lougheed's Progressive Conservative administration (1971–1985), its foundations were set during the later years of Social Credit leadership (1935–1971).[19] We highlight three intersecting initiatives during the 1960s and early 1970s that contributed to the creation of the merged department: i) the preventive health services report; ii) the Preventive Social Service program; and iii) *Mental Health in Alberta: a Report on the Alberta Mental Health Study, 1968* (the Blair Report). These initiatives, summarized below, occurred within the federal context of the Canada Assistance Plan, which was created in 1966 to support the provision of social programs by provinces, territories, and municipalities.

First, in 1965 a special committee was established by the provincial government to review and produce a report containing recommendations on preventive health services in Alberta. In the context of growing concerns about provincial spending on health care, especially hospitals, the committee was explicitly tasked with finding ways to coordinate and integrate preventive health services with other services, including hospitals and other health services, welfare, and special education.[20]

The 144-page preventive health services report was tabled in 1967 and included 247 recommendations.[21] Described in the news media as "explosive," the report recommended significant re-organization of the provincial health department,[22] including to divide the province into nine health regions. While this did not materialize until the mid-1990s,[23] it is relevant to the present discussion because the health region concept underpinned the report's recommendations concerning coordination of health and social services, including that preventive social services be based on the health region (recommendation #161), that the areas served by welfare workers be made coterminous with health regions and health districts (#162), and that the responsibility for the operation and administration of social services be transferred to the boards of health regions (#163).[24] These recommendations, where coordination between sectors involves the social sector falling to the parameters of the health sector rather than the other way around, may illustrate the notion of "health imperialism," a negative term to describe a tendency of the health sector to presumptively take leadership in any intersectoral arrangement.

Another organizational recommendation of the preventive health services report was to replace the Department of Public Health Act (first passed in 1919) with a new Department of Health Act. Under that act, which passed in 1967, the new department was divided into two sections — one for hospital services (responsible for activities under hospital and nursing home legislation) and one for health services (responsible for everything else, such as local health services, vital statistics, environmental health), each of which now had a deputy minister.[25] Concern for the state of public health was evident in the report and echoed in the legislature: "there is great need for active steps to improve the image of public health and raise the standards of operation from the provincial point of view. Otherwise, that branch of the health services known as public health will continue to wane."[26] Moreover, by strengthening a distinction between health and hospitals, the 1967 act seems to have set the stage for the more extensive re-organization that followed in the early 1970s.

The second initiative, which concerned the preventive social service domain, began around the same time. As described in an extensive analysis by Professor of Social Work, Leslie Bella, Alberta's Preventive Social Service program was introduced in 1966 as part of a broader Social Credit reform of welfare services.[27] Embodying the government's philosophy of local autonomy, the program aimed to empower municipalities to deliver preventive social programs, with 80 percent of funding to do so provided by the province.[28] Examples of local programs included counselling, day care, home care, information and referral, youth programs, volunteer recruitment, and community programs.

The Preventive Social Service program had four major — and somewhat morally infused — goals: i) to prevent welfare dependence; ii) to prevent marriage breakdown, which was seen to lead to welfare dependence; iii) to reduce child welfare intake; and iv) to promote general social and physical well-being. An important insight from Bella was that the goals were interpreted differently by politicians on the one hand and administrators on the other. The politicians, in line with the Social Credit's ideological orientation, intended the program to reduce dependency on public assistance and thus prevent the welfare state. The administrators, in contrast, saw the program as a way to strengthen social services and thus expand the welfare state.[29]

Although the preventive health services and preventive social services initiatives were important, Social Credit Health Minister James Henderson argued that the main impetus for the creation of the merged provincial department (Department of Health and Social Development) was the 1969 Blair Report on mental health. The report was released just as Premier Harry Strom was taking over following Ernest Manning's twenty-five-year reign. Set against the broader backdrop of the deinstitutionalization movement, which advocated for replacing residential institutions with community-based services for persons with disabilities,[30] as well as growing concerns by the Alberta government (including as expressed in the preventive health services report) about mental health problems and the costs of treating them,[31] the Blair Commission was asked to make recommendations for a comprehensive and integrated program for diagnosing, treating, caring for, rehabilitating, and preventing mental illness in Alberta.[32] One of the Blair report's key recommendations was to integrate social services and health services at the community level; this was seen as a path to decentralizing mental health services, which were considered to transcend health and social domains. The new provincial Department of Health and Social Development was intended to provide "a common administrative plane" for those community-level services.[33]

CROSS-PARTY OPPOSITION TO THE NEW DEPARTMENT OF HEALTH AND SOCIAL DEVELOPMENT: PEELING BACK THE LAYERS

The Progressive Conservatives, who formed the official opposition starting in 1967, were opposed to the idea of the merged department. Hugh Horner (PC, Lac St. Anne), for example, said "I am totally and absolutely opposed to the amalgamation," arguing that it — along with the hospital commission created around the same time — was "nothing but a bureaucratic expansion out of proportion to what's required." He also insisted on using the word "welfare" because he did not feel that the government was in fact doing anything about "social development."[34] Presciently, Leonard Werry (PC, Calgary-Bowness) expressed concern about whether the amalgamated department would maintain an intended focus on prevention and rehabilitation, and mental health.[35] Nonetheless, the bill to merge the two departments passed in a forced vote in March 1971, marking one element of what was described in the *Hansard* as "the most extensive re-organization of government departments since 1935."[36] The new Department of Health and Social Development was responsible for almost all social services and health programs and for vital statistics.[37]

The department was thus in place when the Progressive Conservatives, under Peter Lougheed, won the 1971 provincial election. Although they had opposed the legislation, they decided to "carry the experiment forward," in part — according to the minister of the new department, Neil Crawford — to reduce additional disruption among departmental staff.[38] The first session of the new legislature (1972) gives some insights into some of the tensions around the new department, both within and between parties. Within the PCs, Dr. Kenneth Paproski (Edmonton-Kingsway), for example, supported the new department's focus on what he termed "total health care," which included "physical, mental and social needs" and emphasized "health maintenance and not disease orientation only."[39] Ernest Jamison (PC, St. Albert), on the other hand, questioned the value of the new department, considering the "many existing agencies and volunteer bodies available" already to deliver these services. This latter comment illustrates the blurred and contested lines of sectoral responsibility — including what services and supports should fall to the public, private or non-profit sectors — that is highly pertinent to a broad vision of public health. Moreover, in strong alignment with a social determinants of health perspective, Jamison also commented "that government can help more by providing employment and housing," arguing that looking after those two needs is key to preventing "social difficulties."[40]

Comments from Roy Farran (PC, Calgary-North Hill) illustrate the difficulty, or unwillingness, of legislators to conceptualize an integrated version of health and social domains. After expressing that consolidation of health and social development would take many years to materialize, he segued into a lengthy commentary about the need to rationalize health programs, focusing on hospital beds. Farran's narrow and downstream view of "health" is illustrated by his comments about the appropriate scope of activities for health departments, specifically the Calgary health department: "The City of Calgary is spending a huge amount of money on an expanding health department . . . . They want to build separate little clinics in each corner of the city that go far beyond the original concept of the medical officer of health who went around and sniffed the drains and tested for typhoid and saw whether the kitchens were clean in the restaurants. Nowadays, they've gotten into the whole broad field of social welfare as well as direct health treatment."[41] Such a viewpoint, which trivialized activities that fall outside of a very narrow version of physical sickness, presented a significant challenge to implementing policy that embraced a broad vision of public health.

Comments from members of the Social Credit opposition, in turn, illustrate some of the long-standing tensions around assistance and deservingness of public support noted earlier in this chapter. Raymond Speaker, the minister of the new department when it was created under SC leadership, for example, questioned whether the PC government saw public assistance as a right or a privilege.[42] Douglas Miller (SC, Taber-Warner) said that "with respect to social development and social assistance . . . I feel strongly that costs and abuses will continue to mount until the entire program is decentralized to the local authority to screen service-development-workout-programs convenient for the needy. As I mentioned, for those who can work, there are plenty of things for them to do."[43] This comment also sheds some light on the reasons for the Social Credit's original focus on decentralization, stemming from the Blair report; namely, they saw it as way to help prevent "abuse of the system" by the undeserving "needy," thus illustrating Alberta's historically punitive approach to public assistance noted by social worker and historian Reichwein.

HOW "HEALTH" WAS CONCEPTUALIZED WITHIN THE DEPARTMENT OF HEALTH AND SOCIAL DEVELOPMENT

Focusing on the period 1971–1972 through 1973–1974, when the department was called Health and Social Development, a few observations can be made about its alignment with the contemporary health-in-all-policies concept. First, in 1971–1972, which was the first full year of the new department, Chief Deputy Minister, Bruce S. Rawson (PC) stated in the department's annual report that the major objective of the new department was "to focus on health and social development needs in the province to bring about better planning and program development, priority setting and the integration and coordination of total service delivery."[44] Although one should be cautious about reading too much into a single sentence in a report from the past, it is interesting that "prevention" is absent from that statement, considering the emphasis on prevention that guided the new department in the first place. Second, the PC government almost immediately added new divisions including community care for those with mental illness.[45] Although this represents a more holistic approach compared to hospitals and residential institutions, it is still quite downstream in its emphasis on illness and treatment. Finally, and of potential concern from the perspective of the "public" in public health, is the report's emphasis on "greater involvement of the private sector" in these new divisions.

Further, for those first few years, annual reports show that the health and social domains within the new department appeared to co-exist rather than to be integrated to any great extent. For example, the summary of "preventive social services" in the 1972–1973 and 1973–1974 annual reports illustrate the ideological and moral underpinnings of the government by emphasizing community initiative, volunteer involvement, and reduction of unwanted outcomes such as "family breakdown," with limited explicit reference to health and well-being, even though promoting well-being was one of the stated goals of the program.[46] Meanwhile, the Provincial Board of Health within the department continued to emphasize health protection-style activities focused on physical illness, such as communicable disease control, food safety, and appropriate waste disposal; and the health units, which had become 100 percent provincially funded starting in 1973, continued to provide preventive public health services throughout the province.[47]

In 1975, in the context of national initiatives such as the Lalonde Report, which recognized a broader array of determinants of health, the department was renamed Social Services and Community Health.[48] The same year, functions related to hospitals and health care insurance were transferred to a separate, newly established provincial Department of Hospitals and Medical Care, which was in place from 1975 to 1988.[49] Conceivably, with downstream, treatment-oriented activities organized separately, this arrangement could permit even more emphasis on social determinants of health by the merged department. Although health and social services appeared to remain organizationally separate during this time, some subtle indications of a shift in overall orientation are apparent in the annual reports. For example, the 1975–1976 report included a section on "prevention":

> In general, preventive services provide support toward developing individual, family and community strengths. These services, provided to all age groups, can touch on the fields of health, education, social welfare, community development, social planning, and even economic development. . . . Most [preventive social services] projects offer services at one or two levels of intervention: primary — where measures are taken to strengthen and support the individual, family and community before any breakdown occurs; [and] secondary — where steps are taken to solve a problem which has just emerged.[50]

Although the program's morally infused focus on "social breakdown" persisted, this description contained words that carry a hint of health promotion (building strengths), intersectoral thinking (health, education, etc.), and universalism (primary prevention).

In the health services section of that same report, the community health section contains the following preamble:

> In contrast with treatment-oriented medicine, community health services are primarily preventive in nature. . . . They are designed to reduce disease and disability, maintain standards of health and promote good health habits. To achieve these goals, community health services must take into account the many factors affecting the health of the individual and the community as a whole [including] . . . the physical and social environment [and] . . . the influences of heredity and lifestyle which may contribute to disease and illness.[51]

In 1977–1978, the preventive social services branch was transferred from the Social Services Division to the Health Services Division of the department. With this transfer, the major preventive programs of the department were grouped together in one division and preventive social services and local health services, including dental, nutrition, home care, immunization, and regulation of day care facilities, were jointly administered.[52]

Overall, this partial analysis of the 1970s, anchored in contemporary health-in-all-policies discourse, suggests that by putting two previously separate policy or service domains into the same government department, integration can increase over time. Importantly, however, this analysis also makes obvious that such service integration — although theoretically consistent with a broad conceptualization of health — by no means ensures an upstream orientation to addressing the social determinants of health as embraced by a broad vision of public health.

Social Services and Community Health was dissolved in 1986 with the creation of the Department of Community and Occupational Health, which absorbed the public health programs, but not the social service programs, from the merged department. The new Department of Social Services, later renamed the Department of Family and Social Services, absorbed the social service programs. With that 1986 legislation, health and social policy domains were once again administratively separate. A few years later, Community and Occupational Health (est. 1986), and Hospitals and Medical Care (est. 1975), were dissolved with the Department of Health Act of 1989.[53] Thus, starting in 1989, all of "health" — including public health, medical care, and hospitals — was once again together under one ministerial roof, and this was the context for our final section.

Mobilization of "Social Determinants of Health" in the Alberta Government: The 1990s–2010s

BACKDROP: THE PROVINCIAL DEPARTMENT OF HEALTH IN THE 1990S

Annual provincial Department of Health reports from the early 1990s suggest some attention to the social determinants of health, including policy antecedents. For example, among the nine health goals identified in Alberta Health's 1991–1992 annual report was "to include a health perspective in public policy," thus aligning with the concept of healthy public policy that had been recently introduced in the Ottawa Charter for Health Promotion.[54] Subsequent annual reports suggest some modest engagement with this goal. For example, the 1993–1994 report stated that "healthy public policy means taking into account the possible impacts on health of a proposed major policy change. It also means consulting with the groups potentially most affected when a policy is changed. As a result of concerns raised by seniors during review of the proposed Alberta Seniors Benefit several changes to the program were suggested."[55] The Alberta Seniors Benefit, a form of social assistance, is administered by a government department other than health, and consulting with seniors is one way to gain insight into its impli-cations for health and well-being.

Considering these initiatives, along with the "Klein Revolution," the 1990s and early 2000s provide an interesting context in which to study mobilization of social determinants of health concepts in the Alberta government.[56] To do so, we searched the *Alberta Hansard* for "social determinants of health"; we summarize some key people and events chronologically in the following pages.[57] To help orient the reader, the individual politicians referenced below are listed in Table 12.2.[58]

TABLE 12.2: List of individuals referenced in our analysis of social determinants of health in Alberta legislative debates, 1990s–2019 (alphabetical by last name).

Name	Party affiliation and constituency (during time period referenced)
Laurie Blakeman	Liberal, MLA for Edmonton-Centre
Heather Forsyth	Progressive Conservative, MLA for Calgary-Fish Creek
Carol Haley	Progressive Conservative, MLA for Airdrie-Chestermere
Dave Hancock	Progressive Conservative, MLA for Edmonton-Whitemud and Minister of Human Services
John Hayden	Progressive Conservative, MLA for Drumheller-Stettler
J.A. Denis Herard	Progressive Conservative, MLA for Calgary-Egmont
Fred Horne	Progressive Conservative, MLA for Edmonton-Rutherford and Minister of Health and Wellness
Ralph Klein	Progressive Conservative, Premier and MLA for Calgary-Elbow
Jim Prentice	Progressive Conservative, Premier and MLA for Calgary-Foothills
Alison Redford	Progressive Conservative, Premier and MA for Calgary-Elbow
Dave Rodney	Progressive Conservative, MLA for Calgary-Lougheed
Linda Sloan	Liberal, MLA for Edmonton Riverview
Ed Stelmach	Progressive Conservative, MLA for Fort Saskatchewan-Vegreville
David Swann	Liberal, MLA for Calgary-Mountain View

SOCIAL DETERMINANTS OF HEALTH IN ALBERTA GOVERNMENT DELIBERATIONS: THE 1990S: EDMONTON-RIVERVIEW MLA, LINDA SLOAN

The first explicit references to "social determinants of health" in the Alberta legislature were made in the late 1990s. Linda Sloan (Liberal; 1997–2001) served as opposition critic for Family and Social Services and stands out as perhaps the only person making such references during the 1990s based on the *Hansard*.[59] For example, in a 1997 debate on Bill 14: The Appropriation Act, which authorized how funds from General Revenue were to be used for the fiscal year, Sloan identified what she saw as a disproportionately low operating allocation to the Department of Labour, compared to other, service-oriented departments such as health and family and social services. This was problematic, she argued, because of what it implied for social determinants of health, namely working conditions:

> That [inadequate funding to the Department of Labour] is reflective, I think, of . . . the subversive means that are taken . . . to undermine the working conditions of people in this province, and to undermine the . . . unions in this province whose existence is to serve, to advocate, and to represent employees and to promote their socioeconomic status. . . . I speak to it knowing the relationship between the social determinants of health . . . not only being defined singularly by accessing services or working within a particular sector but by being able to afford to eat nutritional foods, being able to live in an adequate house . . .[60]

Sloan's recognition of the connections between labour unions and health, and that health is not reducible to health or social services or private income, are indicative of her strong understanding of the social determinants of health. As another illustration, in 1999, Sloan mobilized the social determinants concept in reference to income inequality:

> We saw really late last month the release of a report surrounding income disparity [including] how the gap between rich and poor in the province of Alberta is growing. When that report was released, the Premier heatedly chastised the institution, the Parkland Institute, that had sponsored the conference at which the report was released and proceeded to subliminally suggest that that institute's funding should somehow be undermined. It struck me how arrogant that that approach would be taken when I have not seen a report from this government about income disparity, about the social determinants of health and how their program policy and budget changes have had an impact on the social determinants of health in this province.[61]

Sloan pointed out that, not only was the Klein government failing to address income inequality nor considering how their government's policies were contributing to it, but they tried to undermine an organization for demonstrating that the problem existed.[62]

Overall, an analysis of the social determinants of health concept in Alberta must recognize Linda Sloan as being one of the only voices for this concept in provincial government deliberations in the unfriendly environment of the 1990s Klein government.

THE 2000S: LIBERAL MLA LAURIE BLAKEMAN, THE WELLNESS INITIATIVE, AND THE HEALTHY FUTURES ACT

During the first decade of the 2000s, references to the social determinants of health in the Alberta legislature increased modestly. Standing out amid this growing voice was Laurie Blakeman (Liberal, Edmonton-Centre). From 2004 to 2008, Blakeman served as opposition critic for Health and Wellness. Blakeman effectively mobilized the social determinants concept both in social policy debates (for example, questioning whether health was considered in deliberations concerning the Assured Income for the Severely Handicapped program in 2005) and in health debates.[63]

An example of Blakeman's mobilization of the social determinants concept in health debates is seen in the 2006 debate on Bill 1: Alberta Cancer Prevention Legacy Act, which was broadly intended to position Alberta "to attack cancer at every level, from prevention right through to potential cures." Blakeman skillfully drew attention to the act's limited attention to primary prevention and social determinants of health when she said, "I'm always interested in the juxtapositions that I witness in this House, and there are two of them that I'm seeing come with this bill. On the one hand, we have this bill being tabled in the House on one of the same days that . . . coal-bed methane exploration is resulting in contamination of . . . well water to the point where they can set it on fire. You juxtapose that kind of toxicity in someone's life with this grand bill to deal with ending cancer. You've got to put those two things together, folks."[64] Blakeman used the social determinants of health concept to highlight what she saw as the hypocrisy, gently described as "juxtapositions," of the cancer initiative, considering the limited policy attention to environmental carcinogens.

Two other initiatives during the '00s, both led by Blakeman, were Motion 501 concerning a Wellness Initiative, and Bill 214, the Healthy Futures Act. These are informative in part because of the ensuing debate, which sheds light on points of opposition and informs a broad vision of public health that embraces social determinants of health and their socio-political implications.

Blakeman's 2005 Motion 501, Wellness Initiatives proposed that the government use taxes from tobacco sales to create a wellness fund. The fund was envisioned to contribute to a healthier society and cost containment in the health care system by supporting wellness programs delivered through family and community support services; public health initiatives such as efforts to create healthier environments in schools, hospitals, etc.; and research on how to better integrate social determinants into wellness and health system initiatives.[65]

The motion was defeated (11 for, 31 against). Although some members spoke in favour, commending the motion's focus on investment in the causes of health problems,[66] several others opposed it, drawing on lines of opposition seen in other debates (see Chapters 3 and 8) such as redundancy with existing policies. For example, Carol Haley (PC, Airdrie-Chestermere) argued that she could not support the motion because "there is already a fund dedicated to healthy living initiatives in Alberta. It is called the Department of Health and Wellness. . . . There is another fund. It's . . . called the Alberta Heritage Foundation for Medical Research."[67] These comments reveal a persistent and frustrating conflation of health and health care. Both the Department of Health and Wellness and the Alberta Heritage Foundation for *Medical* Research (italics added) were predominantly focused on biomedical, clinical, and health care-oriented initiatives, which is precisely what the Wellness Initiative was aiming to offset by its broader conceptualization of health and its determinants.

In 2007, Blakeman introduced private member's Bill 214: Healthy Futures Act under the Progressive Conservative Ed Stelmach (2006–2011) government. Recognizing that many important determinants of health have little to do with the health care system, the bill proposed that major policies and funding decisions undergo a health impact assessment, which involves judging the potential health effects of a government initiative with the aim of maximizing the proposal's positive health effects and minimizing its negative effects. The bill, which Blakeman argued aligned with World Health Organization recommendations, would include the appointment of a director of assessment review who would lead and oversee assessment processes.[68]

Although several members voiced support for the bill, several others opposed it, and the bill was defeated at second reading (15 for, 26 against).[69] Once again, opponents argued that the proposed activities were not necessary in light of processes already in place. John Hayden (PC, Drumheller-Stettler), for example, argued that " our government . . . has shown its commitment to continuous improvement in the area of health by creating the Health Quality Council of Alberta. . . . [E]stablishment of a health commissioner [therefore] seems unnecessary."[70] Hayden argued that health impact assessment was not necessary in light of all-party committees and the existing Health Quality Council of Alberta. Importantly, however, the council is entirely focused on the health care system,[71] and thus fundamentally differs in its mandate from the intent of Bill 214, which was to systematically consider the health implications of decisions outside of the health sector.

A second line of opposition was that the proposal was overly broad and thus, by definition, problematic, as argued by Dave Rodney (PC, Calgary-Lougheed): "one of my main concerns with this bill is that it could effectively bring the decision-making apparatus of the government and this Assembly to a grinding halt."[72] Other PC legislators, such as Heather Forsyth (PC, Calgary-Fish Creek), argued that the bill's breadth gave it the potential to be too subjective when she said that "public health impact assessments have the potential to become a public forum of opinion rather than informed decisions on empirical evidence."[73] Health impact assessments *do* involve public consultation and they *are* evidence-based; the comment thus misunderstands that the two can (and should) go together.[74]

Overall, instances where the social determinants of health concept was mobilized in Alberta government during the '00s reveal important challenges for a broad vision of public health, including the need to articulate and defend upstream policies for well-being and health equity in a way that is less vulnerable to predictable and inaccurate, but unfortunately often effective, opposition comments about redundancy, specificity, and conflation with health care.

THE 2010S: ALBERTA'S MINISTRY OF HUMAN SERVICES AND THE SOCIAL POLICY FRAMEWORK

Our final illustration of the mobilization of social determinants of health concepts in the Alberta government is Alberta's Social Policy Framework, which was developed during the PC government of Alison Redford (2011–2014).

To set some context for the framework, we note some relevant comments from the 2012 legislative assembly discussion of budget estimates for the provincial Department of Health and Wellness. In response to a query from David Swann (Liberal, Calgary-Mountain View) around funding for public health, which is a very small proportion of the health and wellness budget, PC Minister of Health and Wellness Fred Horne stated: "To sum up with respect to public health, the expenditure out of the budget formerly under the public health budget for wellness is about 3 percent, but as hopefully I've been able to describe to my colleagues, wellness is embedded throughout not only my ministry in terms of the primary care system but also through many other ministries, including Justice and Attorney General, Human Services, Education, and others that have a direct role in influencing the social determinants of health."[75] In other words, Minister Horne seemed to be justifying a small budget for public health activities (within the health budget) on the basis that other departments were in fact also responsible for policies and services that support the social determinants of health. While accurate, it could also signify "passing the buck" such that no ministry would be responsible for social determinants of health unless there was a framework in place to ensure that they did not fall through cracks of discrete ministries. It was in this context that Alberta's Social Policy Framework was released in 2013 under the leadership of Minister of Human Services, Dave Hancock.

The Ministry of Human Services, created in 2012, consolidated several departments, including Child and Family Services, Housing and Urban Affairs, and Employment and Immigration, and programs, such as Assured Income for the Severely Handicapped and Protection for Persons with Developmental Disabilities. Although it brought many "people-centered" activities into one department, there was some trepidation about how this would play out. Indeed, Hancock himself said that his "biggest concern was whether or not we would have the opportunity to look at it from a holistic basis . . . is this just going to be running programs, or is this going to be an opportunity to reshape how we think about our society and how we think about the role of government in supporting individuals to be successful?"[76]

Other comments, moreover, add nuance around some of the underlying orientations. In reference to flipping pancakes during Social Work Week, Hancock stated that he "got into some exciting conversations with individuals there about . . . how they feel about a minister who says that there are two parameters, the Bible on one side and the Criminal Code on the other. It has to be legal, and it has to be ethical and moral. Within that, we expect you to use judgment. Rules are for when brains run out."[77] The context was the ministry's emphasis on "outcome-based services," where front line professionals such as social workers were to be empowered to use their judgment to achieve a positive outcome for the person or family in front of them. However, the Bible and Criminal Code references seem problematic in the light of their misalignment with a social justice orientation that values inclusion (e.g., diverse religious or spiritual affinities) and that is contrary to a punitive, discriminatory, "tough on crime" approach to societal well-being.[78]

Reminiscent of the health and social merger period of the 1970s, there are indications that the Department of Human Services tended, at least initially, toward a partial and downstream focus on persons living in challenging social and economic conditions, as opposed to a more upstream population-level focus. This is illustrated by a line of questioning from David Swann about the ministry of human services' plans for childcare.

> Effective April 1 the household income that qualifies families to receive the maximum childcare subsidy will increase from $35,000 to

$50,000. This will allow additional low- and middle- income families to receive new or increased funding to offset the cost of accessing childcare, which is a positive development; that is, of course, if they are able to find the childcare space. My understanding is that only about one-fifth of our young parents that are working — that is, about 70 per cent of the mothers that have children of childcare age — can get access to childcare services.[79]

Swann commended the expansion of eligibility for the childcare subsidy but drew attention to the limitations of the current childcare environment for working parents across the population.

Although the health ministry was not part of the new Ministry of Human Services, it was, according to Hancock, integrally involved in the social policy framework itself.[80] Although members could, and did, raise fair questions about what the framework actually meant in practice,[81] the document upon its release in February 2013 showed alignment with a health-in-all-policies approach.[82] For example, included among the main goals was "to coordinate activities within and between government . . . and to ensure that there is policy alignment and consistency." Further, in a section titled "What is social policy," the wording conveys an upstream orientation: "social policy extends beyond a narrow definition of social services and supports: it is about how we work, live, and spend our time, and it helps determine how we come together to meet human needs like housing, employment, education, recreation, leisure, health, safety, and the care of children."[83] Other references to "health" likewise suggest alignment with a social determinants approach; for example, the framework document says that "social, economic, and environmental policies interact and complement each other. For instance . . . land use and development decisions are linked to economic and recreational opportunities at the local level, and the health of the physical environments — from clean air to safe drinking water — is related to the health of the people who live in them."[84]

Overall, these statements illustrate a framework that might have supported an upstream, population-level, social justice-oriented approach to public policy, consistent with a social determinants of health perspective. Unfortunately, we did not get a chance to see whether or to what extent those intentions would have materialized, because the framework disappeared in 2014 with the election of Jim Prentice (PC). This turn was disappointing to many, including Laurie Blakeman, still the Liberal MLA for Edmonton-Centre, who made the following comments in the Prentice throne speech debate in November 2014.

What I want to talk about is what's not in the throne speech. . . . This throne speech had no reference to the social policy framework. . . . Why would you abandon something that so many people have worked on so hard, that was such a buy-in from so many people?

Today we have over 140,000 people in poverty, children in poverty . . . and what are you doing about it? Where is the social policy framework? . . . Like, how many times do you guys have to be given the studies and the facts and the numbers that show you that an investment in social policy pays off over and over and over again? But, no, you guys want to have more police and more ambulance workers and more prisons, because that's where everybody ends up, when you could be investing on the front end.[85]

Conclusions

Anchored in contemporary calls for a health-in-all-policies approach, which is integral to a broad version of public health, in this chapter we considered examples of how the social determinants of health concept has manifested in provincial governments across Alberta's history, including whether or the extent to which an upstream, social justice-oriented approach is evident.

During the first half of the twentieth century, there are examples where formal health structures, such as local boards of health and the provincial Department of Public Health, participated substantively in social assistance initiatives, thus embedding the notion that health and social factors are connected and suggesting subtle but potentially important ways in which governance arrangements matter. And indeed, when health and social policy domains were deliberately placed together in the 1970s in the provincial Department of Health and Social Development, there are indications that, despite some ongoing examples of "turf wars," health and social services seemed to become somewhat more integrated over time. Importantly, however, integrating (or providing a mechanism to integrate) services or policy domains does not in itself ensure an upstream approach as embraced by a social determinants of health perspective. To ensure that health, rather than a narrow focus on illness, and equity, rather than charity, are emphasized, other factors — such as vision, public engagement, leadership, tools for evaluation, and funding — need to be in place.[86]

In their report titled *Health Equity through Intersectoral Action*, the World Health Organization recommended, among other things using political champions to advocate for intersectoral action.[87] This need for political leadership and vision is perhaps best illustrated by our analysis of the most recent period of the

1990s through the 2010s. There were several individuals in the Alberta govern-ment — such as Linda Sloan and Laurie Blakeman — who were highly know-ledgeable, articulate, and passionate about the social determinants of health. Perhaps a main comment of regret is that there were too few of them. Building capacity to mobilize around such voices is an important goal for a united public health community in Alberta that can effectively work toward improving health and well-being for everyone.

NOTES

1   Dennis Raphael, "Part One. Introducing the Social Determinants of Health," in *Social Determinants of Health: Canadian Perspectives* (2nd ed.), ed. Dennis Raphael (Toronto: Canadian Scholars' Press Inc., 2009); Dennis Raphael et al., *Social Determinants of Health: The Canadian Facts* (2nd ed.) (Oshawa: Ontario Tech University Faculty of Health Sciences and Toronto: York University School of Health Policy and Management, 2020), http://www.thecanadianfacts.org/; Katherine L. Frohlich, Nancy Ross, Chantelle Richmond, "Health Disparities in Canada Today: Some Evidence and a Theoretical Framework," *Health Policy* 79, no. 2–3 (2006); Margaret Whitehead, "The Concepts and Principles of Equity in Health," *International Journal of Health Services* 22 (1992).

2   National Collaborating Centre for Determinants of Health (NCCDH), *Let's Talk: Health Equity*, 2nd ed. (Antigonish, NS: NCCDH, St. Francis Xavier University, 2023), https://nccdh.ca/images/uploads/ NCCDH_Lets_Talk_Health_Equity_EN_June5.pdf.

3   For example, Canadian Public Health Association (CPHA), *Public Health: A Conceptual Framework*, Canadian Public Health Association Working Paper (Ottawa: CPHA, 2017), https://www.cpha.ca/ public-health-conceptual-framework; David Butler-Jones, *The Chief Public Health Officer's Report on the State of Public Health in Canada 2008: Addressing Health Inequalities* (Ottawa: Public Health Agency of Canada, 2008), https://www.canada.ca/en/public-health/corporate/publications/chief-public-health-officer-reports-state-public-health-canada/report-on-state-public-health-canada-2008. html); NCCDH, *Alberta Health Services: Establishing a Province-Wide Social Determinants of Health and Health Equity Approach* (Antigonish, NS: NCCDH, St. Francis Xavier University, 2013), http:// nccdh.ca/images/uploads/Alberta_Health_Services_Case_Study_Final_En.pdf.

4   Dennis Raphael, "A Discourse Analysis of the Social Determinants of Health," *Critical Public Health* 21, no. 2 (2011); Amy S. Katz et al., "Vagueness, Power and Public Health: Use of 'vulnerable' in Public Health Literature," *Critical Public Health*, published online 27 August 2019; Lindsay McLaren et al., "Unpacking Vulnerability: Towards Language that Advances Understanding and Resolution of Social Inequities in Public Health," *Canadian Journal of Public Health* 111, no. 3 (2020); Commission on Social Determinants of Health, *Closing the Gap in a Generation: Health Equity through Action on the Social Determinants of Health. Final Report of the Commission on Social Determinants of Health* (Geneva: World Health Organization (WHO), 2008). See also Ron Labonté and David Stuckler, "The Rise of Neoliberalism: How Bad Economics Imperils Health and What to Do About It," *Journal of Epidemiology and Community Health* 70, no. 3 (2016); Fran Baum and Matthew Fisher, "Why Behavioural Health Promotion Endures Despite Its Failure to Reduce Health Inequities," *Sociology of Health & Illness* 36, no. 2 (2014); Fran Baum and Matthew Sanders, "Ottawa 25 Years On: A More Radical Agenda for Health Equity is Still Required," *Health Promotion International* 26, suppl. 2 (2011); Gemma Carey et al., "Can the Sociology of Social Problems Help Us to Understand and Manage 'Lifestyle Drift'?" *Health Promotion International* 32, no. 4 (August 2017); NCCDH, *Let's Talk*.

5   Paul Kershaw, "The Need for Health in All Policies in Canada," *Canadian Medical Association Journal* 190, no. 3 (22 January 2018); Marcello Tonelli, Kwok-Cho Tang and Pierre-Gerlier Forest, "Canada Needs a 'Health in All Policies' Action Plan Now," *Canadian Medical Association Journal* 192, no. 3 (20 January 2020); Evelyne de Leeuw and Carole Clavier, "Healthy Public in All Policies," *Health Promotion International* 26, suppl. 2 (2011).

6   Baldwin Reichwein, *Benchmarks in Alberta's Public Welfare Services: History Rooted in Benevolence, Harshness, Punitiveness and Stinginess* (Edmonton: Alberta College of Social Workers, 2002), https://citeseerx.ist.psu.edu/ document?repid=rep1&type=pdf&doi=84d030e8d1a2d68776e33faed426e6722746d404; Canadian Association of Physicians for the Environment, "Backgrounder: Alberta Coal Plants, Climate Change & Human Health" (2015), https://cape.ca/wp-content/uploads/2018/02/CAPE-Backgrounder-Alberta-Coal-Plants-Climate-Change-Health-2015.pdf; Ann Curry-Stevens, "When Economic

Growth Doesn't Trickle Down: The Wage Dimensions of Income Polarization," in Raphael, *Social Determinants of Health: Canadian Perspectives*, 41–60; Nathalie Auger and Carolyne Alix, "Income, Income Distribution, and Health in Canada," in Raphael, *Social Determinants of Health: Canadian Perspectives*; Richard G. Wilkinson, *Unhealthy Societies: The Afflictions of Inequality* (London: Routledge, 1996); Richard Wilkinson and Kate Pickett, *The Spirit Level: Why Equality is Better for Everyone* (London: Penguin Books, 2009). See also various reports by Parkland Institute (https://www.parklandinstitute.ca).

7   Reichwein, *Benchmarks in Alberta's Public Welfare Services*.

8   "Poor Law – British Legislation," *Encyclopedia Britannica*, accessed 25 November 2020, https://www.britannica.com/event/Poor-Law; Reichwein, *Benchmarks in Alberta's Public Welfare Services*.

9   Robert L. Barker, *The Social Work Dictionary* (Washington, DC: NASW Press, 2003), 474.

10   Reichwein, *Benchmarks in Alberta's Public Welfare Services*. See also Lindsay McLaren, "In Defense of a Population-level Approach to Prevention: Why Public Health Matters Today," *Canadian Journal of Public Health* 110, no. 3 (2019).

11   Gøsta Esping-Andersen, *The Three Worlds of Welfare Capitalism* (Princeton, NJ: Princeton University Press, 1990); Raphael et al., *Social Determinants of Health: The Canadian Facts*. In this context, liberal refers to classical liberalism and its emphasis on individual liberty and equality.

12   Reichwein, *Benchmarks in Alberta's Public Welfare Services*. The single-term leadership of the provincial NDP (2015–2019) represents somewhat of an exception to this broad statement.

13   Kersti Bergqvist, Monica Åberg Yngwe and Olle Lundberg, "Understanding the Role of Welfare State Characteristics for Health and Inequalities," *BMC Public Health* 13, no. 1 (27 December 2013): 1234, https://doi.org/10.1186/1471-2458-13-1234; Gemma Carey and Brad Crammond, "A Glossary of Policy Frameworks: The Many Forms of 'Universalism' and Policy 'Targeting,'" *Journal of Epidemiology and Community Health* 71 (2017); Judith Green et al., "A Model of How Targeted and Universal Welfare Entitlements Impact on Material, Psycho-social and Structural Determinants of Health in Older Adults," *Social Science & Medicine* 187 (2017); Lindsay McLaren and Rachel Petit, "Universal and Targeted Policy to Achieve Health Equity: A Critical Analysis of the Example of Community Water Fluoridation Cessation in Calgary, Canada in 2011," *Critical Public Health* 28, no. 2 (2018).

14   Maureen Riddell and Richard Sherbaniuk, *Towards a Healthier City: A History of the Edmonton Board of Health, 1871–1995* (Edmonton: 1995), 18.

15   Provincial Archives of Alberta (PAA), *Administrative History of the Government of Alberta, 1905–2005* (Edmonton: PAA, 2006); Alvin Finkel, *The Social Credit Phenomenon in Alberta* (Toronto: University of Toronto Press, 1989).

16   Malcolm R. Bow, "Public Health Yesterday, To-Day, and To-Morrow," *Canadian Journal of Public Health* 28, no. 7 (July 1937).

17   The 1971 Speech from the Throne by Harry Strom (SC) can be found in Jack Lucas and Jean-Philippe Gauvin, "Alberta Throne Speeches 1906–2017 (Comparative Agendas Project)," 2019, https://doi.org/10.5683/SP2/0WH5FH, Scholars Portal Dataverse, V1.

18   PAA, *Administrative History of the Government of Alberta, 1905–2005*.

19   For the historical nuances of the lengthy Social Credit leadership in Alberta see Alvin Finkel, *The Social Credit Phenomenon in Alberta* (Toronto: University of Toronto Press, 1989). See also Nancy Kotani and Ann Goldblatt, "Alberta: A Haven for Health Promotion," in *Health Promotion in Canada: Provincial, National & International Perspectives*, eds. Ann Pederson, Michel O'Neill and Irving Rootman (Toronto: W.B. Saunders Canada, 1994).

20   "Boards Inquiry Established," *Edmonton Journal*, 8 April 1965, Alberta Legislature Library, Scrapbook Hansard and "Medical Committee Revived," *Edmonton Journal*, 7 April 1966. Alberta Legislature Library, Scrapbook Hansard. All Scrapbook Hansard references are available at: https://librarysearch.assembly.ab.ca/client/en_CA/scrapbookhansard.

21   The report included recommendations in the following topic areas of preventive services: food safety, occupational health, venereal disease, alcoholism, disability, mental health, home care, tuberculosis, dental health, health services to Indigenous Peoples, lab services, health education, workforce development, and tobacco control. Legislative Assembly of Alberta, *Report of the Special Legislative and Lay Committee*.

22   "Public Health Shake-up Urged," *Edmonton Journal*, 3 March 1967, Alberta Legislature Library, Scrapbook Hansard. The report was tabled in the Legislature on 3 March 1967: "Report Makes 247 Proposals," *Edmonton Journal*, 3 March 1967, Alberta Legislature Library, Scrapbook Hansard.

23   "Plan to Upgrade Health Services," *Edmonton Journal*, 28 March 1968; "Health Bill Divides Opposition," *Edmonton Journal*, 23 April 1968; "Health Region Legislation Held Back for Further Study," *Edmonton Journal*, 5 May 1968; all from Alberta Legislature Library, Scrapbook Hansard.

24 Legislative Assembly of Alberta, *Report of the Special Legislative and Lay Committee*, 109–110.

25 Alberta Department of Public Health, *Annual Report 1967* (Edmonton: Printed by L. S. Wall, Printer to the Queen's Most Excellent Majesty, 1969), 10–11; Legislative Assembly of Alberta, *Report of the Special Legislative and Lay Committee*; *The Department of Health Act*, S.P.A. 1967, c. 27.

26 "Career Service Setting Up Urged," *Edmonton Journal*, 3 March 1967, Alberta Legislature Library, Scrapbook Hansard.

27 Leslie Bella, "The Goal Effectiveness of Alberta's Preventive Social Services Program," *Canadian Public Policy* 8, no. 2 (1982); Leslie Bella, "The Provincial Role in the Canadian Welfare State: The Influence of Provincial Social Policy Initiatives on the Design of the Canada Assistance Plan," *Canadian Public Administration* 22 no. 3 (1979).

28 Some of the provincial funding was shared with the federal government under the Canada Assistance Plan, which was also introduced in 1996. See Bella, "The Provincial Role in the Canadian Welfare State."

29 Bella, "Goal Effectiveness." According to Bella, the program — which was introduced in 1966 — was one of the few to survive into the more fiscally restricted seventies. Further, and based on research by Bella and others, the program was expanded and was renamed Alberta Family and Community Support Services Program.

30 Dustin Galer, "Disability Rights Movement in Canada," in *The Canadian Encyclopedia. Historica Canada*, 4 February 2015; last edited 23 April 2015, https://www.thecanadianencyclopedia.ca/en/article/disability-rights-movement.

31 "Public Health Shake-up Urged," *Edmonton Journal*; "Other Spending," *Edmonton Journal*.

32 Sheila Gibbons, "Alberta Government Creates Blair Commission to Study Mental Health Services in Alberta," *Eugenics Archives*, published 18 October 2013, https://eugenicsarchives.ca/discover/timeline/5260cf02c6813a546900001f.

33 Alberta. Legislative Assembly of Alberta, 16 March 1972. All Alberta Hansard transcripts are available at https://www.assembly.ab.ca/assembly-business/transcripts/transcripts-by-type.

34 "Address in Reply to the Speech from the Throne – Horner," 26 February 1971, Alberta Legislature Library, Scrapbook Hansard.

35 "Budget Debate: Werry," 1 March 1971, Alberta Legislature Library, Scrapbook Hansard.

36 Bob Bell, "Session Ends, MLAs Focus on Election," *Edmonton Journal*, 28 April 1971, Alberta Legislature Library, Scrapbook Hansard.

37 PAA, *Administrative History of the Government of Alberta, 1905–2005.*

38 Alberta. Legislative Assembly of Alberta, 13 March 1972.

39 Alberta. Legislative Assembly of Alberta, 6 March 1972 (throne speech debate).

40 Alberta. Legislative Assembly of Alberta, 13 March 1972.

41 Alberta. Legislative Assembly of Alberta, 16 March 1972.

42 Alberta. Legislative Assembly of Alberta, 3 March 1972.

43 Alberta. Legislative Assembly of Alberta, 14 March 1972.

44 Alberta Health and Social Development, *Annual Report 1971–72* (Edmonton, 1972), 2.

45 Alberta Health and Social Development, *Annual Report 1971–72*, 2.

46 Alberta Health and Social Development, *Annual Report 1972–73* (Edmonton, 1973), and Alberta Health and Social Development, *Annual Report 1973–74* (Edmonton, 1974); Bella, "Goal Effectiveness."

47 Alberta Health and Social Development, *Annual Report 1971–72*; Alberta Health and Social Development, *Annual Report 1972–73*; Alberta Health and Social Development, *Annual Report 1973–74.*

48 Marc Lalonde, *A New Perspective on the Health of Canadians*, Government of Canada (1974), https://www.phac-aspc.gc.ca/ph-sp/pdf/perspect-eng.pdf.

49 PAA, *Administrative History of the Government of Alberta, 1905–2005.* The Department of Hospitals and Medicare absorbed the Hospital Services Commission, an agency that had been created in 1971 that reported to the Minister of Health and Social Development.

50 Alberta Social Services and Community Health, *Annual Report 1975–76* (Edmonton, 1976), 11.

51 Alberta Social Services and Community Health. *Annual Report 1975–76*, 33.

52 Alberta Social Services and Community Health, *Annual Report 1977–78* (Edmonton, 1978).

53 PAA, *Administrative History of the Government of Alberta, 1905–2005.*

54 "Health Promotion Action Means," Health Promotion, WHO, accessed 22 November 2020, https://www.who.int/healthpromotion/conferences/previous/ottawa/en/index1.html.

55 Alberta Health, *Annual Report 1993–1994* (Edmonton, 1994), 8.

56   Kevin Taft, *Shredding the Public Interest* (Edmonton: Parkland Institute, 1997).

57   Although the ideas underlying the social determinants concept are longstanding, the phrase "social determinants of health" arguably started in the 1990s (an early example is the 1998 book by Marmot and Wilkinson: Michael Marmot and Richard G. Wilkinson, *Social Determinants of Health*, 1st ed. [Copenhagen: WHO, 1998]) and expanded significantly in the 2000s. The phrase served as an informative, and fairly specific, search term. We did not systematically search for other terms such as "health in all policies" or "healthy public policy," which is a limitation. However, as seen in our analysis, these ideas did come up in our search, thus speaking to the overlap amongst the terms.

58   There are others who spoke up for social determinants of health but whom we did not feature here, including long-serving Liberal MLA (Edmonton Riverview) Kevin Taft, and David Swann. As one example of Taft's mobilization of the social determinants of health concept, in 2002 Taft spoke in favour of Bill 6: Student Financial Assistance Act, highlighting the benefits of fair access to education not only for individuals but also for society as a whole, including reducing societal inequality and contributing to a healthy, functioning democracy (Alberta. Legislative Assembly of Alberta, 7 March 2002), and during Oral Question Period in 2006 when Taft questioned the government's focus on health reform that would involve out-of-pocket payment in the context of a growing gap between rich and poor in the province (Alberta. Legislative Assembly of Alberta, 14 March 2006).

59   Legislative Assembly of Alberta, member profiles, https://www.assembly.ab.ca/members/members-of-the-legislative-assembly (use search function to locate a particular MLA from any legislative session). Sloan was also a nurse.

60   Alberta. Legislative Assembly of Alberta, 22 May 1997.

61   Alberta. Legislative Assembly of Alberta, 12 April 1999.

62   The Parkland Institute was founded during, and in response to, massive political, economic and cultural changes including those embodied in Alberta by the Klein administration. "About Parkland Institute," Parkland Institute, accessed 22 November 2020, https://www.parklandinstitute.ca/about.

63   Alberta. Legislative Assembly of Alberta, 9 April 2005.

64   Alberta. Legislative Assembly of Alberta, 2 March 2006.

65   Alberta. Legislative Assembly of Alberta, 7 March 2005.

66   These comments came from Dr. Bruce Miller (Liberal), MLA for Edmonton-Glenora, and Dr. David Swann (Liberal), MLA for Calgary-Mountain View. Alberta. Legislative Assembly of Alberta, 7 March 2005.

67   Alberta. Legislative Assembly of Alberta, 7 March 2005.

68   Alberta. Legislative Assembly of Alberta, 26 November 2007.

69   Members who spoke in support of Bill 214 included Harry Chase, Bridget Pastoor, Jack Flaherty, Craig Cheffins, and David Taylor, all Liberals and all of whom spoke to the bill's emphasis on upstream approaches to the well-being of the collective.

70   Alberta. Legislative Assembly of Alberta, 26 November 2007.

71   Alberta. Legislative Assembly of Alberta, 26 November 2007; "Our Mandate," Health Quality Council of Alberta, accessed 22 November 2020, https://hqca.ca/about/our-mandate/.

72   Alberta. Legislative Assembly of Alberta, 26 November 2007.

73   Alberta. Legislative Assembly of Alberta, 3 December 2007.

74   "Health Impact Assessment," Health Topics, WHO, accessed 22 November 2020, https://www.who.int/health-topics/health-impact-assessment#tab=tab_1.

75   Alberta. Legislative Assembly of Alberta, 7 March 2012 (Fred Horne, Progressive Conservative Minister and MLA for Edmonton-Rutherford).

76   Alberta. Legislative Assembly of Alberta, 13 March 2012.

77   Alberta. Legislative Assembly of Alberta, 13 March 2012.

78   Vicki Chartrand, "Broken System: Why is a Quarter of Canada's Prison Population Indigenous?" *The Conversation*, 18 February 2018, https://theconversation.com/broken-system-why-is-a-quarter-of-canadas-prison-population-indigenous-91562.

79   Alberta. Legislative Assembly of Alberta, 13 March 2012.

80   Alberta. Legislative Assembly of Alberta, 13 March 2012.

81   For example, David Swann (Liberal, Calgary-Mountain View) commented: "With respect to the social policy framework . . . I think it's very timely and important for Albertans to be part of that discussion. The minister references the policy framework in broad, vague terms but has yet to tell Albertans in plain language what it's all supposed to mean. I've heard it referred to as an integrated strategy, a comprehensive review, a public consultation, a transition to outcome-based service delivery, and lots of seemingly disparate issues. Can the minister explain what the social policy framework is, how long

its development is expected to take, and what might happen as a result of the framework?" (Alberta. Legislative Assembly of Alberta, 13 March 2012).

82   Alberta Government, *Alberta's Social Policy Framework* (Edmonton, February 2013), https://open. alberta.ca/publications/6214203.

83   Alberta Government, *Alberta's Social Policy Framework*, 4.

84   Alberta Government, *Alberta's Social Policy Framework*, 4–5. See section titled "What is Social Policy?"

85   Alberta. Legislative Assembly of Alberta, 24 November 2014 (evening).

86   Maria Guglielmin et al., "A Scoping Review of the Implementation of Health in All Policies at the Local Level," *Health Policy* 122, no. 3 (2018); Lindsay McLaren and Daniel J. Dutton, "The Social Determinants of Pandemic Impact: An Opportunity to Rethink What We Mean by 'Public Health Spending,'" editorial, *Canadian Journal of Public Health* 111 (2020).

87   Public Health Agency of Canada and WHO, *Health Equity Through Intersectoral Action*.

13

Public Health Leadership: Courage, Conflict, and Evolving Understanding of Power

Donald W.M. Juzwishin and Rogelio Velez Mendoza

Introduction

This chapter showcases twenty-two leaders in public health in Alberta; that is, people who have — over the course of our time period of interest (1919–2019) — been recognized as showing knowledge, courage, commitment, and passion in challenging the status quo and advancing public health science, practice, or policy in Alberta, at times at personal cost to themselves.

Our task in this chapter is somewhat fraught. On the one hand, there are many people who have done important work in public health throughout Alberta's history. From the point of view of the weakening of public health discussed in the introduction to this book, and our goal of contributing to a broad and coherent vision for the field, it is interesting and informative to learn about the accomplishments of key individuals from the past and present. To that end, we assembled the list from various sources, including crowdsourcing nominations from among our (admittedly, mostly professional) Alberta networks.

On the other hand, it would be a grave mistake to consider any historical list of leaders — including this one — uncritically. Who becomes a leader is not arbitrary, nor is it reducible to neoliberal notions of meritocracy. Paths to leadership are situated within social, economic, and political context, which manifest in differential opportunities along dimensions such as class, gender, and ethnicity as they intersect with discipline, sector, and profession. Collectively, these dynamics influence who appears — and who does not appear — in historical records, and why.

These dynamics of power are inherent to a broad vision of public health, and we encourage critical reflection by readers as they read this (inevitably incomplete) list of people who have contributed to public health in Alberta. We conclude our chapter commentary here.

Malcolm Ross Bow, MD (1887–1982)

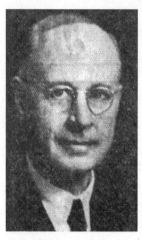

Fig. 13.1: Malcolm Ross Bow. Published in the *Edmonton Journal* (5 October 1944), a Division of Postmedia Network Inc.

For twenty-five years, public health in Alberta was synonymous with Dr. Malcolm Ross Bow. Bow served as deputy minister of public health from 1927 to 1952, and there were few things related to health in the province that did not have his signature during this time (see also Chapters 3 and 4). His contributions shaped government efforts related to mental health, health units, health insurance, tuberculosis treatment, and maternity care, among others. He constantly stressed that investment in prevention, versus cure, was better for Albertans, and cost-beneficial for the province as well.[1]

Born in Ontario in 1887, Bow travelled west after receiving his medical degree and spent fourteen years as chief medical officer of health in Saskatchewan. Under his leadership as deputy minister of public health for Alberta, initiatives included overseeing the expansion of health units in the province following a 1929 amendment to Alberta's Public Health Act; increasing the number of district health nurses from twenty-five in 1939 to thirty-six in 1945; creating rural maternity and "Well Baby" programs around the province; and passing the Tuberculosis Act in 1936, which provided free diagnosis and care for pulmonary tuberculosis.[2] Also during his tenure as deputy minister, Bow oversaw the implementation of the Sexual Sterilization Act (1928), which he openly supported.[3] Bow retained his deputy minister position through the significant change of government in 1935 with the election of the Social Credit party. Bow has been credited with being instrumental in efforts to lower mortality and morbidity from preventable diseases in Alberta.[4]

Bow was also an educator. From 1938 until 1954 he taught public health at the University of Alberta, and he published extensively on the topic, including several papers in the *Canadian Journal of Public Health*. He served as president of the Canadian Public Health Association in 1937. Bow died at the Royal Alexandra Hospital in 1982, at age ninety-four.

Ashbury Somerville, MD (1896-1967)

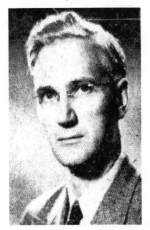

Fig. 13.2: Ashbury Somerville. Published in the *Edmonton Journal* (4 October 1952), a Division of Postmedia Network Inc.

Dr. Ashbury Somerville was born in Hartney, Manitoba and served overseas with the Canadian Army in World War I. Following the war, and after graduating from the University of Manitoba, he practised medicine for several years in Eckville, Alberta. Somerville subsequently obtained his diploma in public health from the University of Toronto in 1932 and served successively in three Alberta Institutions: the Red Deer Health Unit, the Baker Memorial Sanatorium in Calgary, and the Provincial Mental Hospital in Ponoka.

In 1936, Somerville became the medical officer of health of the Foothills Health Unit in High River, Alberta, and in 1942, he was appointed director of communicable disease control, director of health units, and inspector of hospitals for the provincial Department of Public Health.[5] In 1952, Somerville became acting assistant deputy minister of health, succeeding Malcolm Bow upon his retirement, and subsequently served as deputy minister of health until 1961.[6]

While serving on the Nursing Education Committee of the University of Alberta's General Faculty Council, Somerville chaired a committee to study and report on the nursing education facilities and programs of the schools of nursing in Alberta. He also contributed to the work of the Canadian Public Health Association, including serving for several years on the executive council and as president during 1954-1955. In 1965, the Canadian Public Health Association awarded him with an Honorary Life Membership.[7]

Although Somerville retired from active involvement in public health in 1961, he continued to contribute his time. In 1965, he was appointed chair of the newly formed Legislative and Lay Committee to study preventive health services in Alberta (see Chapter 12).[8]

Laura Margaret Attrux, LLD (1909-1987)

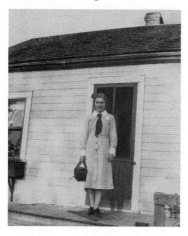

Fig. 13.3: Laura Margaret Attrux. "Laura Attrux, district nurse, Whitecourt, Alberta," 1944, NA-3953-6, Courtesy of Glenbow Archives, Archives and Special Collections, University of Calgary.

Laura Attrux was born in Duck Lake, Saskatchewan, on 29 June 1909. For her contributions to nursing, she was recognized with an honorary doctor of laws degree from the University of Alberta in 1970.

Attrux enrolled at St. Paul's Hospital School of Nursing in Saskatoon, graduating in 1930. Postgraduate training took her to the Vancouver General Hospital, where she trained in obstetrics followed by more intense training at the New York Maternity Centre and the Kentucky Frontier Centre. She received her certificate in advanced obstetrics for nurses from the University of Alberta and a diploma in public health nursing from the University of Toronto.[9]

Attrux started her career in obstetrics at the Holy Cross Hospital in Calgary in 1933. Her heart, however, was in public health, and in 1939 she accepted a post in Valleyview, Alberta, a small rural community where she served for two years. Next, she moved to Whitecourt, Alberta, where she applied her public health skills in areas ranging from dentistry to veterinary work. In 1949, Attrux moved to Smith, Alberta and set up monthly clinics in surrounding communities. By that time, Slave Lake was large enough to have its own district nursing service, and Attrux accepted the position of district nurse in 1951. Ten years later, she took a position in Wabasca, north of Slave Lake, Alberta and convinced the Minister of Health, Donovan Ross, to provide a four-wheel drive vehicle for getting around the community.

Attrux served the Indigenous Peoples of the Wabasca region where her focus included tuberculosis control. In the fall of 1962, Attrux went to Swan Hills to establish the municipal nursing service and once complete she moved to High Level to set up the municipal nursing service in 1964, which was Alberta's most northerly post and from where she served many surrounding communities, including Paddle Prairie, Keg River Cabins, Keg River Post, Rainbow Lake, and Carcajou. Serving such a large area and in the context of the oil boom in Alberta, Attrux enrolled in the local flying school and purchased a Cessna 150. When Rainbow Lake needed nursing service, she served the area by flying in. Attrux loved serving her communities and was proud of having delivered 1,031 babies and having helped to set up nursing stations across the province. Attrux retired in 1974, after thirty-five years of public health service.[10]

Attrux died in 1987 and is buried near her childhood home in Hafford, Saskatchewan.

Helen Griffith Wylie Watson, BSc, MA (1911–1974)

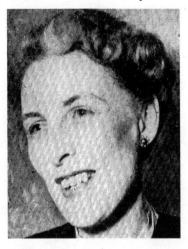

Helen Watson made substantial contributions to public health at local, provincial, national, and international levels through her leadership as a district nurse, university educator, and director of public health nursing in Alberta.[11] Born in Stettler, Alberta, Watson graduated from the University of Alberta with a BSc degree in nursing in 1934, and she subsequently earned a major in public health nursing from the University of British Columbia.

Watson began working as a nurse in 1931 with the Okotoks/High River Rural Health Unit, one of Alberta's first experiments to establish health units to serve a rural population. In 1937 she joined the provincial Division of Public Health Nursing and served as a district nurse carrying out midwifery and emergency medical services in Alberta communities that had neither a hospital nor a physician, including Stanmore, Peers, Valleyview, Kinuso, and Bow Island.

Fig. 13.4: Helen Griffith Wylie Watson (née McArthur). Published in the *Vancouver Sun* (12 December 1946), a Division of Postmedia Network Inc.

Recognizing the need for midwifery services in rural Alberta, Watson attended Columbia University, graduating in 1940. For her MA thesis, she developed a midwifery course for Alberta's district nurses. On her return to Alberta, Watson assumed the post of acting director of the School of Nursing at the University of Alberta, where she implemented the course. She continued to expand the provincial nursing service in her capacity as director of the Public Health Nursing Division in the provincial Department of Public Health, a position that she held from 1944 to 1946. During her time as director, seven "One-Nurse" health units were established in rural Alberta. Watson served as president of the Alberta Public Health Association in 1944–1945.

In 1946, Watson was appointed the first national director of Red Cross Nursing Services, a position she held for twenty-four years. She served on the International Council of Nurses where she chaired a nursing advisory committee, and she was president of the Canadian Nurses Association from 1950 to 1954. In 1957, the Red Cross awarded Watson the Florence Nightingale Award for her years of service, and in 1964 the University of Alberta bestowed an honorary doctor of laws degree. Watson was named an Officer of the Order of Canada just before her death in 1974.[12]

Edward Stuart Orford Smith, MSc, MB, DPH, FRCPC (1911–1983)

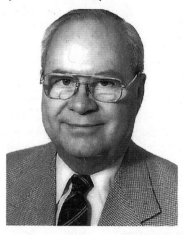

Fig. 13.5: E.S.O. Smith. Photo courtesy of family of Dr. Smith.

Edward Stuart Orford Smith was born in London, England on 10 July 1919. He grew up in London and attended Marlborough College, Cambridge University, and the University of London in England, followed by the School of Hygiene at the University of Toronto, earning a total of eleven academic degrees and fellowships.

In July 1940, Smith entered medical school at the London Hospital Medical College just as the World War II bombing of London began. The experience exposed him to more trauma victims than would have been the case during peacetime. He joined the army in 1943 as an officer for the First Battalion of the Manchester Regiment and landed in Normandy on 27 June 1944, twenty-one days after D-Day.[13] Interested in public health, Smith enrolled in 1946 at the London School of Hygiene and Tropical Medicine. After graduation he worked in England and in the French zone of Germany with the International Refugee Organization until 1951.

Smith's public health service in Alberta began in 1953 as medical officer of health in the Sturgeon Health Unit. He also served as director of local health services (1956–1966) and as director of epidemiology for the departments of Health (1967–1971), Health and Social Development (1971–1975), and Social Services and Community Health (1975–1979).[14] Smith developed and taught a course in epidemiology at the University of Alberta. He was president of the Canadian Public Health Association in 1974–1975, where he served on numerous committees including as chair of the Canadian Public Health Association's task force on fluoride. He was a member of the Alberta Public Health Association for more than twenty-five years, serving sixteen years in executive offices, including as president in 1965–1966.[15]

Smith wrote over thirty scientific publications on topics such as poliomyelitis, rabies, cancer, hypertension, smoking, alcohol, traffic accidents, venereal disease, heart disease, family planning, epidemiology, reporting and contact tracing methods, and occupational health. He served in Alberta as commanding officer of the #23 Medical Company in the militia and as provincial commissioner of the St. John Ambulance Brigade.[16]

A few of the honours awarded to Dr. Smith over his life include the Canadian Forces Decoration and Clasp; Knight of Grace, Order of St. Lazarus; Serving Brother and Officer Brother, Order of St. John; and Her Majesty the Queen's Silver Jubilee Medal. Smith died in 1983.

James Howell, MD, FRCPC, FFPHM (1934–2012)

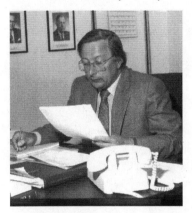

Fig. 13.6: James Howell. "Dr. Howell. Edmonton Board of Health," 1981, City of Edmonton Archives ET-28-262.

James Howell was born in Farnworth, Lancashire, England in 1934. He graduated with a degree in medicine from St. Mary's Hospital Medical School at the University of London in 1957. Howell was aware of and concerned about the social determinants of health, which led to his contributions to establishing programs to address health status inequities, child poverty, and community solidarity.

Howell immigrated with his family to Canada in 1967 to take the post of medical officer of health for the Sturgeon Health Unit in Alberta. Howell led the health unit in thinking about how it could best serve its community and address emerging public health challenges. In 1975, Howell became the medical officer of health for the Edmonton Board of Health, which was succeeded by the Capital Health Region. Howell oversaw the food and lodging regulations when Edmonton hosted the Commonwealth Games in 1978 as well as the immunization programs during the swine flu scare of 1976–1977. In the latter situation, Howell had to make a difficult decision to abandon the vaccination effort when he heard of the possible harmful side effects of the vaccine.[17]

Howell devoted his career to promoting and protecting health. One of his most important initiatives was the creation of the inner-city Boyle McCauley Health Centre, Edmonton's only community health centre.[18] As described by health units historian Adelaide Schartner, the centre served thousands of people living in significantly challenging circumstances, and "from the beginning, the goal of the health centre was to look at the whole person and include that person in decisions about their care."[19]

Howell was also a clinical professor in the Faculty of Medicine at the University of Alberta. In 1994, he was awarded the Canadian Public Health Association's R.D. Defries Award, their highest award, as well as Honorary Life Membership. Howell was an avid writer and historian of public health. He wrote a short history of the Edmonton Board of Health on the occasion of its 100th anniversary, which was published in the *Canadian Journal of Public Health*. Howell served the Capital Health Region for twenty-eight years. He died in 2012 after a brief illness.

John Waters, MD (1943–2001)

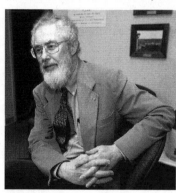

Fig. 13.7: John Waters. Edmonton Journal, 6 February 2001. Reproduced with the permission of the *Edmonton Journal*, a Division of Postmedia Network Inc.

Born in Edmonton in 1943, John Waters grew up in Winnipeg where he graduated from medical school in 1966. After some work in northern Manitoba, he was named Manitoba's chief medical officer. This experience brought him back to Alberta, where in 1980, he was named chief provincial health officer, a role he fulfilled for twenty-one years. Described by the *Globe and Mail* newspaper as "Alberta's low-profile lifesaver,"[20] Waters is credited as the driving force behind numerous provincial immunization programs that contributed to a decrease in the incidence of communicable diseases. Waters was passionate about child health, communicable disease control, and preventive medicine.

Waters established the Alberta Advisory Committee on Communicable Disease Control. He initiated the first provincial program for routine prenatal hepatitis B screening and introduced universal immunization programs including vaccines for measles, mumps, and rubella; haemophilus influenza type B; and hepatitis B, and he introduced a new whooping cough vaccine. He was regarded as one of Canada's top experts in communicable disease. Waters held clinical posts in departments of pediatrics, medicine, and community health sciences, at the University of Calgary and the University of Alberta.

Waters established a Council of Medical Officers of Health. He also served on various committees dedicated to immunization and infectious disease control, including the National Advisory Committee on Immunization, the Canadian Pediatric Society's Infectious Disease and Immunization Committee, the Canadian Working Group on Polio Eradication, and the Canadian Working Group on Measles Elimination.[21]

Waters was awarded the Canadian Public Health Association's R.D. Defries Award in 2002 and a scholarship in his name is administered by the Alberta Public Health Association. Waters died in 2001 at the age of fifty-eight.

Shirley M. Stinson, MNA, EdD, LLD (1929–2020)

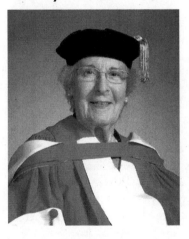

Fig. 13.8: Shirley Stinson. Photo courtesy of Shirley Stinson.

Shirley Stinson is recognized as a visionary leader, teacher, administrator, and researcher whose contributions are described as having changed the face of nursing in Canada.[22] Born in Arlee, Saskatchewan, in 1929, Stinson's nursing career began when she graduated from the University of Alberta with a BSc degree in nursing. Stinson earned her master's degree from the University of Minnesota and a doctor of education degree from Teacher's College, Columbia University, NY, making her the first Alberta nurse to complete a doctoral program.

Stinson spent her early career as a public health staff nurse before becoming a University of Alberta faculty member in 1969, where she held joint professor positions in the Faculty of Nursing and the Department of Public Health Sciences in the Faculty of Medicine. Her vision and belief that graduate nursing students require knowledge of advanced clinical nursing practice, theory, research, and history were the basis for Stinson's work in the establishment of western Canada's first master's in nursing program in 1975 at the University of Alberta. Stinson also designed the first funded Canadian PhD in nursing program. She played key roles in convincing the Alberta government to support nursing research, and the 1982 establishment of the Alberta

Foundation for Nursing Research — with Stinson as founding chair — made Alberta the first jurisdiction in the western world to earmark funds for nursing research.[23]

Stinson published extensively in scientific and professional literatures; lectured and advised professional organizations and institutions worldwide; served on advisory and development committees for international nursing conferences; and served as a consultant to organizations such as the Pan American Health Organization, the World Health Organization, and the Colombian Nurses Association in Bogotá.

Stinson received many awards, including the Senior National Health Scientist Research Award, which she was the first nurse and woman to receive. She also received Canada's two highest nursing awards: the Ross Award in Nursing Leadership and the Canadian Nurses Association's Jeanne Mance Award. Stinson was honoured by several lifetime memberships and four honorary doctorates. In 1999, she was awarded the Alberta Order of Excellence and in 2001, she was awarded Officer of the Order of Canada and invested in 2002.[24] Stinson died in 2020 at the age of ninety.

Karen Mills, DipNu, BScN, MHSA (b. 1932)

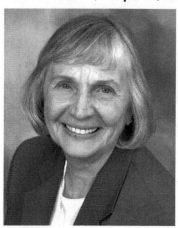

Fig. 13.9: Karen Mills. Photo by 2003 Wells Photographic Design for University of Alberta. Courtesy of Karen Mills.

Karen Mills was born and raised in Edmonton. Mills chose the public health nursing path because of an understanding that prevention, early intervention, and health promotion were essential ingredients in a healthy public.[25] Mills received her diploma in nursing from the University of Alberta Hospital in 1956, and subsequently completed her bachelor of science in nursing and master's in health services administration degrees at the University of Alberta.

Her career in public health spanned diverse roles, including public health staff nurse, associate director then director of nursing for the Edmonton Board of Health, and associate professor in the Faculty of Nursing at the University of Alberta. Mills served on a multitude of boards and organizations that focused on advancing the role of public health. Among her many honours are several lifetime memberships, including to the Alberta Public Health

Association and the Canadian Public Health Association. In 1989, Mills received the R.D. Defries Award from the Canadian Public Health Association. In 1993, she co-chaired the world's first International Conference on Community Health Nursing Research, which was held in Edmonton.[26]

In her nursing director capacity, Mills' management philosophy included encouraging further education and continuous learning and fostering supportive environments that enhanced staff skills, abilities, and approaches. Initiatives under her leadership, aside from vital basic public health nursing programs, were many and varied. In 1979, for example, nurses were called on to collaborate with other agencies to develop an effective response to the impact of refugees arriving from Indochina. Mills led a collaborative, immediate, and supportive response to survivors of the 1987 Edmonton tornado. Finally, a pilot Short Stay Maternity Program launched with the Royal Alexandra Hospital in 1989 led to the establishment of the Alberta Health Services Health Link program.

In her own words, Mills said of her work: "what is positive today is the heightened interest and attention to the need for prevention and promotion strategies. There seems a greater recognition and understanding of the complex interplay of factors that create and challenge health and well-being. Public health nurses practise in this environment, entering people's lives through a range of vital programs that serve the broad spectrum of community life. Working in public health has been a privilege."[27]

Doug Wilson, MD FRCPC (b. 1935)

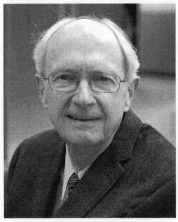

Fig. 13.10: Doug Wilson. Photo courtesy of the School of Public Health, University of Alberta.

Doug Wilson was born in Toronto in 1935. He graduated from the Faculty of Medicine at the University of Toronto in 1959 and trained in internal medicine and nephrology in Vancouver, Toronto, Boston, and London, England. In 1967, Wilson joined the staff of the Toronto General Hospital where he launched the kidney transplant program; he also practised, taught, and conducted research, and became professor of medicine and director of the Division of Nephrology. In 1984, he joined the University of Alberta as dean of the Faculty of Medicine, a position he held for ten years.[28]

After his deanship of the University of Alberta's Faculty of Medicine, Wilson's interest shifted toward public and population health and health promotion. He was instrumental in establishing the interdisciplinary Centre for Health Promotion Studies in 1996, which focused on the social and behavioural determinants of population health. He contributed substantially to the establishment of Canada's first stand-alone faculty dedicated to public health, at the University of Alberta, in the context of the post-Severe Acute Respiratory Syndrome crisis of the early 2000s (see Chapter 6).

Wilson is a Fellow of the Royal College of Physicians and Surgeons of Canada and of the American College of Physicians. He has received many awards for his contributions to public health including the Canadian Public Health Association Honorary Life Membership Award (2002) and Certificate of Merit (2006), and the Alberta Centennial Medal (2005). Wilson is a long-time supporter of the Alberta Public Health Association and is described by colleagues as a wise and respected leader. For him, public health's interdisciplinary focus and its strong connection to the community are critical elements to its success.[29]

Muriel Stanley Venne CM, BA (b. 1937)

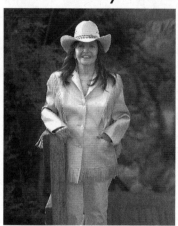

Fig. 13.11: Muriel Stanley Venne. Photo courtesy of the Alberta Order of Excellence.

Muriel Stanley Venne, a member of the Métis Nation, was born in Lamont, Alberta in 1937. Through her advocacy she has advanced fairness and justice in the treatment of Indigenous Peoples in Alberta, Canada, and internationally, for which she was inducted into the Alberta Order of Excellence in 2019. Having suffered and survived tuberculosis in her adolescence, Venne empathized with the suffering of others. A strong advocate against the abuse of Indigenous women, she started the Native Outreach program at the Métis Association of Alberta. In 1973, Premier Peter Lougheed appointed her to the Alberta Human Rights Commission where she advocated for Indigenous human rights issues. In 1984, Venne established the Institute for the Advancement of Aboriginal Women which serves to build community and educate people on the accomplishments of Indigenous women across Alberta. Instrumental in the publication of *The Rights Path – Alberta*, Venne raised awareness and understanding of Indigenous Peoples' human rights.[30]

Venne is strongly committed to bringing attention to and changing how the Canadian law and criminal justice systems respond to systemic violence against Indigenous women. Her work resulted in 231 Calls for Justice from the National Inquiry into Missing and Murdered Indigenous Women and Girls in Canada.

Venne understands the importance of recognizing and celebrating successes.[31] In 1995, she introduced the Esquao Awards, which honour the strength, resilience, and beauty of Indigenous women. Over 480 adult women from over ninety towns and cities across Alberta have received an Esquao Award.

Venne was honoured with the Alberta Human Rights Award in 1998, and she was the first Métis person to receive the Order of Canada in 2005.

Anne Fanning Binder, CM, MD, FRCPC (b. 1939)

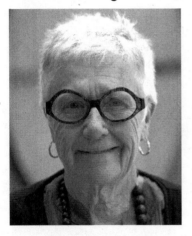

Fig. 13.12: Anne Fanning. Photo courtesy of University of Alberta Hospital photography department.

Anne Fanning was born in London, Ontario, in 1939 and studied medicine at the University of Western Ontario, graduating in 1963. Although she developed an early interest in public health, shaped by her mother's work as a school physician, Fanning chose to study internal medicine and infectious disease under the tutelage of George Goldsand, who saw the importance of bringing together the practices of medicine and public health.

Fanning's early work with tuberculosis patients revealed to her the threat that a manageable disease posed for populations living in oppressive conditions. To facilitate her effectiveness in treatment of tuberculosis at the Aberhart Hospital, she employed three Indigenous health workers to increase communication between patients and staff and to alleviate the devastating effect of long-term hospitalization. In 1987, Fanning was appointed director of Tuberculosis Services for Alberta, a position she held until 1995 when she was, in her words, "downsized." In her teaching role in the Division of Infectious Diseases at the University of Alberta, Fanning emphasized the unique health issues of Canada's Indigenous Peoples. She helped to create the Indigenous Health Care careers program to encourage Indigenous students to study medicine.[32]

Fanning's work at the University of Alberta drew her into the small but vigorous national and international community of experts involved in the prevention and treatment of tuberculosis. She has been an active member of the International Union Against Tuberculosis and Lung Disease since 1987, where she served ten years as a board member, including one term as president. She was the founder of the Union's North American Region, and she continues to be involved in the Global Indigenous STOP TB initiative and the working group on Ethics and Social Justice in Lung Health. Although she retired in 2007, Fanning remains strongly committed to issues of social justice, giving occasional lectures on tuberculosis and global health, and working with the Alberta Council for Global Cooperation to advance the United Nations Sustainable Development Goals. She received the Order of Canada in 2006 and the Alberta Order of Excellence in 2017.[33]

Wilton Littlechild CM, AOE, MSC, QC, IPC (b. 1944)

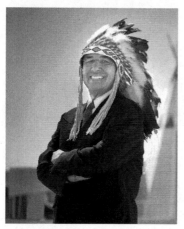

Fig. 13.13: Wilton Littlechild. Photo courtesy of the Alberta Order of Excellence.

Chief Wilton Littlechild was born on 1 April 1944 on the Ermineskin Reserve in Maskwacis, Alberta. He was taken from his family at age six and spent fourteen years at three different residential schools. Having experienced and borne witness to many sad and tragic abuses, Littlechild chose to focus on his positive experiences.[34] He gained resilience and confidence from sports, which he applied to education. While attending the University of Alberta, Littlechild played on the Golden Bears hockey and swimming teams and managed the basketball and football teams. He graduated with a bachelor's degree in 1967 and a master's degree in 1975, both in physical education.

Littlechild started the first all-Indigenous junior hockey team and many other sports programs in Alberta. He encouraged athletes to pursue their education by making that a prerequisite to play on teams he coached. A serious sports injury, coupled with a paucity of Indigenous lawyers, prompted Littlechild to pursue global Indigenous law as a career. In 1976, the Cree Nation honoured him as an Honorary Chief for being the first person with Indian Status from Alberta to graduate with a law degree.

His grandparents were strong influences on his life — they expected him to fulfill his responsibility to make his community better and stronger. After establishing his law practice on the reserve, he initiated — on his Elders' requests — a global Indigenous rights movement at the United Nations and several other international forums that advocate for sports and for the United Nations Declaration on the Rights of Indigenous Peoples.

As the first member of Parliament with Status and a member of the Truth and Reconciliation Commission of Canada, Littlechild has been active in promoting health and well-being for youth in the physical, spiritual, and mental domains. For his achievements, he has received several honours, including five honorary doctorate degrees, induction as a Member of the Order of Canada, and eight honours in sports including induction into Canada's Sports Hall of Fame.

Bretta Maloff, RD, MEd (b. 1945)

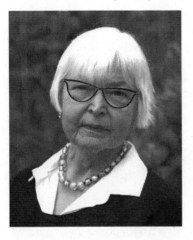

Fig. 13.14: Bretta Maloff. Photo by Moreley Maloff; courtesy of Bretta Maloff.

Bretta Maloff was born in Pine Falls, Manitoba, in 1945 and graduated from the University of Manitoba in 1966 with a bachelor of home economics degree, followed by a graduate diploma in public health from the University of Toronto and a master's degree in education from the University of Calgary in 1982. Maloff started her career in public health nutrition in 1966 in Saskatchewan, initially in a summer job in medical services, and then with the Prince Albert Health Region, providing nutrition services in rural and Indigenous communities.

Maloff's career in Alberta began as a public health nutritionist with the Edmonton and Calgary Boards of Health. In those roles, Maloff led the development of several important initiatives, including nutrition services and in-home care for high-risk prenatal groups, provincial guidelines for infant feeding, and day care nutrition; the Canadian Heart Health Initiative demonstration project, which was a precursor to the comprehensive school health model in Alberta, and the successful 1989 Calgary water fluoridation plebiscite campaign (see Chapter 9).[35]

When the Calgary Regional Health Authority was established in 1994, Maloff's role expanded to include leadership in community development and responsibility for developing the Strengthening Community Action and Public Participation Frameworks for the region. These led to collaborations with the University of Calgary in two research initiatives, funded by the Alberta Heritage Foundation for Medical Research and the Canadian Health Services Research Foundation. In 2005, her role expanded again to include managing several health promotion programs in areas of maternal health, child health, Indigenous health, oral health, tobacco, injury, policy, community development, and nutrition. When Alberta Health Services was established in 2009, Maloff became the provincial executive director for health promotion. During that time, she served as a member of Health Canada's National Sodium Working Group and initiated Alberta Health Services' childhood obesity strategy. Toward the later years of her career, Maloff transitioned her focus to system-wide clinical quality improvement in the areas of diabetes; nutrition; obesity; and maternal, infant, and child health.[36]

Maloff served as president of the Alberta Public Health Association in 1977–1978. She has served on the boards of the Canadian Public Health Association, Dietitians of Canada, and the Heart and Stroke Foundation, and is currently an active volunteer with Alberta Health Services' Cancer Strategic Clinical Network Core Committee and the Canadian Cancer Society Board.

David Swann, MD, FRCP(C); MLA (b. 1949)

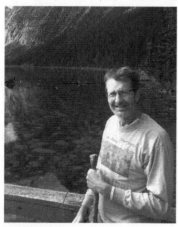

Fig. 13.15: David Swann. Photo by Dave Dunn; courtesy of David Swann.

David Swann was born in Taber, Alberta, in 1949. He describes his career as fruitful and filled with unexpected turns. After receiving his doctor of medicine degree from the University of Alberta in 1975, Swann worked for three years in mission hospitals in South Africa. He subsequently moved to Pincher Creek, Alberta, where he was discouraged by the absence of preventive health measures in practice. He returned to the University of Calgary in 1984 and completed his fellowship in community medicine. After graduation, Swann worked in a health development project in the Philippines for a year and a half, where he was demoralized by corrupt politics, poverty, and environmental destruction. After two years back in Canada, he confronted medicine's impotence in challenging weak public policy, and assumed the role of consulting medical officer of health in southern Alberta, while also teaching part-time at the University of Calgary's medical school. In his medical officer of health role, he tackled contentious issues related to urban oil and gas activity, gun control, air and water pollution, game ranching, and feedlot operations.[37]

Swann's career took a hard turn in 2002. As president of the Society of Alberta Medical Officers, he challenged the Alberta Conservative government to take action on climate warming after the society had formally supported the international Kyoto Protocol to reduce greenhouse gas emissions. He was abruptly terminated from his chief medical officer of health role with the Palliser Health Region. The public and medical communities were outraged at the dismissal, and Swann ran in the next provincial election in Calgary and became a Liberal MLA in 2004 (see Chapter 8).[38]

An issue in public health today, Swann attests, is the reluctance of professionals to mobilize the political will for healthy public policy in areas such as the social determinants of health, gun control, and improving prevention and support for mental health and addictions. He attributes some of his success in politics and public health to "courageous individuals — regular citizens — who inspired me to think deeply about underlying causes [of ill health], organize, gather evidence, and courageously and persistently press elected officials to do their jobs — act in the long-term public interest."[39]

Jan Reimer, BA (b. 1952)

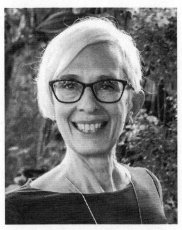

Fig. 13.16: Jan Reimer. Photo by Megan Kemshead Photography; courtesy of Megan Kemshead and Jan Reimer.

Jan Reimer was elected Edmonton's first female mayor at the age of thirty-seven. During her time as mayor (1989–1995) and since leaving office, she has worked to build stronger communities and support those experiencing abuse in their relationships.

Born in 1952, Reimer received her bachelor of arts degree from the University of Alberta. After a short period working in the welfare field in Australia and then community development in Edmonton, she served as an Edmonton alderman (now known as city councillors) for nine years. Her 1989 Edmonton mayoral campaign was unusual in that her platform emphasized environmental issues and social development and she was elected in spite of running a low-budget campaign. She also disclosed her biggest financial supporters; something that the other candidates did not do.[40] One of her biggest public health initiatives was a comprehensive waste management system for Edmonton, including curbside recycling that led to reduced use of the Edmonton landfill.

During her two terms in office, Reimer undertook several strategic initiatives, including the Mayor's Task Force on Safer Cities, a youth advisory committee, a diversity initiative, and an economic development strategy. After leaving office, she worked on the Senior Friendly initiative with the Alberta Council on Aging to create programs and guidelines to meet the needs of the growing population of seniors.

Since 2001, Reimer has worked as the executive director of the Alberta Council of Women's Shelters, a non-profit organization representing women's and seniors' shelters across the province. In that capacity, she has helped the organization to be an active voice on issues of family violence in Alberta through awareness and advocacy.

Reimer was recognized as Edmontonian of the Century in 2004, and she was a recipient of the Governor General's Award in Commemoration of the Persons Case in 2006 for her contributions to women's equality. Jan Reimer School in Edmonton, named in her honour, opened in 2017.[41]

Louis Hugo Francescutti, MD, PhD, MPH, FRCPC, CCFP(PC) (b. 1953)

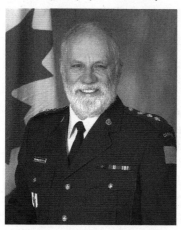

Fig. 13.17: Louis Francescutti. Photo courtesy of the Department of National Defence.

Louis Hugo Francescutti was born in Montréal in 1953. He was of the firm belief, and would not be satisfied, until the general public and political leaders finally understand that injury is a disease that can be prevented.

Francescutti completed his MD and PhD in immunology at the University of Alberta. While training as a resident in general surgery, he became interested in injury prevention. He understood that treating trauma was always a losing battle and that an emphasis on prevention should be the first step in trying to prevent trauma in the first place. Convinced of the value of prevention, Francescutti went on to complete his master's of public health and preventive medicine residency at Johns Hopkins University in Baltimore.[42]

One of Francescutti's contributions to public health include starting the Alberta Centre for Injury Control and Research and securing ongoing funding for that centre from the Alberta government. Prior to that, he created the

Injury Awareness and Prevention Centre at the University of Alberta. In 2005, Francescutti founded the Alberta Coalition for Cellphone-Free Driving. His sights were always set on health policy that would reduce injuries in Alberta.[43]

As president of the Royal College of Physicians and Surgeons of Canada (2010–2013), and then president of the Canadian Medical Association (2012–2014), Francescutti advocated for and became a voice for injury control. He advocated for helmets for cyclists, mandatory seatbelts and child restraints, prohibitions on riding in the back of pickup trucks, and banning the use of cellphones while driving. To see success in public health, Francescutti believes it is crucial to be persistent and motivated, to set a target, and to persevere until that target is reached, all while not being afraid of being controversial.[44]

In 2017, the governor general of Canada awarded Francescutti with a prestigious military meritorious service medal for "heightening the medical community's support of the [Canadian Armed Forces] and their representation in activities under his purview."[45] In 2010, he was acknowledged as one of the most influential Albertans by *Venture Magazine*, and in 2012 he was awarded the Queen Elizabeth II Diamond Jubilee Medal. Francescutti was named one of the hundred physicians of the century by the Alberta Medical Association / College of Physicians and Surgeons of Alberta in 2005.

At the time of writing, Francescutti is a professor in the School of Public Health at the University of Alberta, and an emergency physician at the Royal Alexandra Hospital, Edmonton.

Jim Talbot, MD, PhD (b. 1953)

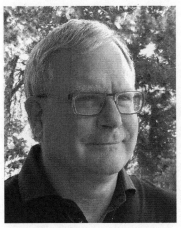

Fig. 13.18: James Talbot. Photo courtesy of James Talbot.

Jim Talbot was born in Ottawa, Ontario, in 1953. Talbot believes that public health always wins, perhaps not in the time frame one expects, and not in the way one might hope, but public health is always victorious. Talbot thinks of public health as the best job in the world because the mission of those in practice is to help people they have never met. He calls it the ultimate humanitarian vocation.[46]

Talbot received his BSc degree (1975) and his PhD (1980) in biochemistry from the University of Alberta prior to entering medical school at the University of Toronto, from where he graduated in 1985.[47] His experience in public health includes his work as the director of the Provincial Laboratory of Public Health for Northern Alberta, a position that he held for ten years. Talbot served as a medical officer of health for Alberta Health Services in Edmonton, chief medical officer of health for Nunavut and Alberta, and is a founding member of two health surveillance networks: the Sistema Regional de Vacunas surveillance network in Latin America, and the Alberta Real-Time Syndromic Surveillance Network.[48]

In June 2013, Talbot was responsible for the province's public health response following the southern Alberta floods, for which he received the Premier's Letter of Commendation. He also put together a provincial plan to address the fentanyl and opioid crises by adding treatment spaces in Alberta and distributing thousands of doses of the antidote naloxone.

Talbot's public health interests include surveillance and epidemiology to gather the evidence needed to guide action to prevent or mitigate disease and injury. He is also interested in the history of public health, public health leadership, advocacy, Indigenous and women's health and wellness, and emergency preparedness and management. He has written on the current state of public health, including serving as the sole Alberta coauthor on a 2017 commentary published in the *Canadian Journal Public Health* titled "The Weakening of Public Health: A Threat to Population Health and Health Care System Sustainability."[49]

Karen M. Grimsrud, BMedSc, MD, MHSc (b. 1954)

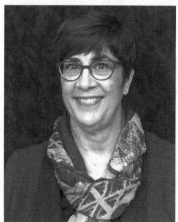

Fig. 13.19: Karen Grimsrud. Photo courtesy of Karen Grimsrud.

Karen Grimsrud was born in Edmonton, Alberta, in 1954. Grimsrud is a graduate of the University of Alberta; she completed her public health training at the University of Toronto. Grimsrud served in Alberta's public health system, holding the position of deputy medical officer of health with the Edmonton Board of Health from 1986 to 1995. Grimsrud then served with the Government of Alberta, first as deputy provincial health officer and then acting provincial health officer from 1996 to 2008, returning as chief medical officer of health from 2016 to 2019. From 2009 to 2016, Grimsrud worked with the Public Health Agency of Canada, where she led efforts in evidence-based public health methodology and guideline development for the Canadian Task Force on Preventive Health Care.

Grimsrud's work has focused on immunization, communicable disease control, public health emergency preparedness, environmental health, chronic disease prevention, and public health guideline development. She oversaw the introduction of new vaccines in the Alberta Childhood Immunization Schedule, and she managed several major disease events including invasive meningococcal disease, measles, hantavirus, Severe Acute Respiratory Syndrome, and West Nile Virus. During her time as provincial health officer of Alberta, she provided provincial leadership in the risk assessment and response to several significant infection control circumstances, including an incident in a Vegreville hospital in 2007 when an outbreak revealed that hospital equipment had not been properly sterilized.[50] Grimsrud also led the development of provincial emergency preparedness plans, most notably the pandemic influenza response, and she co-chaired the Federal/Provincial/Territorial Pandemic Influenza Committee. Soon after re-joining the Government of Alberta in April 2016, Grimsrud led the public health response to the Fort McMurray wildfires (see Chapter 11). More recently she has brought attention to and implemented harm reduction strategies to address the opioid crisis. Grimsrud was the co-chair of the provincial minister's Opioid Emergency Response Commission, which was instrumental in advancing health policy and programs.

Petra Schulz, MEd (b. 1958)

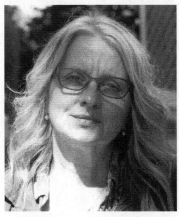

Fig. 13.20: Petra Shultz. Photo by Richard Shultz; courtesy of Petra Schultz.

Petra Schulz was born in Germany in 1958 and studied special education at the Philipps Universität in Marburg, Germany. Since 2000, Schulz has taught in the Faculty of Health and Community Studies at MacEwan University, where she has advocated for equal citizen rights for children and adults with diverse learning needs.

Schulz is a highly visible and effective advocate who is committed to the introduction and implementation of harm reduction strategies and practices to reduce the death toll from drug overdoses. Schulz co-founded the volunteer parent and family advocacy group Moms Stop the Harm following the 2014 death of her son Danny, a talented chef, to an accidental fentanyl overdose. Moms Stop the Harm advocates locally, nationally, and internationally for implementing evidence-based, public health and human rights responses to drug use and the opioid crisis, including support for harm reduction as a key component of a comprehensive response and support for the decriminalization of possession of drugs for personal use as essential to a public health approach.[51]

Schulz presents to researchers, clinicians, and community stakeholders and decision makers at provincial and national levels, advocating for the introduction of, and reducing access barriers to, naloxone kits; wider acceptance of supervised consumption sites; greater availability of evidence-based treatment for substance use disorders; reducing the social stigma of people who use substances; and the need for more research to understand the full social, political, and economic dimensions of drug overdoses, stressing that a multi-faceted societal approach is necessary.

Schulz points to the war on drugs as an utter political, policy, economic, program, and moral failure. In respect to the future of public health, she points to lessons learned from the opioid and fentanyl crises and failure of the public health response to them. She implores governments and public health officials to garner valuable insights into how society might address future social issues. She wants policy-makers to answer key questions: What went wrong in the response to the crises? How can we raise awareness of harmful drug use in society? How could we have prevented the crises? How do we remove the stigma associated with addressing drug use?[52]

Kim D. Raine, BSc, RD, MA, PhD, FCHAS (b. 1961)

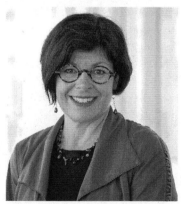

Fig. 13.21: Kim Raine. Photo by Virginia Quist, Visual Communications Associates, School of Public Health, University of Alberta. Courtesy of Kim Raine.

Kim Raine was born in Halifax in 1961. A dietitian, Raine says that she did not choose public health; it chose her. She studied nutrition and practised as a dietitian but recognized that the factors that influence people's nutrition were far greater than what many people understood and talked about. During her PhD studies in education at Dalhousie University in Halifax, Nova Scotia, she started studying the social determinants of health before they were called that, including talking with women living in low-income circumstances about feeding their children and trying to understand the relationship between health and income.

When she moved to Alberta in 1997, Raine became the principal investigator of the Alberta Heart Health Project, the objective of which was to build capacity for health promotion in health systems. She was the first faculty member hired in the University of Alberta Centre for Health Promotion Studies, which was created in 1996. The centre was interdisciplinary and focused on promoting health through addressing social determinants (see Chapter 6). She was the director of the centre from 2002 to 2008, during which time she led the Healthy Alberta Communities initiative, a community-based health promotion intervention. Then, she became an applied public health chair funded by the Canadian Institutes of Health Research and the Heart and Stroke Foundation. The focus of that work was community and policy interventions to prevent obesity and chronic diseases. In 2009, Raine co-led the creation of the Alberta Policy Coalition for Chronic Disease Prevention, which was, at the time of writing, in its tenth year of advocating for healthy public policy. In 2018, she was appointed associate dean of research in the School of Public Health at the University of Alberta. Raine believes that although public health as a system is weakening, public health principles are slowly being integrated within health and social systems. Initiatives that create health-promoting environments in schools and policies that promote a guaranteed basic income, for example, may not be part of the health system but are helping to reduce inequities and improve public health.[53]

Raine considers herself an optimist, which she believes to be an essential ingredient for success in the field of public health. Her proudest achievement is advocating for healthy public policy, which she attributes to following her passion for addressing the social determinants of health.[54]

Les Hagen, MSM (b. 1963)

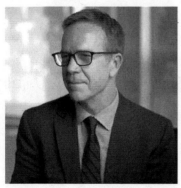

Fig. 13.22: Les Hagen. Photo courtesy of Les Hagen.

Les Hagen was born in Lethbridge, Alberta, in 1963. Hagen is an example of how commitment to one cause and persistent advocacy can lead to change. Over his thirty-year career, he has contributed substantially to tobacco reduction efforts in Alberta, which have contributed to a marked decrease in tobacco consumption in the province (see Chapter 9). Hagen has been part of important changes in public health and tobacco control in Alberta. As he describes it, in the 1970s, Canadian health charities focused on education and were not actively engaged in meaningful public policy measures. The mid-1980s saw organizations become more political, including hiring lobbyists to engage lawmakers and advance public policy measures to address chronic diseases, including via tobacco reduction.[55]

Hagen joined the Group Against Smokers Pollution in Edmonton as a volunteer in 1987. Shortly thereafter, the group was renamed Action on Smoking & Health, and Hagen was hired as its executive director in 1989. Hagen led Action on Smoking & Health toward becoming more politically engaged; moving beyond addressing smoking in public places and realigning itself to confronting the tobacco industry and taking a broader mandate in tobacco control, including restrictions on advertising and promotion.

One of the biggest challenges for Action on Smoking & Health has been to overcome barriers resulting from Alberta's historical "cowboy" culture of limited regulation, low taxes, and a work hard/play hard lifestyle. A succession of governments in Alberta were not necessarily sympathetic to bringing forward comprehensive policy measures to address public health issues like smoking. However, thanks in large part to Action on Smoking & Health, Alberta is now leading the country on several important tobacco policy initiatives, including becoming the first jurisdiction in North America to pass legislation to ban flavoured tobacco.[56]

Action on Smoking & Health and its partners have engaged actively with provincial and local policy-makers, and they have focused on creating publicity and shaping public opinion around tobacco control. Hagen attributes the group's successes to three factors: strategic efforts to keep the issue on the public agenda in a deliberate and systematic way; ongoing interaction with key policy-makers to advance the policy agenda; and working with other prominent health organizations that lend credibility and respect to the anti-tobacco cause while mobilizing thousands of members and supporters when required.

NOTES

1 "Regina's First Medical Health Officer Dies in Edmonton at 94," *Leader-Post*, 29 July 1982, A20.

2 *Act respecting the Prevention and Treatment of Tuberculosis*, Statutes of the Province of Alberta, 1936, c. 50.

3 Alberta Department of Public Health, *Annual Report 1931* (Edmonton: Printed by W.D. McLean, King's Printer, 1932), 20–21; Alberta Department of Public Health, *Annual Report 1932* (Edmonton: Printed by W.D. McLean, King's Printer, 1933), 19.

4 Robert Lampard, *Alberta's Medical History: Young and Lusty, and Full of Life* (Red Deer: Robert Lampard, 2008), 297.

5 "Report of the Committee on Honorary Life Membership, The Canadian Public Health Association 1964-1965, Annual Report – Part I," *Canadian Journal of Public Health* 56, no. 6 (June 1965), 261.

6 Provincial Archives of Alberta (PAA), *An Administrative History of the Government of Alberta, 1905–2005* (Edmonton: PAA, 2006), 292.

7 CPHA Resources, "Alberta Deputy Minister of Health and Supporter of CPHA."

8 "News Notes: Alberta," *Canadian Journal of Public Health* 56, no. 5 (1965): 225.

9   Archives Society of Alberta, "Attrux, Laura Margaret," Alberta on Record, College & Association of Registered Nurses of Alberta Museum and Archives collection, accessed 24 November 2018, https://albertaonrecord.ca/attrux-laura-margaret-1909-1987.

10   Kay Sanderson and Elda Hauschildt, *Remarkable Alberta Women* (Calgary: Famous Five Foundation, 1999), 200.

11   Sharon Richardson, "Helen Griffith McArthur – 1911–1974," in *American Nursing: A Biographical Dictionary*, ed. Vern Bullough and Lilli Sentz (New York: Springer Publishing Company, 2000), 3:196–198.

12   "Unlock the Past with CARMN," Unlock the past with Central Alberta Regional Museum Network, accessed 02 April 2024, https://centralmuseumsab.ca/view/153/helen-griffith-wylie-mcarthur; Bullough and Sentz, *American Nursing*, 198.

13   Jeff Titterington, "From London to Yellowknife: 40 Years a Doctor," *The Yellowknifer*, 2 February 1983.

14   "Years of Service to Public Health in Alberta and CPHA," Profiles in Public Health: E.S.O. Smith, CPHA Resources, accessed 24 November 2018, http://resources.cpha.ca/CPHA/ThisIsPublicHealth/profiles/item.php?l=E&i=1326.

15   CPHA Resources, "Years of Service to Public Health in Alberta and CPHA."

16   CPHA Resources, "Years of Service to Public Health in Alberta and CPHA."

17   *Edmonton Journal*, "James Howell," obituaries, 4 July 2012, http://edmontonjournal.remembering.ca/obituary/james-howell-1066049623.

18   Christopher Rutty and Sue C. Sullivan, *This is Public Health: a Canadian History* (Ottawa: CPHA, 2010), 8.18, https://cpha.ca/sites/default/files/assets/history/book/history-book-print_all_e.pdf.

19   Adelaide Schartner, *Health Units of Alberta* (Edmonton: Health Unit Association of Alberta, 1983), 42.

20   Jill Mahoney, "John Waters: Alberta's Low-profile Lifesaver," *The Globe and Mail*, 19 July 2001, R7.

21   Mahoney, "Alberta's Low-profile Lifesaver."

22   "Dr. Shirley M. Stinson," The Alberta Order of Excellence, 1999, accessed 7 April 2024, https://www.alberta.ca/aoe-shirley-stinson.

23   Shirley Stinson, interview by Don Juzwishin, 28 September 2018.

24   "Shirley Marie Stinson, O.C., A.O.E., Ed.D., LL.D., R.N." Honours: Order of Canada, The Governor General of Canada, accessed 7 April 2024, https://www.gg.ca/en/honours/recipients/146-306.

25   Karen Mills, interview by Don Juzwishin, 28 September 2018.

26   Margaret King et al., *Proceedings of the First International Conference on Community Health Nursing Research: Health Promotion, Illness & Injury Prevention, Edmonton, Alberta, September 26th–29th, 1993* (Edmonton: Edmonton Board of Health, 1993).

27   Karen Mills, interview.

28   "Douglas R. Wilson Lecture series," School of Public Health, University of Alberta, accessed 5 June 2019, https://www.ualberta.ca/public-health/about/academic-events/douglas-r-wilson-lecture/.

29   "Douglas R. Wilson Lecture series," School of Public Health.

30   "Muriel Stanley Venne, CM, BA (Hon)," Alberta Order of Excellence, 2019, accessed 7 April 2024, https://www.alberta.ca/aoe-muriel-stanley-venne; "Esquao Awards Programs," Institute for the Advancement of Aboriginal Women, accessed 28 July 2020, http://iaaw.ca/programs-services/esqua-awards-programs/; Institute for the Advancement of Aboriginal Women, *The Rights Path – Alberta, 3rd ed.* (2001), accessed 28 July 2020, https://12e01dc8-2416-76ba-c3b5d01ce01e03b3.filesusr.com/ugd/b2f015_c99b319fa17149cc804ae4617a0aeebf.pdf.

31   Muriel Stanley Venne, personal communication with Don Juzwishin, 13 December 2019.

32   Anne Fanning, interview by Don Juzwishin and Rogelio Velez Mendoza, 30 August 2018.

33   Anne Fanning, interview.

34   Chief Wilton Littlechild, personal communication with Don Juzwishin, 12 December 2019.

35   Bretta Maloff, interview by Temitayo Famuyide, 11 November 2018.

36   Bretta Maloff, interview.

37   David Swann, interview by Rogelio Velez Mendoza, 20 September 2018.

38   Brad Mackay, "Firing Public Health MD over Pro-Kyoto Comments a No-No, Alberta Learns," *Canadian Medical Association Journal* 167, no. 10 (Nov 2002): 1156-1156-a.

39   David Swann, interview.

40   Jack Masson and Edward C. LeSage Jr., *Alberta's Local Governments: Politics and Democracy* (Edmonton: University of Alberta Press, 1994), 310.

41   Paula Simons, "Former Mayor Jan Reimer on Women, Politics and Misogyny," *Edmonton Journal*, updated 31 January 2018.

42   Louis Francescutti, interview by Rogelio Velez Mendoza, 24 September 2018.

43   Louis Francescutti, interview.

44   "Louis Francescutti CV," The World Medical Association, accessed 7 April 2014, https://www.wma.net/wp-content/uploads/2018/09/Louis-Francescutti-CV-FINAL-50-page.pdf.

45   "Honorary Colonel Louis Hugo Francescutti, M.S.M," Meritorious Service Decorations – Military Division, The Governor General of Canada, accessed 5 June 2019, https://www.gg.ca/en/honours/recipients/139-1136.

46   James "Jim" Talbot, PhD, MD, FRCPC Profile, *Alberta Public Health Association Newsletter*, Alberta Public Health Association (APHA) History Archives (Currently in transition to the PAA).

47   "James Talbot," Faculty and Staff, University of Alberta, accessed 4 June 2019, https://www.ualberta.ca/public-health/about/faculty-staff/adjunct-emeritus-faculty/talbot.

48   "James Talbot," Faculty and Staff.

49   Ak'ingabe Guyon et al., "The Weakening of Public Health: A Threat to Population Health and Health Care System Sustainability," *Canadian Journal of Public Health* 108, no. 1 (2017).

50   "Alberta Hospital Closed after Superbug, Sterilization Problems," *CBC News*, 20 March 2007, https://www.cbc.ca/news/canada/edmonton/alberta-hospital-closed-after-superbug-sterilization-problems-1.668781.

51   Petra Shultz, interview by Don Juzwishin and Rogelio Velez Mendoza, 31 August 2018.

52   Petra Shultz, interview.

53   Kim Raine, interview by Rogelio Velez Mendoza, 31 August 2018.

54   Kim Raine, interview.

55   Les Hagen, interview by Rogelio Velez Mendoza, 30 November 2018.

56   Les Hagen, interview.

Conclusion

Lindsay McLaren

> *"History does not lie in the material alone, but in the identification, selection, organization and shaping of that information into some kind of product"*
>
> —Heritage Note Series: Conducting Historical Research,
>   Alberta Historical Resources Foundation[1]

Our overall objective for this volume was to commemorate, critique, and learn from Alberta's public health history. This objective was informed and prompted by our concerns about the limited contemporary coherence and visibility, and thus impact, of a broad public health perspective, which has only been confirmed by the COVID-19 pandemic. That broad perspective is conveyed by our working definition of public health as the science and art of preventing sickness and promoting health through organized efforts of society, where health refers to well-being and health equity in populations and their structural causes. Dedicating focused attention to the field's history in Alberta, we reasoned, offered one way to illustrate public health's enduring core features and unique contributions to society. Doing so, in turn, allows us to think about a version of public health — as a field of applied policy, practice, and scholarly inquiry — that maintains its historical strengths while also adapting to contemporary health challenges and their structural causes. This is imperative if public health is to remain an important and relevant societal institution.

With respect to the opening quotation to this chapter, this volume's objective and positioning as described above strongly influenced our "identification, selection, organization and shaping" of materials, from which we now draw several concluding points.

Governance Arrangements Matter, Even if [or When] the Extent is Unknown

As an institution with a strong state element, a historical study of public health demands careful attention to government and governance. This includes the ways in which government administrative arrangements have supported or hindered a broad version of public health that is fundamentally concerned with upstream determinants of well-being and health equity in populations.

To this end, we framed some chapters using a health-in-all-policies perspective, which foregrounds the fundamental understanding that key determinants of well-being and health equity reflect policy decisions outside of the formal health sector.[2] Chapter 8 and Chapter 12, for example, highlight historical circumstances in Alberta where public health was administratively coupled with other policy domains — environment and social services respectively — within provincial government departments. Such administrative coupling offers one mechanism for breaking the entrenched conflation of health and health care, and working toward an intersectoral approach to supporting the public's health by improving social and ecological determinants of health.[3] By studying these examples in their socio-historical contexts, however, the importance of ideological and political economic factors becomes clear: supportive administrative structure is insufficient to offset dominant, indeed hegemonic, narratives that privilege physical dimensions of disease, reductive and downstream solutions to health problems, and inadequate attention to root causes of social and health inequity including the regime of obstruction created by the intersection of mainstream economics and colonial, extractive industry.[4]

Concerning legislative elements, our historical tracking of the provincial Public Health Act (see Chapter 4) provided a different kind of window onto public health practice over time, including its scope and lines of authority.[5] The origins of the act in communicable disease control and health protection / environmental health activities are not unique to Alberta, and they make sense in the light of the early twentieth century disease context (see Chapter 3). They present, however, a challenging legacy for our field. This is despite decades of efforts — dating at least to the Ottawa Charter for Health Promotion of 1986 — to advance a broader version of public health that emphasizes well-being; health equity; and upstream, intersectoral thinking about root causes of health problems. From this perspective, although the act provides an important foundation for certain organized efforts of society (a phrase contained in many definitions of public health), it also presents — through its contents and its omissions — an institutionalized barrier that constrains how we, as a society, think about and operationalize public health.

Notwithstanding this legacy, there have been shifts over time in the Public Health Act that potentially shed some light on the who, what, and how of public health today. One example is a 1970 amendment that removed the provincial medical officer of health as chair of the Provincial Board of Health and replaced it with deputy minister of health. From the perspective of the COVID-19 pandemic, where the legislative versus political elements of the provincial chief medical officers of health's role and authority have been vigorously debated,[6] this early change seems — in hindsight — potentially significant to understanding the diffuse and poorly understood version of public health seen today. Moreover, the 1984 rewrite of the Public Health Act instituted many changes, including the elimination of the Provincial Board of Health, which had existed since 1907, and — in the context of evolving human rights legislation — its replacement with a board that was advisory in nature and focused on appeals; the removal of topics such as milk pasteurization and community water fluoridation, which were moved to other pieces of legislation; and the relaxing of parameters around the membership of local boards of health, such that having members from municipal government was no longer required. We found limited if any specific commentary on these changes in the public domain, and thus it is difficult to judge their meaning and significance. However, from our contemporary vantage point, where public health is lacking in coherence and unity, one can speculate how a succession of seemingly innocuous changes to a key piece of provincial legislation could have contributed to the weak and narrow version of public health that we have today.

Downstream Drift Is Insidious

A persistent and significant challenge for public health is downstream drift, or the tendency of policy and practice to focus on individual-level behavioural or clinical/biomedical factors, rather than an upstream approach, which embraces root causes of poor health and health inequity that lie in harmful and inequitable social, economic, political, and colonial systems and structures.[7]

The reasons for downstream drift are multiple, complex, and insidious. A historical perspective can shed light on the drift, including when and in what circumstances it occurred. In Chapter 2, we sought such insights via an analysis of one hundred years of provincial government throne speeches. By considering references to "health," "public health," and "prevention" in the speeches, we showed subtle but important changes over the course of the twentieth and early twenty-first century. First, policy attention to public health activities of prevention and health protection declined, while attention to downstream disease treatment and management increased. Second, we observed that references to "prevention" shifted from primary prevention in whole populations toward greater emphasis on secondary prevention for those deemed "high-risk" or "vulnerable," which often, although not necessarily, have a more downstream orientation. Third, references to "public health" changed over time, a shift that was especially apparent during the lengthy period of Social Credit government under Ernest Manning (1943-1968). Starting in the late 1950s, this government's use of "public health" appeared to drift from a broad concept that included primary prevention in populations, toward a narrower emphasis on treatment, management, diagnostics, and rehabilitation activities within the context of health care. This narrower version of public health largely continued, with the occasional exception and nuance, in subsequent Alberta governments. Because this narrow version is not aligned with public health's stated goals of providing conditions for population well-being and health equity, these shifts over time in the meaning of key terms and concepts seem significant.

Social Justice and Health Equity: One Step Forward, Two Steps Back

Public health communities have long voiced concern about unfair social and economic conditions and their relation to unequal health outcomes, yet substantive efforts to redress inequities including their structural, social, political, economic, ecologic, and colonial determinants have not been forthcoming.

A historical lens can illuminate areas of progress, setbacks, and inactivity in Alberta in this regard. On the one hand, we have repealed some forms of egregiously discriminatory legislation such as the Sexual Sterilization Act (see Chapter 1); although this took us until 1972 and has not eliminated involuntary sterilization.[8] There has been some important recent progress in data infrastructure, including strengthening data ownership and control and facilitating disaggregated data (e.g., data broken down by race or ethnicity) to show inequities in health outcomes like COVID-19 infection and mortality by social and economic identities and circumstances.[9] However, while better approaches to data collection and analysis can illuminate inequities, they are insufficient on their own. For example, despite extensive statistical documentation of health inequities and their root causes in neoliberal, extractive and colonial systems and structures; those systems and structures persist and public health communities

– on the whole – do not engage deeply toward dismantling them. Instead, we continue to accept and perpetuate what can only be described as unacceptable social and economic conditions and health outcomes, for many Indigenous communities in Alberta (Chapter 7). We also, with very few exceptions, continue to elect, and thus shift power to, neoliberally-oriented provincial governments that mobilize a market justice rather than a social justice orientation to health and well-being (Chapter 8 and Chapter 12). And finally, also with few exceptions, we do not engage substantively with climate justice and ecological determinants of health including their political and economic drivers, despite these representing enormously significant threats to health equity (see Chapter 6 and Chapter 8). Connecting the dots between these issues, and strengthening critical engagement around them, are urgent tasks for public health communities.

Points of Opposition to Healthy Public Policy Are Consistent and Predictable

In several chapters we examined the nature of contention and debate around public health policy, including how these manifested in provincial government deliberations.[10] This included seatbelt legislation (Chapter 3), tobacco control, community water fluoridation, and workers' health (Chapter 9), climate change (Chapter 8), and social determinants of health (Chapter 12).

Across these debates we observed some consistency in terms of key points and strategies of opposition. For seatbelt legislation and community water fluoridation, which represent relatively discrete, although not simple, preventive policies, opponents consistently and often effectively mobilized several arguments. These included 1) skepticism about policy effectiveness; for example, questioning or raising doubts about whether or not seat belts saved lives; 2) concern about possible harms; for example, drawing on personal stories where someone was injured by a seatbelt; and 3) agreement with the goal of the policy but not with the mechanism; for example, accepting that seat belts were beneficial but opposing the use of mandates, instead preferring an educational approach to encourage voluntary use.

Consistent points and strategies of opposition were also apparent for more complex policies that transcend sectors, such as those to address climate change (Chapter 8) and to strengthen workers' health (Chapter 9) and social determinants of health (Chapter 12); all of which are obstructed by mobilization of powerful capitalist and colonial interests. One point of opposition was to express concern about the administrative burden associated with complex policy; for example, a proposal to implement health impact assessment of policy in sectors other than health was considered unacceptable because it would "bring the decision-making apparatus of the government to a grinding halt." Another strategy was to (mis) characterize a policy as redundant or as duplicating policies or activities already in place in a way that obscured or glossed over the substantive differences between the weak legislation that was already in place and the stronger and more upstream legislation that was being proposed. A third point of opposition mobilized the isolated nature of government departments; for example, opponents to climate change legislation asserted that the health impacts of climate change fall outside of the purview of the health ministry. This latter point reflects and perpetuates the significant challenge for public health noted earlier; namely, a hegemonic narrative that conflates health and medical care. Working to decouple the two is fundamental to a broad vision of public health.[11]

Although the capitalist and colonial barriers to healthy public policy are immense, we may perhaps see some way forward around the consistency of these specific points of opposition — which we observed repeatedly, at different points in time and for different policies — and thus their predictability. With respect to representational advocacy, or strategies for generating support for public health goals among broader publics,[12] these points present an opportunity for public health communities to mobilize around articulating and advancing concise and compelling counter-narratives. Provincial/territorial and national public health associations (see Chapter 5) offer a platform for this.[13] From the perspective of a broad vision of public health, which is concerned with root causes of population well-being and health equity, it is essential to also include facilitational advocacy; that is, listening to and working with members of publics who are most affected by these decisions and whose voices are under-represented in policy debates.[14] As discussed in Chapter 6, there is a significant need and opportunity to embed all of these issues, and most importantly critical thinking around them, within public health education programs.

Crises Can Prompt Deep and Substantive Change for the Better

This volume was submitted, and in fact much of the research and writing completed, during the global COVID-19 pandemic, which offered many privileged academics, including the authors of this volume, the gift of time. With respect to our concerns about the state of public health, including its visibility and impact, the pandemic has indeed prompted important changes. It has, for example, placed public health in the spotlight, with one early example being chief public health / medical officers — who are usually mostly invisible to the public — attaining the status of household names across the country. On the other hand, and significantly, the pandemic has reinforced a narrow, reductive, and medicalized version of public health that is focused on communicable disease control and the health care system, led by certain kinds of scientists and health care professionals, such as physicians, epidemiologists, and virologists.[15]

As articulated in a growing amount of thoughtful commentary,[16] the pandemic has unambiguously demonstrated the need for a broad and coherent version of public health that gives voice to a much broader range of experts in collective well-being and health equity, including those communities who are most affected, and social science and humanities scholars who are experts in critically contextualizing societal institutions and their underlying dimensions of power. The pandemic has shown us, in no uncertain terms, that health cannot be separated from the economy, nor from any other aspects of our lives, identities, and contexts. It has magnified inequities along axes such as income, employment circumstances, gender, race, ethnicity, and ability, which are in no sense natural or inevitable divides — rather they are "the result of a toxic combination of poor social policies and programs, unfair economic arrangements, and bad politics."[17] The COVID-19 pandemic, moreover, is only one example of a much broader, deeper, and intersecting set of threats to the integrity of our collective well-being, ecosystems, and democracies.

What might a coherent alternative look like, at this important crossroads? We humbly conclude with a few thoughts about this, which place Alberta in its broader national and international context.[18]

An Integrated, Coherent Version of Public Health

In the light of our concerns that the field of public health lacks coherence and thus vision, a key goal of this volume has been to characterize, or articulate the contours of, a broad version of public health. In fact, in some ways this is the easy part since several visions have already been articulated. Three have appeared throughout this book.[19] The first is the Ottawa Charter for Health Promotion of 1986, which was ahead of its time in characterizing health as a resource for everyday life, and for identifying prerequisites for health, including peace, shelter, education, food, income, a stable ecosystem, sustainable resources, social justice, and equity. Strengthening health and health equity, according to the charter, requires efforts to build healthy public policy; create supportive environments for health; strengthen community action, including from under-represented voices; develop personal skills to make choices conducive to health; and reorient health services so they are more attuned to prevention and health promotion.

A second vision occurred more than twenty years later when the World Health Organization Commission on Social Determinants of Health identified three overarching recommendations to improve population health and health equity, a goal it described as "closing the gap in a generation."[20] Those overarching recommendations were to improve daily living conditions; tackle the inequitable distribution of money, power, and resources; and measure the problem (of health inequity) and assess the impact of action.

In 2015, a third vision appeared when the Truth and Reconciliation Commission released its final report and recommendations following a multi-year process of information gathering and public discussions concerning Canadian government policies of cultural genocide, which have caused unacceptable social and economic conditions for Indigenous Peoples in Canada. The social and ensuing health inequities that continue,[21] which provide a dramatic example of the social determinants of health, may only be addressed through a foundation of reconciliation, defined as commitment by *all* Canadians to an ongoing process of establishing and maintaining respectful relationships. Canada must fully implement and work toward substantive realization of the United Nations Declaration on the Rights of Indigenous Peoples.[22]

Although leadership within the health sector is critical,[23] it goes without saying that the goals expressed in these three visions go well beyond the scope and mandate of the health sector. Moreover, the health sector in practice frequently refers to a narrow set of professional actors with a largely biomedical orientation, which serves to obstruct meaningful efforts to support well-being and health equity for all. One potential way to operationalize the fundamental understanding that the primary determinants of well-being and health equity reflect public policy decisions outside of the health sector, within government, is a health-in-all-policies approach, which we have referenced throughout this volume.[24] Indeed, such an approach has been implemented in Canadian jurisdictions. Importantly, however, critical commentary has identified that intersectoral collaboration may come at the expense of a sustained and meaningful focus on upstream determinants of injustices.[25]

Another framework is a well-being economy, or an economy that pursues human and ecological well-being rather than a narrow version of economic growth. A well-being economy — which is not a new idea but is gaining recent national and international momentum — begins with the recognition that our current economic system of neoliberal capitalism does not support the health and well-being of all people and the planet. The benefits of economic growth accrue mostly to the wealthiest individuals and corporations, while incomes at the bottom have stagnated or declined. A narrow focus on economic growth, moreover, underpins activities that permit and encourage destruction of our ecosystems, such as subsidies to polluting industries. There are several examples of an alternative vision offered by a well-being economy, such as the Wellbeing Economy

Alliance, a global collaboration of organizations, alliances, movements, and individuals working to transform the economic system into one that delivers social justice for a healthy planet; New Zealand's well-being budget, which is based on recognition that "just because a country is doing well economically does not mean all of its people are"; Wales's Wellbeing of Future Generations legislation and commissioner, which enshrines long-term thinking in government; and important work toward an alternative to the GDP in British Columbia that centres First Nations concepts of well-being.[26]

Although health-in-all-policies and a well-being economy are being advanced by different communities, sectors, and disciplines, they potentially have important common ground which, when coupled with a strong critical perspective, offer exciting opportunities for thinking about a broader vision of the public's health.

Coordinating a Wider Public Health Vision Across Political Jurisdictions

Having identified contours of an integrated vision for public health, a second step is to find ways for governments to coordinate their leadership. This requires engaging with Canadian federalism as well as the inherent jurisdictions and authority of Indigenous Peoples.

The Canadian federal government's economic support mobilization during the COVID-19 pandemic was significant. Massive amounts of money were invested in people, and some jurisdictional boundaries were overcome to do so. The challenge is to transition those activities from a singular emergency protection response to one element of an integrated, longer-term approach to coherent investment in the broader determinants of health. There are some modest hints of a shift in that direction. The federal government's structural supports shifted, in some cases, into medium-term solutions such as a more flexible and inclusive system of employment insurance. In its 2021 federal budget, the Trudeau government announced significant support for a national childcare system with emphasis on quality and affordability.[27] Stemming from a supply and confidence agreement with the NDP, the federal government has committed to working toward redressing the historical omission of dental care from our national health care system. These signals follow the federal government's 2019 mandate letters, which referenced well-being budgeting, that is, finding ways to ensure that program spending and taxation decisions support people's well-being (rather than private profit accumulation).[28] While potentially promising, the extent to which these initiatives meaningfully work to redress the inequities in power and resources which constitute root causes of health inequities in Canada remains to be seen.[29]

In our federated country, coordinated leadership demands provincial cooperation, the absence of which has been clear in the pandemic. However, for some elements of public health, there is a working guide to better coordination, in the form of the Declaration on Promotion and Prevention, which was signed by Canada's federal, provincial, and territorial health ministers in 2010.[30] As discussed throughout this volume, health portfolios across the country are overwhelmingly focused on treatment-oriented medical care. In this declaration, however, ministers from different political parties committed to principles of prevention, health promotion, and social determinants of health. Imagine how different the COVID-19 pandemic experience might have been had the potential of that declaration been translated into robust governance structures and public policy that is guided by the well-being of all people (for example, generous, accessible, and ongoing social protections like paid sick days, a living wage, and alternative sources of income for essential workers such as grocery store workers) rather than the interests of a privileged minority (for example, the food retail corporations that profited amid the suffering).[31]

Creating supportive governance for well-being and health equity does not stop with Canadian federalism, however. A future that is healthy and just for all people and the planet demands that Canada meet its government-to-government agreements with First Nations and the Métis and Inuit. Although the federal government has endorsed and is implementing the United Nations Declaration on the Rights of Indigenous Peoples, this action will not be effective until or unless Canada concedes that the Inherent Rights of Indigenous Peoples, including the rights to self-determination and free, prior, and informed consent before adopting and implementing legislative or administrative measures that may affect them, are not subordinate to the Canadian constitution, and that colonial sovereignty and authority are not superior to Indigenous sovereignty and authority. As described by Cree and Saulteaux scholar Gina Starblanket and published in important work by Cree scholar Angele Alook and colleagues, a framework for dual governance and shared control is laid out in the historic treaties; it generally involves the establishment of separate governments and jurisdictions in distinct spaces and dual governance and jurisdiction in shared spaces and matters of mutual concern.[32]

Health Uncoupled from Health Care

Underpinning the success of the first two steps, a third step is to work from the ground up to break down the pernicious and entrenched conflation, especially in colonial society, of health, health care, and public health — and to help people to embrace a broad vision of health as well-being that is fundamentally shaped by the circumstances in which we are born, grow, live, work, and age; including the quality and integrity of our natural environments and our relationships therewith. Popular discourse about health is dominated by a focus on medical care and individual lifestyle behaviours.[33] This conflation is also pervasive — as shown throughout this volume — within our key decision-making structures, both within and outside of the health sector. We need to find better ways to broaden our vision, integrate sectors and government departments around that broader vision, and connect the dots between health and its broader social determinants on a large scale.

Inward Vision

An important challenge that we encountered in writing this volume stems from the observation that public health is a multi-faceted field that includes applied practice and policy, scholarly inquiry, and community activism. However, these different aspects of public health are not on equal footing. Power and politics result in some elements and perspectives rising to the top and becoming the visible face of our field. This was well illustrated during the pandemic, as noted earlier in this chapter.

One way of organizing our thinking about public health is in terms of mainstream and critical perspectives. In general, mainstream perspectives are those that privilege dominant ways of thinking that focus on behavioural and biomedical perspectives; knowing, which are the "scientific" and mostly reductive quantitative approaches anchored in epidemiology and biostatistics; and doing, or top-down, expert driven approaches, which tend to underpin much practice and policy. In contrast, critical perspectives are those which challenge the status quo by situating it within political and historical contexts and making visible the embedded but often hidden elements of power. Critical approaches look outward, illuminating the health-damaging effects of social structures. At the same time, they look inward, asking difficult questions about successes and failures in public health and to expose and question assumptions in our field.[34]

Both perspectives have strengths and weaknesses. Critical perspectives are essential for uncovering root causes of poor health and health inequities because they illuminate structures and processes of power and exclusion that obstruct a just world. A drawback is that they sometimes critique or criticize elements of public health without necessarily articulating constructive alternatives.[35] Because mainstream approaches tend to be depoliticized and ahistorical, they have the considerable drawback of obscuring root causes and thereby perpetuating downstream individualized approaches to solving problems. However, they are more likely than critical scholarship to be solution-focused, and this should be mobilized to good purpose. Underpinning our work in this volume, and toward a broad vision of public health focused on population well-being and health equity and their root causes in systems and structures, is a desire to try to bring together the best of both perspectives. As a way forward, we humbly conclude with the following two, related thoughts.

First, we see value in public health communities coming together to envision and work toward, a social democratic public health framework. In a recent paper published in the *European Journal of Social Policy*, author Sylvia Walby considers the question of social theory as it relates to public health, specifically in the context of the COVID-19 pandemic.[36] She identifies that, among the political philosophies that have been mobilized to explain the relationship between the individual and society in the context of the pandemic, social democracy has been "curiously absent." This is a problem, she argues, for at least two reasons. First, public health and social democracy are, at least theoretically, aligned; as Walby says, "social democracy is the model of society that informs the public health project, in which 'if one is sick, we are all potentially sick.'. . . [Moreover] it is a social model which insists that justice and efficiency are linked together, rather than being opposed in a zero-sum trade-off."[37]

Another reason why it is problematic to omit social democracy is because it provides a strong counter-philosophy to neoliberalism. In Walby's words, "interventionist social democratic practices can be contrasted with neoliberal policies that pursue more minimal intervention to (mistakenly) reduce damage to the economy."[38] Walby's social democratic public health is highly consistent with the broad vision of public health that we embrace in this volume. Its interventionist orientation, underpinned by social democratic visions of justice and inclusion, aligns with strengths of some historical (mainstream) public health policy and practice. And its underpinnings in political philosophy and robust social theory respect the essential contributions of critical perspectives, which are considerably more recent as applied to public health.

Second, and toward a social democratic public health, we suggest that public health communities find ways to overcome tensions between practice and scholarly communities, by working toward what health sociologist Mykhalovskiy and colleagues call "critical social science *with* public health," where public health refers to applied (mainstream) policy and practice.[39] These authors distinguish between critical social science *in*, *of*, and *with* public health (see Table 14.1). Briefly, while critical perspectives *in* and *of* public health relationships are common and have strengths, they also have drawbacks that are emblematic of the tensions found between scholarship and practice in the field. One common example is the situation where critical perspectives are positioned outside of, and thus secondary to, the aims of mainstream public health.

To bring the best of mainstream/applied and critical perspectives together, as per critical social science *with* public health, the power and epistemological tensions between scholarship and practice cannot be ignored or avoided but rather must become a site of productive inquiry for which time and effort are carved out. It requires deep epistemic, disciplinary, and sectoral humility by all.[40] In our view, attention to these issues could present an exciting and truly collective and justice-oriented post-pandemic era of public health that is for, and in the interest of, the public's health.

TABLE 14.1: Critical perspectives in, of, and with public health practice.

Type of relationship	Description	Opportunities	Drawbacks
Critical perspectives *in* public health	Critical scholars work within the institutional and discursive spaces of public health (e.g., within a university School of Public Health or a public health department in the health care system).	Can provide a way for critical scholars to contribute to applied concerns in public health.	Can erode the unique analytic contributions and scholarly autonomy of critical scholars, because social science theories, concepts, and methods are used in service of public health aims.
Critical perspectives *of* public health	Critical scholars are situated outside of public health, which becomes an object of critical inquiry (e.g., illuminating a tendency to overlook fundamental causes of poor health).	Can identify and yield significant insights into built-in and implicit flaws of public health practices, forms of reasoning, politics, concerns, modes of organization, etc.	Can turn into an entirely negative critique, which points out the failings of public health but does not pursue constructive alternatives.
Critical perspectives *with* public health	A relationship between critical perspectives and public health practice that recognizes sources of difference and tension and works productively with those differences and tensions.	Begins to address inadequacies of *in* and *of* orientations; may permit productive channelling of conflict towards tackling key problems such as politics of austerity.	Risk of devolving into a superficial and uncomplicated space of shared interests. Requires commitment to reflexivity on both sides (rare), and ongoing engagement.

Source: adapted from Eric Mykhalovskiy et al., "Critical Social Science with Public Health: Agonism, Critique and Engagement," *Critical Public Health* 29, no. 5 (October 20, 2019), https://doi.org/10.1080/09581596.2018.1474174.

NOTES

1   Alberta Historical Resources Foundation, *Heritage Note Series: Conducting Historical Research* (Edmonton: Government of Alberta, 2019), https://open.alberta.ca/dataset/025851a2-f4b8-4b4c-b1c1-351233ef5eb9/resource/23c504b7-d62b-40c0-9cff-5b08048b7d32/download/heritage-note-conducting-historical-research-2019-final.pdf.

2   Paul Kershaw, "The Need for Health in All Policies in Canada," *Canadian Medical Association Journal* 190, no. 3 (2018): E64–E65, https://doi.org/10.1503/cmaj.171530; World Health Organization, "Ottawa Charter for Health Promotion – Charte D'ottawa pour la Promotion de la Santé," *Canadian Journal of Public Health / Revue Canadienne de Santé Publique* 77, no. 6, Special Health Promotion Issue (November/December 1986): 425; Trevor Hancock, "Beyond Health Care: From Public Health Policy to Healthy Public Policy," *Canadian Journal of Public Health* 76, Suppl 1 (June 1985): 9.

3   Commission on Social Determinants of Health (CSDH), *Closing the Gap in a Generation: Health Equity through Action on the Social Determinants of Health. Final Report of the Commission on Social Determinants of Health* (Geneva: World Health Organization, 2008), https://www.who.int/publications/i/item/WHO-IER-CSDH-08.1; Dennis Raphael et al., *Social Determinants of Health: The Canadian Facts*, 2nd ed. (Oshawa: Ontario Tech University Faculty of Health Sciences and Toronto: York University School of Health Policy and Management, 2020), http://www.thecanadianfacts.org/.

4   Fran Baum and Matthew Fisher, "Why Behavioural Health Promotion Endures Despite Its Failure to Reduce Health Inequities," *Sociology of Health & Illness* 36, no. 2 (February 2014): 213, https://doi.org/10.1111/1467-9566.12112; William K. Carroll, ed., *Regime of Obstruction: How Corporate Power Blocks Energy Democracy* (Edmonton: Athbasca University Press, 2021).

5   Canadian Public Health Association, (CPHA) *Public Health: A Conceptual Framework*, Canadian Public Health Association Working Paper (Ottawa: CPHA, 2017), https://www.cpha.ca/public-health-conceptual-framework. We recognize that these changes are not necessarily reducible to the Public Health Act alone, but they often appeared in one form or another in that piece of legislation, making the act a useful historical anchor.

6   Patrick Fafard et al., "Contested Roles of Canada's Chief Medical Officers of Health," *Canadian Journal of Public Health* 109 (2018); Nate Pike, host, "Episode 2.26 – Dr. Ubaka Ogbogu," The Breakdown with Nate Pike (podcast), 17 November 2020, https://podcasts.apple.com/ca/podcast/the-breakdown-with-nate-pike/id1493155854?i=1000499092482.

7   Frances Elaine Baum and David M Sanders, "Ottawa 25 Years On: A More Radical Agenda for Health Equity is Still Required," *Health Promotion International* 26, supplement 2 (2011): ii253; National Collaborating Centre for Determinants of Health, *Let's Talk: Moving Upstream* (Antigonish, NS: National Collaborating Centre for Determinants of Health, St. Francis Xavier University, 2014), https://nccdh.ca/images/uploads/Moving_Upstream_Final_En.pdf.

8   Fakiha Baig, "Indigenous women still forced, coerced into sterilization: Senate report," *Global News*, 3 June 2021, https://globalnews.ca/news/7920118/indigenous-women-sterilization-senate-report/.

9   Kwame McKenzie, "Socio-Demographic Data Collection and Equity in Covid-19 in Toronto," *eClinicalMedicine* 34 (1 April 2021), https://doi.org/10.1016/j.eclinm.2021.100812; "Interactive Health Data Application," Alberta Health, Government of Alberta, accessed 12 December 2020, http://www.ahw.gov.ab.ca/IHDA_Retrieval/; "Welcome to the Alberta First Nations Information Governance Centre!," Alberta First Nations Information Governance Centre, accessed 12 December 2020, http://www.afnigc.ca/main/index.php?id=home.

10   Our examination of debates within the provincial legislature relied heavily on the *Alberta Hansard*, and we express considerable gratitude to former premier Peter Lougheed for initiating that valuable data source (in its current printed form) in 1972. Provincial Archives of Alberta (PAA), *An Administrative History of the Government of Alberta, 1905–2005* (Edmonton: PAA, 2006), 450; Allan Tupper and Roger Gibbins, eds., *Government and Politics in Alberta* (Edmonton: The University of Alberta Press, 1992), 150.

11   Lindsay McLaren, "What We Need Is a Political-Economic Public Health," letter to the editor, *Health Promotion and Chronic Disease Prevention in Canada* 43, no. 4 (April 2023): 199, https://doi.org/10.24095/hpcdp.43.4.05.

12   Katherine E. Smith and Ellen A. Stewart, "Academic Advocacy in Public Health: Disciplinary 'Duty' or Political 'Propaganda?'" *Social Science & Medicine* 189 (2017): 35.

13   Canadian Networks of Public Health Associations, "A Collective Voice for Advancing Public Health: Why Public Health Associations Matter Today," *Canadian Journal of Public Health* 110. no. 3 (2019).

14   Smith and Stewart, "Academic Advocacy in Public Health."

15   Hancock et al., "There Is Much More to Public Health than COVID-19," healthydebate, 15 June 2020, https://healthydebate.ca/2020/06/topic/more-to-public-health-than-covid/.

16   For example, see Nancy Krieger, "ENOUGH: COVID-19, Structural Racism, Police Brutality, Plutocracy, Climate Change — and Time for Health Justice, Democratic Governance, and an Equitable, Sustainable Future," *American Journal of Public Health* 110, no. 11 (November 1, 2020).

17   CSDH, *Closing the Gap in a Generation,* 1.

18   Adapted from Lindsay McLaren and Trish Hennessy, "A Broader Vision of Public Health," *The Monitor* (Canadian Centre for Policy Alternatives), January/February 2021, https://www.policyalternatives.ca/publications/monitor/broader-vision-public-health.

19   World Health Organization, "Ottawa Charter for Health Promotion;" CSDH, *Closing the Gap in a Generation*; Truth and Reconciliation Commission of Canada, *Honouring the Truth, Reconciling for the Future, Summary of the Final Report of the Truth and Reconciliation Commission of Canada* (Winnipeg, MB: Truth and Reconciliation Commission of Canada, 2015), https://web.archive.org/web/20200513112354/https://trc.ca/index-main.html.

20   CSDH, *Closing the Gap in a Generation,* 1.

21   For a profound example of enduring inequities, see the National Inquiry into Missing and Murdered Indigenous Women and Girls website, accessed 20 December 20202, https://www.mmiwg-ffada.ca.

22   "Implementing the United Nations Declaration on the Rights of Indigenous Peoples in Canada," Department of Justice, Government of Canada, last modified 12 April 2021, https://www.justice.gc.ca/eng/declaration/index.html. There is a growing amount of important work that considers how to do this; for example, Angele Alook et al., *The End of This World: Climate Justice in So-Called Canada* (Toronto: Between the Lines, 2023).

23   Theresa W. S. Tam, "Preparing for Uncertainty During Public Health Emergencies: What Canadian Health Leaders Can Do Now to Optimize Future Emergency Response," *Healthcare Management Forum* 33, no. 4 (July 1, 2020), https://doi.org/10.1177/0840470420917172.

24   Paul Kershaw, "The Need for Health in All Policies in Canada."

25   Lindsay McLaren and Temitayo Famuyide, "What We Can Learn from Québec's Health in All Policies Approach," *Think Upstream* (blog), 15 February 2023, https://www.thinkupstream.ca/post/what-we-can-learn-from-québec-s-health-in-all-policies-approach.

26   Lindsay McLaren, "A Well-Being Economy: A New Paradigm for Health Equity in Alberta," *Parkland Institute* (blog), 18 August 2022, https://www.parklandinstitute.ca/well_being_economy.

27   "Budget 2021: A Canada-wide Early Learning and Child Care Plan," Department of Finance Canada, Government of Canada, last modified 19 April 2021, https://www.canada.ca/en/department-finance/news/2021/04/budget-2021-a-canada-wide-early-learning-and-child-care-plan.html; David Macdonald et al., "Budget 2021 Analysis: Does It Deliver?," *The Monitor* (Canadian Centre for Policy Alternatives), 19 April 2021, https://monitormag.ca/articles/budget-2021-analysis-does-it-deliver.

28   Trish Hennessy, "After the Throne Speech: A Test of Our Resolve," *The Monitor* (Canadian Centre for Policy Alternatives), 24 September 2020; Lindsay McLaren, "What does the Federal Throne Speech Mean for Public Health?," *The Monitor* (Canadian Centre for Policy Alternatives), 30 September, 2020; David Macdonald et al., "A Fiscal Update for Hard Times: Is it Enough?," *Behind the Numbers* (Canadian Centre for Policy Alternatives), 30 November 2020, https://behindthenumbers.ca/2020/11/30/a-fiscal-update-for-hard-times-is-it-enough/; Kelsey Lucyk, "Intersectoral Action on the Social Determinants of Health and Health Equity in Canada: December 2019 Federal Government Mandate Letter Review," *Health Promotion and Chronic Disease Prevention in Canada* 40, no. 10 (2020).

29   "About the AFB," Canadian Centre for Policy Alternatives, accessed 6 July 2023, https://policyalternatives.ca/projects/alternative-federal-budget/about.

30   Public Health Agency of Canada, *Creating a Healthier Canada: Making Prevention a Priority* (Public Health Agency of Canada, 2010), https://www.phac-aspc.gc.ca/hp-ps/hl-mvs/declaration/pdf/dpp-eng.pdf.

31   Jim Stanford, "New Data on Continued Record Profits in Canadian Foot Retail," Centre for Future Work, 10 December 2023, https://centreforfuturework.ca/2023/12/10/new-data-on-continued-record-profits-in-canadian-food-retail/

32   Alook et al., *The End of This World.*

33   Michael Hayes et al., "Telling Stories: News Media, Health Literacy and Public Policy in Canada," *Social Science & Medicine* 64, no. 9 (2007).

34   Ted Schrecker, "What Is Critical about Critical Public Health? Focus on Health Inequalities," *Critical Public Health* 32, no. 2 (2021), https://doi.org/10.1080/09581596.2021.1905776; Judith Green and Ronald Labonté, eds., *Critical Perspectives in Public Health* (New York and Abingdon, UK: Routledge, 2008).

35   Ewen Speed and Lindsay McLaren, "Towards a Theoretically Grounded, Social Democratic Public Health," editorial, *Critical Public Health* 32, no. 5 (2022).

36   · Sylvia Walby, "The COVID Pandemic and Social Theory: Social Democracy and Public Health in the Crisis," *European Journal of Social Theory* 24, no. 1 (February 2021), https://doi.org/10.1177/1368431020970127. See also Ewen Speed and Lindsay McLaren, "Towards a Theoretically Grounded, Social Democratic Public Health."

37   Walby, "The COVID Pandemic and Social Theory."

38   Walby, "The COVID Pandemic and Social Theory."

39   Eric Mykhalovskiy- et al., "Critical Social Science with Public Health: Agonism, Critique and Engagement," *Critical Public Health* 29, no. 5 (2019), https://doi.org/10.1080/09581596.2018.1474174.

40   Lindsay McLaren, *Wellbeing Budgeting: A Critical Public Health Perspective* (Montreal, QC: National Collaborating Centre for Healthy Public Policy, 2022), https://ccnpps-ncchpp.ca/docs/2022-Wellbeing-Budgeting-A-Critical-Public-Health-Perspective.pdf; Sean A. Valles, *Philosophy of Population Health: Philosophy for a New Public Health Era* (London and New York: Routledge, 2018).

Appendix A

Alberta-relevant papers published in the *Canadian Journal of Public Health*, 1919–2019

This list includes publications that present findings specific to Alberta or parts of Alberta (other provinces may also be featured). It excludes articles by Alberta-based researchers where the research focus is not specific to Alberta.

	Year	Author(s)	Title
1.	1928	T.H. Whitelaw	Alberta Health Officials' Association
2.	1929	R.B. Jenkins	Some Findings in the Epidemic of Poliomyelitis in Alberta, 1927
3.	1930	M.R. Bow	Public Health Services in Alberta
4.	1931	A.C. McGugan	Anterior Poliomyelitis in Alberta in 1930
5	1934	A.C. McGugan	Alberta State Health Insurance Report
6.	1935	M.R. Bow	Municipal Hospitals in Alberta
7.	1935	M.R. Bow	Essential Features of a Health Program: as seen by a Provincial Medical Officer of Health
8.	1935	M.R. Bow & F.T. Cook	The History of the Department of Public Health of Alberta
9.	1935	A.C. McGugan	The Alberta Health Insurance Act
10.	1936	F.W. Jackson, R.O. Davison, M.R. Bow	Co-ordination of Medical Practice with Public Health in Manitoba, Saskatchewan, and Alberta
11.	1937	M.R. Bow	Physical Examination of Nurses before and during Employment
12.	1937	M.R. Bow	Public Health Yesterday, To-Day, and To-Morrow
13.	1938	R.D. DeFries	Recent Health Legislation in Canada
14.	1938	A. Stewart & W.D. Porter	Food Purchases by Families in Edmonton and Lacombe, Alberta
15.	1939	Mary Sandin, Mabel Patrick, and Andrew Stewart	Food Consumption of Twenty-Nine Families in Edmonton, Alberta
16.	1941	George Hunter and L. Bradley Pett	A Dietary Survey in Edmonton
17.	1941	A.C. McGugan	Acute Anterior Poliomyelitis in Alberta in 1941
18.	1942	A.C. McGugan	Equine Encephalomyelitis (Western Type) in Humans in Alberta, 1941
19.	1944	Malcolm R. Bow	The Maternity Hospitalization Act of Alberta 1944
20.	1945	W. H. Hill	Recording Child Hygiene Activities in Calgary

APPENDIX A: (*continued*)

	Year	Author(s)	Title
21.	1945	G.M. Little	Scarlet Fever Immunization in Edmonton, Alberta: A Further Study
22.	1946	G.M. Little	Pertussis Immunization in Edmonton
23.	1947	Harold Orr	The Compulsory Premarital Serological Test in Alberta
24.	1948	John H. Brown	Alberta: The Only Rat-Free Province in Canada
25.	1948	G.M. Little	An Outbreak of Paratyphoid Fever in Edmonton, Alta
26.	1952	Malcolm R. Bow and J.T. Brown	Rocky Mountain Spotted Fever in Alberta, 1935–1950
27.	1952	Helen G. McArthur	Nursing Today and in the Future
28.	1953	J.H. Brown, Margaret H. O'Meara, M.L. Friend, H. Dean	The Public Health Importance of Domestic Flies and Their Control on a District Basis in Alberta
29.	1954	John H. Brown	The Mosquito Problem in Relation to Irrigation Developments in Alberta
30.	1954	E.S. Orford Smith and Beatrice E. Cole	A Winter Outbreak of Poliomyelitis in Northern Alberta
31.	1955	W. Bramley-Moore	The Alberta Medical Insurance Plan
32.	1956	F.W. Ings	A Challenge to the Alberta Division
33.	1956	M.G. McCallum	Alberta's Provincial-Municipal Hospitalization Plan
34.	1958	E.J. Thiessen	The Alberta Tuberculosis Association Rehabilitation Program
35.	1959	A. Somerville and R.D. DeFries	The Alberta Department of Public Health
36.	1961	E.S.O. Smith	A Review of the Effectiveness of Salk Vaccine in Alberta with Special Reference to the Outbreak of Poliomyelitis in 1960
37.	1961	M.G. McCallum	The Alberta Rheumatic Fever Prophylaxis Program
38.	1962	Gordon Nikiforuk	The fluoridation dilemma
39.	1962	C.H. Bigland	Salmonella Reservoirs in Alberta
40.	1965	P.B. Rose	The Alberta Medical Plan
41.	1966	John H. Brown and John A. Marken	Western Equine Encephalitis in Alberta
42.	1966	H.L. Hogge, G.H. Ball, S.L. Dobko . . . R.H. Ferguson	Air and Water Pollution Control Programs in Alberta: A Panel Presentation
43.	1968	Amy M. Elliott	Production of low budget television programs in Alberta
44.	1970	Beryl Ebert and Marguerite Macalister	A Study of the Activities of Nursing Personnel in Ten Health Units and One City Health Department in the Province of Alberta, 1968

	Year	Author(s)	Title
45.	1970	V.W. Kadis, W.E. Breitkreitz and O.J. Jonasson	Insecticide Levels in Human Tissues of Alberta Residents
46.	1971	J.O. Iversen, G. Seawright and R.P. Hanson	Serologic Survey for Arboviruses in Central Alberta
47.	1971	Stanley Greenhill	Alberta Health Care Utilization Study (1968 and 1970): Some Preliminary Data on the 1968 Pre-Medicare Phase
48.	1973	Marlene Mackie	Lay Perception of Heart Disease in an Alberta Community
49.	1973	J.M. Howell and E.S.O. Smith	An Agricultural Accident Survey in Alberta, 1970
50.	1973	John B. Newton	Screening the Preschool and School Child: The Leduc-Strathcona Health Unit Program
51.	1973	Irving Rootman and Jack Oakey	School and Community Correlates of Alcohol Use and Abuse Among Alberta Junior High School Students
52.	1975	J. Mark Elwood and Janice R. Rogers	The Incidence of Congenital Abnormalities in British Columbia, Alberta, Manitoba and New Brunswick, 1966–1969
53.	1976	Herbert Buchwald	Alberta's New Look for Occupational Health and Safety
54.	1977	Gerda Bako, Walter C. Mackenzie, E.S.O. Smith	Drivers in Alberta with Previous Impaired Driving Records Responsible for Fatal Highway Accidents: A Survey, 1970–1972
55.	1978	Agnes O'Neil	The Measles Epidemic in Calgary, 1974–1975: The Duration of Protection Conferred by Vaccine
56.	1979	Judy E. Peacoke	The Epidemiology of Influenza in Canada, 1977–78
57.	1980	Helen M. Ready and Phyllis M. Craig	Evaluation of Tuberculin Testing by Jet Injection
58.	1980	Donald T. Wigle, Yang Mao and Michael Grace	Relative Importance of Smoking as a Risk Factor for Selected Cancers
59.	1980	Elly Bollegraaf	An Overview of the Salmonella Surveillance System in Canada
60.	1980	Marjorie Baskin, Louise Levesque, Alexander S. Macpherson . . . David L. Sackett	Canada's Health Care Evaluation Seminars: An Epilogue and Evaluation
61.	1981	R. Khakhria and H. Lior	Phage Typing of Salmonella typhi in Canada (1967–1976)
62.	1981	R.A. Morgan	Orthoptists: Paramedical Specialists and Their Role in Eye Care
63.	1981	L.E and F.A. Rozovsky	The Disabled and the Law
64.	1981	Carol A. Ewasechko	Prevalence of Head Lice (Pediculus capitis [De Geer]) Among Children in a Rural, Central Alberta School
65.	1981	F.M.M. White, B.A. Lacey, B.A. Lacy, P.D.A. Constance	An Outbreak of Poliovirus Infection in Alberta — 1978

	Year	Author(s)	Title
66.	1981	Lawrence J. Nestman and Kyung S. Bay	A Coordinated Home Care Program and its Patients
67.	1981	Herbert C. Northcott and George K. Jarvis	Government Influence, Media Influence, and Quitting Smoking
68.	1982	S. Wadhera and C. Nair	Trends in Cesarean Section Deliveries, Canada, 1968–1977
69..	1982	Martha E. Smith and Howard B. Newcombe	Use of the Canadian Mortality Data Base for Epidemiological Follow-up
70.	1982	Gerda Bako, E.S.O. Smith . . . Ron Dewar	The Geographical Distribution of High Cadmium Concentrations in the Environment and Prostate Cancer in Alberta
71.	1982	Earler L. Sinder	The Needs of Health and Related Community Agencies Serving Elderly Families
72.	1982	D.J. Hosking, C.A. Raddojevic and J.R Seaborn	Effects of a Four-Day Work Week Experiment on the Provision of Community Health Services
73.	1982	Donald G. Somers and Louise Favreau	Newborn Screening for Phenylketonuria: Incidence and Screening Procedures in North America
74.	1982	Richard N. Nuttall	The Development of Indian Boards of Health in Alberta
75.	1982	Patrick C.W. Lai, John Z. Garson and Catherine A. Hankins	The Prevalence of Breast Feeding in Calgary, 1979–1980
76.	1983	Theresa Gyorkos	Estimation of Parasite Prevalence based on Submissions to Provincial Laboratories
77.	1983	Norma E. Thurston and Janet C. Kerr	A Nutritional Knowledge Questionnaire for the Elderly
78.	1983	Kyung s. Bay, Lawrence Nestman and Brian Bayda	Attitudes and Opinions of Physicians Toward a Coordinated Home Care Program
79.	1984	John W. Shaw	A Retrospective Comparison of the Effectiveness of Bromination and Chlorination in Controlling Pseudomonas Aeruginosa in Spas (Whirlpools) in Alberta
80.	1984	Gerda Bako, Ron Dewar, John Hanson and Gerry Hill	Population Density as an Indicator of Urban-Rural Differences in Cancer Incidence, Alberta, Canada, 1969–73
81.	1984	R. Sauve, K. Buchan, A. Clyne, and D. McIntosh	Mothers' Milk Banking: Microbiologic Aspects
82.	1984	Paul Fieldhouse	A Revival in Breastfeeding
83.	1984	Gerald N. Predy	A Brief History of Public Health in Alberta
84.	1984	Ian D. McIntosh and Donnie Ure	Maternity Early Discharge in a Local Health Authority

	Year	Author(s)	Title
85.	1985	Harvey Krahn, Graham S. Lowe, and Julian Tanner	The Social-Psychological Impact of Unemployment in Edmonton
86.	1985	Agnes E. O'Neil, Daniel Richen and Philip Lundrie	A Waterborne Epidemic of Acute Infectious Non-bacterial Gastroenteritis in Alberta, Canada
87.	1987	Mabel L. Halliday and W. Harding Le Riche	Regional Variation in Surgical Rates, Alberta, 1978, and the Relationship to Characteristics of Patients, Doctors Performing Surgery and Hospitals where the Surgery was Performed
88.	1988	Katherine Cormie, Joy Edwards, James Howell (...) Helen Ready	The Edmonton Tornado Disaster: The Role of the Health Department
89.	1988	Penelope J. MacDonald and James M. Howell	Community-Based Surveys: A Component of the Measurement of Health in Edmonton
90.	1989	Peter C. Berger, R. Wayne Elford, Maryann Yeo . . . Chandar M. Anand	Pharyngitis 1987: A Survey of Physicians' Attitudes and Practices in Southern Alberta
91.	1989	Cornelia J. Baines, Andrée Christen, Antoine Simard . . . Anthony B. Miller	The National Breast Screening Study: Pre-recruitment Sources of Awareness in Participants
92.	1989	Janice M. Morse, Joan L. Bottorff, and Jeanette Boman	Patterns of Breastfeeding and Work: The Canadian Experience
93.	1989	Wendy L. Neander and Janice M. Morse	Tradition and Change in the Northern Alberta Woodlands Cree: Implications for Infant Feeding Practices
94.	1990	Thomas J. Abernathy and Donna M. Lentjes	A Three-year Census of Dependent Elderly
95.	1990	Delmarie T. Sadoway, Tichard H.M. Plain, and Colin L. Soskolne	Infant and Preschool Immunization Delivery in Alberta and Ontario: A Partial Cost-Minimization Analysis
96.	1990	Lawrence W. Svenson and Connie K. Varnhagen	Knowledge, Attitudes and Behaviours Related to AIDS Among First-Year University Students
97.	1990	Martin T. Schechter, Walter O. Spitzer, Marian E. Hutcheon . . . Nicolas Steinmetz	A Study of Mortality Near Sour Gas Refineries in Southwest Alberta: An Epidemic Unrevealed
98.	1990	Yang Mao, Paul Hasselback, John W. Davies . . . Donald T. Wigle	Suicide in Canada: An Epidemiological Assessment
99.	1990	Lawrence W. Svenson	Mental Health Services in Edmonton – An Assessment of Service Availability
100.	1990	Barbara J. Cobbie and Betty J. Tucker	The Perceived Health Needs of Abused Women
101.	1990	Steve E. Hrudey, Colin L. Soskolne, Johannes Berkel, and Shirley Fincham	Drinking Water Fluoridation and Osteosarcoma
102.	1991	Reg S. Sauve and J.H. Geggie	Growth and Dietary Status of Preterm and Term Infants during the First Two Years of Life
103.	1991	Herbert C. Northcott and Linda Reutter	Public Opinion Regarding AIDS Policy: Fear of Contagion and Attitude Toward Homosexual Relationships

	Year	Author(s)	Title
104.	1991	Margaret Leora Russell, and Edgar J. Love	Contraceptive Prescription: Physician Beliefs, Attitudes and Socio-demographic Characteristics
105.	1991	Ian Robertson, David W. Megran, Maire A. Duggan . . . Gavin C.E. Stuart	Cervico-Vaginal Screening in an STD Clinic
106.	1991	Heather E. Bryant, William M. Csokonay, M. Love, and E.J. Love	Self-reported Illness and Risk Behaviours Amongst Canadian Travellers While Abroad
107.	1991	Paul Cappon	HIV: The Debate Over Isolation as a Measure of Personal Control
108.	1991	Allison L. McKinnon, John W. Gartrell, Linda A. Derksen, and George K. Jarvis	Health Knowledge of Native Indian Youth in Central Alberta
109.	1991	Tom J Paton, Nonie J. Lee, Wadieh R. Yacoub, and Bruce Angus	A Health Centre Survey of Childhood Injury in Edmonton
110.	1992	Thomas J. Abernathy and Lorne D. Bertrand	The Prevalence of Smokeless Tobacco and Cigarette Use Among Sixth, Seventh and Eighth Grade
111.	1992	Karen White, Ardene Vollman and Arlene Ritchie	Meningococcal Disease and Death in Rural Alberta December 1991
112.	1992	Judy M. Birdsell, H. Sharon Campbell, S. Elizabeth McGregor and Gerry B. Hill	Steve Fonyo Cancer Prevention Program: Description of an Innovative Program
113.	1992	Thomas J. Abernathy and Lorne D. Bertrand	Preventing Cigarette Smoking Among Children: Results of a Four-Year Evaluation of the PAL Program
114.	1992	Janice M. Morse, Gail Ewing, Diane Gamble and Patricia Donahue	The Effect of Maternal Fluid Intake on Breast Milk Supply: A Pilot Study
115.	1992	Martha C. Piper, Lynn E. Pinnell, Johanna Darrah . . . Paul J. Byrne	Construction and Validation of the Alberta Infant Motor Scale (AIMS)
116.	1992	Charlene M.T. Robertson and Michael G.A. Grace	Validation of Prediction of Kindergarten-age School-readiness Scores of Nondisabled Survivors of Moderate Neonatal Encephalopathy in Term Infants
117.	1992	Cynthia M. Mathieson, Peter D. Faris, Henderikus J. Stam and Lori A. Egger	Health Behaviours in a Canadian Community College Sample: Prevalence of Drug Use and Interrelationships Among Behaviours
118.	1992	Lawrence W. Svenson, Connie K. Varnhagen, Anne Marie Godin and Tracy L. Salmon	Rural High School Students' Knowledge, Attitudes and Behaviours Related to Sexually Transmitted Diseases
119.	1992	S. Elizabeth McGregor, Ellen Murphy and Jeff Reeve	Attitudes about Cancer and Knowledge of Cancer Prevention Among Junior High Students in Calgary, Alberta
120.	1992	J. Howard Brunt and Edgar J. Love	Hypertension and Its Correlates in the Hutterite Community of Alberta

	Year	Author(s)	Title
121.	1992	Marja J. Verhoef and Edgar J. Love	Women's Exercise Participation: The Relevance of Social Roles Compared to Non-role-related Determinants
122.	1992	Lawrence W. Svenson	Breast Self-examination Behaviours Among Female University Students
123.	1993	Linda L. Smith and Linda M. Lathrop	AIDS and Human Sexuality
124.	1993	R.D. Egedahl, M. Fair and R. Homik	Mortality Among Employees at a Hydrometallurgical Nickel Refinery and Fertilizer Complex in Fort Saskatchewan, Alberta
125.	1993	Pamela A. Ratner	The Incidence of Wife Abuse and Mental Health Status in Abused Wives in Edmonton, Alberta
126.	1993	Len Chernichko, L. Duncan Saunders and Suzanne Tough	Unintentional House Fire Deaths in Alberta 1985–1990: A Population Study
127.	1993	Nonie J. Fraser-Lee, Penelope J. Macdonald, James M. Howell and Patrick A. Hessel	The Hopes and Hazards of Health Goals Development
128.	1994	Delmarie T. Sadoway, Jennifer R. Loucraft and Bonnie A. Johnston	Public Health Practice: Maximizing Influenza Immunization in Edmonton: A Collaborative Model
129.	1994	Tanis R. Fenton and Jayne E. Thirsk	Twin Pregnancy: The Distribution of Maternal Weight Gain of Non-smoking Normal Weight Women
130.	1994	R. Anne Dow-Clarke, Lynn MacCalder and Patrick A. Hessel	Health Behaviours of Pregnant Women in Fort McMurray, Alberta
131.	1994	Tammy E. Horne	Predictors of Physical Activity Intentions and Behaviour for Rural Homemakers
132.	1994	Cathy E. Leinweber, J. Morag Macdonald and H. Sharon Campbell	Community Smoking Cessation Contests: An Effective Public Health Strategy
133.	1994	Thomas J. Abernathy	Compliance for Kids: A Community-based Tobacco Prevention Project
134.	1994	Nonie J. Fraser-Lee and Patrick A. Hessel	Acute Respiratory Infections in the Canadian Native Indian Population: A Review
135.	1994	Barbara Romanowski and Patricia Campbell	Sero-epidemiologic Study to Determine the Prevalence and Risk of Hepatitis B in a Canadian Heterosexual Sexually Transmitted Disease Population
136.	1994	Robert M. Semenciw, Howard I. Morrison, Dierdre Morison and Yang Mao	Leukemia Mortality and Farming in the Prairie Provinces of Canada
137.	1994	Theresa W. Gyorkos, Terry N. Tannenbaum, Michal Abrahamowicz ... Steven A. Grover	Evaluation of the Effectiveness of Immunization Delivery Methods
138.	1994	Theresa W. Gyorkos, Eliane D. Franco, Terry N. Tannenbaum ... Steven A. Grover	Practice Survey of Immunization in Canada

	Year	Author(s)	Title
139.	1994	Philippe Duclos, Martin L. Tepper, John Weber and Raymond G. Marusyk	Seroprevalence of Measles- and Rubella-Specific Antibodies Among Military Recruits, Canada, 1991
140.	1994	Norman R.C. Campbell, David B. Hogan and Donald W. McKay	Pitfalls to Avoid in the Measurement of Blood Pressure in the Elderly
141.	1994	Sherri Kashuba, Gordon Flowerdew, Patrick A. Hessel . . . Richard Musto	Acute Care Hospital Morbidity in the Blood Indian Band, 1984–87
142.	1994	Marja J. Verhoef, Margaret L. Russell and Edgar J. Love	Alternative Medicine Use in Rural Alberta
143.	1994	Elisabeth J. Thompson and Margaret L. Russell	Risk Factors for Non-Use of Seatbelts in Rural and Urban Alberta
144.	1994	Randy N. Ross and Brian Phillips	Twenty Questions for Tanning Facility Operators: A Survey of Operator Knowledge
145.	1995	Margaret E. King, Margaret J. Harrison and Linda Reutter	Public Health Nursing or Community Health Nursing: Examining the Debate
146.	1995	Joy L. Johnson, Pamela A. Ratner and Joan L. Bottorff	Urban-Rural Differences in the Health-Promoting Behaviours of Albertans
147.	1995	Wendy Benson	Strategies and Willingness of Rural Restaurateurs to Promote Healthy Foods
148.	1995	Philip Jacobs, Ed Hall, Isabel Henderson and Debra Nichols	Episodic Acute Care Costs: Linking Inpatient and Home Care
149.	1995	C. Anthony Ryan, Suzanne Tough and Graeme Dowling	Less Common Causes of Accidental Drownings in Alberta
150.	1995	Cathy E. Leinweber, H. Sharon Campbell and Darcy L. Trottier	Is a Health Promotion Campaign Successful in Retail Pharmacies?
151.	1996	Margaret I. Wanke and L. Duncan Saunders	Survey of Local Environmental Health Programs in Alberta
152.	1996	W. Kerry Mummery and Les C. Hagen	Tobacco Pricing, Taxation, Consumption and Revenue: Alberta 1985-1995
153.	1996	M.L. Russell	Denominators for Estimation of Influenza Vaccine Coverage Among High Risk Persons Aged 15 to 64 Years
154.	1996	Penny A. Jennett and Kalyani Premkumar	Technology-based Dissemination
155.	1996	Patrick A. Hessel, Terry Sliwkanich, Dennis Michaelchuk . . . Thu-Ha Nguyen	Asthma and Limitation of Activities in Fort Saskatchewan, Alberta
156.	1997	Kenneth C. Johnson and Jocelyn Rouleau	Temporal Trends in Canadian Birth Defects Birth Prevalences, 1979–1993

	Year	Author(s)	Title
157.	1997	Gerry Predy, Bill Carney and Joy Edwards	Effectiveness of Recorded Messages to Communicate the Risk of Acquiring Hantavirus Pulmonary Syndrome
158.	1997	Penny A. Sutcliffe, Raisa B. Deber and George Pasut	Public Health in Canada: A Comparative Study of Six Provinces
159.	1997	Jennifer M. Medves and Beverley A.C. O'Brien	Cleaning Solutions and Bacterial Colonization in Promoting Healing and Early Separation of the Umbilical Cord in Healthy Newborns
160.	1998	Elaine Grandin, Eugen Lupri and Merlin B. Brinkerhoff	Couple Violence and Psychological Distress
161.	1998	W. Kerry Mummery, John C. Spence, Joanne A. Vincenten and Donald C. Voaklander	A Descriptive Epidemiology of Sport and Recreation Injuries in a Population-Based Sample: Results from the Alberta Sport and Recreation Injury Survey (ASRIS)
162.	1998	Ted M. Birse and Janice Lander	Prevalence of Chronic Pain
163.	1998	Deanna L. Williamson and Janet E. Fast	Poverty and Medical Treatment: When Public Policy Compromises Accessibility
164.	1998	Shi Wu Wen, Shiliang Liu and Dawn Fowler	Trends and Variations in Neonatal Length of In-hospital Stay in Canada
165.	1998	Zhiqiang Wang and Reg S. Sauve	Assessment of Postneonatal Growth in VLBW Infants: Selection of Growth References and Age Adjustment for Prematurity
166.	1998	Richard T. Burnett, Sabit Cakmak and Jeffrey R. Brook	The Effect of the Urban Ambient Air Pollution Mix on Daily Mortality Rates in 11 Canadian Cities
167.	1998	Lawrence W. Svenson, Donald P. Schopflocher, R.S. Sauve and Charlene M.T. Robertson	Alberta's Infant Mortality Rate: The Effect of the Registration of Live Newborns Weighing Less Than 500 Grams
168.	1998	Christiane Poulin, Pamela Fralick, Elizabeth M. Whynot . . . Joseph Rinehart	The Epidemiology of Cocaine and Opiate Abuse in Urban Canada
169.	1998	W. Kerry Mummery and John C. Spence	Stages of Physical Activity in the Alberta Population
170.	1999	Linda Reutter, Anne Neufeld and Margaret J. Harrison	Public Perceptions of the Relationship between Poverty and Health
171.	1999	Diane Doering, Rose Kocuipchyk and Shelley Lester	A Tuberculosis Screening and Chemoprophylaxis Project in Children from a High-Risk Population in Edmonton, Alberta
172.	1999	David M. Patrick, Michael L. Rekart, Darrel Cook . . . A. Rees	Non-Nominal HIV Surveillance: Preserving Privacy While Tracking an Epidemic
173.	1999	Philip Jacobs, Peter Calder, Marliss Taylor . . . Terry Albert	Cost Effectiveness of Streetworks' Needle Exchange Program of Edmonton
174.	1999	Jat S. Sandhu, Patricia M. Campbell, Jutta K. Preiksaitis . . . Patrick A. Hessel	Validation of Self-reported Transfusion Histories in Renal Dialysis Patients

APPENDIX A: (*continued*)

	Year	Author(s)	Title
175.	1999	Judith A. Leech, Kerri Wilby and Edmund McMullen	Environmental Tobacco Smoke Exposure Patterns: A Subanalysis of the Canadian Human Time-Activity Pattern Survey
176.	1999	A. Casebeer, K. Deis and S. Doze	Health Indicator Development in Alberta Health Authorities: Searching for Common Ground
177.	2000	Daniel W.L. Lai	Prevalence of Depression Among the Elderly Chinese in Canada
178.	2000	David Lester, PhD	Gun Availability and the Use of Guns for Suicide and Homicide in Canada
179.	2000	Shi Wu Wen, Jocelyn Rouleau, Robert Brian Lowry . . . Tanya Turner	Congenital Anomalies Ascertained by Two Record Systems Run in Parallel in the Canadian Province of Alberta
180.	2000	Greg D. Appleyard and Alvin A. Gajadhar	A Review of Trichinellosis in People and Wildlife in Canada
181.	2000	Stephen R. Manske, Chris Y. Lovato, Jean Shoveller and Kelly A. Velle	Public Health Capacity and Interest in Using Electronic Communication for Staff Training and Resource Dissemination: A National Survey
182.	2000	Wendy L. Maurier and Herbert C. Northcott	Self-reported Risk Factors and Perceived Chance of Getting HIV/AIDS in the 1990s in Alberta
183.	2000	Margaret L. Russell and Colleen J. Maxwell	The Prevalence and Correlates of Influenza Vaccination Among a Home Care Population
184.	2001	Elan C. Paluck, Deanna L. Williamson, C. Dawne Milligan and C. James Frankish	The Use of Population Health and Health Promotion Research by Health Regions in Canada
185.	2001	Frederick A. Leighton, Harvey A. Artsob, May C. Chu and James G. Olson	A Serological Survey of Rural Dogs and Cats on the Southwestern Canadian Prairie for Zoonotic Pathogens
186.	2001	Don D. Sin, Larry W. Svenson and S.F. Paul Man	Do Area-Based Markers of Poverty Accurately Measure Personal Poverty?
187.	2001	Jean-Pierre Grégoire, Pierre MacNeil, Kevin Skilton . . . Bryan Ferguson	Inter-Provincial Variation in Government Drug Formularies
188.	2001	Laura McLeod and Wendy W. Lau	Decreasing Influenza Impact in Lodges: 1997–2000 Calgary Regional Health Authority
189.	2001	Suzanne C. Tough, Lawrence W. Svenson, David W. Johnston and Don Schopflocher	Characteristics of Preterm Delivery and Low Birthweight Among 113,994 Infants in Alberta: 1994–1996
190.	2001	Nico M. Trocmé, Bruce J. MacLaurin, Barbara A. Fallon . . . Diane A. Billingsley	Canadian Incidence Study of Reported Child Abuse and Neglect: Methodology
191.	2001	Linda I. Reutter, Diane N. Dennis and Douglas R. Wilson	Young Parents' Understanding and Actions Related to the Determinants of Health

	Year	Author(s)	Title
192.	2001	M.L. Russell and Cheryl A. Ferguson	Improving Population Influenza Vaccine Coverage Through Provider Feedback and Best Practice Identification
193.	2001	Scott B. Patten	Descriptive Epidemiology of a Depressive Syndrome in a Western Canadian Community Population
194.	2002	Kathleen Steel O'Conner, Susan E. MacDonald, Lisa Hartling . . . Michael L. Rekart	The Influence of Prevalence and Policy on the Likelihood that a Physician will Offer HIV Screening in Pregnancy
195.	2002	Sharon Yanicki, Paul Hasselback, Mark Sandilands and Chris Jensen-Ross	The Safety of Canadian Early Discharge Guidelines: Effects of Discharge Timing on Readmission in the First Year Post-discharge and Exclusive Breastfeeding to Four Months
196.	2002	Corrine D. Truman and Linda Reutter	Caregiving and Care-seeking Behaviours of Parents Who Take Their Children to an Emergency Department for Non-urgent Care
197.	2002	Judith C. Kulig, Cathy J. Meyer, Shirley A. Hill . . . Sharon L. Myck	Refusals and Delay of Immunization Within Southwest Alberta: Understanding Alternative Beliefs and Religious Perspectives
198.	2002	Wilma M. Hopman, Claudie Berger, Lawrence Joseph . . . Emmanuel A. Papadimitropoulos	Is There Regional Variation in the SF-36 Scores of Canadian Adults?
199.	2002	Linda I. Reutter, Margaret J. Harrison and Anne Neufeld	Public Support for Poverty-related Policies
200.	2002	David Johnson, Yan Jin and Corrine Truman	Early Discharge of Alberta Mothers Post-delivery and the Relationship to Potentially Preventable Newborn Readmissions
201.	2002	Richard Long	Tuberculosis Control in Alberta: A Federal, Provincial and Regional Public Health Partnership
202.	2002	John C. Spence, Ronald C. Plotnikoff and W. Kerry Mummery	The Awareness and Use of Canada's Physical Activity Guide to Healthy Active Living
203.	2002	Judee E. Onyskiw	Health and Use of Health Services of Children Exposed to Violence in Their Families
204.	2002	Roy West, E. Keith Borden, Jean-Paul Collet . . . Robert S. Tonks	"Cost-effectiveness" Estimates Result in Flawed Decision-making in Listing Drugs for Reimbursement
205.	2002	Niko Yiannakoulias, Karen E. Smoyer-Tomic, John Hodgson . . . Donald C. Voaklander	The Spatial and Temporal Dimensions of Child Pedestrian Injury in Edmonton
206.	2002	Danielle A. Southern, William A. Ghali, Peter D. Faris . . . Merril L. Knudtson	Misclassification of Income Quintiles Derived from Area-based Measures: A Comparison of Enumeration Area and Forward Sortation Area
207.	2003	Suzanne C. Tough, Alexandra J. Faber, Lawrence W. Svenson and David W. Johnston	Is Paternal Age Associated with an Increased Risk of Low Birthweight, Preterm Delivery, and Multiple Birth?

	Year	Author(s)	Title
208.	2003	Angus H. Thompson, Arif Alibhai, L. Duncan Saunders . . . Narmatha Thanigasalam	Post-maternity Outcomes Following Health Care Reform in Alberta: 1992–1996
209.	2003	Kathy Nykolyshyn, Jackie A. Petruk, Natasha Wiebe . . . Brian H. Rowe	The Use of Bicycle Helmets in a Western Canadian Province Without Legislation
210.	2003	Joan D. Ing and Linda Reutter	Socioeconomic Status, Sense of Coherence and Health in Canadian Women
211.	2003	Yan Jin, Keumhee C. Carriere, Gerry Predy . . . Thomas J. Marrie	The Association Between Influenza Immunization Coverage Rates and Hospitalization for Community-acquired Pneumonia in Alberta
212.	2003	Donald P. Schopflocher and Margaret L. Russell	Method for Ascertaining Denominators for Evaluation of Population Coverage with Pneumococcal Vaccine
213.	2003	Juanita Hatcher and Douglas C. Dover	Trends in Histopathology of Lung Cancer in Alberta
214.	2003	Brent E. Hagel, I. Barry Pless and Robert W. Platt	Trends in Emergency Department Reported Head and Neck Injuries Among Skiers and Snowboarders
215.	2003	Lynn M. Meadows and Linda A. Mrkonjic	Breaking – Bad News: Women's Experiences of Fractures at Midlife
216.	2004	Paul J. Villeneuve, Kenneth C. Johnson, Yang Mao and Anthony J. Hanley	Environmental Tobacco Smoke and the Risk of Pancreatic Cancer: Findings from a Canadian Population-based Case-control Study
217.	2004	Caroline D. McAllister and Margaret L. Russell	Travel Counsellors and Travel Health Advice
218.	2004	T. Cameron Wild, Amanda B. Roberts, John Cunningham . . . Hannah Pazderka-Robinson	Alcohol Problems and Interest in Self-help: A Population Study of Alberta Adults
219.	2004	Mats Ramstedt	Alcohol Consumption and Alcohol-related Mortality in Canada, 1950–2000
220.	2004	Samantha L. Bowker, Colin L. Soskolne, Stan C. Houston . . . Gian S. Jhangri	Human Immunodeficiency Virus (HIV) and Hepatitis C Virus (HCV) in a Northern Alberta Population
221.	2004	Hude Quan, William A. Ghali, Stafford Dean . . . Merril L. Knudtson	Validity of using surname to define Chinese ethnicity
222.	2004	Richard Long, Denise Whittaker, Krista Russell . . . Ravi Bhargava	Pediatric Tuberculosis in Alberta First Nations (1991–2000): Outbreaks and the Protective Effect of Bacille Calmette-Guérin (BCG) Vaccine
223.	2004	Teresa To, Astrid Guttmann, Paul T. Dick . . . Jennifer K. Harris	What Factors Are Associated with Poor Developmental Attainment in Young Canadian Children?
224.	2004	Donna M. Wilson and Corrine D. Truman	Long-Term-Care Residents: Concerns Identified by Population and Care Trends

	Year	Author(s)	Title
225.	2004	Alyssa D. Reed, Robert J. Williams, Patricia A. Wall and Paul Hasselback	Waiting Time for Breast Cancer Treatment in Alberta
226.	2004	Ronald C. Plotnikoff, Kim Bercovitz and Constantinos A. Loucaides	Physical Activity, Smoking, and Obesity Among Canadian School Youth: Comparison Between Urban and Rural Schools
227.	2005	Philip Jacobs, Arto Ohinmaa, Kamran Golmohammadi . . . Scott Klarenbach	Public Investment in Providing Information for Chronic Disease Prevention for Adults in Alberta
228.	2005	Shainoor Virani, Heather Young, David Strong . . . Ellen Toth	Rationale and Implementation of the SLICK Project: Screening for Limb, I-Eye, Cardiovascular and Kidney (SLICK) Complications in Individuals with Type 2 Diabetes in Alberta's First Nations Communities
229.	2005	Michele T. Guerin, S. Wayne Martin and Gerarda A. Darlington	Temporal Clusters of Salmonella Serovars in Humans in Alberta, 1990–2001
230.	2006	Suzanne Tough, Karen Benzies, Christine Newburn-Cook . . . Reg Sauve	What Do Women Know About the Risks of Delayed Childbearing?
231.	2006	Shainoor Virani, Heather Young, David Strong . . . Ellen Toth	Rationale and Implementation of the SLICK Project Screening for Limb, I-Eye, Cardiovascular and Kidney (SLICK) Complications in Individuals with Type 2 Diabetes in Alberta's First Nations Communities
232.	2006	Jennifer A. Beaulac, Richard N. Fry and Jay Onysko	Lifetime and Recent Prostate Specific Antigen (PSA) Screening of Men for Prostate Cancer in Canada
233	2006	Philip Jacobs, Arto Ohinmaa, Kamran Golmohammadi . . . Scott Klarenbach	Public Investment in Providing Information for Chronic Disease Prevention for Adults in Alberta
234.	2006	Danielle A. Southern, Peter D. Faris, Merril L. Knudtson and William A. Ghali	Prognostic Relevance of Census-derived Individual Respondent Incomes Versus Household Incomes
235.	2006	Ronald C. Plotnikoff, John C. Spence, Leonor S. Tavares . . . Linda McCargar	Characteristics of Participants Visiting the "Canada on the Move" Website
236.	2006	Lori J. Curtis and Michael Pennock	Social Assistance, Lone Parents and Health: What Do We Know, Where Do We Go?
237.	2006	Stephanie J. Knaak	The Problem with Breastfeeding Discourse
238.	2006	Sean A. Kidd and Larry Davidson	What Is the Evidence for Parenting Interventions Offered in a Canadian Community?
239.	2006	Pascal Michel, Leah J. Martin, Carol E. Tinga and Kathryn Doré	Regional, Seasonal, and Antimicrobial Resistance Distributions of Salmonella Typhimurium in Canada: A Multi-Provincial Study
240.	2007	Anwar T. Merchant, Mahshid Dehghan and Noori Akhtar-Danesh	Seasonal Variation in Leisure time Physical Activity Among Canadians
241.	2007	Lise Gauvin, Éric Robitaille, Mylène Riva . . . Louise Potvin	Conceptualizing and Operationalizing Neighbourhoods: The Conundrum of Identifying Territorial Units

	Year	Author(s)	Title
242.	2007	Sabrina S. Plitt, Ali M. Somily and Ameeta E. Singh	Outcomes from a Canadian Public Health Prenatal Screening Program for Hepatitis B: 1997–2004
243.	2007	Julie A. Bettinger, David W. Scheifele, Scott A. Halperin . . . Gregory Tyrrell	Invasive Pneumococcal Infections in Canadian Children, 1998–2003: Implications for New Vaccination Programs
244.	2007	Sandy Jacobs, Andrea Warman, Natalie Roehrig . . . Richard Long	Mycobacterium tuberculosis Infection in First Nations Preschool Children in Alberta: Implications for BCG (bacille Calmette-Guérin) Vaccine Withdrawal
245.	2007	Katherine L.W. Smith, Flora I. Matheson, Rahim Moineddin and Richard H. Glazier	Gender, Income and Immigration Differences in Depression in Canadian Urban Centres
246.	2007	C. James Frankish, Glen E. Moulton, Darryl Quantz . . . Brian E. Evoy	Addressing the Non-medical Determinants of Health: A Survey of Canada's Health Regions
247.	2007	Mark S. Tremblay and Sarah Connor Gorber	Canadian Health Measures Survey: Brief Overview
248.	2007	Sharlene Wolbeck Minke, Kim D. Raine, Ronald C. Plotnikoff . . . Cynthia Smith	Resources for Health Promotion: Rhetoric, Research and Reality
249.	2007	Hude Quan, Fu-Lin Wang, Donald Schopflocher and Carolyn De Coster	Mortality, Cause of Death and Life Expectancy of Chinese Canadians in Alberta
250.	2007	Tracey L. O'Sullivan, Carol A. Amaratunga, Jill Hardt . . . D. Gibson	Are We Ready? Evidence of Support Mechanisms for Canadian Health Care Workers in Multi-jurisdictional Emergency Planning
251.	2007	David Yip, Ravi Bhargava, Yin Yao, (. . . .) Richard Long	Pediatric Tuberculosis in Alberta: Epidemiology and Case Characteristics (1990–2004)
252.	2008	Kimberly A. Godwin, Barbara Sibbald, Tanya Bedard . . . Laura Arbour	Changes in Frequencies of Select Congenital Anomalies since the Onset of Folic Acid Fortification in a Canadian Birth Defect Registry
523.	2008	M. Anne Harris, Adrian R. Levy and Kay E. Teschke	Personal Privacy and Public Health: Potential Impacts of Privacy Legislation on Health Research in Canada
254.	2008	Ronald C. Plotnikoff, Nandini D. Karunamuni, Jeffrey A. Johnson . . . Lawrence W. Svenson	Health-related Behaviours in Adults with Diabetes: Associations with Health Care Utilization and Costs
255.	2008	Melissa L. Potestio, Lindsay McLaren, Ardene Robinson Vollman and P.K. Doyle-Baker	Childhood Obesity: Perceptions Held by the Public in Calgary, Canada
256.	2008	Joy Edwards, Judy Evans and Angela D. Brown	Using Routine Growth Data to Determine Overweight and Obesity Prevalence Estimates in Preschool Children in the Capital Health Region of Alberta

	Year	Author(s)	Title
257.	2008	M.L. Russell, D.P. Schopflocher and L.W. Svenson	Health Disparities in Chickenpox or Shingles in Alberta?
258.	2008	Catherine P. Gladwin, John Church and Ronald C. Plotnikoff	Public Policy Processes and Getting Physical Activity into Alberta's Urban Schools
259.	2008	Lance Honish, Colin L. Soskolne, Ambikaipakan Senthilselvan and Stan Houston	Modifiable Risk Factors for Invasive Meningococcal Disease During an Edmonton, Alberta Outbreak, 1999–2002
260.	2009	Catherine A. Worthington and Bruce J. MacLaurin	Level of Street Involvement and Health and Health Services Use of Calgary Street Youth
261.	2009	Heather L. Kehler, Katie H. Chaput and Suzanne C. Tough	Risk Factors for Cessation of Breastfeeding Prior to Six Months Postpartum among a Community Sample of Women in Calgary, Alberta
262.	2009	Hude Quan, Fu-Lin Wang, Donald Schopflocher and Carolyn De Coster	Mortality, Cause of Death and Life Expectancy of Chinese Canadians in Alberta
263.	2009	Leia M. Minaker, Linda McCargar, Irene Lambraki . . . Rhona M. Hanning	School Region Socio-economic Status and Geographic Locale is Associated with Food Behaviour of Ontario and Alberta Adolescents
264.	2009	Svetlana Popova, Jayadeep Patra, Satya Mohapatra . . . Jürgen Rehm	How Many People in Canada Use Prescription Opioids Non-medically in General and Street Drug Using Populations?
265.	2009	Doris Sturtevant, Jutta Preiksaitis, Ameeta Singh . . . Richard Long	The Feasibility of Using an 'Opt-Out' Approach to Achieve Universal HIV Testing of Tuberculosis Patients in Alberta
266.	2009	Raphaël Bize, Ronald C. Plotnikoff, Shannon D. Scott . . . Wendy Rodgers	Adoption of the Healthy Heart Kit by Alberta Family Physicians
267.	2009	Eileen Schmidt, Susan Mide Kiss and Wendi Lokanc-Diluzio	Changing Social Norms: A Mass Media Campaign for Youth Ages 12-18
268.	2009	R. Brian Lowry	Congenital Anomalies Surveillance in Canada
269.	2009	Dick Menzies, Megan Lewis and Olivia Oxlade	Costs for Tuberculosis Care in Canada
270.	2009	Xiaoyan Guo, Noreen Willows, Stefan Kuhle . . . Paul J. Veugelers	Use of Vitamin and Mineral Supplements among Canadian Adults
271.	2009	Jeffrey A. Johnson, Stephanie U. Vermeulen, Ellen L. Toth . . . Lynden Crowshoe	Increasing Incidence and Prevalence of Diabetes among the Status Aboriginal Population in Urban and Rural Alberta, 1995–2006
272.	2009	Leia M. Minaker, Kim D. Raine and Sean B. Cash	Measuring the Food Service Environment: Development and Implementation of Assessment Tools
273.	2009	Feng Xiao Li, Paula J. Robson, Fredrick D. Ashbury . . . Heather E. Bryant	Smoking Frequency, Prevalence and Trends, and Their Socio-demographic Associations in Alberta, Canada
274.	2009	Feng Xiao Li and Juanita Hatcher	Update on prevalence, trend and socio-demographic association of five modifiable lifestyle risk factors for cancer in Alberta and Canada

	Year	Author(s)	Title
275.	2010	Catharine T. Chambers, Jane A. Buxton and Mieke Koehoorn	Consultation with Health Care Professionals and Influenza Immunization among Women in Contact with Young Children
276.	2010	Sabrina S. Plitt, Jennifer Gratrix, Sharyn Hewitt . . . Ameeta E. Singh	Seroprevalence and Correlates of HIV and HCV among Injecting Drug Users in Edmonton, Alberta
277.	2010	Jordana Linder, Lindsay McLaren, Geraldine Lo Siou . . . Paula J. Robson	The Epidemiology of Weight Perception: Perceived Versus Self-reported Actual Weight Status among Albertan Adults
278.	2010	Danielle A. Southern, Barbara Roberts, Alun Edwards . . . William A. Ghali	Validity of Administrative Data Claim-based Methods for Identifying Individuals with Diabetes at a Population Level
279.	2010	Pamela J. Cameron, David C. Este and Catherine A. Worthington	Physician Retention in Rural Alberta: Key Community Factors
280.	2010	S. Jody Heymann, Megan Gerecke and Martine Chaussard	Paid Health and Family Leave: The Canadian Experience in the Global Context
281.	2010	Nicola M. Cherry, Fortune Sithole, Jeremy R. Beach and Igor Burstyn	Second WCB Claims: Who is at Risk?
282.	2010	Glenn Keays and I.B. Pless	Impact of a Celebrity Death on Children's Injury-related Emergency Room Visits
283.	2010	Valerie Carson, Stefan Kuhle, John C. Spence and Paul J. Veugelers	Parents' Perception of Neighbourhood Environment as a Determinant of Screen Time, Physical Activity and Active Transport
284.	2010	Aline Simen-Kapeu, Stefan Kuhle and Paul J. Veugelers	Geographic Differences in Childhood Overweight, Physical Activity, Nutrition and Neighbourhood Facilities: Implications for Prevention
285.	2010	Igor Burstyn, Nitin Kapur and Nicola M. Cherry	Substance Use of Pregnant Women and Early Neonatal Morbidity: Where to Focus Intervention?
286.	2010	Shireen Surood and Daniel W.L. Lai	Impact of Culture on Use of Western Health Services by Older South Asian Canadians
287.	2010	Richard Long and Jody Boffa	High HIV-TB Co-infection Rates in Marginalized Populations: Evidence from Alberta in Support of Screening TB Patients for HIV
288.	2010	Anne Aspler, Huey Chong, Dennis Kunimoto . . . Richard Long	Sustained Intra- and Inter-jurisdictional Transmission of Tuberculosis within a Mobile, Multi-ethnic Social Network: Lessons for Tuberculosis Elimination
289.	2010	Catherine Paradis, Andrée Demers and Elyse Picard	Alcohol Consumption: A Different Kind of Canadian Mosaic
290.	2010	Loraine D. Marrett, David A. Northrup, Erin C. Pichora . . . Cheryl F. Rosen	The Second National Sun Survey: Overview and Methods

	Year	Author(s)	Title
291.	2010	Loraine D. Marrett, Erin C. Pichora and Michelle L. Costa	Work-time Sun Behaviours Among Canadian Outdoor Workers: Results From the 2006 National Sun Survey
292.	2010	Katerina Maximova and Harvey Krahn	Health Status of Refugees Settled in Alberta: Changes Since Arrival
293.	2010	Erica Frank, Carolina Segura, Hui Shen and Erica Oberg	Predictors of Canadian Physicians' Prevention Counseling Practices
294.	2010	Richard T. Oster, Sandra Shade, David Strong and Ellen L. Toth	Improvements in Indicators of Diabetes-related Health Status Among First Nations Individuals Enrolled in a Community-driven Diabetes Complications Mobile Screening Program in Alberta, Canada
295.	2010	Aline Simen-Kapeu and Paul J. Veugelers	Socio-economic Gradients in Health Behaviours and Overweight Among Children in Distinct Economic Settings
296.	2010	Marni D. Brownell, Shelley A. Derksen, Douglas P. Jutte . . . Lauren Yallop	Socio-economic Inequities in Children's Injury Rates: Has the Gradient Changed Over Time?
297.	2010	Shihe Fan, Corinne Blair, Angela Brown . . . James Talbot	A Multi-function Public Health Surveillance System and the Lessons Learned in Its Development: The Alberta Real Time Syndromic Surveillance Net
298.	2011	Jonathan M. Dawrant, Daniele Pacaud, Andrew Wade . . . Fiona J. Bamforth	Informatics of Newborn Screening for Congenital Hypothyroidism in Alberta 2005–08: Flow of Information from Birth to Treatment
299.	2011	Leah J. Martin, Stan Houston, Yutaka Yasui . . . L. Duncan Saunders	All-cause and HIV-related Mortality Rates Among HIV-infected Patients After Initiating Highly Active Antiretroviral Therapy: The Impact of Aboriginal Ethnicity and Injection Drug Use
300.	2011	Mohammad Karkhaneh, Brian H. Rowe, L. Duncan Saunders . . . Brent Hagel	Bicycle Helmet Use After the Introduction of All Ages Helmet Legislation in an Urban Community in Alberta, Canada
301.	2011	Ellen Moffatt, Lorraine G. Shack, Graham J. Petz . . . Ron Colman	The Cost of Obesity and Overweight in 2005: A Case Study of Alberta, Canada
302.	2011	Christine L. Heidebrecht, Jennifer A. Pereira, Susan Quach . . . Jeffrey C. Kwong	Approaches to Immunization Data Collection Employed Across Canada During the Pandemic (H1N1) 2009 Influenza Vaccination Campaign
303.	2012	Agnieszka A. Kosny and Marni E. Lifshen	A National Scan of Employment Standards, Occupational Health and Safety and Workers' Compensation Resources for New Immigrants to Canada
304.	2012	Nancy Hanusaik, Katerina Maximova, Natalie Kishchuk . . . Jennifer O'Loughlin	Does Level of Tobacco Control Relate to Smoking Prevalence in Canada: A National Survey of Public Health Organizations
305.	2012	Cheryl E. Peters, Anne-Marie Nicol and Paul A. Demers	Prevalence of Exposure to Solar Ultraviolet Radiation (UVR) on the Job in Canada

APPENDIX A: (continued)

	Year	Author(s)	Title
306.	2012	Kerry A. Vander Ploeg, Katerina Maximova, Stefan Kuhle . . . Paul J. Veugelers	The Importance of Parental Beliefs and Support for Physical Activity and Body Weights of Children: A Population-based Analysis
307.	2012	Brendan T. Smith, Peter M. Smith, Jacob Etches and Cameron A. Mustard	Overqualification and Risk of All-cause and Cardiovascular Mortality: Evidence from the Canadian Census Mortality Follow-up Study (1991–2001)
308.	2012	Danusia Moreau, Jennifer Gratrix, Dennis Kunimoto . . . Rabia Ahmed	A Shelter-associated Tuberculosis Outbreak: A Novel Strain Introduced Through Foreign-born Populations
309.	2012	Donald Schopflocher, Eric VanSpronsen, John C. Spence . . . Candace I.J. Nykiforuk	Creating Neighbourhood Groupings Based on Built Environment Features to Facilitate Health Promotion Activities
310.	2012	Candace I.J. Nykiforuk, Laura M. Nieuwendyk, Shaesta Mitha and Ian Hosler	Examining Aspects of the Built Environment: An Evaluation of a Community Walking Map Project
311.	2013	Richard Long and Deanne Langlois-Klassen	Increase in multidrug-resistant tuberculosis (MDR-TB) in Alberta among foreign-born persons: implications for tuberculosis management
312.	2013	Leah J. Martin, Stan Houston, Yutaka Yasui . . . L. Duncan Saunders	Poorer Physical Health-related Quality of Life Among Aboriginals and Injection Drug Users Treated with Highly Active Antiretroviral Therapy
313.	2013	Kristen M. Jacklin, Jennifer D. Walker and Marjory Shawande	The Emergence of Dementia as a Health Concern Among First Nations Populations in Alberta, Canada
314.	2013	Seanna E. McMartin, Noreen D. Willows, Ian Colman . . . Paul J. Veugelers	Diet Quality and Feelings of Worry, Sadness or Unhappiness in Canadian Children
315.	2013	Tharsiya Nagulesapillai, Sheila W. McDonald, Tanis R. Fenton . . . Suzanne C. Tough	Breastfeeding Difficulties and Exclusivity Among Late Preterm and Term Infants: Results from the All Our Babies Study
316.	2013	Charlene D. Elliott, Rebecca Carruthers Den Hoed and Martin J. Conlon	Food Branding and Young Children's Taste Preferences: A Reassessment
317.	2013	Ewa Makvandi, Louise Bouchard, Pierre-Jerôme Bergeron and Golnaz Sedigh	Methodological Issues in Analyzing Small Populations Using CCHS Cycles Based on the Official Language Minority Studies
318.	2013	Amy L. Hall, Hugh W. Davies, Paul A. Demers . . . Cheryl E. Peters	Occupational Exposures to Antineoplastic Drugs and Ionizing Radiation in Canadian Veterinary Settings: Findings from a National Surveillance Project
319.	2013	Laura E. Forbes, Shawn N. Fraser, Shauna M. Downs . . . Linda J. McCargar	Changes in Dietary and Physical Activity Risk Factors for Type 2 Diabetes in Alberta Youth Between 2005 and 2008

	Year	Author(s)	Title
320.	2014	Perry Hystad, Michael Brauer, Paul A. Demers . . . Anne-Marie Nicol	Geographic variation in radon and associated lung cancer risk in Canada
321.	2014	Chantal R.M. Nelson, Juan Andres Leon and Jane Evans	The relationship between awareness and supplementation: Which Canadian women know about folic acid and how does that translate into use?
322.	2014	Megan E. Lefebvre, Christine A. Hughes, Yutaka Yasui . . . Stan Houston	Antiretroviral treatment outcomes among foreign-born and Aboriginal peoples living with HIV/AIDS in northern Alberta
323.	2014	Stephen Wood, Debbie McNeil, Wendy Yee . . . Sarah Rose	Neighbourhood socio-economic status and spontaneous premature birth in Alberta
324.	2014	Cynthia K. Colapinto, Melissa Rossiter, Mohammad K.A. Khan . . . Paul J. Veugelers	Obesity, lifestyle and socio-economic determinants of vitamin D intake: A population-based study of Canadian children
325.	2015	Rhonda J. Rosychuk, Amanda S. Newton, Xiaoqing Niu and Liana Urichuk	Space and time clustering of adolescents' emergency department use and post-visit physician care for mood disorders in Alberta, Canada: A population-based 9-year retrospective study
326.	2015	Hmwe Hmwe Kyua, Katholiki Georgiades, Harriet L. MacMillan and Michael H. Boyle	Community- and individual-level factors associated with smoking and heavy drinking among Aboriginal people in Canada
327.	2015	Jennifer L. Black and Jean-Michel Billette	Fast food intake in Canada: Differences among Canadians with diverse demographic, socio-economic and lifestyle characteristics
328.	2015	Hans Krueger, Joshua Krueger and Jacqueline Koot	Variation across Canada in the economic burden attributable to excess weight, tobacco smoking and physical inactivity
329.	2015	Nicholas Kuzik, Dawne Clark, Nancy Ogden . . . Valerie Carson	Physical activity and sedentary behaviour of toddlers and preschoolers in childcare centres in Alberta, Canada
330.	2015	Urshila Sriram and Valerie Tarasuk	Changes in household food insecurity rates in Canadian metropolitan areas from 2007 to 2012
331.	2015	Kristin M. Eccles and Stefania Bertazzon	Applications of geographic information systems in public health: A geospatial approach to analyzing MMR immunization uptake in Alberta
332.	2015	David M. Stieb, Stan Judek, Aaron van Donkelaar . . . Marc H. Smith-Doiron	Estimated public health impacts of changes in concentrations of fine particle air pollution in Canada, 2000 to 2011
333.	2015	Cheryl Currie, T. Cameron Wild, Donald Schopflocher and Lory Laing	Racial discrimination, post-traumatic stress and prescription drug problems among Aboriginal Canadians
334.	2015	Paulina C. Podgorny and Lindsay McLaren	Public perceptions and scientific evidence for perceived harms/risks of community water fluoridation: An examination of online comments pertaining to fluoridation cessation in Calgary in 2011

	Year	Author(s)	Title
335.	2016	Yan Yuan, Qian Shi, Maoji Li . . . Faith G. Davis	Canadian brain cancer survival rates by tumour type and region: 1992–2008
336.	2016	Aynslie Hinds, Lisa M. Lix, Mark Smith . . . Claudia Sanmartin	Quality of administrative health databases in Canada: A scoping review
337.	2016	Kate L. Bassil, Junmin Yang, Laura Arbour . . . Erik D. Skarsgard	Spatial variability of gastroschisis in Canada, 2006–2011: An exploratory analysis
338.	2016	Patricia A. Collins, Megan Gaucher, Elaine M. Power and Margaret H. Little	Implicating municipalities in addressing household food insecurity in Canada: A pan-Canadian analysis of newsprint media coverage
339.	2016	C. Andrew Basham and Carolyn Snider	Homicide mortality rates in Canada, 2000–2009: Youth at increased risk
340.	2016	Erin A. Bampton, Steven T. Johnson and Jeff K. Vallance	Correlates and preferences of resistance training among older adults in Alberta, Canada
341.	2016	Sabrina S. Plitt, Mariam Osman, Vanita Sahni . . . Kimberley Simmonds	Examination of a prenatal syphilis screening program, Alberta, Canada: 2010–2011
342.	2016	Katya M. Herman and Travis J. Saunders	Sedentary behaviours among adults across Canada
343.	2016	Mariane Sentenac, Geneviève Gariepy, Britt McKinnon and Frank J. Elgar	Hunger and overweight in Canadian school-aged children: A propensity score matching analysis
344.	2016	Armita Dehmoobadsharifabadi, Sonica Singhal and Carlos Quiñonez	Investigating the "inverse care law" in dental care: A comparative analysis of Canadian jurisdictions
345.	2016	Lisa Eisenbeis, Zhiwei Gao, Courtney Heffernan . . . Geetika Verma	Contact investigation outcomes of Canadian-born adults with tuberculosis in Indigenous and non-Indigenous populations in Alberta
346.	2017	Nonsikelelo Mathe, Terry Boyle, Fatima Al Sayah . . . Jeffrey A. Johnson	Correlates of accelerometer-assessed physical activity and sedentary time among adults with type 2 diabetes
347.	2017	Bita Imam, William C. Miller, Heather C. Finlayson . . . Tal Jarus	Incidence of lower limb amputation in Canada
348.	2017	Christoffer Dharma	Understanding sexual orientation and health in Canada: who are we capturing and who are we missing using the statistics Canada sexual orientation question?
349.	2017	Michelle M. Vine, Daniel W. Harrington, Alexandra Butler . . . Scott T. Leatherdale	Compliance with school nutrition policies in Ontario and Alberta: an assessment of secondary school vending machine data from the COMPASS study
350.	2017	W.I. Andrew Bonner, Mustafa Andkhoie, Charlene Thompson . . . Michael Szafron	Patterns and factors of problematic marijuana use in the Canadian population: Evidence from three cross-sectional surveys

	Year	Author(s)	Title
351.	2017	Phongsack Manivong, Sam Harper, Erin Strumpf	The contribution of excise cigarette taxes on the decline in youth smoking in Canada during the time of the Federal Tobacco Control Strategy (2002–2012)
352.	2017	Vineet Saini, Shannon E. MacDonald, Deborah A. McNeil . . . Suzanne Tough	Timeliness and completeness of routine childhood vaccinations in children by two years of age in Alberta, Canada
353.	2017	Lynn McIntyre, Xiuyun Wu, Cynthia Kwok and J.C. Herbert Emery	A natural experimental study of the protective effect of home ownership on household food insecurity in Canada before and after a recession (2008–2009)
354.	2017	Hans Krueger, Jacqueline Koot and Ellie Andres	The economic benefits of fruit and vegetable consumption in Canada
355.	2017	Cynthia Huber, Sylvia Baran, Cindi de Graaff . . . Rafael Figueiredo	Redirecting public oral health fluoride varnish intervention to low socio-economic status children in Alberta
356.	2017	Nonsikelelo Mathe, Terry Boyle, Fatima Al Sayah . . . Jeffrey A. Johnson	Correlates of accelerometer-assessed physical activity and sedentary time among adults with type 2 diabetes
357.	2017	Bita Imam, William C. Miller, Heather C. Finlayson . . . Tal Jarus	Incidence of lower limb amputation in Canada
358.	2018	Amanda Raffoul, Scott T. Leatherdale, Sharon I. Kirkpatrick	Dieting predicts engagement in multiple risky behaviours among adolescent Canadian girls: a longitudinal analysis
359.	2018	Sarah Brennenstuhl	Health of mothers of young children in Canada: identifying dimensions of inequality based on socio-economic position, partnership status, race, and region
360.	2018	Peter Warrington, Gregory Tyrrell, Kimberley Choy . . . Ryan Cooper	Prevalence of latent tuberculosis infection in Syrian refugees to Canada
361.	2018	Jessica Moe, Carlos A. Camargo, Susan Jelinski . . . Brian H. Rowe	Epidemiologic trends in substance and opioid misuse-related emergency department visits in Alberta: a cross-sectional time-series analysis
362.	2018	Erica Phipps & Jeffrey R. Masuda	Towards equity-focused intersectoral practice (EquIP) in children's environmental health and housing: the transformational story of RentSafe
363.	2018	Laura A. Rivera, Matthew T. Henschke, Edwin Khoo . . . Michael H. Forseth	A modeling study exploring the impact of homelessness on rostered primary care utilization in Calgary, Canada
364.	2018	Maegan V. Mazereeuw, Diana R. Withrow, E. Diane Nishri . . . Loraine D. Marrett	Cancer incidence among First Nations adults in Canada: follow-up of the 1991 Census Mortality Cohort (1992–2009)
365.	2018	Patrick Fafard, Brittany McNena, Agatha Suszek, Steven J. Hoffman	Contested roles of Canada's Chief Medical Officers of Health
366.	2018	Sonja Senthanar	Work-related musculoskeletal risk among refugees: recommendations for improvement to promote health and well-being

	Year	Author(s)	Title
367.	2019	Adam G. Cole, Sarah Aleyan, Wei Qian, Scott T. Leatherdale	Assessing the strength of secondary school tobacco policies of schools in the COMPASS study and the association to student smoking behaviours
368.	2019	Jonathan Simkin, Gina Ogilvie, Brendan Hanley & Catherine Elliott	Differences in colorectal cancer screening rates across income strata by levels of urbanization: results from the Canadian Community Health Survey (2013/2014)
369.	2019	David M. Stieb, Jiayun Yao, Sarah B. Henderson . . . Jeffrey R. Brook	Variability in ambient ozone and fine particle concentrations and population susceptibility among Canadian health regions
370.	2019	Sholeh Rahman, Katerina Maximova, Valerie Carson . . . Paul J. Veugelers	Stay in or play out? The influence of weather conditions on physical activity of grade 5 children in Canada
371.	2019	Stacey Bourque, Em M. Pijl, Erin Mason . . . Takara Motz	Supervised inhalation is an important part of supervised consumption services
372.	2019	Karmpaul Singh, Shelly Russell-Mayhew, Kristin von Ranson & Lindsay McLaren	Is there more to the equation? Weight bias and the costs of obesity
373.	2019	Jennifer S. Hermann, Kimberley A. Simmonds, Christopher A. Bell . . . Shannon E. MacDonald	Vaccine coverage of children in care of the child welfare system
374.	2019	Conar R. O'Neil, Emily Buss, Sabrina Plitt . . . Stephen Shafran	Achievement of hepatitis C cascade of care milestones: a population-level analysis in Alberta, Canada
375.	2019	Christine McKernan, Genevieve Montemurro, Harneet Chahal . . . Kate E. Storey	Translation of school-learned health behaviours into the home student insights through photovoice
376.	2019	Erica Y. Lau, Negin A. Riazi, Wei Qian . . . Guy Faulkner	Protective or risky? The longitudinal association of team sports participation and health-related behaviours in Canadian adolescent girls
377.	2019	Katrina Milaney, Stacy Lee Lockerbie, Xiao Yang Fang, Kaylee Ramage	The role of structural violence in family homelessness
378.	2019	Diana C Sanchez-Ramirez, Yan Chen, Jason R. Randall . . . Don Voaklander	Injury-related health services use and mortality among Métis people in Alberta
379.	2019	Phillip Quon, Kelcie Lahey, Mackenzie Grisdale . . . April Elliott	Prevalence of distracted walking with mobile technology: an observational study of Calgary and Edmonton high school students

Appendix B

Details and Sources for "Leading," "Selected," and "Certain" Causes of Death presented in Table 3.1 and Figure 3.1

Year and classification system	Diseases of the Heart	Malignant Tumors	Cerebrovascular Disease
1915 Classification system is not named but cause numbers match ICD-2 codes[1]	[77] "Pericarditis" [78] "Acute Endocarditis" [79] "Other Diseases of the Heart"	[39] "Cancer and Other Malignant Tumors of the Buccal Cavity" [40] "Cancer and Other Malignant Tumors of the Stomach, Liver" [41] "Cancer and Other Malignant Tumors of the Peritoneum, Intestines, Rectum" [42] "Cancer and Other Malignant Tumors of the Female Genital Organs" [43] "Cancer and Other Malignant Tumors of the Breast" [44] "Cancer of the Skin" [45] "Cancer and other malignant tumors of other organs or of organs not specified"	[64] "Cerebral Hemorrhage"
1920 Classification system is not named but cause numbers match ICD-2 codes[2]	[77] "Pericarditis" [78] "Acute Endocarditis" [79] "Other Diseases of the Heart" (Collectively reported as "Organic Disease of the Heart")	[39] "Cancer and Other Malignant Tumors of the Buccal Cavity" [40] "Cancer and Other Malignant Tumors of the Stomach, Liver" [41] ""Cancer and Other Malignant Tumors of the Peritoneum, Intestines, Rectum" [42] "Cancer and Other Malignant Tumors of the Female Genital Organs" [43] "Cancer and Other Malignant Tumors of the Breast" [44] "Cancer of the Skin" [45] "Cancer and Other Malignant Tumors of Other Organs or of Organs Not Specified" (Collectively reported as "Cancer and Malignant Tumors")	[64] "Cerebral Hemorrhage"

Violent Deaths (Excluding Suicide)	Pneumonia (All Forms)	Pulmonary Tuberculosis	Influenza
[164] "Poisoning by Food" [165] "Other Acute Poisonings" [166] "Conflagration" [167] "Burns" [168] "Absorption of Deleterious Gases" [169] "Accidental Drowning" [170] "Traumatism by Firearms" [171] "Traumatism by Cutting or Piercing Instruments" [172] "Traumatism by Falls" [173] "Traumatism in Mines and Quarries" [174] "Traumatism by Machines" [175] "Traumatism by Other Crushing (Vehicles, Railways, Landslides, etc.)" [176] "Injuries by Animals" [178] "Excessive Cold" [179] "Effects of Heat" [180] "Lightning" [181] "Electricity (Lightning excepted)" [184] "Homicide (Murder or Manslaughter)" [185] "Fractures (Causes Not Specified)" [186] "Other External Causes, Legal Hanging"	[91] "Broncho-Pneumonia" [92] "Pneumonia"	[28] "Tuberculosis of the Lungs"	[10] "Influenza"
[164] "Poisoning by Food" [165] "Other Acute Poisonings" [166] "Conflagration" [167] "Burns" [168] "Absorption of Deleterious Gases" [169] "Accidental Drowning" [170] "Accidents by Firearms" [171] "Accidents by Cutting or Piercing Instruments" [172] "Accidental Falls" [173] "Accidents in Mines and Quarries" [174] "Accidents by Machines" [175] "Accidents by Other Crushing (Vehicles, Railways, Landslides, etc.)" [176] "Injuries by Animals" [178] "Excessive Cold" [179] "Effects of Heat" [180] "Lightning" [181] "Electricity (Lightning excepted)" [184] "Homicide (Murder or Manslaughter)" [185] "Fractures (causes not specified)" [186] "Other External Causes, Legal Hanging" [186a] "Results of Wounds, etc. in War"	[91] "Broncho-Pneumonia" [92] "Pneumonia" (Collectively reported as "Pneumonia & Broncho-Pneumonia")	[28] "Tuberculosis of the Lungs" (Reported as "Tuberculosis of the Lungs")	[10] "Influenza" [10a] "Influenza (Epidemic)" (Collectively reported as "Influenza")

Year and classification system	Diseases of the Heart	Malignant Tumors	Cerebrovascular Disease
1925 Classification system is not named but cause numbers match ICD-3 codes[3]	[87] "Pericarditis" [88] (a) "Acute Endocarditis" (b) "Acute Myocarditis" [89] "Angina Pectoris" [90] "Other Diseases of the Heart" (Collectively reported as "Heart Disease")	[43] "Cancer and Other Malignant Tumors of the Buccal Cavity" [44] "Cancer and Other Malignant Tumors of the Stomach and Liver" [45] "Cancer and Other Malignant Tumors of the Peritoneum, Intestines and Rectum" [46] "Cancer and Other Malignant Tumors of the Female Genital Organs" [47] "Cancer and Other Malignant Tumors of the Breast" [48] "Cancer and Other Malignant Tumors of the Skin" [49] "Cancer and Other Malignant Tumors of Other or Unspecified Organs" (Collectively reported as "Cancer")	[74] (a) "Apoplexy" (b) Cerebral Haemorrhage" (c) "Cerebral Thrombosis and Embolism" (Collectively reported as "Apoplexy")

Violent Deaths (Excluding Suicide)	Pneumonia (All Forms)	Pulmonary Tuberculosis	Influenza
[175] "Poisoning by Food" [177] "Other Acute Accidental Poisonings" [178] "Conflagration" [179] "Accidental Burns and Scalds" [180] "Accidental Mechanical Suffocation" [181] "Accidental absorption of irrespirable or poisonous Gas" [182] "Accidental Drowning" [183] "Accidental Traumatism by firearms" [184] "Accidental Traumatism by cutting or piercing instruments" [185] "Accidental Traumatism by fall" [186] (a) "Accidental Traumatism by Mines" [187] "Accidental Traumatism by Machines" [188] (a) "Railroad Accidents" (b) "Street-car Accidents" (c) "Automobile Accidents" (e) "Injuries by other vehicles" (f) "Other Crushing" [189] "Injuries by Animals (Not poisoning)" [190] "Wounds of War" [192] "Starvation" [193] "Excessive Cold" [194] "Excessive Heat" [195] "Lighting" [196] "Other Accidental Electric Shocks" [197] "Homicide by firearms" [198] "Homicide by cutting or piercing instruments" [199] "Homicide by other means" [200] "Infanticide" [202] "Other External Violence (Cause Specified)" [203] "External Violence (Cause not Specified)" (Collectively reported as "Violent Deaths")	[100] (a) "Bronchopneumonia" (b) "Capillary Bronchitis" [101] (a) "Lobar Pneumonia" (b) "Pneumonia (not otherwise defined)" (Collectively reported as "Pneumonia (All Forms)")	[31] "Tuberculosis of the Respiratory System" (Reported as "Pulmonary Tuberculosis")	[11] "Influenza" (Reported as "Influenza")

Year and classification system	Diseases of the Heart	Malignant Tumors	Cerebrovascular Disease
1930 Classification system is not named but cause numbers match ICD-3 codes[4]	[87] "Pericarditis" [88] (a) "Acute endocarditis" (b) "Acute myocarditis" [89] "Angina pectoris" [90] (a) "Valvular disease" (b) "Fatty degeneration of the heart" (c) "Aortic insufficiency" (d) "Chronic endocarditis" (e) "Chronic myocarditis" (f) "Other diseases of the heart" (Collectively Reported as "Diseases of the Heart")	[43] "Cancer of the buccal cavity" [44] "Cancer of the stomach and liver" [45] "Cancer of the peritoneum, intestines and rectum" [46] "Cancer of the female genital organs" [47] "Cancer of the breast" [48] "Cancer of the skin" [49] (a) "Cancer of eye and ear" (b) "Cancer of circulatory system" (c) "Cancer of respiratory system" (d) "Cancer of digestive system" (e) "Cancer of genito-urinary system" (f) "Cancer of bones and joints" (g) other specified organs (h) "Generalized cancer (i) "Unspecified" (Collectively reported as "Malignant Tumors")	[74] (a) "Apoplexy" (b) Cerebral haemorrhage" (c) "Cerebral thrombosis and embolism" (Collectively reported as "Apoplexy")

Violent Deaths (Excluding Suicide)	Pneumonia (All Forms)	Pulmonary Tuberculosis	Influenza
[175] "Poisoning by food" [176] "Poisoning by venomous animals" [177] "Other acute accidental poisonings" [178] "Conflagration" [179] "Accidental burns and scalds" [180] (a) "Accidental suffocation by overlaying" (b) "Accidental asphyxia" [181] "Accidental absorption of irrespirable or poisonous gas" [182] "Accidental drowning" [183] "Accidental traumatism by firearms" [184] "Accidental traumatism by cutting or piercing instruments" [185] "Accidental traumatism by fall" [186] (a) "Accidental traumatism by mines" [187] "Accidental traumatism by machines" [188] (a) "Railroad accidents" (b) "Street-car accidents" (c) "Automobile accidents" (e) "Injuries by other vehicles" (f) "Other crushing" [189] "Injuries by animals (not poisoning)" [192] "Starvation" [193] "Excessive cold" [194] "Excessive heat" [195] "Lighting" [196] "Other accidental electric shocks" [197] "Homicide by firearms" [198] "Homicide by cutting or piercing instruments" [199] "Homicide by other means" [201] "Fracture (cause not specified)" [202] "Other external violence (cause Specified)" (Collectively reported as "Violent Deaths (excluding suicide)")	[100] (a) "Bronchopneumonia" (b) "Capillary bronchitis" [101] (a) "Lobar pneumonia" (b) "Pneumonia (not otherwise defined)" (Collectively reported as "Pneumonia (All Forms)")	[31] "Tuberculosis of the respiratory system" (Reported as "Pulmonary Tuberculosis")	[11] "Influenza" (Reported as "Influenza")

Year and classification system	Diseases of the Heart	Malignant Tumors	Cerebrovascular Disease
1935 Classification system is not named but cause numbers match ICD-4 codes[5]	[90] "Pericarditis" [91] "Acute Endocarditis" [92] "Chronic endocarditis, valvular diseases" [93] "Diseases of the myocardium" [94] "Diseases of the coronary arteries and angina pectoris" [95] "Other diseases of the heart" (Collectively reported as "Diseases of the Heart")	[45] "Cancer of the buccal cavity and pharynx" [46] (a) "Of the oesophagus" (b) "Of the stomach and duodenum" (c) "Of the rectum" (d) "Of the liver and biliary ducts" (e) "Of the pancreas" (f) "Of the peritoneum" (g) "Of other organs" [47] (a) "Of the larynx" (b) "Of the lung" (c) "Of the mediastinum" (d) "Of other organs of the respiratory systems" [48] (a) "Of the uterus" (b) "Of the cervix uteri" [49] "Cancer of other female genital organs" [50] "Cancer of the breast" [51] (a) "Of the bladder (male)" (b) "Of the kidney (male)" (c) "Of the prostate gland" (d) "Of the testicles and annexa" (e) "Of the male genito-urinary organs" [52] "Cancer of the skin" [53] (a) "Of the eye and orbit" (b) "Of the circulatory system" (c) "Of the glandular system" (d) "Of the female urinary organs" (e) "Of the bones and joints" (f) "of the brain" (g) "Of the spine and spinal cord" (h) "Of the neck" (i) "Of the abdomen" (j) "Of other specified organs (k) "Multiple cancer" (m) "Of unspecified or unknown location" (Collectively reported as "Cancer")	[82] "Cerebral haemorrhage, cerebral embolism and thrombosis" (Collectively reported as "Cerebral Haemorrhage")

Violent Deaths (Excluding Suicide)	Pneumonia (All Forms)	Pulmonary Tuberculosis	Influenza
[173] "Homicide by firearms" [174] "Homicide by cutting or piercing instruments" [175] "Homicide by other means" [176] "Attack by venomous animals" [177] "Food poisoning" [178] "Accidental absorption of toxic gas" [179] "Other acute accidental poisonings (except by gas)" [180] "Conflagration" [181] "Accidental burns (conflagration excepted)" [182] "Accidental mechanical suffocation" [183] "Accidental drowning" [184] "Accidental injuries by firearms" [185] "Accidental injuries by cutting or piercing instruments" [186] "Accidental injury by fall, crushing or landslide" [188] "Injuries by animals" [189] "Hunger or thirst" [190] "Excessive cold" [191] "Excessive heat" [192] "Lighting" [193] "Accidents due to electric currents" [194] "Other accidents" [195] "Violent deaths of which the nature is (accident, suicide, homicide) is unknown" [198] "Capital punishment" (Collectively reported as "Violent Deaths (Suicide Excepted)")	[107] (a) "Broncho-pneumonia" (b) "Capillary bronchitis" [108] "Lobar pneumonia" [109] "Pneumonia, unspecified" (Collectively reported as "Pneumonia (All Forms)")	[23] "Tuberculosis of the respiratory System" (Reported as "Pulmonary Tuberculosis")	[11] "Influenza" (Reported as "Influenza")

Year and classification system	Diseases of the Heart	Malignant Tumors	Cerebrovascular Disease
1940 Classification system is not named but cause numbers match ICD-4 codes[6]	[90] "Pericarditis" [91] "Acute Endocarditis" [92] "Chronic endo-carditis, valvular diseases" [93] "Diseases of the myocardium" [94] "Diseases of the coronary arteries and angina pec-toris" [95] "Other diseases of the heart" (Collectively reported as "Diseases of the Heart")	[45] "Cancer of the buccal cavity and pharynx" [46] (a) "Of the oesophagus" (b) "Of the stomach and duodenum" (c) "Of the rectum" (d) "Of the liver and biliary ducts" (e) "Of the pancreas" (f) "Of the peritoneum" (g) "Of other organs" [47] (a) "Of the larynx" (b) "Of the lung" (c) "Of the mediastinum" (d) "Of other organs of the respiratory systems" [48] (a) "Of the uterus" (b) "Of the cervix uteri" [49] "Cancer of other female genital organs" [50] "Cancer of the breast" [51] (a) "Of the bladder (male)" (b) "Of the kidney (male)" (c) "Of the prostate gland" (d) "Of the testicles and annexa" (e) "Of the male genito-urinary organs" [52] "Cancer of the skin" [53] (a) "Of the eye and orbit" (b) "Of the circula-tory system" (c) "Of the glandular system" (d) "Of the female urinary organs" (e) "Of the bones and joints" (f) "of the brain" (g) "Of the spine and spinal cord" (h) "Of the neck" (i) "Of the abdomen" (j) "Of other specified organs (k) "Multiple cancer" (m) "Of unspecified or unknown location" (Collectively reported as "Cancer")	[82] "Cerebral haem-orrhage, cerebral embolism and thrombosis" (Collectively re-ported as "Cerebral Haemorrhage")

Violent Deaths (Excluding Suicide)	Pneumonia (All Forms)	Pulmonary Tuberculosis	Influenza
[173] "Homicide by firearms" [174] "Homicide by cutting or piercing instruments" [175] "Homicide by other means" [176] "Attack by venomous animals" [177] "Food poisoning" [178] "Accidental absorption of toxic gas" [179] "Other acute accidental poisonings (except by gas)" [180] "Conflagration" [181] "Accidental burns (conflagration excepted)" [182] "Accidental mechanical suffocation" [183] "Accidental drowning" [184] "Accidental injuries by firearms" [185] "Accidental injuries by cutting or piercing instruments" [186] "Accidental injury by fall, crushing or landslide" [188] "Injuries by animals" [189] "Hunger or thirst" [190] "Excessive cold" [191] "Excessive heat" [192] "Lightning" [193] "Accidents due to electric currents" [194] "Other accidents" [195] "Violent deaths of which the nature is (accident, suicide, homicide) is unknown" [198] "Capital punishment" (Collectively reported as "Violent Deaths (Suicide Excepted)")	[107] (a) "Bronchopneumonia" (b) "Capillary bronchitis" [108] "Lobar pneumonia" [109] "Pneumonia, unspecified" (Collectively reported as "Pneumonia (All Forms)")	[23] "Tuberculosis of the respiratory System" (Reported as "Pulmonary Tuberculosis")	[11] "Influenza" (Reported as "Influenza")

Year and classification system	Diseases of the Heart	Malignant Tumors	Cerebrovascular Disease
1945 Classification system is labelled "Int. List No.," which corresponds to ICD-5 codes[7]	[90] "Pericarditis (acute rheumatic excluded)" [91] "Acute Endocarditis (non-rheumatic)" [92] "Chronic affections of the valves and endocardium" [93] "Diseases of the myocardium" [94] "Diseases of the coronary arteries and angina pectoris" [95] "Other diseases of the heart" (Collectively reported as "Diseases of the Heart")	[45] "Cancer of the buccal cavity and pharynx" [46] "Cancer of the digestive organs and peritoneum" [47] "Cancer of the respiratory system" [48] "Cancer of the uterus" [49] "Cancer of other female genital organs" [50] "Cancer of the breast" [51] "Cancer of the male genital organs" [52] "Cancer of the urinary organs" [53] "Cancer of the skin" [54] "Cancer of the brain" [55] "Cancer of other and unspecified organs" (Collectively reported as "Cancer")	[83] "Intracranial lesions of vascular origin" (Reported as "Cerebral Haemorrhage")

Violent Deaths (Excluding Suicide)	Pneumonia (All Forms)	Pulmonary Tuberculosis	Influenza
[166] "Homicide by firearms"	[107] "Broncho-pneumonia"	[13] "Tuberculosis of the Respiratory System"	[33] "Influenza"
[167] "Homicide by cutting or piercing instruments"	[108] "Lobar pneumonia"		Reported as "Influenza"
[168] "Homicide by other unspecified means"	[109] "Pneumonia (unspecified)"	Reported as "Pulmonary Tuberculosis"	
[169] "Railway accidents (excluding motor vehicles)"	(Collectively reported as "Pneumonia (All Forms)")		
[170] "Motor vehicle accidents"			
[171] "Street-car and other road transport accidents"			
[172] "Water transport accidents"			
[173] "Air transport accidents"			
[174] "Accidents in Mines and Quarries"			
[175] "Agricultural and forestry accidents"			
[176] "Other accidents involving machinery"			
[177] "Food poisoning"			
[178] "Accidental absorption of poisonous gas"			
[179] "Acute accidental poisonings by solids or liquids"			
[180] "Conflagration"			
[181] "Accidental burns (conflagration excepted)"			
[182] "Accidental mechanical suffocation"			
[183] "Accidental drowning"			
[184] "Accidental injuries by firearms"			
[185] "Accidental injuries by cutting or piercing instruments"			
[186] "Accidental injury by fall or crushing"			
[188] "Injuries by animals"			
[189] "Hunger or thirst"			
[190] "Excessive cold"			
[191] "Excessive heat"			
[192] "Lightning"			
[193] "Accidents due to electric currents"			
[194] "Attack by venomous animals (non-occupational)"			
[195] "Other accidents"			
[196] "Deaths of persons in military service during operations of war"			
[197] "Death of civilians due to operations of war"			
[198] "Legal executions"			
(Collectively reported as "Violent Deaths (Suicide excepted)")			

Year and classification system	Diseases of the Heart	Malignant Tumors	Cerebrovascular Disease
1950 Classification system is the "Intermediate List" of ICD-6 (also known as List A)[8]	[A79] "Rheumatic fever" [A80] "Chronic rheumatic heart disease" [A81] "Arteriosclerotic and degenerative heart disease" [A82] "Other diseases of heart" [A83] "Hypertension with heart disease" (Collectively reported as "Diseases of the Heart")	[A44] "Malignant neoplasm of buccal cavity and pharynx" [A45] "Malignant neoplasm of oesophagus" [A46] "Malignant neoplasm of stomach" [A47] "Malignant neoplasm of intestine, except rectum" [A48] "Malignant neoplasm of rectum" [A49] "Malignant neoplasm of larynx" [A50] "Malignant neoplasm of trachea, and of bronchus and lung not specified as secondary" [A51] "Malignant neoplasm of breast" [A52] "Malignant neoplasm of cervix uteri" [A53] "Malignant neoplasm of other and unspecified parts of the uterus" [A54] "Malignant neoplasm of prostate" [A55] "Malignant neoplasm of skin" [A56] "Malignant neoplasm of bone and connective tissue" [A57] "Malignant neoplasm of all other and unspecified sites" [A58] "Leukaemia and aleukaemia" [A59] "Lymphosarcoma and other neoplasms of lymphatic and haematopoietic system" (Collectively reported as "Cancer")	[A70] "Vascular lesions affecting central nervous system" (Reported as "Cerebral Haemorrhage")
1955 Classification system is the "Intermediate List" of ICD-6 (also known as List A)[9]	[A79] "Rheumatic fever" [A80] "Chronic rheumatic heart disease" [A81] "Arteriosclerotic and degenerative heart disease" [A82] "Other diseases of heart" [A83] "Hypertension with heart disease" (Collectively reported as "Diseases of the Heart")	[A44] "Malignant neoplasm of buccal cavity and pharynx" [A45] "Malignant neoplasm of oesophagus" [A46] "Malignant neoplasm of stomach" [A47] "Malignant neoplasm of intestine, except rectum" [A48] "Malignant neoplasm of rectum" [A49] "Malignant neoplasm of larynx" [A50] "Malignant neoplasm of trachea, and of bronchus and lung not specified as secondary" [A51] "Malignant neoplasm of breast" [A52] "Malignant neoplasm of cervix uteri" [A53] "Malignant neoplasm of other and unspecified parts of the uterus" [A54] "Malignant neoplasm of prostate" [A55] "Malignant neoplasm of skin" [A56] "Malignant neoplasm of bone and connective tissue" [A57] "Malignant neoplasm of all other and unspecified sites" [A58] "Leukaemia and aleukaemia" [A59] "Lymphosarcoma and other neoplasms of lymphatic and haematopoietic system" (Collectively reported as "Cancer")[10]	[A70] "Vascular lesions affecting central nervous system" (Reported as "Cerebral Haemorrhage")

Violent Deaths (Excluding Suicide)	Pneumonia (All Forms)	Pulmonary Tuberculosis	Influenza
[AE138] "Motor vehicle accidents" [AE139] "Other transport accidents" [AE140] "Accidental poisoning" [AE141] "Accidental falls" [AE142] "Accident cause by machinery" [AE143] "Accidents caused by fire and explosion of combustible material" [AE144] "Accident caused by hot substance, corrosive liquid, steam, and radiation" [AE145] "Accident caused by firearm" [AE146] "Accidental drowning and submersion" [AE147] "All other accidental causes" [AE149] "Homicide and injury purposely inflicted by other persons (not in war)" (Collectively reported as "Violent Deaths (Suicide excepted)")	[A89] "Lobar pneumonia" [A90] "Broncho-pneumonia" [A91] "Primary atypical, other and unspecified pneumonia" (Collectively reported as "Pneumonia (All Forms)")	[A1] "Tuberculosis of the Respiratory System" Reported as "Pulmonary Tuberculosis"	[A88] "Influenza" Reported as "Influenza"
[AE138] "Motor vehicle accidents" [AE139] "Other transport accidents" [AE140] "Accidental poisoning" [AE141] "Accidental falls" [AE142] "Accident cause by machinery" [AE143] "Accidents caused by fire and explosion of combustible material" [AE144] "Accident caused by hot substance, corrosive liquid, steam, and radiation" [AE145] "Accident caused by firearm" [AE146] "Accidental drowning and submersion" [AE147] "All other accidental causes" [AE149] "Homicide and injury purposely inflicted by other persons (not in war)" (Collectively reported as "Violent Deaths (Suicide excepted)")	[A89] "Lobar pneumonia" [A90] "Broncho-pneumonia" [A91] "Primary atypical, other and unspecified pneumonia" (Collectively reported as "Pneumonia (All Forms)")	[A1] "Tuber-culosis of the respiratory System" (Reported as "Pulmonary Tuberculosis")	[A88] "Influenza" Reported as "Influenza"

Year and classification system	Diseases of the Heart	Malignant Tumors	Cerebrovascular Disease
1960 Classification system is the "Intermediate List" of ICD-7 (also known as List A)[11]	[A79] "Rheumatic fever" [A80] "Chronic rheumatic heart disease" [A81] "Arteriosclerotic and degenerative heart disease" [A82] "Other diseases of heart" [A83] "Hypertension with heart disease" (Collectively reported as "Diseases of the Heart")	[A44] "Malignant neoplasm of buccal cavity and pharynx" [A45] "Malignant neoplasm of oesophagus" [A46] "Malignant neoplasm of stomach" [A47] "Malignant neoplasm of intestine, except rectum" [A48] "Malignant neoplasm of rectum" [A49] "Malignant neoplasm of larynx" [A50] "Malignant neoplasm of trachea, and of bronchus and lung not specified as secondary" [A51] "Malignant neoplasm of breast" [A52] "Malignant neoplasm of cervix uteri" [A53] "Malignant neoplasm of other and unspecified parts of the uterus" [A54] "Malignant neoplasm of prostate" [A55] "Malignant neoplasm of skin" [A56] "Malignant neoplasm of bone and connective tissue" [A57] "Malignant neoplasm of all other and unspecified sites" [A58] "Leukaemia and aleukaemia" [A59] "Lymphosarcoma and other neoplasms of lymphatic and haematopoietic system" (Collectively reported as "Cancer")	[A70] "Vascular lesions affecting central nervous system" Reported as "Cerebral Haemorrhage"
1965 Classification system is the "Intermediate List" of ICD-7 (also known as List A)[12]	[A79] "Rheumatic fever" [A80] "Chronic rheumatic heart disease" [A81] "Arteriosclerotic and degenerative heart disease" [A82] "Other diseases of heart" [A83] "Hypertension with heart disease" (Collectively reported as "Diseases of the Heart")	[A44] "Malignant neoplasm of buccal cavity and pharynx" [A45] "Malignant neoplasm of oesophagus" [A46] "Malignant neoplasm of stomach" [A47] "Malignant neoplasm of intestine, except rectum" [A48] "Malignant neoplasm of rectum" [A49] "Malignant neoplasm of larynx" [A50] "Malignant neoplasm of trachea, and of bronchus and lung not specified as secondary" [A51] "Malignant neoplasm of breast" [A52] "Malignant neoplasm of cervix uteri" [A53] "Malignant neoplasm of other and unspecified parts of the uterus" [A54] "Malignant neoplasm of prostate" [A55] "Malignant neoplasm of skin" [A56] "Malignant neoplasm of bone and connective tissue" [A57] "Malignant neoplasm of all other and unspecified sites" [A58] "Leukaemia and aleukaemia" [A59] "Lymphosarcoma and other neoplasms of lymphatic and haematopoietic system" (Collectively reported as "Cancer")[13]	[A70] "Vascular lesions affecting central nervous system" Reported as "Cerebral Haemorrhage"

Violent Deaths (Excluding Suicide)	Pneumonia (All Forms)	Pulmonary Tuberculosis	Influenza
[AE138] "Motor vehicle accidents" [AE139] "Other transport accidents" [AE140] "Accidental poisoning" [AE141] "Accidental falls" [AE142] "Accident cause by machinery" [AE143] "Accidents caused by fire and explosion of combustible material" [AE144] "Accident caused by hot substance, corrosive liquid, steam, and radiation" [AE145] "Accident caused by firearm" [AE146] "Accidental drowning and submersion" [AE147] "All other accidental causes" [AE149] "Homicide and injury purposely inflicted by other persons (not in war)" (Collectively reported as "Violent Deaths (Suicide excepted)")	[A89] "Lobar pneumonia" [A90] "Broncho-pneumonia" [A91] "Primary atypical, other and unspecified pneumonia" (Collectively reported as "Pneumonia (All Forms)")	[A1] "Tuber-culosis of the respiratory System" Reported as "Pulmonary Tuberculosis"	[A88] "Influenza" Reported as "Influenza"
[AE138] "Motor vehicle accidents" [AE139] "Other transport accidents" [AE140] "Accidental poisoning" [AE141] "Accidental falls" [AE142] "Accident cause by machinery" [AE143] "Accidents caused by fire and explosion of combustible material" [AE144] "Accident caused by hot substance, corrosive liquid, steam, and radiation" [AE145] "Accident caused by firearm" [AE146] "Accidental drowning" [AE147] "All other accidental causes" [AE149] "Homicide and injury purposely inflicted by other persons (not in war)" (Collectively reported as "Violent Deaths (Suicide excepted)")	[A89] "Lobar pneumonia" [A90] "Broncho-pneumonia" [A91] "Primary atypical, other and unspecified pneumonia" (Collectively reported as "Pneumonia (All Forms)")	[A1] "Tuber-culosis of the respiratory System" Reported as "Pulmonary Tuberculosis"	[A88] "Influenza" Reported as "Influenza"

Year and classification system	Diseases of the Heart	Malignant Tumors	Cerebrovascular Disease
1970 Classification system is the "Intermediate List A" of ICD-8 (also known as List A)[14]	[A80] "Active rheumatic fever" [A81] "Chronic rheumatic heart disease" [A82] "Hypertensive disease" [A83] "Ischaemic heart disease" [A84] "Other forms of heart diseases" (Collectively reported as "Heart Disease")	Malignant Neoplasms [A45] "Buccal cavity and pharynx" [A46] "Oesophagus" [A47] "Stomach" [A48] "Intestine, except rectum" [A49] "Rectum and rectosigmoid junction" [A50] "Larynx" [A51] "Trachea, and of bronchus and lung" [A52] "Bone" [A53] "Skin" [A54] "Breast" [A55] "Cervix uteri" [A56] "Uterus, other" [A57] "Prostate" [A58] "Other and unspecified sites" [A59] "Leukaemia" [A60] "Lymphatic and haemotopoietic tissue" (Collectively reported as "Cancer")	[A85] Cerebrovascular Disease
1975 Classification system is "Eighth revisions [sic] of the ICD and A-code, Causes for Tabulation of Morbidity and Mortality" (corresponds to ICD-8 List A)[15]	[A80] "Active rheumatic fever" [A81] "Chronic rheumatic heart disease" [A82] "Hypertensive disease" [A83] "Ischaemic heart disease" [A84] "Other forms of heart diseases"	[A45] "Malignant neoplasm of buccal cavity and pharynx" [A46] "Malignant neoplasm of oesophagus" [A47] "Malignant neoplasm of stomach" [A48] "Malignant neoplasm of intestine, except rectum" [A49] "Malignant neoplasm of rectum and rectosigmoid junction" [A50] "Malignant neoplasm of larynx" [A51] "Malignant neoplasm of trachea, and of bronchus and lung" [A52] "Malignant neoplasm of bone" [A53] "Malignant neoplasm of skin" [A54] "Malignant neoplasm of breast" [A55] "Malignant neoplasm of cervix uteri" [A56] "Other malignant neoplasm of uterus" [A57] "Malignant neoplasm of prostate" [A58] "Malignant neoplasm of other and unspecified sites" [A59] "Leukaemia" [A60] "Other neoplasms of lymphatic and haemotopoietic tissue"	[A85] "Cerebrovascular Disease"

Violent Deaths (Excluding Suicide)	Pneumonia (All Forms)	Pulmonary Tuberculosis	Influenza
[AE138] "Motor vehicle accidents" [AE139] "Other transport accidents" [AE140] "Accidental poisoning" [AE141] "Accidental falls" [AE142] "Accidents caused by fire" [AE143] "Accidental drowning" [AE144] "Accident caused by firearm missiles" [AE145] "Accidents mainly of industrial type" [AE146] "All other accidents" [AE148] "Homicide; legal intervention" [AE149] "Injury undetermined if accidentally or purposely inflicted" [AE150] "War injuries"	Pneumonia [A91] "Viral" [A92] "Other"	Tuberculosis [A6] "Respiratory System"	[A90] "Influenza"
[AE138] "Motor vehicle accidents" [AE139] "Other transport accidents" [AE140] "Accidental poisoning" [AE141] "Accidental falls" [AE142] "Accidents caused by fire" [AE143] "Accidental drowning and submersion" [AE144] "Accident caused by firearm missiles" [AE145] "Accidents mainly of industrial type" [AE146] "All other accidents" [AE148] "Homicide and injury purposely inflicted by other persons; legal intervention" [AE149] "Injury undetermined whether accidentally or purposely inflicted" [AE150] "Injuries resulting from operations of war"	[A91] "Viral pneumonia" [A92] "Other pneumonia"	[A6] "Tuberc-ulosis of respiratory System"	[A90] "Influenza"

Year and classification system	Diseases of the Heart	Malignant Tumors	Cerebrovascular Disease
1980 Classification system is "List of 72 Selected Causes of Death" which correspond to ICD-9 numbers. List number is in (round brackets); corresponding ICD-9 code is in [square brackets][16]	(28) [390-398] "Rheumatic fever and rheumatic heart disease" (29) [402] "Hypertensive heart disease" (30) [404-414] "Ischaemic heart disease" (31) [410] "Acute myocardial infarction" (32) [411] "Other acute and subacute forms of ischaemic heart disease" (33) [413] "Angina pectoris" (34) [412,414] "Other forms of chronic ischaemic heart disease" (35) [424] "Other diseases of endocardium" (36) [415-423,425-429] "All other forms of heart disease" (Collectively reported as "Diseases of the Heart"[17])	(14) [140-149] "Malignant neoplasm of lip, oral cavity and pharynx" (15) [150-159] "Malignant neoplasm of digestive organs and peritoneum" (16) [160-165] "Malignant neoplasm of respiratory and intrathoracic organs" (17) [174-175] "Malignant neoplasm of female breast" (18) [179-187] "Malignant neoplasm of genital organs" (19) [188-189] "Malignant neoplasm of urinary organs" (20) [170-173,190-199] "Malignant neoplasm of other and unspecified sites" (21) [204-208] "Leukaemia" (22) [200-203] "Other malignant neoplasm of lymphatic and haematopoietic tissue" (Collectively reported as "Malignant Neoplasms")	(38) [431-432] "Intracerebral haemorrhage and other intracranial haemorrhage" (39) [434.0,434.9] "Cerebral thrombosis and unspecified occlusion of cerebral arteries" (40) [434.1] "Cerebral embolism" (41) [430,433,435-438] "All other and late effects of cerebrovascular disease" (Collectively reported as "Cerebrovascular Disease")

Violent Deaths (Excluding Suicide)	Pneumonia (All Forms)	Pulmonary Tuberculosis	Influenza
(68) [E810-E825] "Motor vehicle accidents" (69) [E800-E807, E826-949] "All other accidents and adverse effects" (71) [E960-E978] "Homicide and legal intervention" (72) [E980-E999] "All other external causes"	(45) [480-486] "Pneumonia" (Reported in "Pneumonia and Influenza")	(3) [010-012] "Tuberculosis of the respiratory system" (Reported as "Tuberculosis of the Respiratory System")	(46) [487] "Influenza" (Reported in "Pneumonia and Influenza")

Year and classification system	Diseases of the Heart	Malignant Tumors	Cerebrovascular Disease
1985 Classification system is reported to be ICD-9 (list of "282 selected causes of death, from the International Classification of Disease (ICD9)"; however, numbers do not match ICD-9 codes[18]	[127] "Acute rheumatic fever" [128] "Diseases of mitral valve" [129] "Diseases of aortic valve" [130] "Diseases of mitral and aortic valves" [131] "All other rheumatic heart disease" [133] "Hypertensive heart disease" [135] "Hypertensive heart and renal disease" [136] "Acute myocardial infarction" [137] "Other acute and subacute forms of ischemic heart disease" [138] "Angina pectoris" [139] "All Other forms of chronic ischemic heart disease" [140] "Diseases of pulmonary circulation" [141] "Acute and subacute endocarditis" [142] "Acute pericarditis, acute myocarditis, and other diseases of pericardium" [143] "Mitral valve disorder" [144] "Aortic valve disorder" [145] "All other diseases of endocardium" [146] "Heart failure" [147] "Myocarditis, unspecified and myocardial degeneration" [148] All other and ill-defined forms of heart disease" (Collectively reported as "Diseases of the Heart")[19]	Malignant Neoplasms [37] "Of lip" [38] "Of tongue" [39] "Of pharynx" [40] "Of other and ill-defined sites within the lip, oral cavity and pharynx" [41] "Of esophagus" [42] "Of stomach" [43] "Of small intestine" [44] "Hepatic and splenic flexures and transverse colon" [45] "Descending colon" [46] "Sigmoid colon" [47] "Cecum, appendix and ascending colon" [48] "Hepatic and splenic flexures and transverse other and colon, unspecified" [49] "Of rectum, rectosigmoid junction and anus" [50] "Liver, primary" [51] "Intrahepatic bile ducts" [52] "Liver, not specified as primary or secondary" [53] "Of gallbladder and extrahepatic bile ducts" [54] "O pancreas" [55] "Of retroperitoneum, peritoneum, and other and ill-defined sites" [56] "Of Larynx" [57] "Of trachea, bronchus, and lung" [58] "Of all other ill-defined sites" [59] "Of bone and articular cartilage" [60] "Of consecutive and other soft tissue" [61] "Melanoma of skin" [62] "Other malignant neoplasm of skin" [63] "Of female breast" [64] "Of male breast" [65] "Of cervix uteri" [66] "Of other parts of uterus" [67] "Of ovary and other uterine adnexa" [68] "Of other and unspecified female organs" [69] "Of prostate" [70] "Of testis" [71] "Of penis and other male genital organs" [72] "Of bladder" [73] "Of kidney and other and unspecified urinary organs" [74] "Of eye" [75] "Of brain" [76] "Of other and unspecified parts of nervous system" [77] "Of thyroid gland and other endocrine glands and related structures" [78] "Of all other and unspecified sites" [79] "Lymphosarcoma and reticulosarcoma" [80] "Hodgkin's disease" [81] "Other malignant neoplasms of lymphoid and histiocytic tissue" [82] "Multiple myeloma and immunoproliferative neoplasms" [83] "Lymphoid leukaemia" [84] "Myeloid leukaemia" [85] "Monocytic leukaemia" [86] "Other and unspecified leukaemia" (Collectively reported as "Malignant Neoplasms")	[149] "Subarachnoid haemorrhage" [150] "Intracerebral and other intercranial haemorrhage" [151] "Occlusion and stenosis of precerebral arteries" [152] "Cerebral thrombosis and unspecified occlusion of cerebral arteries" [153] "Cerebral embolism" [154] "Acute but ill-defined cerebrovascular disease" [155] "Other and late effects of cerebrovascular disease" (Collectively reported as "Cerebrovascular Disease (Strokes)")

Violent Deaths (Excluding Suicide)	Pneumonia (All Forms)	Pulmonary Tuberculosis	Influenza
[234] "Railway accidents"	[164] "Viral pneumonia"	[A7] "Tuberculosis of the respiratory system"	[A168] "Influenza"
[235] Motor vehicle accidents "Involving collision with train"	[165] "Pneumococcal and other bacterial pneumonia"		(Reported in "Pneumonia and Influenza")
[236] Motor vehicle accidents "Involving collision with another motor vehicle"	[166] "Broncho-pneumonia, organism unspecified"		
[237] Motor vehicle accidents "Involving collision with pedestrian"	[167] "Pneumonia due to other and unspecified organism"		
[238] Motor vehicle accidents "Involving collision with other vehicle or object"			
[239] Motor vehicle accidents "Not involving collision on highway"	(Collectively reported in "Pneumonia and Influenza")		
[240] "Motor vehicle traffic accident of unspecified nature"			
[241] "Motor vehicle nontraffic accidents"			
[242] "Other road vehicle accidents"			
[243] "Water transport accidents"			
[244] "Air and space transport accidents"			
[245] "Vehicle accidents not elsewhere classifiable"			
[246] "Accidental poisoning by drugs, medicaments, and biologicals"			
[247] "Accidental poisoning by other solid or liquid substances"			
[248] "Accidental poisoning by gases and vapors"			
[249] "Misadventures during medical care, abnormal reactions & late complications"			
[250] "Fall from one level to another"			
[251] "Fall on the same level"			
[252] "Fracture, cause unspecified, and other unspecified falls"			
[253] "accidents caused by fires and flames"			
[254] "Lightning"			
[255] "Accidental drowning and submersion"			
[256] "Suffocation caused by inhalation or ingestion of food or other object"			
[257] "Accident caused by handgun"			
[258] "Accidents cause by all other and unspecified firearms"			
[259] "Accident caused by explosive material"			
[260] "Accidents caused by hot, caustic, or corrosive substances and radiation"			
[261] "Accident caused by electric current"			
[262] "All other accidents and late effects of accidental injury"			
[263] "Adverse effects of drugs, medicaments and biologicals in therapeutic use"			
[271] "Assault by handgun"			
[272] "Assault by all other and unspecified firearms"			
[273] "Assault by cutting and piercing instrument"			
[274] "Assault by all other means and late effect of injury"			
[275] "Legal execution"			
[276] "Other legal intervention and late effects"			
Injury undetermined whether accidental or inflicted"			
[277] "From poisoning by drugs, medicaments, and biologicals"			
[278] "From poisoning by other solid or liquid substances"			
[279] "From injury by handgun"			
[280] "From injury by all other and unspecified firearms"			
[281] "From injury by all other means and late effects of injury"			
[282] "Injury resulting from operations of war"			

APPENDIX B: (*continued*)

Year and classification system	Diseases of the Heart	Malignant Tumors	Cerebrovascular Disease
1990 Classification system is reported to be ICD-9 ("ICD-9 282 Selected Causes of Death"); however, numbers do not match ICD-9 codes[20]	[127] "Acute rheumatic fever" [128] "Diseases of mitral valve" [129] "Diseases of aortic valve" [130] "Diseases of mitral and aortic valves" [131] "All other rheumatic heart disease" [133] "Hypertensive heart disease" [135] "Hypertensive heart and renal disease" [136] "Acute myocardial infarction" [137] "Other acute and subacute forms of ischemic heart disease" [138] "Angina pectoris" [139] "All Other forms of chronic ischemic heart disease" [140] "Diseases of pulmonary circulation" [141] "Acute and subacute endocarditis" [142] "Acute pericarditis, acute myocarditis, and other diseases of pericardium" [143] "Mitral valve disorder" [144] "Aortic valve disorder" [145] "All other diseases of endocardium" [146] "Heart failure" [147] "Myocarditis, unspecified and myocardial degeneration" [148] All other and ill-defined forms of heart disease" (Collectively reported as "Diseases of the Heart")	Malignant Neoplasms [37] "Of lip" [38] "Of tongue" [39] "Of pharynx" [40] "Of other and ill-defined sites within the lip, oral cavity and pharynx" [41] "Of esophagus" [42] "Of stomach" [43] "Of small intestine" [44] "Hepatic and splenic flexures and transverse colon" [45] "Descending colon" [46] "Sigmoid colon" [47] "Cecum, appendix and ascending colon" [48] "Hepatic and splenic flexures and transverse other and colon, unspecified" [49] "Of rectum, rectosigmoid junction and anus" [50] "Liver, primary" [51] "Intrahepatic bile ducts" [52] "Liver, not specified as primary or secondary" [53] "Of gallbladder and extrahepatic bile ducts" [54] "O pancreas" [55] "Of retroperitoneum, peritoneum, and other and ill-defined sites" [56] "Of Larynx" [57] "Of trachea, bronchus, and lung" [58] "Of all other ill-defined sites" [59] "Of bone and articular cartilage" [60] "Of consecutive and other soft tissue" [61] "Melanoma of skin" [62] "Other malignant neoplasm of skin" [63] "Of female breast" [64] "Of male breast" [65] "Of cervix uteri" [66] "Of other parts of uterus" [67] "Of ovary and other uterine adnexa" [68] "Of other and unspecified female organs" [69] "Of prostate" [70] "Of testis" [71] "Of penis and other male genital organs" [72] "Of bladder" [73] "Of kidney and other and unspecified urinary organs"" [74] "Of eye" [75] "Of brain" [76] "Of other and unspecified parts of nervous system" [77] "Of thyroid gland and other endocrine glands and related structures" [78] "Of all other and unspecified sites" [79] "Lymphosarcoma and reticulosarcoma" [80] "Hodgkin's disease" [81] "Other malignant neoplasms of lymphoid and histiocytic tissue" [82] "Multiple myeloma and immunoproliferative neoplasms" [83] "Lymphoid leukaemia" [84] "Myeloid leukaemia" [85] "Monocytic leukaemia" [86] "Other and unspecified leukaemia" (Collectively reported as "Malignant Neoplasms"	[149] "Subarachnoid haemorrhage" [150] "Intracerebral and other intercranial haemorrhage" [151] "Occlusion and stenosis of precerebral arteries" [152] "Cerebral thrombosis and unspecified occlusion of cerebral arteries" [153] "Cerebral embolism" [154] "Acute but ill-defined cerebrovascular disease" [155] "Other and late effects of cerebrovascular disease" (Collectively reported as "Cerebrovascular Disease (Strokes)")

Violent Deaths (Excluding Suicide)	Pneumonia (All Forms)	Pulmonary Tuberculosis	Influenza
[234] "Railway accidents"	[164] "Viral pneumonia"	[A7] "Tuberculosis of the respiratory system"	[A168] "Influenza"
[235] Motor vehicle accidents "Involving collision with train"	[165] "Pneumococcal and other bacterial pneumonia"		(Reported in "Pneumonia and Influenza")
[236] Motor vehicle accidents "Involving collision with another motor vehicle"	[166] "Broncho-pneumonia, organism unspecified"		
[237] Motor vehicle accidents "Involving collision with pedestrian"	[167] "Pneumonia due to other and unspecified organism"		
[238] Motor vehicle accidents "Involving collision with other vehicle or object"			
[239] Motor vehicle accidents "Not involving collision on highway"	(Collectively reported as "Pneumonia and Influenza")		
[240] "Motor vehicle traffic accident of unspecified nature"			
[241] "Motor vehicle nontraffic accidents"			
[242] "Other road vehicle accidents"			
[243] "Water transport accidents"			
[244] "Air and space transport accidents"			
[245] "Vehicle accidents not elsewhere classifiable"			
[246] "Accidental poisoning by drugs, medicaments, and biologicals"			
[247] "Accidental poisoning by other solid or liquid substances"			
[248] "Accidental poisoning by gases and vapors"			
[249] "Misadventures during medical care, abnormal reactions & late complications"			
[250] "Fall from one level to another"			
[251] "Fall on the same level"			
[252] "Fracture, cause unspecified, and other unspecified falls"			
[253] "accidents caused by fires and flames"			
[254] "Lightning"			
[255] "Accidental drowning and submersion"			
[256] "Suffocation caused by inhalation or ingestion of food or other object"			
[257] "Accident caused by handgun"			
[258] "Accidents cause by all other and unspecified firearms"			
[259] "Accident caused by explosive material"			
[260] "Accidents caused by hot, caustic, or corrosive substances and radiation"			
[261] "Accident caused by electric current"			
[262] "All other accidents and late effects of accidental injury"			
[263] "Adverse effects of drugs, medicaments and biologicals in therapeutic use"			
[271] "Assault by handgun"			
[272] "Assault by all other and unspecified firearms"			
[273] "Assault by cutting and piercing instrument"			
[274] "Assault by all other means and late effect of injury"			
[275] "Legal execution"			
[276] "Other legal intervention and late effects"			
Injury undetermined whether accidental or inflicted"			
[277] "From poisoning by drugs, medicaments, and biologicals"			
[278] "From poisoning by other solid or liquid substances"			
[279] "From injury by handgun"			
[280] "From injury by all other and unspecified firearms"			
[281] "From injury by all other means and late effects of injury"			
[282] "Injury resulting from operations of war"			

Year and classification system	Diseases of the Heart	Malignant Tumors	Cerebrovascular Disease
1995 Classification system is reported to be ICD-9 ("Selected Causes of Death ICD 9"); however, numbers do not match ICD-9 codes[21]	[127] "Acute rheumatic fever" [128] "Diseases of mitral valve" [129] "Diseases of aortic valve" [130] "Diseases of mitral and aortic valves" [131] "All other rheumatic heart disease" [133] "Hypertensive heart disease" [135] "Hypertensive heart and renal disease" [136] "Acute myocardial infarction" [137] "Other acute and subacute forms of ischemic heart disease" [138] "Angina pectoris" [139] "All Other forms of chronic ischemic heart disease" [140] "Diseases of pulmonary circulation" [141] "Acute and subacute endocarditis" [142] "Acute pericarditis, acute myocarditis, and other diseases of pericardium" [143] "Mitral valve disorder" [144] "Aortic valve disorder" [145] "All other diseases of endocardium" [146] "Heart failure" [147] "Myocarditis, unspecified and myocardial degeneration" [148] All other and ill-defined forms of heart disease" (Collectively reported as "Diseases of the Heart")	Malignant Neoplasms [37] "Of lip" [38] "Of tongue" [39] "Of pharynx" [40] "Of other and ill-defined sites within the lip, oral cavity and pharynx" [41] "Of esophagus" [42] "Of stomach" [43] "Of small intestine" [44] "Hepatic and splenic flexures and transverse colon" [45] "Descending colon" [46] "Sigmoid colon" [47] "Cecum, appendix and ascending colon" [48] "Hepatic and splenic flexures and transverse other and colon, unspecified" [49] "Of rectum, rectosigmoid junction and anus" [50] "Liver, primary" [51] "Intrahepatic bile ducts" [52] "Liver, not specified as primary or secondary" [53] "Of gallbladder and extrahepatic bile ducts" [54] "O pancreas" [55] "Of retroperitoneum, peritoneum, and other and ill-defined sites" [56] "Of Larynx" [57] "Of trachea, bronchus, and lung" [58] "Of all other ill-defined sites" [59] "Of bone and articular cartilage" [60] "Of consecutive and other soft tissue" [61] "Melanoma of skin" [62] "Other malignant neoplasm of skin" [63] "Of female breast" [64] "Of male breast" [65] "Of cervix uteri" [66] "Of other parts of uterus" [67] "Of ovary and other uterine adnexa" [68] "Of other and unspecified female organs" [69] "Of prostate" [70] "Of testis" [71] "Of penis and other male genital organs" [72] "Of bladder" [73] "Of kidney and other and unspecified urinary organs"" [74] "Of eye" [75] "Of brain" [76] "Of other and unspecified parts of nervous system" [77] "Of thyroid gland and other endocrine glands and related structures" [78] "Of all other and unspecified sites" [79] "Lymphosarcoma and reticulosarcoma" [80] "Hodgkin's disease" [81] "Other malignant neoplasms of lymphoid and histiocytic tissue" [82] "Multiple myeloma and immunoproliferative neoplasms" [83] "Lymphoid leukaemia" [84] "Myeloid leukaemia" [85] "Monocytic leukaemia" [86] "Other and unspecified leukaemia" (Collectively reported as "Malignant Neoplasms")	[149] "Subarachnoid haemorrhage" [150] "Intracerebral and other intercranial haemorrhage" [151] "Occlusion and stenosis of precerebral arteries" [152] "Cerebral thrombosis and unspecified occlusion of cerebral arteries" [153] "Cerebral embolism" [154] "Acute but ill-defined cerebrovascular disease" [155] "Other and late effects of cerebrovascular disease" (Collectively reported as "Cerebrovascular Disease (Strokes)")

Violent Deaths (Excluding Suicide)	Pneumonia (All Forms)	Pulmonary Tuberculosis	Influenza
[234] "Railway accidents"	[164] "Viral pneumonia"	[A7] "Tuberculosis of the respiratory system"	[A168] "Influenza"
[235] Motor vehicle accidents "Involving collision with train"	[165] "Pneumococcal and other bacterial pneumonia"		
[236] Motor vehicle accidents "Involving collision with another motor vehicle"	[166] "Broncho-pneumonia, organism unspecified"		(Reported in "Pneumonia and Influenza")
[237] Motor vehicle accidents "Involving collision with pedestrian"	[167] "Pneumonia due to other and unspecified organism"		
[238] Motor vehicle accidents "Involving collision with other vehicle or object"			
[239] Motor vehicle accidents "Not involving collision on highway"	(Collectively reported as "Pneumonia and Influenza")		
[240] "Motor vehicle traffic accident of unspecified nature"			
[241] "Motor vehicle nontraffic accidents"			
[242] "Other road vehicle accidents"			
[243] "Water transport accidents"			
[244] "Air and space transport accidents"			
[245] "Vehicle accidents not elsewhere classifiable"			
[246] "Accidental poisoning by drugs, medicaments, and biologicals"			
[247] "Accidental poisoning by other solid or liquid substances"			
[248] "Accidental poisoning by gases and vapors"			
[249] "Misadventures during medical care, abnormal reactions & late complications"			
[250] "Fall from one level to another"			
[251] "Fall on the same level"			
[252] "Fracture, cause unspecified, and other unspecified falls"			
[253] "accidents caused by fires and flames"			
[254] "Lightning"			
[255] "Accidental drowning and submersion"			
[256] "Suffocation caused by inhalation or ingestion of food or other object"			
[257] "Accident caused by handgun"			
[258] "Accidents cause by all other and unspecified firearms"			
[259] "Accident caused by explosive material"			
[260] "Accidents caused by hot, caustic, or corrosive substances and radiation"			
[261] "Accident caused by electric current"			
[262] "All other accidents and late effects of accidental injury"			
[263] "Adverse effects of drugs, medicaments and biologicals in therapeutic use"			
[271] "Assault by handgun"			
[272] "Assault by all other and unspecified firearms"			
[273] "Assault by cutting and piercing instrument"			
[274] "Assault by all other means and late effect of injury"			
[275] "Legal execution"			
[276] "Other legal intervention and late effects"			
Injury undetermined whether accidental or inflicted			
[277] "From poisoning by drugs, medicaments, and biologicals"			
[278] "From poisoning by other solid or liquid substances"			
[279] "From injury by handgun"			
[280] "From injury by all other and unspecified firearms"			
[281] "From injury by all other means and late effects of injury"			
[282] "Injury resulting from operations of war"			

Year and classification system	Diseases of the Heart	Malignant Tumors	Cerebrovascular Disease
2000 Classification system is ICD-10 codes from Statistics Canada's selected group causes[22]	[I00-I02] "Acute rheumatic fever" [I05-I09] "Chronic rheumatic heart disease" [I11] "Hypertensive heart disease" [I13] "Hypertensive heart and renal disease" [I20-I25] "Ischaemic heart diseases" [I26-I28] "Pulmonary heart disease and diseases of pulmonary circulation" [I30-I52] "Other forms of heart disease" (Collectively reported as "Diseases of heart")	[C00-C14] "Malignant neoplasms of lip, oral cavity and pharynx" [C15-C26] "Malignant neoplasms of digestive organs" [C30-C39] "Malignant neoplasm of respiratory and intrathoracic organs" [C40-C41] "Malignant neoplasm of bone and articular cartilage" [C43-C44] "Melanoma and other malignant neoplasms of skin" [C45-C49] "Malignant neoplasms of mesothelial and soft tissue" [C50-C50] "Malignant neoplasm of breast" [C51-C58] "Malignant neoplasms of female genital organs" [C60-C63] "Malignant neoplasms of male genital organs" [C64-C68] "Malignant neoplasm of urinary tract" [C69-C72] "Malignant neoplasms of eye, brain and other parts of central nervous system" [C73-C75] "Malignant neoplasms of thyroid and other endocrine glands" [C76-C80] "Malignant neoplasms of ill-defined, secondary and unspecified sites" [C81-C96] "Malignant neoplasm of lymphoid, haematopoietic and related tissue" [C97-C97] "Malignant neoplasms of independent (primary) multiple sites" (Collectively reported as "Malignant Neoplasms")	[I60] "Subarachnoid haemorrhage" [I61] "Intracerebral haemorrhage" [I62] "Other nontraumatic intracranial haemorrhage" [I63] "Cerebral infarction" [I64] "Stroke, not specified as haemorrhage or infarction" [I65] "Occlusion and stenosis of precerebral arteries, not resulting in cerebral infarction" [I66] "Occlusion and stenosis of cerebral arteries, not resulting in cerebral infarction" [I67] "Other cerebrovascular diseases" [I68] "Cerebrovascular disorders in diseases classified elsewhere" [I69] "Sequelae of cerebrovascular disease" (Collectively reported as "Cerebrovascular diseases")

Violent Deaths (Excluding Suicide)	Pneumonia (All Forms)	Pulmonary Tuberculosis	Influenza
[V01-V99, Y85] "Transport accidents" [W00-X59, Y86] "Nontransport accidents" [X93-X95] "Assault (homicide) by discharge of firearms" [X85-X92, X96-Y09, Y87.1] "Assault (homicide) by other and unspecified means and their sequelae" [Y35, Y89.0] "Legal intervention" [Y22-Y24] "Discharge of firearms, undetermined intent" [Y10-Y21, Y25-Y34, Y87.2, Y89.9] "Other and unspecified events of undetermined intent and their sequelae" [Y36, Y89.1] "Operations of war and their sequelae"	[J12] "Viral pneumonia, not elsewhere classified" [J13] "Pneumonia due to Streptococcus pneumoniae" [J14] "Pneumonia due to Haemophilus influenzae" [J15] "Bacterial pneumonia, not elsewhere classified" [J16] "Pneumonia due to other infectious organisms, not elsewhere classified" [J17] "Pneumonia in diseases classified elsewhere" [J18] "Pneumonia, organism unspecified" (Collectively reported as "Pneumonia")	[A16] "Respiratory tuberculosis, not confirmed bacteriologically or histologically"	[J09] "Influenza due to identified zoonotic or pandemic influenza virus" [J10] "Influenza due to identified seasonal influenza virus" [J11] "Influenza, virus not identified" (Collectively reported as "Influenza")

Year and classification system	Diseases of the Heart	Malignant Tumors	Cerebrovascular Disease
2005 Classification system is ICD-10 codes from Statistics Canada's selected group causes[23]	[I00-I02] "Acute rheumatic fever" [I05-I09] "Chronic rheumatic heart disease" [I11] "Hypertensive heart disease" [I13] "Hypertensive heart and renal disease" [I20-I25] "Ischaemic heart diseases" [I26-I28] "Pulmonary heart disease and diseases of pulmonary circulation" [I30-I52] "Other forms of heart disease" (Collectively reported as "Diseases of heart")	[C00-C14] "Malignant neoplasms of lip, oral cavity and pharynx" [C15-C26] "Malignant neoplasms of digestive organs" [C30-C39] "Malignant neoplasm of respiratory and intrathoracic organs" [C40-C41] "Malignant neoplasm of bone and articular cartilage" [C43-C44] "Melanoma and other malignant neoplasms of skin" [C45-C49] "Malignant neoplasms of mesothelial and soft tissue" [C50-C50] "Malignant neoplasm of breast" [C51-C58] "Malignant neoplasms of female genital organs" [C60-C63] "Malignant neoplasm of male genital organs" [C64-C68] "Malignant neoplasm of urinary tract" [C69-C72] "Malignant neoplasms of eye, brain and other parts of central nervous system" [C73-C75] "Malignant neoplasms of thyroid and other endocrine glands" [C76-C80] "Malignant neoplasms of ill-defined, secondary and unspecified sites" [C81-C96] "Malignant neoplasm of lymphoid, haematopoietic and related tissue" [C97-C97] "Malignant neoplasms of independent (primary) multiple sites" (Collectively reported as "Malignant Neoplasms")	[I60] "Subarachnoid haemorrhage" [I61] "Intracerebral haemorrhage" [I62] "Other nontraumatic intracranial haemorrhage" [I63] "Cerebral infarction" [I64] "Stroke, not specified as haemorrhage or infarction" [I65] "Occlusion and stenosis of precerebral arteries, not resulting in cerebral infarction" [I66] "Occlusion and stenosis of cerebral arteries, not resulting in cerebral infarction" [I67] "Other cerebrovascular diseases" [I68] "Cerebrovascular disorders in diseases classified elsewhere" [I69] "Sequelae of cerebrovascular disease" (Collectively reported as "Cerebrovascular diseases")

Violent Deaths (Excluding Suicide)	Pneumonia (All Forms)	Pulmonary Tuberculosis	Influenza
[V01-V99, Y85] "Transport accidents" [W00-X59, Y86] "Nontransport accidents" [X93-X95] "Assault (homicide) by discharge of firearms" [X85-X92, X96-Y09, Y87.1] "Assault (homicide) by other and unspecified means and their sequelae" [Y35, Y89.0] "Legal intervention" [Y22-Y24] "Discharge of firearms, undetermined intent" [Y10-Y21, Y25-Y34, Y87.2, Y89.9] "Other and unspecified events of undetermined intent and their sequelae" [Y36, Y89.1] "Operations of war and their sequelae"	[J12] "Viral pneumonia, not elsewhere classified" [J13] "Pneumonia due to Streptococcus pneumoniae" [J14] "Pneumonia due to Haemophilus influenzae" [J15] "Bacterial pneumonia, not elsewhere classified" [J16] "Pneumonia due to other infectious organisms, not elsewhere classified" [J17] "Pneumonia in diseases classified elsewhere" [J18] "Pneumonia, organism unspecified" (Collectively reported as "Pneumonia")	[A16] "Respiratory tuberculosis, not confirmed bacteriologically or histologically"	[J09] "Influenza due to identified zoonotic or pandemic influenza virus" [J10] "Influenza due to identified seasonal influenza virus" [J11] "Influenza, virus not identified" (Collectively reported as "Influenza")

Year and classification system	Diseases of the Heart	Malignant Tumors	Cerebrovascular Disease
2010 Classification system is ICD-10 codes from Statistics Canada's selected group causes[24]	[I00-I02] "Acute rheumatic fever" [I05-I09] "Chronic rheumatic heart disease" [I11] "Hypertensive heart disease" [I13] "Hypertensive heart and renal disease" [I20-I25] "Ischaemic heart diseases" [I26-I28] "Pulmonary heart disease and diseases of pulmonary circulation" [I30-I52] "Other forms of heart disease" (Collectively reported as "Diseases of heart")	[C00-C14] "Malignant neoplasms of lip, oral cavity and pharynx" [C15-C26] "Malignant neoplasms of digestive organs" [C30-C39] "Malignant neoplasm of respiratory and intrathoracic organs" [C40-C41] "Malignant neoplasm of bone and articular cartilage" [C43-C44] "Melanoma and other malignant neoplasms of skin" [C45-C49] "Malignant neoplasms of mesothelial and soft tissue" [C50-C50] "Malignant neoplasm of breast" [C51-C58] "Malignant neoplasms of female genital organs" [C60-C63] "Malignant neoplasms of male genital organs" [C64-C68] "Malignant neoplasm of urinary tract" [C69-C72] "Malignant neoplasms of eye, brain and other parts of central nervous system" [C73-C75] "Malignant neoplasms of thyroid and other endocrine glands" [C76-C80] "Malignant neoplasms of ill-defined, secondary and unspecified sites" [C81-C96] "Malignant neoplasm of lymphoid, haematopoietic and related tissue" [C97-C97] "Malignant neoplasms of independent (primary) multiple sites" (Collectively reported as "Malignant Neoplasms")	[I60] "Subarachnoid haemorrhage" [I61] "Intracerebral haemorrhage" [I62] "Other nontraumatic intracranial haemorrhage" [I63] "Cerebral infarction" [I64] "Stroke, not specified as haemorrhage or infarction" [I65] "Occlusion and stenosis of precerebral arteries, not resulting in cerebral infarction" [I66] "Occlusion and stenosis of cerebral arteries, not resulting in cerebral infarction" [I67] "Other cerebrovascular diseases" [I68] "Cerebrovascular disorders in diseases classified elsewhere" [I69] "Sequelae of cerebrovascular disease" (Collectively reported as "Cerebrovascular diseases")

Violent Deaths (Excluding Suicide)	Pneumonia (All Forms)	Pulmonary Tuberculosis	Influenza
[V01-V99, Y85] "Transport accidents" [W00-X59, Y86] "Nontransport accidents" [X93-X95] "Assault (homicide) by discharge of firearms" [X85-X92, X96-Y09, Y87.1] "Assault (homicide) by other and unspecified means and their sequelae" [Y35, Y89.0] "Legal intervention" [Y22-Y24] "Discharge of firearms, undetermined intent" [Y10-Y21, Y25-Y34, Y87.2, Y89.9] "Other and unspecified events of undetermined intent and their sequelae" [Y36, Y89.1] "Operations of war and their sequelae"	[J12] "Viral pneumonia, not elsewhere classified" [J13] "Pneumonia due to Streptococcus pneumoniae" [J14] "Pneumonia due to Haemophilus influenzae" [J15] "Bacterial pneumonia, not elsewhere classified" [J16] "Pneumonia due to other infectious organisms, not elsewhere classified" [J17] "Pneumonia in diseases classified elsewhere" [J18] "Pneumonia, organism unspecified" (Collectively reported as "Pneumonia")	[A16] "Respiratory tuberculosis, not confirmed bacteriologically or histologically"	[J09] "Influenza due to identified zoonotic or pandemic influenza virus" [J10] "Influenza due to identified seasonal influenza virus" [J11] "Influenza, virus not identified" (Collectively reported as "Influenza")

Year and classification system	Diseases of the Heart	Malignant Tumors	Cerebrovascular Disease
2015 Classification system is ICD-10 codes from Statistics Canada's selected group causes[25]	[I00-I02] "Acute rheumatic fever" [I05-I09] "Chronic rheumatic heart disease" [I11] "Hypertensive heart disease" [I13] "Hypertensive heart and renal disease" [I20-I25] "Ischaemic heart diseases" [I26-I28] "Pulmonary heart disease and diseases of pulmonary circulation" [I30-I52] "Other forms of heart disease" (Collectively reported as "Diseases of heart")	[C00-C14] "Malignant neoplasms of lip, oral cavity and pharynx" [C15-C26] "Malignant neoplasms of digestive organs" [C30-C39] "Malignant neoplasm of respiratory and intrathoracic organs" [C40-C41] "Malignant neoplasm of bone and articular cartilage" [C43-C44] "Melanoma and other malignant neoplasms of skin". [C45-C49] "Malignant neoplasms of mesothelial and soft tissue" [C50-C50] "Malignant neoplasm of breast" [C51-C58] "Malignant neoplasms of female genital organs" [C60-C63] "Malignant neoplasms of male genital organs" [C64-C68] "Malignant neoplasm of urinary tract" [C69-C72] "Malignant neoplasms of eye, brain and other parts of central nervous system" [C73-C75] "Malignant neoplasms of thyroid and other endocrine glands" [C76-C80] "Malignant neoplasms of ill-defined, secondary and unspecified sites" [C81-C96] "Malignant neoplasm of lymphoid, haematopoietic and related tissue" [C97-C97] "Malignant neoplasms of independent (primary) multiple sites" (Collectively reported as "Malignant Neoplasms")	[I60] "Subarachnoid haemorrhage" [I61] "Intracerebral haemorrhage" [I62] "Other nontraumatic intracranial haemorrhage" [I63] "Cerebral infarction" [I64] "Stroke, not specified as haemorrhage or infarction" [I65] "Occlusion and stenosis of precerebral arteries, not resulting in cerebral infarction" [I66] "Occlusion and stenosis of cerebral arteries, not resulting in cerebral infarction" [I67] "Other cerebrovascular diseases" [I68] "Cerebrovascular disorders in diseases classified elsewhere" [I69] "Sequelae of cerebrovascular disease" (Collectively reported as "Cerebrovascular diseases")

Violent Deaths (Excluding Suicide)	Pneumonia (All Forms)	Pulmonary Tuberculosis	Influenza
[V01-V99, Y85] "Transport accidents" [W00-X59, Y86] "Nontransport accidents" [X93-X95] "Assault (homicide) by discharge of firearms" [X85-X92, X96-Y09, Y87.1] "Assault (homicide) by other and unspecified means and their sequelae" [Y35, Y89.0] "Legal intervention" [Y22-Y24] "Discharge of firearms, undetermined intent" [Y10-Y21, Y25-Y34, Y87.2, Y89.9] "Other and unspecified events of undetermined intent and their sequelae" [Y36, Y89.1] "Operations of war and their sequelae"	[J12] "Viral pneumonia, not elsewhere classified" [J13] "Pneumonia due to Streptococcus pneumoniae" [J14] "Pneumonia due to Haemophilus influenzae" [J15] "Bacterial pneumonia, not elsewhere classified" [J16] "Pneumonia due to other infectious organisms, not elsewhere classified" [J17] "Pneumonia in diseases classified elsewhere" [J18] "Pneumonia, organism unspecified" (Collectively reported as "Pneumonia")	[A16] "Respiratory tuberculosis, not confirmed bacteriologically or histologically"	[J09] "Influenza due to identified zoonotic or pandemic influenza virus" [J10] "Influenza due to identified seasonal influenza virus" [J11] "Influenza, virus not identified" (Collectively reported as "Influenza")

NOTES

1 Source: Table: "Death During the Year 1915, by Ages and Sexes," Alberta Department of Agriculture, *Annual Report 1915* (Edmonton: 2016), 264–270. Codes match ICD-2. Includes deaths at all ages. For the history of the ICD and an explanation of its several revisions, see Iwao M. Moriyama, Ruth M. Loy and Alastair H.T. Robb-Smith, *History Of The Statistical Classification of Diseases and Causes Of Death*, edited by Harry M. Rosenberg and Donna L. Hoyert (Hyattsville, MD: National Center for Health Statistics; 2011), https://www.cdc.gov/nchs/data/misc/classification_diseases2011.pdf

2 Source: "Diagram Showing Number of Deaths from Eight Selected Causes" and "Causes of Death during the Year 1920, by ages and sexes (for the whole province)," Alberta Department of Public Health, *Annual Report of the Vital Statistics Branch 1920* (Edmonton: Printed by J.W. Jeffery, King's Printer, 1921), 23 and 28–43. Codes match ICD-2. Includes deaths at all ages.

3 Source: Table: "Causes of death which during the two previous years accounted for at least one per cent of total of the death," (a) "Deaths during the Year 1925—by Ages and Sexes for the Whole Province (Indians Excepted)," and (b) "Deaths during the Year 1925, by ages and sexes, of Indians Living on Reserves," Alberta Department of Public Health, *Annual Report 1925* (Edmonton: Printed by W.D. McLean, King's Printer, 1926), 68, 96–109, and 142–144. Codes match ICD-3. Includes deaths at all ages. In this particular year, the causes of deaths for Indigenous and non-Indigenous people were published in two separate tables. We added the numbers from the two tables to present a total sum for the province. This was to be consistent with other years, where a single table presents causes of death for Indigenous and non-Indigenous peoples. Importantly, statistics for Indigenous peoples are at best incomplete.

4 Source: "Causes of Death" and "Table 17. Causes of Death by Sex and Age for the Whole Province, 1930," Alberta Department of Public Health, *Annual Report of the Vital Statistics Branch 1930* (Edmonton: Printed by W.D. McLean, King's Printer, 1931), 6 and 44–57. Codes match ICD-3. Includes deaths at all ages.

5 Source: "Certain principal causes of death" and "Table 17. Causes of Death by Sex and Age for the Whole Province, 1935," Alberta Department of Public Health, *Annual Report of the Vital Statistics Branch 1935* (Edmonton: Printed by A. Shnitka King's Printer, 1936), 8 and 48–65. Codes match ICD-4. Includes deaths at all ages.

6 Source: "Certain principal causes of death" and "Table 17. Causes of Death by Sex and Age for the Whole Province, 1940," Alberta Department of Public Health, *Annual Report of the Vital Statistics Branch 1940* (Edmonton: Printed by A. Shnitka King's Printer, 1941), 7 and 48–65. Codes match ICD-4. Includes deaths at all ages.

7 Source: "Table 16. Causes of Death by Sex, Age and Residence for the Whole Province, 1945" and "Table 25. Principal Causes of Death by Numbers and Rates for each Years of the Last Decennial Period" Alberta Department of Public Health, *Annual Report of the Vital Statistics Branch 1945* (Edmonton: Printed by A. Shnitka King's Printer, 1947), 33–53 and 117. Codes match *International List of Causes of Death* numbers in its fifth revision (ICD5). Includes deaths at all ages.

8 Source: "Table 18: Certain Causes of Death, by Numbers and Rates for each year of the last Decennial Period," Alberta Department of Public Health, *Annual Report of the Bureau of Vital Statistics 1955* (Edmonton: Printed by A. Shnitka King's Printer, 1956), 62 and Table "TABLE 58. Causes of death (Intermediate List) by sex and age in Canada, by provinces, by place of residence, 1950 – continued Alberta," in Vital Statistics Section, Health and Welfare Division, Dominion Bureau of Statistics, *Vital Statistics 1950 Statistiques Vitales* (Ottawa, 1953), 340–349. Codes match "Intermediate List" numbers published in the *International List of Causes of Death* in its sixth revision (ICD-6). List is also known as "List A: Intermediate list of 150 causes for tabulation of morbidity and mortality." Includes deaths at all ages.

9 Source: "Table 8: Deaths, by Cause and Sex, by Age, Alberta 1955" and "Table 18: Certain Causes of Death, by Numbers and Rates for each year of the last Decennial Period," Alberta Department of Public Health, *Annual Report of the Bureau of Vital Statistics 1955* (Edmonton: Printed by A. Shnitka King's Printer, 1956), 22–29 and 62. Codes match ICD-6 Intermediate List. Includes deaths at all ages.

10 There is a discrepancy in the number of deaths due to "Cancer," between the number reported in "Table 18: Certain Causes of Deaths" (1,234) and the sum that is obtained by adding the number of deaths from Cancer's constituent codes in "Table 8: Death, by Cause and Sex, by Age, Alberta 1955" (1,266). We used the number in Table 18.

11 Source: "Table 8: Deaths, by Cause and Sex, by Age, Alberta 1960" and "Table 18: Certain Causes of Death, by Numbers and Rates for each year of the last Decennial Period," Alberta Department of Public Health, *Annual Report of the Division of Vital Statistics 1960* (Edmonton: Printed by L.S. Wall, Queen's Printer, 1962), 27–35 and 72. Codes match ICD-7 Intermediate List. Includes deaths at all ages.

12   Source: "Table 8: Deaths, by Cause and Sex, by Age, Alberta 1965" and "Table 19: Certain Causes of Death, by Numbers and Rates for each year of the last Decennial Period," Alberta Department of Public Health, *Annual Report of the Vital Statistics Division 1965* (Edmonton: Printed by L.S. Wall, Printer to the Queen Most Excellent Majesty, 1967), 29–37 and 72. Codes match ICD-7 Intermediate List of 150 Causes. Includes deaths at all ages.

13   There is a discrepancy in the number of deaths due to "Cancer", between the number reported in "Table 19: Certain Causes of Deaths" (1,625) and the sum that is obtained by adding the number of deaths from Cancer's constituent codes in "Table 8: Death, by Cause and Sex, by Age, Alberta 1965" (1,659). We used the number in Table 19.

14   Source: "Summary" and "Table 6: Deaths, by Cause and Sex, by Age, Alberta 1970," Alberta Department of Health, *Annual Report of the Division of Vital Statistics 1970* (Edmonton: Printed by L.S. Wall, Printer to the Queen Most Excellent Majesty, 1972), 7 and 45–54. Codes match ICD-8's "List A: List of 150 causes for tabulation of morbidity and mortality." Includes deaths at all ages.

15   Source: "Table 11b: Deaths occurring in Alberta, cause by Sex, 1975," Alberta Social Services and Community Health, *Vital Statistics Annual Review 1975 and 1976* (Edmonton: 1978), 37–47. Codes match ICD-8 Intermediate List A: List of 150 Causes for Tabulation of Morbidity and Mortality. Includes deaths at all ages for residents and non-residents.

16   The number in round brackets () indicates the number from the list of seventy-two causes selected for the province's Vital Statistics Annual Review. The number in square brackets [] indicates the corresponding ICD-9 codes. Source: "Table 11: Deaths Occurring in Alberta, Cause by Sex and Age, 1980" and "Summary of Vital Statistics" Alberta Social Services and Community Health, *Vital Statistics Annual Review 1980* (Edmonton: 1983), 22–27 and 30. In the "Summary of Vital Statistics" only rates are given for the Leading Causes of Death. Includes deaths at all ages for residents and non-residents.

17   See Note in Vital Statistics Annual Review 1985: "In Vital Statistics Annual Reviews for the years 1979 through 1983, the category 'Diseases of the Heart' has been understated. Deaths which should have been classified in Condition 34 (Other Chronic Ischemic Heart Diseases) were included in Condition 67 (All Other Diseases)." Alberta Community and Occupational Health, *Vital Statistics Annual Review 1985* (Edmonton: 1986), 58.

18   Source: "Table 11: Deaths, Cause by Sex and Age, 1985" and "Vital Statistics Summary, Alberta 1985" Alberta Community and Occupational Health, *Vital Statistics Annual Review 1985* (Edmonton: 1986), 18–49 and 55. Causes include 282 Selected Causes of Death from ICD-9. The "List of 282 Selected Causes of Death" (and the list of "72 Selected Causes of Death" used in 1980) was constructed based on the WHO Basic Tabulation List and developed by the National Center for Health Statistics (NCHS) of the Centre of Disease Control and Prevention (CDC) of the United States. See U.S. Department of Health and Human Service, National Center for Health Statistics, *Technical Appendix from Vital Statistics of the United States 1989* (Lanham, Md.: Bernan Associates, 1993), 9. Includes deaths at all ages for residents and non-residents.

19   The grouped cause of death, "Diseases of the Heart," defined by Alberta (and others) as the sum of ICD-9 codes 390–398, 402, 404, 410–429, does not match the sum of the figures of the heart-related causes reported individually in the Annual Review's "Table 11: Deaths, Cause by Sex and Age, 1985." We believe that the reason for this is that the combined causes reported in the Annual Review do not strictly correspond to the ICD codes included in "Diseases of the Heart", and the figures for "Diseases of the Heart" are constructed from available death reports and files, and not from the sum of the combined causes published that year. This applies to the years 1985, 1990, and 1995. See Public Health Surveillance and Environmental Health Branch, Public Health Division, Alberta Health & Wellness, *ICD-9 to ICD-10 Coding with Reference to Causes of Death Grouping in Alberta*, Health Surveillance System Series Working Document (July, 2006), https://open.alberta.ca/dataset/5bbd50c0-ed15-4dc8-b51f-affa45b82a17/resource/c69757b3-7bb2-49ed-b7a9-9cfa560ad7e3/download/icd-death-grouping-2007.pdf; Leslie Geran, Patricia Tully, Patricia Wood (Health Statistics Division), Brad Thomas (Household Survey Methods Division), Statistics Canada, *Comparability of ICD-10 and ICD-9 for Mortality Statistics in Canada* (Ottawa, Minister of Industry, 2005), see "Table 4. Bridge-coding of 1999 deaths: ICD-10/ICD-9 comparability ratios," https://www150.statcan.gc.ca/n1/en/pub/84-548-x/84-548-x2005001-eng.pdf?st=SYGBFzcN

20   Source: "Table 11: Deaths, Cause by Sex and Age, 1990" and "Vital Statistics Summary, Alberta 1990" Alberta Health, *Vital Statistics Annual Review 1990* (Edmonton: 1991), 22–46 and 62. Causes include 282 Selected Causes of Death from ICD-9. Includes deaths at all ages for residents and non-residents. See note above concerning inconsistencies for deaths from heart-related causes in 1985, 1990, and 1995.

21   "Causes of death are based on the International Classification of Diseases 9th Edition; and for reporting purposes are combined into 282 causes." Source: "Table 11: Deaths, Cause by Sex and Age, 1995" and "Vital Statistics Summary, Alberta 1995" Alberta Health, *Vital Statistics Annual Review 1995* (Edmonton: 1996), 18–40, 58 and 62. Causes include 282 Selected Causes of Death from ICD-9. Includes deaths at all ages for residents and non-residents. See note above concerning inconsistencies for deaths from heart-related causes in 1985, 1990, and 1995.

22   Source: Statistics Canada. Deaths and mortality rate (age standardization using 2011 population), by selected grouped causes. Table: 13-10-0800-01 (formerly CANSIM 102-0553). Including crude rate per 100,000 population. https://doi.org/10.25318/1310080001-eng. Includes deaths at all ages. Causes match the "Table B. List of 113 Selected Causes of Death," from the Centers for Disease Control and Prevention / National Center for Health Statistics, "Instruction Manual; Part 9; ICD-10 Cause-of-Death Lists for Tabulating Mortality Statistics." Codes correspond to ICD-10.

23   Source: Statistics Canada. Deaths and mortality rate (age standardization using 2011 population), by selected grouped causes. Table: 13-10-0800-01 (formerly CANSIM 102-0553). Including crude rate per 100,000 population. https://doi.org/10.25318/1310080001-eng. Includes deaths at all ages. Codes correspond to ICD-10.

24   Source: Statistics Canada. Deaths and mortality rate (age standardization using 2011 population), by selected grouped causes. Table: 13-10-0800-01 (formerly CANSIM 102-0553). Including crude rate per 100,000 population. https://doi.org/10.25318/1310080001-eng. Includes deaths at all ages. Codes correspond to ICD-10.

25   Source: Statistics Canada. Deaths and mortality rate (age standardization using 2011 population), by selected grouped causes. Table: 13-10-0800-01 (formerly CANSIM 102-0553). Including crude rate per 100,000 population. https://doi.org/10.25318/1310080001-eng. Includes deaths at all ages. Codes correspond to ICD-10.

Index

Page numbers followed by *t* indicate tables and *f* indicate figures. Pages numbers followed by *n* and a number indicate the note number in the chapter endnotes.

Alberta Public Health Association, 137–156, 371; governance, 142, 371; incorporation, 138; membership trends, 150, 151*t*; non-profit sector, 138–142; overview, 137–138, 154; resolution trends, 142–144, 155–156; 1940s, 144–145; 1950s, 145–146; 1960s, 146–147; 1970s, 147–148; 1980s, 148–150, 272; 1990s, 150–152; 2000 to present, 152–154
Alberta Safety Council, 76
Alberta Seniors Benefit, 351–352
Alberta's First Nations consultation guidelines on land management and resource development (Alberta Government), 198*t*
Alberta Teachers' Association, 285–286
Alberta Union of Public Employees, 285
Alberta Women's Bureau, 140
alcohol and drug abuse/dependence: Department of Health services, 121; First Nations programs, 197*t*; in throne speeches, 44, 49, 52, 53
Alexander First Nation (kipohtakaw), 205, 206
Alma Ata Declaration, 299–300
Alook, Andy, 216
Alook, Angele, 400
Amrhein, Carl, 169–170
Anderson, Dennis L., 81–82
Anderson, Wayne, 249*t*
antibiotics, 71, 72
Applied Public Health Chairs program, 168–169
Arcand, Ella, 204, 205, 206, 207–208, 210–211
Assembly of First Nations, 197*t*, 213
Assembly of Treaty Chiefs in Alberta, 199*t*
Attrux, Laura Margaret, 368–369
Auger, Gordon T., 212, 216
automobile industry, 76, 150

B

Babiuk, Elke, 278*f*
bacteriologists, 114, 115
Banff National Park, 241*t*, 243
Baragar, C. A., 71
Batiuk, John, 78
Bayliss, Nicholas, 101*t*
behaviour: in health promotion strategies and campaigns, 40–41, 52, 300, 301, 303, 313–314; *vs.* social determinants of health, 176–177, 393–394
Bella, Leslie, 346
Benevolent Societies Act (later Societies Act), 139
Berger, Lawrence, 309

Berger Report *(Report of the Advisory Committee on Indian and Inuit Health Consultation)*, 197*t*
Betkowski, Nancy, 100*t*, 111*t*, 151, 272
Bigstone Cree Nation (Mistassini Nehewiyuk), 212–217
Bill of Rights (Alberta), 124
Blackfoot Nation (Niitsitapi), 218, 220, 223
Blair Report on mental health, 344*t*, 346–347
Blakeman, Laurie, 249*t*, 253, 352*t*, 354–355, 358
Blood Tribe (Kainai Nation), 217–222
Board of Industrial Relations, 283
boards of health, 113, 117, 119–120. *See also* Edmonton Board of Health; local boards of health; Provincial Board of Health
Bogle, Robert, 99*t*
Bonko, William, 249*t*
Bow, Malcolm Ross: career, 96–97*t*, 109*t*, 366; comments by, 3, 11–12, 70, 144–145, 302–303, 305, 343
Bowden Public School District, 312
Boyle McCauley Health Centre (Edmonton), 372
Braithwaite, Edward, 114
Brantford experiment on fluoridation, 274
Bringing the Spirit Home detoxification centre, 222
British Columbia GDP alternatives, 399
Broda, David, 249*t*, 252
Brownlee goverment, 46
Bryce, Peter, 195*t*, 199–200
Buck, Walter A., 81
budgeting, 399
building codes, 329, 335
Building Communities from the Inside Out: A Path Toward Finding and Mobilizing a Community's Assets (Kretzmann and McKnight), 214
Bureau of Public Welfare, 140, 343, 344*t*
Buse, Chris G., 240

C

Calgary: public health administration, 113, 118, 120, 122, 348; riot against Chinese immigrants, 22; smoking legislation, 270; water fluoridation, 276, 277–279, 379
Calgary Health Services, 277
Calgary Herald, 308
Calgary Regional Health Authority, 278–279, 379
Campus Alberta Health Outcomes and Public Health, 176, 180*t*
Canada: Department of Health, 7; emergency operations, 324; environmental policy,

Communicable Diseases Regulation, 63
community: in cancer prevention, 78; in
emergency responses, 330–331; in health
promotion strategy, 299; in preventive
social services, 349, 350. *See also* First
Nation community experiences
Community Health Representatives program:
accreditation and deployment, 208–210;
concept and development, 197t, 204–205,
206–207; Ella Arcand's reflections on,
210–211
Community Health Sciences (University of
Calgary), 165, 166, 171, 173, 180t
community health services, 350
Community Medicine specialty, 165, 180t
Comparative Agendas coding scheme, 34
comprehensive school health approach,
314–315, 379
Constitution Act (1982), 197t
construction workers, 281, 285
contact tracing, 80
Co-Operative Commonwealth Federation
party, 282
corporate sponsorships, 271
Corriveau, Andre, 101t
Council on Education for Public Health, 169,
170
COVID-19 pandemic, 6, 93–94, 286–287, 309,
393, 396–397, 399, 402
Cowan, Kevin, 220, 223
Crawford, Neil, 98t, 347
Cross, Wallace Warren, 96–97t, 144, 145, 275,
276
cultural loss, 194, 224
Cyr, Scott, 249t, 256, 257

D

dairy industry, 119, 124–125
data collection and analysis, 394
Dawson, Angus, 20
deaths. *See* diseases and deaths
Declaration on Promotion and Prevention,
400
Declaration on the Rights of Indigenous
Peoples, 198t, 199t
deinstitutionalization movement, 346
Dental Association Act, 118
dental health and services, 70, 215–217, 273,
399
Department of Agriculture (1905-1917),
62–63, 95t, 114–115, 117, 324
Department of Community & Occupational
Health (1986-1989), 99–100t, 344t, 351
Department of Crown-Indigenous Relations
and Northern Affairs Canada, 199t

Department of Education, 312–313
Department of Environment (Alberta), 245t,
246–247, 259–260
Department of Environment (Canada), 244
Department of Family and Social Services, 351
Department of Health (1967-1971, 1989-2000,
2012-2014, 2017-2019): annual reports,
351; jurisdictions with Welfare, 146–147;
leadership and administration, 98t,
100–101t, 101–102t, 301–302, 344t; and
school curricula, 312–313
Department of Health Act, 345–346, 351
Department of Health (Canada), 7
Department of Health & Seniors (2015-2016),
102t
Department of Health & Social Development
(1971-1975), 98t, 110t, 343, 344t, 345–349
Department of Health and Welfare (Canada).
See Department of National Health and
Welfare
Department of Health & Wellness (2000-
2012), 101t, 301–302, 355, 356
Department of Hospitals and Medical Care,
344t, 349–350, 351
Department of Indian Affairs (Canada), 202
Department of Indigenous and Northern
Affairs (Canada), 199t
Department of Indigenous Services Canada,
199t
Department of Labour, 353
Department of Municipal Affairs (1918-1919),
95t, 116, 324, 334
Department of National Health and Welfare
(Canada), 27–28, 196t, 202, 207, 274
Department of Neglected Children, 70
Department of Provincial Secretary (1918),
95t, 116
Department of Public Health (1919-1967):
annual reports, 11, 304; disease
branches, 68; drug distributions, 72;
establishment and organization, 7, 40,
63, 117–118, 120–121, 259, 307, 343, 344t;
eugenics program, 19, 20; historical
accounts, 3; and immigrants, 23–24;
leadership, 95–98t; mental health,
70; nutrition division, 74; and school
curricula, 313; in throne speeches, 38; on
tuberculosis in Indigenous population,
28; water fluorine and tooth decay
research, 273
Department of Public Welfare, 120, 146–147,
324, 343
Department of Social Services & Community
Health (1975-1986), 98–99t, 343, 344t,
349–351

sex education, 146, 313
Sexual Sterilization Act (Alberta), 19–20, 25, 118, 366, 394
Shah, Nayan, 22
Shandro, Tyler, 102t
Shiell, Alan, 169, 171
Short Stay Maternity Program, 375
Shredding the Public Interest (Taft), 127
Shulz, Petra, 385–386
Simmons, Helen, 147
Sinclair, Niigaanwewidam James, 203
Skans, Oskar N., 309
Skinner, Daniel, 176
Slater, Dennis, 239
Slave Lake: district nursing, 368; wildfire, 329–331, 335
Sloan, Linda, 352–353
smallpox, 22, 113, 311–312
Smith, Edward Stuart Orford, 370–371
Smith, George P., 95t, 116
Smoke-free Places (Tobacco Reduction) Amendment Act, 272–273
smoking and tobacco control, 150, 152
Smorang, Jackie, 277
Smylie, Janet, 21, 191–192
social assistance programs: concerns about abuse, 348; and health program administration, 146–147, 342–343; in history, 120–121, 341–342; non-profit delivery, 140–142; workfare, 126. *See also* preventive social service programs
social cohesion, 335
Social Credit (SC) governments: labour legislation, 282–284; social policy and services, 343, 345, 346; and universal health insurance, 120; water fluoridation, 275. *See also* Manning government; Strom government
social democracy, 402
social determinants of health: and disaster vulnerability, 334; early childhood, 302; and human intervention, 166; in Ottawa Charter, 122; political and economic factors, 4–5, 224, 256–257, 260, 280, 282; in public health education, 176–178; and public policy, 339–341, 349–351; and public spending, 10–12; resolutions of Alberta Public Health Association, 144, 148, 149, 153; and Social Policy Framework, 356–359; speeches and debates, 40, 352–356
Social Determinants of Health (Raphael), 21
social justice: *vs.* market justice, 258; and Notley government, 128; and public health, 5, 394–395; in Social Policy

Framework, 357, 358; in Truth and Reconciliation Calls to Action, 193
social movements, 146
social policy and services administration, 146–147, 339–360; in Alberta Public Health Association resolutions, 146–147; early years, 342–343; milestone events, 344t; overview, 339–341, 359–360, 392; Social Policy Framework, 356–359; societal responses to poverty and need, 341–342; 1970s and 1980s, 342, 345–351; 1990s to 2010s, 351–356
social workers, 80, 357
Societies Act, 139
Somerville, Ashbury, 3, 97–98t, 367; *Report of the Special Legislative and Lay Committee Inquiring into Preventive Health Services in the Province of Alberta*, 110t
Speaker, Raymond, 348
Spencer, Harrison, 172, 174
Spirit of Healing initiative, 211
sports promotion, 378
Stachenko, Sylvie, 170
Stahnisch, Frank W., 1, 163; *Public Health Advocacy: Lessons Learned from the History of the Alberta Public Health Association*, 3
Stanley, George D., 68
Starblanket, Gina, 400
state medicine, 109t, 110t, 120
"Statement of the Government of Canada on Indian Policy, 1969" (White Paper), 196t, 203
Stelmach, Ed, 250t, 352t
Stelmach government (2006-2011), 50, 128, 272, 355–356
Steve Fonyo Cancer Prevention Program, 78
Stewart, Charles, 23
Stewart, Miriam, 167
Stewart government (1917-1921), 39–40, 46
Stinson, Shirley M., 373–374
Stone, Deborah: *Policy Paradox: The Art of Political Decision Making*, 5–6
strikes, 282, 285–286
Strom government (1968-1971), 49, 247, 343, 344t
Sullivan, Sue C.: *This is Public Health: A Canadian History*, 3–4
surveillance, 63, 80
A Survey of the Contemporary Indians of Canada: Economic, Political, Educational Needs and Policies (Hawthorn), 196t
surveys, 25, 74, 77
Suzuki, David, 272

victim assistance, 329, 330
Victorian Order of Nurses, 140
violence protections advocacy and support, 377, 382
Vital Statistics Act, 7, 62, 118
vital statistics reporting processes, 62–63

W

wait times, 39, 111*t*
Walby, Sylvia, 402
Wales, Wellbeing of Future Generations legislation, 399
waste management, 381
water fluoridation, 119, 273–279, 395
water pollution and waterworks regulations, 119, 245–246
Waters, John, 99–100*t*, 101*t*, 372–373
Watson, Helen Griffith Wylie, 369–370
Weaselhead, Charles, 217, 218, 220, 223, 224
Webber, Neil, 99*t*
Weber, Barret, 141
Weingarten, Harvey, 171
Welch-Rose report (1915), 164, 180*t*
welfare, 339–342. *See also* social assistance programs
Welfare of Children Act (1925), 139–140
Wellbeing Economy Alliance, 398–399
Wellness Initiatives proposal, 354–355
Werry, Leonard, 347
Western Canada Medical Journal, 26
What Makes Health Public? (Coggon), 21
White, Fred: *Report of the Inquiry into Systems of State Medicine*, 109*t*
Whitelaw, Thomas H., 311
White Paper (Statement of the Government of Canada on Indian Policy), 196*t*, 203
Why are Some People Healthy and Others Not? The Determinants of Health of Populations (Evans et al), 214
wildfires, 329–333, 385
Wilson, Doug, 167, 169, 375–376
Winnipeg General Strike of 1919, 282
Winslow, Charles-Edward, 1, 4–5, 11
Winter Counts, 223
Wolfe, Ruth, 165
women: advocacy organizations, 76, 288*n*12; eugenics targets, 26; workers, 282, 283, 307
women's shelters, 139, 382
Wood Buffalo wildfire, 329, 331–333, 335
workers: and childcare, 357–358; disparities, 121, 353; early immigrants, 280–281; health and political economy, 279–287; in public health sector, 38, 143, 144,

145–146, 147, 168, 181*t*; World War I era, 281–282
"workfare," 126
working conditions, 39, 239, 279–280, 299
Working People in Alberta: A History (Finkel), 280
Workmen's Compensation Act (1908), 139
World Health Organization: Commission on Social Determinants of Health, 339–340, 397398; 1946 Constitution, 5; definition of health, 61, 299; framework conventions and studies, 256, 272; *Health Equity through Intersectoral Action*, 359

Y

Yanicki, Sharon, 174–175
Yassi, Annalee, 177
Yellowhead Tribal Council, 206, 211
Young, Kue, 170
YWCA, 139

Z

Zander, Rudolph, 78
Zaozirny, John B., 81
Zernicke, Ron, 171–172
Zwozdesky, Gene, 101*t*